TNM
Staging Atlas

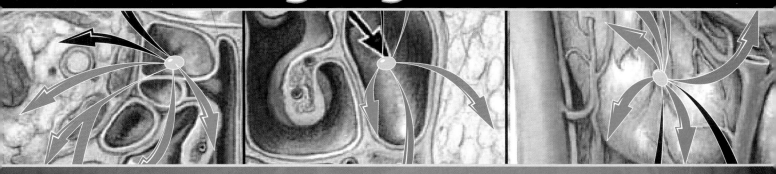

Philip Rubin, MD
Professor and Chair Emeritus
Department of Radiation Oncology
University of Rochester Medical School
Former Associate Director
Senior Associate in Surgery and Medicine
James P. Wilmot Cancer Center
University of Rochester Medical Center
Rochester, New York

John T. Hansen, PhD
Professor of Neurobiology and Anatomy
and Associate Dean
University of Rochester
School of Medicine and Dentistry
Rochester, New York

Wolters Kluwer | Lippincott Williams & Wilkins
Health
Philadelphia • Baltimore • New York • London
Buenos Aires • Hong Kong • Sydney • Tokyo

Acquisitions Editor: Jonathan Pine
Managing Editor: Stacey Sebring
Project Manager: Rosanne Hallowell
Manufacturing Manager: Kathleen Brown
Marketing Manager: Sharon Zinner
Art Director: Risa Clow
Cover Designer: Mike Pottman
Production Services: Aptara, Inc.

Library of Congress Cataloging-in-Publication Data

Rubin, Philip, 1927-
  TNM staging atlas / Philip Rubin, John T. Hansen.
    p. ; cm.
  Includes bibliographical references and index.
  ISBN-13: 978-0-7817-6021-8 (alk. paper)
  ISBN-10: 0-7817-6021-6 (alk. paper)
  1. Tumors—Classification—Atlases. 2. Cancer—Classification—Atlases. I. Hansen, John T.
  II. Title. [DNLM: 1. Neoplasm Staging—methods—Atlases. 2. Neoplasms—Atlases.
  QZ 17 R896t 2008]
  RC258.R83 2008
  616.99′4–dc22

                              2007030638

RAMSL

Les Cinq amours

Rebecca, Amanda, Madelyn, Sara, Lisa

My beautiful and bright granddaughters

Philip Rubin

To my wife Paula, my children Amy and Sean,

and my granddaughter Abigail,

for their love, inspiration and support

John T. Hansen

Table of Contents

SECTION 6: GENERALIZED ANATOMIC PRIMARY SITES

SECTION 7: OPHTHALMIC PRIMARY SITES

Preface

Since its inception, the TNM system has embraced the concept of determining the true anatomic extent of a cancer at the time of its initial diagnosis. The surgeon Pierre Denoix introduced the cancer language, the alphabet was simple, T: local tumor spread, N: regional lymph node involvement, and M: distant hematogenous seeding or metastases. The subscript of 1, 2, 3, or 4 delineated cancer advancement. The addition of stage-grouping different TNM combinations allowed for simplification to four stages: I, II, III, and IV. Once cancer staging and classification became universally adopted by multidisciplinary oncologists, it resulted in a more uniform design of clinical trial target groups for their randomization. Prognosis is more accurate and, most importantly, end-results reporting of survival and outcomes following treatment has allowed for comparisons between cancer centers for the sake of therapeutic improvements and gains.

The first edition of the *Cancer Staging Manual (CSM)* by the American Joint Committee on Cancer (AJCC) arrived in 1976, following a national conference first devoted to the concept of cancer staging. By the third edition in the 1980s, all major cancer sites were included, and both the AJCC and International Union Against Cancer/Union Internationale Contre le Cancer (UICC) agreed to a joint publication leading to its international usage. In the 1990s, a number of revisions of the TNM staging system began and were made to adopt staging systems of major surgical and medical oncology cooperative investigative groups, including the International Federation of Gynecology and Obstetrics (FIGO), among others.

As we herald the new millennium, the sixth edition of *CSM*, printed in 2002, has numerous revisions, and raises the issue of consistency versus change and its impact on assessing the oncology literature. The first dilemma is use of the same TNM designations, whereby the stage has been redefined and assigned to different degrees of tumor advancement. Second, improvements in diagnostic techniques such as CT, MRI, and PET can lead to more accurate staging and, with it, stage migration. Finally, the oncology literature, which spans the past 5 decades, has constantly shown improvements in survival rates at different anatomic sites, but may reflect both revisions and modifications in staging rather than pure therapeutic gains.

A picture is worth a thousand words; a well-designed illustration is worth even more. This *TNM Staging Atlas* is intended to be a companion volume to major multidisciplinary oncology textbooks providing a visual reference with clear full color diagrams of TNM stages by organ site and their TNM anatomy to augment the verbal detailed anatomic descriptions at the beginning of each chapter of the CSM. It is designed to enable practicing oncologists and physicians to access the data they need in oncologic diagnostic, prognostic, and treatment decision-making. For consistency, chapters are arranged in the same sequence, and when possible related figures, tables, and text appear together on the same two-page spread to minimize the need to flip back and forth. For medical students and residents, the volume is central to understanding 3D human anatomy by cancer spread patterns. The primary site oncoanatomy is presented in 3D/3-Planar fashion as is the regional nodal anatomy, followed by a review of vascular spread patterns.

Our continued interest in the staging and classification of cancers dates back to the first edition (1977) of the AJCC Cancer Staging Manual, which was the first compilation of all primary sites staged to that time. At that time, I (Philip Ruben) was privileged to be one of the editors along with Ollie Beahrs (Surgery) and David Carr (Medicine) to organize and establish this important endeavor. In *Clinical Oncology and Oncoimaging*, through its numerous editions, we have illustrated cancer staging. The medical illustrations of cancer staging were introduced into our oncology textbook, *Clinical Oncology for Medical Students and Physicians*, sponsored and printed by the American Cancer Society, and reprinted in color in *Oncologic Imaging* as well as in the numerous editions of *Principles and Practice of Radiation Oncology*.

Philip Rubin
John Hansen

Acknowledgments

Each and every book places high demands on creative processes to produce a unique and singular volume. The seminal concept of providing an oncoanatomy as the paradigm for understanding the basis for the TNM staging of cancer extent was germinated, with John Hansen, as a learning elective for medical students. The inspiration thereby provided has been translated by a wonderful team of medical illustrators, Tiffany Gagnon and Kristen Johnson, who rallied to actualize this demanding assignment. The major burden of assemblage of text, figures, and tables, which became a Sisyphean chore, was carried by Heike Kross, my editorial and research assistant, with dedication and devotion. Her colleague, Frank Stock, a gifted artist, undertook the final task of refining the art to meet publication requirements for high resolution illustrations.

The blooming and blossoming of the concept of utilizing cancer spread patterns to provide a scaffold for appreciating 3D anatomy is in large part due to the enthusiastic response of medical students and radiation oncology residents. The term *oncoanatomy* embodies the idea of the cancer crab's six basic directions of invasion and was endorsed by our faculty in our teaching seminars. Of special note are Alvin Ureles, George Uschold, and Pat Fultz, but in addition, Sandy Constine, Yuhchyau Chen, Ralph Brasacchio, and Arvin Soni. Of my colleagues, who have reviewed this text and offered their encouragement to pursue this venture, I need to recognize Robert Sagerman, Luther Brady, and Carlos Perez for their critique and recommendations. Stuart Byer and James Afferton have provided keen advice from the perspective of clinical oncology applications.

We are grateful to our publisher, Lippincott Williams & Wilkins, for their encouragement and support to produce this endeavor. Specifically, Jonathan Pine provided a generous grant for the artwork essential to foster the initial phase of the project. Stacey Sebring, Senior Managing Editor, was responsible for coordinating the editorial and illustrative aspects to produce the book. Thanks to Donna Kessler for attentiveness to page proofs and timely turnaround. Also, we are indebted to the LWW policy of allowing us to use their publishing assets and copyrights for producing medical illustrative material from *Grant's Atlas of Anatomy*, *Ereschenko's Atlas of Histology* and *Ross's Histology*.

Finally, my beautiful and bright RAMSL granddaughters, to whom this book is dedicated, have all participated actively in numerous draft versions of this volume. Of particular comment are Madelyn and Amanda, who actively participated in formulating and configuring 3planar anatomy during college breaks, holidays, and past summers. A special note for survival rate figures at the end of chapters based on SEER 5 year survival rates for individual cancer sites over the past 5 decades (1950–2000), illustrated by Madelyn.

Philip Rubin
John T. Hansen

How to Use the Atlas

The Concept of TNM Oncoanatomy

- The oncoanatomy is the paradigm for the oncotaxonomy, that is, the anatomic extent of cancer spread is the basis for cancer classification and staging.
- The oncoanatomy refers to the normal tissue organization of a specific anatomic site that determines the clinical behavior of the cancer that originates there and its pattern of spread.
- The cancer crab invades the anatomic site of origin in six basic directions: anterior-posterior, superior-inferior, medial-lateral. Although the cancer can infiltrate in a myriad number of directions, it usually follows the path of least resistance around these six vectors. The tumor infiltrates along fascial and muscle planes, invading fatty areolar spaces, and enters low pressure lymphatics and venous channels.
- The 3 dimensional anatomic aspects and construct of a region is readily appreciated by utilizing the model of cancer spread patterns. That is, each manifestation of the cancer clinically is based upon a specific vector of tumor involvement providing a geographic, anatomic-physiologic basis as its explanation.
- The organization of this *TNM Staging Atlas* is based on a 3D/3-Planar cross sectional presentations of the Regional Anatomy. Each diagram is referenced to *Grant's Atlas of Anatomy*.
- The most important decision in cancer treatment is the *first decision* once the neoplasm is definitely diagnosed as to its histopathologic type and grade.
- Knowing the *anatomic extent of the cancer* or its stage is most often the key determinant in achieving a successful outcome.

These concepts were developed over a 20 year span in which the authors introduced first year medical students to 3D/3-planar anatomy using cancer spread patterns. The anatomic surgical dissection of cadavers was reinforced by viewing the anatomy on CT and MRI planar views. We provided "neoplasm" to provide "new life" to cadaver dissection learning.

Organization Rationale

- The oncoanatomy is presented as Regional Sections (7), which then are divided into Primary Cancer Sites (63). Then each regional section is presented first as an orientation diagram in an anterior and lateral projection, with surface anatomy landmarks and a radiographic osseous feature, the vertebral level.
- Each anatomic region is presented in 3D/3-planar sections; a coronal, a sagittal, and a transverse axial section of anatomy. There are seven anatomic regions, each with several primary cancer sites, which are ordered from cephalad to caudad.
- This "companion volume" to major multidisciplinary multiauthored oncology textbooks is designed for the oncologist to have a visual illustrated reference to TNM staging to complement the associated verbal descriptive anatomy that begins each chapter in the latest edition of the AJCC and UICC (sixth edition).
- Each cancer site is introduced by a diagram of anatomic features identifiable on physical or radiographic examination.
- The derivative normal cellular and histologic features of each site provide a basis for the WHO histopathologic classification of cancers at each anatomic site.
- The patterns of cancer spread at the primary site (T), to regional nodes (N), and to a distant target organ of first metastases (M), often based on venous drainage, are concisely presented as the logic built into the TNM system of tumor progression.
- The 3D/3-Planar Oncoanatomy of the primary site and the regional nodes along with its venous drainage are presented in succession.
- The first-station lymph nodes (N) are shown for each primary site with emphasis on the sentinel lymph node.
- Hematogenous spread via draining venous channels (M) will often determine the target metastatic organ.
- The clinical imaging criteria for staging with onco-imaging annotations are emphasized in the rules for TNM classification.
- The cancer survival results over the past 5 decades are presented as Surveillance Epidemiology and End Results (SEER) 5-year survival data (1950–2000).
- In reviewing the staging systems that have been designed, adopted, and modified over time, there is a need to utilize the international anatomical terminology (Terminologia Anatomica) to improve the

accuracy of reporting by oncologic disciplines to supplement the numbering of lymph node stations in a region.

Special Features: Color Code

A unifying feature of this Atlas is a color code that portrays the spectrum of cancer progression at primary sites (T) and lymph node regions (N), and of stage grouping.

1. For the primary (T), color-coded arrows on the cancer crab spread patterns allow the reader to immediately appreciate cancer progression and advancement. Each arrow points to specific structures that advance the stage when invaded. Arrow color changes and length increases as stage advances.

T0 or Tis	yellow
T1	green
T2	blue
T3	purple
T4a	red
T5b	black

2. For regional nodes, the designation of nodal progression N1, N2, N3 is colored the same as T1, T2, and T3. Beyond N3 refers to second station or echelon of nodes. We are suggesting M_N for such regional lymph nodes, which are considered truly juxtaregional but not placed in M1. Such juxtaregional nodes are quite distant and rarely curable.

N0	yellow
N1	green
N2	blue
N3	purple
N4 N_m	red
N4 M_1	black

3. For TNM Stage Grouping (the second figure in each chapter), the color code remains the same. Horizontal color bars encompass T and N categories, which vary in each stage group. Variations in cancer staging, A and B, when applied to stages III and IV, in effect creates 5 or 6 stages. In such situations, color coding may vary but is designed to show progression.

0	yellow
I	green
II	blue
III	purple
IVA	red
IVB	black

4. The vertical arrangement of TNM is to allow the reader to read across the page to check T and N definitions on left with pictorial display and stage groupings on right. When stage group is not shown, an asterisk alerts the reader and is annotated in the legend.
5. The anatomy presented throughout the text is based on or modified from *Grant's Atlas* and is accordingly cross referenced to *Grant's Atlas*, 6th edition, 2004.
6. The histologic sections presented are from both Ereschenko (10th Edition) or *Ross Histology* (4th Edition).

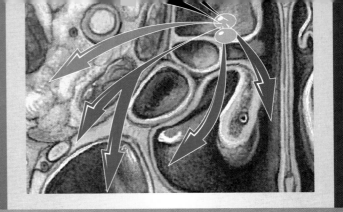

SECTION 1

HEAD AND NECK PRIMARY SITES

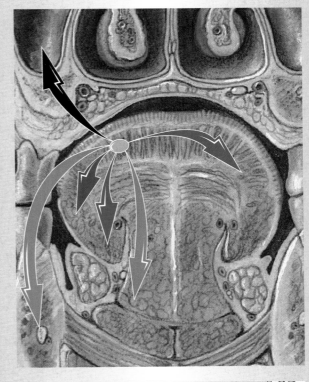

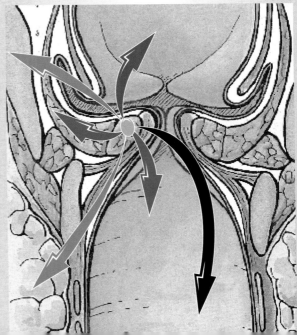

1

Introduction and Orientation

The study of the patterns of tumor spread and their invasive behavior provides a unique spyglass, through which one can view and understand this regional anatomy three dimensionally.

Perspective and Patterns of Spread

The head and neck area is a very complex region consisting of a series of mazes and channels that constitute the upper aerodigestive passages. A large variety of tumors arise from the different tissues that constitute the various structures of the head and neck sites. This section focuses on malignancies arising from the surface epithelium, which are the most frequently encountered cancers. They are very destructive if allowed to progress, and because of the resultant functional disabilities, their impact on social presentation, particularly with regard to self-image, speech, and communication, can be extremely detrimental. The challenge is not only to be able to control these cancers, but also to maintain normal anatomic relationships and structure. *The TNM staging reflects the patterns of spread and the oncologic anatomy (Fig. 1.1).* The common cancers arising in the upper aerodigestive passages are mainly in the pharyngeal and laryngeal tubes (Table 1.1).

Although head and neck cancers are clustered together, they are a very diverse group of tumors. If facial and scalp skin cancers and melanomas were included with extracranial head and neck tumors, this would be the most common anatomic site for malignancy. When typically limited to mucosal cancers of the upper aerodigestive tract, it accounts for 3% of all cancers and ranks 6th worldwide—7th for men and 11th for women. The classic patient population presenting with head and neck cancers consists of those with excessive smoking and alcohol habits. Essential to success are programs designed for posttreatment abstinence to avoid a recurrence of malignant tumors.

Cancers in the head and neck region are similar in terms of their biologic behavior; it is the differences in primary site anatomy that define the uniqueness of their clinical manifestations. The conceptualization of three-dimensional anatomy of the head and neck region is therefore appreciated through cancer spread (Fig. 1.1). *The cancer crab can spread in six basic directions: superiorly–inferiorly, medially–laterally, and anteriorly–posteriorly.* There are an infinite number of possible patterns around these six basic vectors; however, these are predetermined by the arrangement of muscle and fascial planes. Cancers of the head and neck tend to follow the path of least resistance, invading fatty areolar spaces, which are particularly vulnerable; along nerves through perineural invasion; and entering bony ostia and foramena. Lymphatics and vessels also provide low-pressure flow channels of minimal resistance.

TNM Staging Criteria

The "head and neck" area is generally considered one anatomic and physiologic unit because their boundaries are not well defined. Cancers arising in the different sites of the upper aerodigestive passages spread into the neck nodes as first station nodes. The specific site of the first node to be affected varies according to the origin of the primary tumor. *In fact, every primary site drains into the cervical nodes as noted, but each site has a preference for a specific sentinel node.* This is often the first evidence of cancer somewhere in the head, of an unknown primary. Because many midline areas drain bilaterally, both sides of the neck are vulnerable to cancer spread. Bilateral and contralateral lymphatic involvement also are common. *Once one node is affected, the entire complex of lymph nodes in the neck is at risk because of altered flow into collateral channels.*

The classification and staging of head and neck cancers is an excellent prototype for the classification and staging of cancer in general. There has always been a guiding principle to maintain uniform criteria across all anatomic primary sites. Two major modifications of T and N categories and stage grouping have been made based on survival data of clinical trials. Major changes in nodal criteria occurred with the third edition (1987) when criteria as N2 mobility versus N3 fixation of lymph nodes were changed to size. Size of nodes was adopted as the criterion to be more objective. *A fixed node to the carotid artery was replaced by >6 cm in greatest diameter and the N definitions N1 ≤3 cm, N2 3 to 6 cm, and N3 >6 cm have been uniformly applied across all head and neck sites except for the nasopharynx. In the sixth edition (2002), a major change in all sites was dividing the primary cancer into stage IVA T4a resectable, stage IVB T4b N2 unresectable, and stage IVC is for distant metastases.*

In general, every effort has been made to bring the stage groupings of the head and neck to a relatively

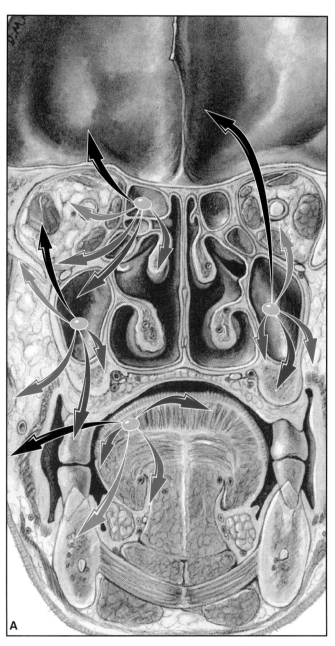
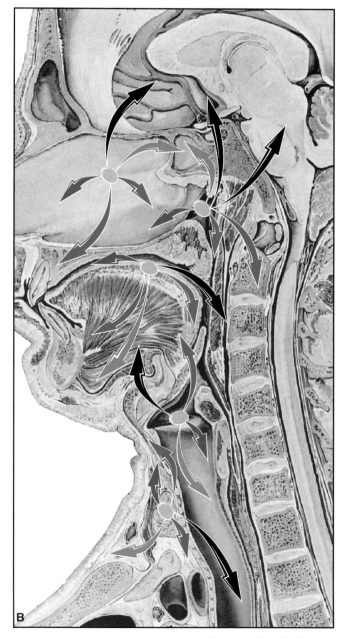

Figure 1.1 **Collage of patterns of spread.** The different head and neck primary cancer sites are presented cephalad to caudad. **A.** Coronal: Ethmoid, maxillary antrum, and oral cavity. **B.** Sagittal: maxillary antral, nasopharynx, oral cavity, larynx, and thyroid. There are six basic directions or vectors (*arrows*): anterior-posterior, medial-lateral, superior-inferior. The *arrows* are color-coded for T stage category: Tis yellow, T1 green, T2 blue, T3 purple, T4a red, T4b black.

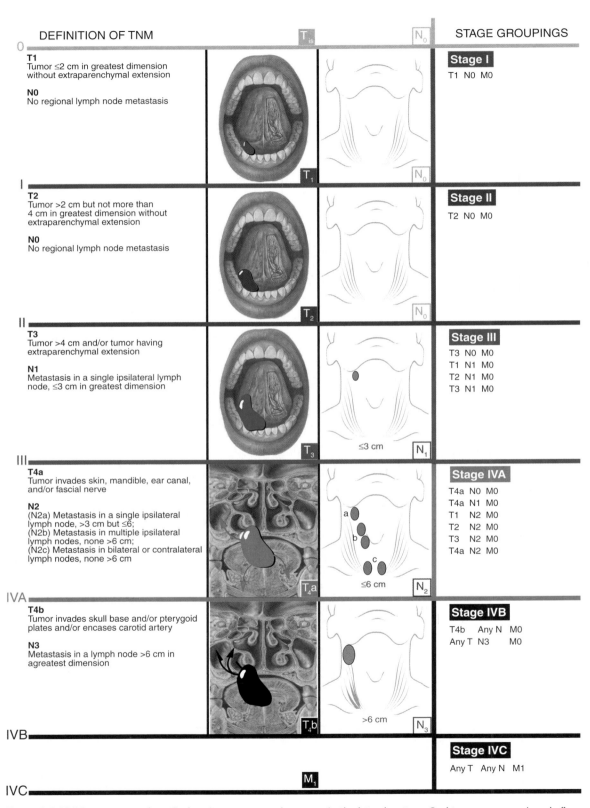

DEFINITION OF TNM

T1
Tumor ≤2 cm in greatest dimension without extraparenchymal extension

N0
No regional lymph node metastasis

T2
Tumor >2 cm but not more than 4 cm in greatest dimension without extraparenchymal extension

N0
No regional lymph node metastasis

T3
Tumor >4 cm and/or tumor having extraparenchymal extension

N1
Metastasis in a single ipsilateral lymph node, ≤3 cm in greatest dimension

T4a
Tumor invades skin, mandible, ear canal, and/or fascial nerve

N2
(N2a) Metastasis in a single ipsilateral lymph node, >3 cm but ≤6;
(N2b) Metastasis in multiple ipsilateral lymph nodes, none >6 cm;
(N2c) Metastasis in bilateral or contralateral lymph nodes, none >6 cm

T4b
Tumor invades skull base and/or pterygoid plates and/or encases carotid artery

N3
Metastasis in a lymph node >6 cm in agreatest dimension

STAGE GROUPINGS

Stage I
T1 N0 M0

Stage II
T2 N0 M0

Stage III
T3 N0 M0
T1 N1 M0
T2 N1 M0
T3 N1 M0

Stage IVA
T4a N0 M0
T4a N1 M0
T1   N2 M0
T2   N2 M0
T3   N2 M0
T4a N2 M0

Stage IVB
T4b   Any N M0
Any T N3   M0

Stage IVC
Any T Any N M1

Figure 1.2 TNM stage grouping. Oral cavity cancers tend to occur in the lateral gutters. Oral tongue cancers invade floor of mouth because of interdigitation of intrinsic and extrinsic musculature. Vertical presentations of stage groupings, which follow same color code for cancer stage advancement are organized in horizontal lanes: Stage 0, yellow; I, green; II, blue; III, purple; IVA, red; and IVB, black. Definitions of TN on left and stage grouping on right.

TABLE 1.1 Histopathologic Type: Common Cancers of the Upper Aerodigestive Tract

Squamous Cell Carcinoma Microscopic Variants	Adenocarcinoma Major or Minor Salivary Gland
Keratinizing; well differentiated; moderately well differentiated; poorly differentiated	Low-grade adenocarcinoma
Nonkeratinizing; anaplastic squamous carcinoma	Adenoid cystic carcinoma
Lymphoepithelioma	Mucoepidermoid (low or high grade)
Transitional cell carcinoma	Carcinoma expleomorphic adenoma
Spindle cell squamous carcinoma	Poorly differentiated adenocarcinoma

uniform combination of TNM criteria for all sites. This useful attribute would be beneficial to adopt at other anatomic cancer sites.

Summary of Changes

The T stage determines the stage grouping with modification by N stage. Size implying depth of invasion is the key criterion for primary tumors: T1 is <2 cm, T2 is >2 cm and <4 cm, and T3 >4 cm. A uniform description of advanced tumors has been recommended: T4 lesions are divided into T4a resectable, T4b unresectable, and assignment to stage IVA

and stage IVB, respectively. Stage IVC is metastatic disease (Fig. 1.2).

No major changes have been made in nodal classification staging; however, N2 is stage IVA, N3 is stage IVB, and for a notation as to an upper and lower neck node (supraclavicular, Fig. 1.2).

Overview of Oncoanatomy

The mucosal surfaces of the two major sectors differ (Fig. 1.3; Table 1.2). The respiratory passage is a ciliated columnar or pseudocolumnar epithelium (Fig. 1.3B–D) and the

TABLE 1.2 Overview of the Histogenesis at Primary Cancer Sites

Primary Site Structure	Derivative Normal Cell	Cancer Histopathology	Axial Level
Ethmoid sinus, nasal cavity	Ciliated pseudocolumnar epithelial Olfactory bipolar neurons	Adenocarcinoma Esthesioneuroblastoma	Sphenoid Sinus
Maxillary sinus	Ciliated pseudocolumnar epithelial	Squamous cell cancer, undifferentiated	Clivus
Nasopharynx	Ciliated pseudocolumnar epithelial Waldeyer's lymphoid cells	Lymphoepithelioma	C1
Oral cavity	Stratified squamous epithelial Minor salivary gland epithelial	Squamous cell cancer Adenocarcinoma	C2/3
Parotid gland	Serous acini cuboidal epithelial	Acini adenocarcinoma Adenoid cystic cancer	C3
Oropharynx	Stratified squamous epithelial	Squamous cell cancer	C3
Hypopharynx	Stratified squamous epithelial	Squamous cell cancer, more differentiated	C4
Supraglottis	Ciliated pseudocolumnar epithelial	Squamous cell cancer Less differentiated	C4
Glottis	Stratified squamous epithelial	Squamous cell cancer Very differentiated	C5
Subglottis	Ciliated columnar and pseudocolumnar epithelium	Squamous cell cancer Less differentiated	C6
Thyroid	Lining cuboidal epithelium of follicles	Adenocarcinomas Follicular, papillary, medullary	C7

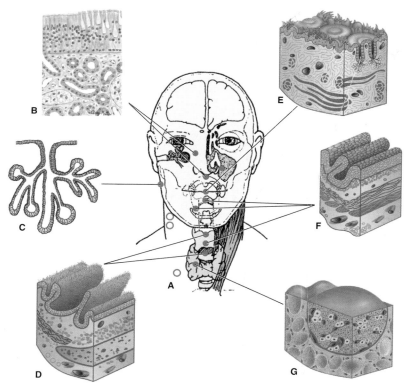

Figure 1.3 **Oncoanatomy overview.** (A) Histologic sections indicate the type of mucosa present in different primary sites in the head and neck. In the upper respiratory system, paranasal sinus, nasopharynx (B) and supraglottic and subglottic larynx (D) are ciliated columnar and pseudocolumnar epithelium. Stratified squamous epithelium covers the upper digestive system (E, oral cavity and tongue; F, orohypopharynx); in contrast, the cuboidal epithelium lines the follicles of the thyroid gland (G) and the glandular component of the salivary gland which becomes columnar epithelium in the duct (C). **A.** Primary cancer site isocenters. **B.** Paranasal sinus and nasopharynx. **C.** Salivary gland. **D.** Supraglottic and subglottic larynx. **E.** Oral cavity and tongue. **F.** Oropharynx and hypopharynx. **G.** Thyroid.

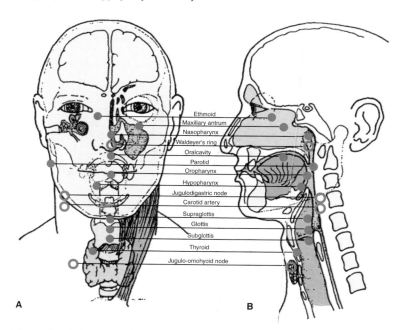

Figure 1.4 Orientation of three-planar T-oncoanatomy. The locations of 11 primary cancer sites are indicated at their anatomic isocenters with red bullets. Open circles are important lymph nodes. **A.** Coronal. **B.** Sagittal. **C.** Bone and cartilage frame for head and neck primary sites. **D.** Sagittal view. Sectors are upper respiratory (*blue*) and upper digestive (*pink*) systems. Green fasciae are continuous inferiorly in chest and to the skull. **E.** Cervical fascial planes. *Note:* prevertebral.

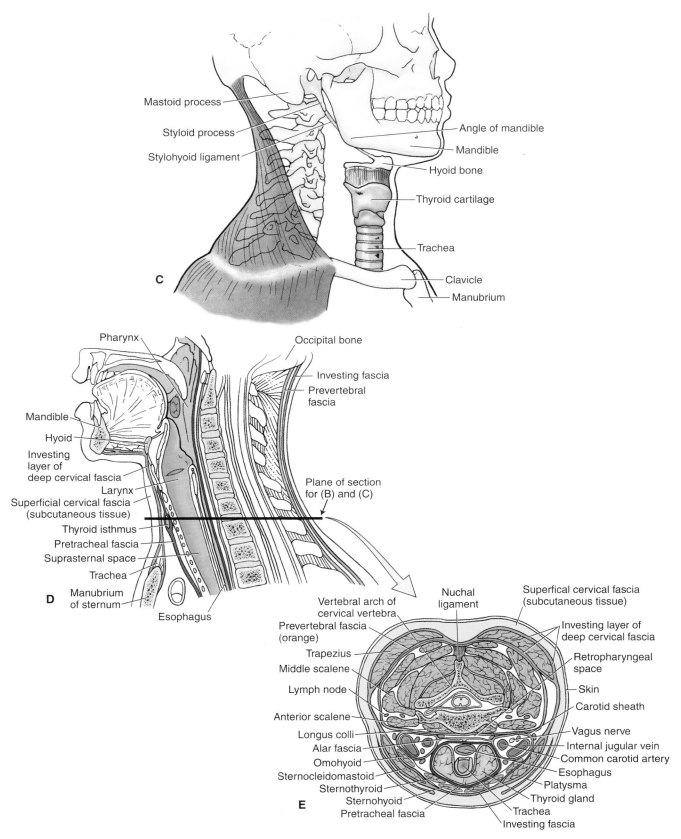

Mastoid process
Styloid process
Stylohyoid ligament
Angle of mandible
Mandible
Hyoid bone
Thyroid cartilage
Trachea
Clavicle
Manubrium
C

Pharynx
Occipital bone
Investing fascia
Prevertebral fascia
Mandible
Hyoid
Investing layer of deep cervical fascia
Larynx
Superficial cervical fascia (subcutaneous tissue)
Thyroid isthmus
Pretracheal fascia
Suprasternal space
Trachea
Manubrium of sternum
Esophagus
Plane of section for (B) and (C)
D

Vertebral arch of cervical vertebra
Prevertebral fascia (orange)
Trapezius
Middle scalene
Lymph node
Anterior scalene
Longus colli
Alar fascia
Omohyoid
Sternocleidomastoid
Sternothyroid
Sternohyoid
Pretracheal fascia
Nuchal ligament
Superfical cervical fascia (subcutaneous tissue)
Investing layer of deep cervical fascia
Retropharyngeal space
Skin
Carotid sheath
Vagus nerve
Internal jugular vein
Common carotid artery
Esophagus
Platysma
Thyroid gland
Trachea
Investing fascia
E

Figure 1.4 (*Continued*)

TABLE 1.3	Anatomic Isocenters of Primary Cancer Sites		
Primary Site Structure	**Coronal**	**Sagittal**	**Transverse**
Ethmoid sinus, nasal cavity	Right/left of midline, orbit	Zygomatic arch	Sphenoid sinus/base of skull
Maxillary sinus	Right/left bridge of nose	Zygomatic arch	Clivus
Nasopharynx	Hard palate	External auditory meatus	C1
Oral cavity	Lips	Teeth	C2/3
Parotid gland	Ramus mandible	Angle of mandible	C3
Oropharynx	Lips/teeth	Angle of mandible	C3
Hypopharynx	Hyoid	Greater horn of hyoid bone	C4
Supraglottis	Thyroid cartilage notch	Horn of thyroid cartilage	C5
Glottis	Below thyroid cartilage notch	Horn of thyroid cartilage	C5
Subglottis	Cricoid cartilage	Cricoid cartilage	C7
Thyroid	Right/left paratracheal	Paratracheal	C6/7

TABLE 1.4	Sentinel Nodes		
		Level/Location of Node(s)[a]	
Primary Site Structure	**Sentinel Node(s)**	**Axial Level**	**AJCC Level**
Ethmoid sinus, nasal cavity	Retropharyngeal	C1	nl
Maxillary sinus	Submandibular	C3	I
Nasopharynx	Retropharyngeal	C1	nl
Oral cavity	Submandibular Jugulodigastric	C3 C3	I II
Parotid gland	Parotid nodes	C2/C3	I
Oropharynx	Jugulodigastric, superior deep cervical	C3	II
Hypopharynx	Mid deep cervical	C4	III
Supraglottis	Jugulodigastric, superior/mid deep cervical	C4/5	II
Glottis	Prelaryngeal	C5	VI
Subglottis	Jugulo-omohyoid, inferior deep cervical	C7	IV
Thyroid	Jugulo-omohyoid Inferior/mid/superior deep cervical	C3–I1	IV III/II

[a]Sentinel nodes transfer axial level; they may not be at the same level as the primary site.
Abbreviation: nl, not listed.

TABLE 1.5	Imaging Modalities and Strategies for Diagnosis and Staging for Head and Neck	
Modality	**Strategy**	**Recommended**
Primary tumor and nodes		
Computed tomography	Excellent for defining extent of primary depth of invasion and enlargement of involved nodes. Preferred for bone invasion.	Yes—3–5 mm cuts, 3 mm for primary site, 5 mm for neck
Magnetic resonance imaging	Offers best 3-D or 3-planar views of primary and nodes, especially soft tissue extensions. Gadolinium contrast for extensions and perineuronal spread.	Yes—≤4 cm slices Gd—for intracranial and perineuronal spread
Magnetic resonance spectroscopy	Provides metabolic and biochemical analysis of tumor, choline/creatinine ratio elevated in tumor vs. normal tissues.	No
Positron emission tomography	Functional and metabolic imaging of ^{18}FDG is based on 2-deoxy modification inhibits the molecule from subsequent enzymatic conversion and is "metabolically trapped" in tumor cells.	No—potential exists for distinguishing Recurrence from tissue necrosis
Single photon emission computed tomography	^{201}Thallium used to detect tumor recurrence vs. normal tissue imaging, especially central nervous system.	No—high uptake normally in salivary and thyroid glands
Metastases		
Chest film	Search for metastases.	Yes
Radionuclide scan	^{99m}Tc for bone metastases	Yes—if symptomatic

Abbreviations: 3D, three dimensional; FDG, fluorodeoxyglucose.
From Bragg DG, Rubin P, Hricak H. *Oncologic imaging.* 2nd Ed. Philadelphia: WB Saunders; 2002.

digestive passage is a stratified squamous epithelium (Fig. 1.3E,F). Both give rise mainly to squamous cell cancers. Most cancers are epithelial in origin, arising from the surface and evolving into four general patterns of invasion: shallow, mucosal, premalignant leukoplakia-like warty lesions often become submucosal.

- *Verrucous growths:* Wartlike, spreading on the surface rather than in depth;
- *Exophytic and exuberant growth:* An polyploid mushroom in appearance that undergoes;
- *Fungation, necrosis of growth:* This type of tumor usually, but not always, undergoes ulceration; and
- *Endophytic invasive growth:* Infiltration into muscle or erosion of bone and cartilage, and invasion perineurally of the cranial nerves and their branches.

Adenocarcinomas arise from the endocrine thyroid gland and the exocrine salivary glands (Fig. 1.3C–G).

Because most of the sites consist of different tissue layers (an epithelial surface, underlying muscle and/or bone with an air-containing cavity), the study of primary tumor sites, where neoplasms commonly arise, requires an appreciation of the surrounding structures. Fat collections in specific pockets in and about the face, pharynx and larynx, and the areolar spaces, which are normally collapsed, are pre-established planes for cancer spread and infection. These spaces allow for mobility and the sliding of muscles during deglutition and speech. The various foramena are particularly vulnerable to spread. Because nerves pass through these openings in their course, perineural infiltration is often a problem.

Orientation of T-oncoanatomy: Odyssey of Primary Sites

The anatomic isocenter of a primary cancer site is the intersection of the three planar T-oncoanatomy views: coronal, sagittal, and transverse taken from *Grant's Atlas of Human Anatomy.* The axial orientation of the vertebral level is an important imaging reference point. Surface anatomy can vary from patient to patient; however, it is presented as a guide for the localization of the cancer in both accessible and internal anatomic sites that cannot be assessed on routine physical examination. The red bullets in our multilayered coronal

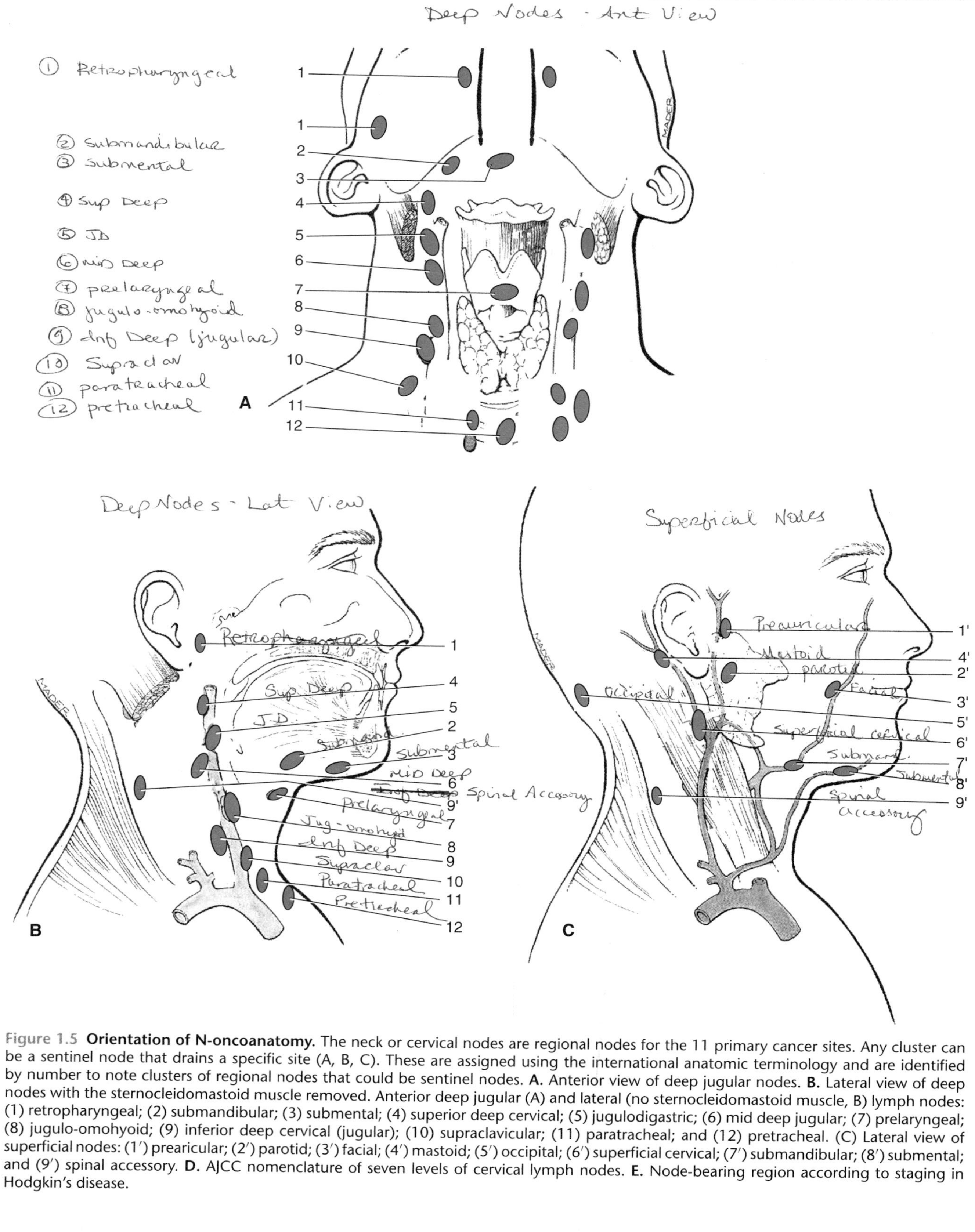

Figure 1.5 Orientation of N-oncoanatomy. The neck or cervical nodes are regional nodes for the 11 primary cancer sites. Any cluster can be a sentinel node that drains a specific site (A, B, C). These are assigned using the international anatomic terminology and are identified by number to note clusters of regional nodes that could be sentinel nodes. **A.** Anterior view of deep jugular nodes. **B.** Lateral view of deep nodes with the sternocleidomastoid muscle removed. Anterior deep jugular (A) and lateral (no sternocleidomastoid muscle, B) lymph nodes: (1) retropharyngeal; (2) submandibular; (3) submental; (4) superior deep cervical; (5) jugulodigastric; (6) mid deep jugular; (7) prelaryngeal; (8) jugulo-omohyoid; (9) inferior deep cervical (jugular); (10) supraclavicular; (11) paratracheal; and (12) pretracheal. (C) Lateral view of superficial nodes: (1′) preauricular; (2′) parotid; (3′) facial; (4′) mastoid; (5′) occipital; (6′) superficial cervical; (7′) submandibular; (8′) submental; and (9′) spinal accessory. **D.** AJCC nomenclature of seven levels of cervical lymph nodes. **E.** Node-bearing region according to staging in Hodgkin's disease.

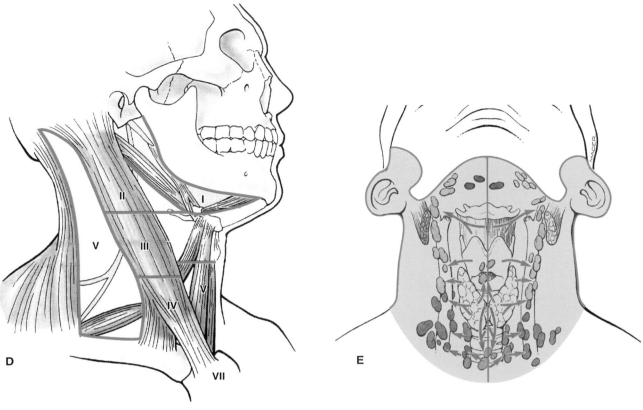

Figure 1.5 (*Continued*)

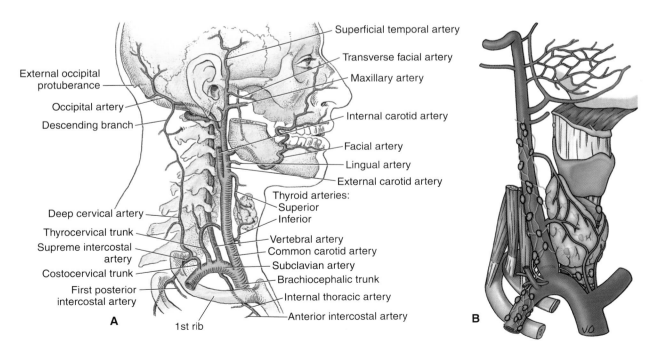

Figure 1.6 **Orientation of M-oncoanatomy. A.** Carotid artery with major branches shown. **B.** Pterygoid plexus of veins drains most of head and neck sites into internal deep jugular. Note green small normal lymph nodes are juxtaposed. The jugular vein drains into the superior vena cava and then into the right heart making lung the target organ.

(Fig. 1.4A) and sagittal (Fig. 1.4B) planes are a combination of both superficial and deep landmarks to identify primary sites. The tabulation of oncologic anatomy in the head and neck region starts at the base of the skull, and primary sites of head and neck cancers are noted in an axial fashion from cephalad to caudad and are arranged along planes anterior to the entire cervical spine from C1 to C7.

There are two major anatomic sectors with 11 distinct cancer primary sites currently staged (Fig. 1.4C–E; Table 1.3). These sectors are the upper aerorespiratory passage consisting of the nasal cavity, paranasal sinuses, the nasopharynx and the larynx; and the upper digestive passage, which contains the oral cavity, lips, oropharynx, and hypopharynx. Taken together, the anatomic physiologic complexity lies in the oropharynx, which is common to both systems.

Cervical fascial planes are important for compartmentalizing the neck and have a major impact on staging. To appreciate the neck compartments an axial and sagittal views (Fig. 1.4D,E) is required. The anterior compartment is defined by an investing fascia that envelopes the sternocleidomastoid muscle, and superficial muscles which are usually considered resectable (stage IVA), and houses the pharynx, larynx, and thyroid gland. Therefore, when pharyngeal cancer spread is anterior and inferior, it is more often amenable to surgical removal. With posterior and superior invasion patterns, pharyngeal cancers penetrate the prevertebral fascia into the prevertebral space, which is not resectable (stage IVB). Lateral spread into the carotid sheath is also an ominous sign; fixation of lymph nodes to the carotid artery renders the cancer unresectable. Clinically, it is difficult to diagnose cancer fixation to arteries; therefore, cancer node size >6 cm makes the evaluation more objective and has been shown to correlate with carotid artery involvement. The retropharyngeal space is ideal for pharyngeal cancer (Fig. 1.3C) spread vertically, but once the prevertebral fascia is invaded the cancer is no longer resectable. A concise overview (odyssey) of the 11 primary sites follows:

1. Cancers of the ethmoid sinus are the most superior in the head and neck region, whereas frontal sinuses and the sphenoid sinus tumefaction are rare and secondary to other neoplastic processes. Esthesioneuroblastoma can arise in the roof of the nasal cavity and involve the cribriform plate. Paranasal sinus cancer spread into other sinuses and orbital invasion are common.

2. Cancers of the nasopharynx can be insidious in onset and highly metastatic to lymph nodes. Cranial nerve involvement is due to cancer entry of the cavernous sinus via the foramen lacerum involving cranial nerves III, IV, V, and VI. In contrast, enlarging cervical metastatic lymph nodes, the highest in the deep cervical chain (Rouviere's node), can compress cranial nerves IX, X, XI, and XII.

3. Cancers of the maxillary antra can masquerade as a unilateral sinusitis and only become evident as erosion of their paper thin bones (lamina papyracea) occurs, loosening molar teeth, eroding into the cheek destroying the zygomatic arch, and most catastrophically into the orbit. The sentinel node tends to be submaxillary and therefore misleading.

4. Cancer of the lips and oral cavity can arise at numerous subsites that initiate the upper digestive passage. The common sites of malignancies are the food gutters, namely the floor of mouth and lateral border of the tongue. The sentinel nodes are often a function of the exact anatomic location of the primary cancer. With 10 different oral cavity subsites, anterior cancers lead to submental and submaxillary nodal invasion, whereas posterior neoplasms result in jugulodigastric nodes.

5. Neoplasms of the parotid gland are highly varied, and even benign mixed pleomorphic adenomas tend to recur, as can low-grade mixed mucoepidermoid cancers. Perineural invasion of cranial nerves VII, V, or both is a characteristic of cylindromas. The parotid gland lymph nodes are both the regional and sentinel nodes in location. Prolonged survival even in the face of pulmonary metastasis is a peculiarity of some salivary gland cancers.

6. Cancer of the oropharynx arises at the isocenter of the upper aerodigestive passage, which houses Waldeyer's ring, a favored site for malignant transformation. The underlying muscular planes predetermine spread patterns. The sentinel node is the jugulodigastric. Odynophagia referred to the middle ear is due to Jacobson's branch of cranial nerve IX.

7. Cancers of the hypopharynx may surround the larynx and block the food bolus, leading to aspiration into the larynx. Dysphagia can be caused by local invasion as well as cranial nerve involvement. The jugulo-omohyoid is often the sentinel node and can be invaded in contiguity with a primary.

8–10. Cancers of the larynx are divided into three parts: the supraglottis, glottis, and subglottis. Vocal cord involvement can be an early sign of malignancy. The malignant gradient varies with true glottic cancers being most readily detected in the earlier stages and therefore highly curable, whereas both the supraglottic and especially the subglottic cancers can be silent and more egregious in onset. Transglottic cancers advance as the cancer crosses the vocal cords. Paratracheal or paralaryngeal nodes can be the sentinel nodes. Odynophagia referred to the outer external ear is due to Arnold's nerve, a branch of the vagus (cranial nerve X), which supplies sensation to the larynx.

11. Thyroid cancers, although considered part of head and neck tumors, are unique because they arise from an endocrine gland and not an epithelial surface. The cancers can be well-differentiated colloid or papillary adenocarcinomas compatible with long survival despite lymph node invasion. Although the Delphic lymph node located above the isthmus can be the sentinel node, more often the inferior deep jugulo-omohyoid nodes are at risk. Anaplastic cancers can be highly lethal and metastasize early to the lungs.

Orientation of Regional Lymph Nodes: N-oncoanatomy

Understanding the complex anatomy of the neck is essential to appreciate the many nuances and evolution of changes. *Most important is an appreciation that the major regional nodal areas are divided into superficial and deep cervical node chains; the latter includes the high retropharyngeal and parapharyngeal nodes.* Each of the major head and neck cancer sites drain into a specific region of neck nodes—sentinel nodes (Fig. 1.5; Table 1.4). Some have unilateral drainage, others bilateral. The most commonly involved lymph nodes are those along the internal jugular vein, which are subdivided into superior, mid, and inferior deep cervical node chains. They include the jugulodigastric and jugulo-omohyoid, and the scalene nodes in the anterior aspect of the supraclavicular fossae. A series of two planar orientation diagrams of regional lymph nodes and their lymphatics are shown in anterior and lateral views (Fig. 1.5A–C). Each primary anatomic site or subsite has a sentinel node or favored nodes to which it drains preferentially. This can be determined clinically by injecting a radiocolloid such as Au[198] or methylene blue dye at the primary site and dissecting the node that concentrates the most radioactivity. It is equally important to be aware of all the lymph nodes at risk. The clinician needs to locate first station nodes in three planes to determine if they are accessible for physical examination.

Traditionally, the triangles of the neck are used to define the topographic anatomy that consists of anterior and posterior triangles (Fig. 1.5D). *The sternocleidomastoid muscle divides the neck into these two major triangles; many other small triangles exist.* The external jugular vein and the platysma muscle are superficial to the sternocleidomastoid muscle. Deep to the sternocleidomastoid are the carotid artery, internal jugular vein, and some cranial nerves. Deep cervical lymph nodes also surround the carotid sheath. The lymphatic channels and lymph nodes are located more anteriorly as they follow the sternocleidomastoid muscle inferiorly. The nodes in the neck make up one of the most important sec-

tions of oncologic anatomy. The lymphatics of the head are, in essence, the lymphatic channels in the neck and their lymph nodes. Regional nodes are not always the closest anatomically to the primary site nor are the sentinel nodes solely involved with cancers of the head and neck. Distant primary sites both above and below the diaphragm can spread to neck nodes, especially supraclavicular nodes (Virchow's node).

The nomenclature we use is that of *The International Anatomic Terminology*, and this correlates with various staging systems and terms proposed by the American Joint Committee on Cancer (AJCC). The AJCC has grouped regional lymph nodes in the neck into seven levels and subdivided specific anatomic subsites (Fig. 1.5D). Each level is designated by a Roman numeral (I–VII). *Lymph node-bearing region* is promulgated by Hodgkin's disease and lymphoma staging rather than anatomic physiologic considerations and deserves to be reconsidered in terms of cancer spread. According to AJCC/International Union Against Cancer clinical staging for Hodgkin's disease, each side of the neck is one lymph node-bearing region (Fig. 1.5E). The lymphoid tissue of Waldeyer's ring is an extranodal lymphoid collection that forms the palatine tonsils. The lymphoid tissue extends superiorly into the pharyngeal wall and the roof of the nasopharynx and inferiorly into the base of the tongue. Midline anatomic sites such as Waldeyer's ring drain bilaterally, whereas paired or parallel structures drain unilaterally to their respective deep jugular nodes, right or left.

M-oncoanatomy of Regional Veins and the Neurovascular Bundle

The head and neck is generally considered one anatomic and physiologic unit; all sites share a common regional arterial blood supply and venous drainage (Fig. 1.6A). Most of the upper aerodigestive passages are supplied by the branches of the carotid artery. Their venous drainage is through the pterygoid venous plexus deep to the masseter muscle and is retropharyngeal, next to the posterior aspect of the parotid gland and then by way of the jugular veins. Cancer can disseminate hematogenously through vascular routing most often to the superior vena cava to the right side of the heart and lung via the pulmonary circulation and then to other organs systemically. Lung is the target organ for the first signs of distant metastases for the majority of head and neck cancers.

The cranial nerves become peripheral as they exit the skull to innervate the head and neck region. Cranial nerves IX, X, XI, and XII descend in the neck with the carotid artery and internal jugular vein and constitute the major neurovascular bundle in the head and neck region (Fig. 1.6B). Metastatic cancer to the deep chain of jugular lymph nodes can produce cranial neuropathy. Rouviere's node is the highest cervical node; it is clinically inaccessible and retropharyngeal in location.

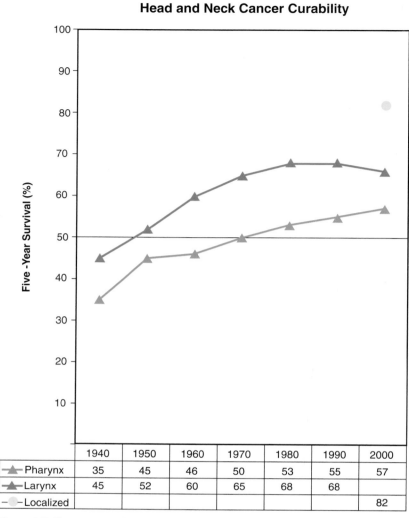

Head and Neck Cancer Curability

	1940	1950	1960	1970	1980	1990	2000
▲ Pharynx	35	45	46	50	53	55	57
▲ Larynx	45	52	60	65	68	68	
● Localized							82

Figure 1.7 **Five-year survival curve.** There has been a steady increase in 5-year survival for oral cavity, pharynx, and larynx cancers from 1950 to 2000.

TABLE 1.6	**Head and Neck: Cancer Statistics**				
			5-Year Survival Rates (%)		
Site	**Incidence**	**Mortality**	**1950**	**2000**	**Percent Gain**
Oral cavity and pharynx	28,260	7,230	46	60	+14
Larynx	10,270	3,830	52	67	+15
Thyroid	23,600	1,460	80-	96	+16

From Ries LAG, Eisner MP, Kosary CL, et al, eds. *SEER Cancer Statistics Review, 1975–2001* [Tables XII-4 and XIX-4]. Bethesda, MD: National Cancer Institute. Available at: http://seer.cancer.gov/csr/1975_2001/.

TABLE 1.7	Cancer Curability by Stages at Diagnosis (1992–1998)			
	5-Year Survival Rate (%)			
Site	All Stages	Local	Regional	Distant
Oral cavity and pharynx	56	95	81	31
Larynx	64	82	51	38
Thyroid	96	99	95	44

From Ries LAG, Eisner MP, Kosary CL, et al, eds. *SEER Cancer Statistics Review, 1975–2001* [Tables XII-4 and XIX-4]. Bethesda, MD: National Cancer Institute. Available at: http://seer.cancer.gov/csr/1975_2001/.

Jugular foramen syndrome is characterized by loss of the gag reflex (cranial nerve IX), vocal cord paralysis (cranial nerve X), atrophy of the trapezius muscle (cranial nerve XI), and deviation of the uvula (cranial nerve X) and tongue on protrusion (cranial nerve XII).

Rules for Classification and Staging

Clinical Staging and Imaging

Clinical staging is an essential step in establishing meaningful data. Physical examination includes visualization of upper aerodigestive passage whenever possible and is often combined with mirror or direct endoscopy. Palpation is critical to define endophytic induration whenever feasible. Imaging is important, particularly spiral computed tomography (CT) and magnetic resonance imaging (MRI), which can provide superb visualization of the three-planar anatomy. MRI provides better visualization of soft tissue cancer infiltration; CT better detects bone destruction. The difference in density of tissue planes allows for viewing fat as black on CT and white on MRI, in contrast to the grey of muscles and viscera in contrasting these diagnostic modes. Cancer can be enhanced by contrast administration owing to a greater degree of tumor neovascularization versus normal tissue vascularity. However, MRI is better than CT in that tumorous infiltrates appear intensely white. Identification of enlarged lymph nodes (>1 cm^2) requires contrast visualization of arteries and veins (white) on CT; blood flow allows for a black image of the neck vessels on MRI. Each anatomic site is discussed for nuances, imaging highlights, and notations. Suspicious neck nodes need fine needle aspiration for confirmation (Table 1.5). An excellent reference from which oncoimaging notations highlight important aspects of cancer spread and staging at each primary site is by Bragg, Rubin, and Hricak (2002).

Pathologic Staging

Gross specimen should be evaluated for margins. Unresected gross residual tumor must be reported and marked with clips. All resected lymph node specimens should describe size, number, and level of involved nodes and whether there is extracapsular spread. Specimens postradiation and/or chemotherapy need to so noted. Specimen shrinkages may occur up to 30% after resection itself. Designations pT and pN should be used after histopathologic evaluation. Perineural invasion deserves special notation.

Cancer Statistics and Survival

Cancers of the oral cavity and pharynx—the upper digestive passage—account for 28,000 new cases per year. In addition, cancers of the larynx provide another 10,000 patients and thyroid cancers 23,600. Approximately 25% of head and neck cancer patients die annually, often from other causes. For long-term survival, thyroid cancers, with only 1,500 deaths (5%), are the exception. The improvement in oral cavity and pharyngeal tumors from 1950 to 2000 was modest (14%) and matches larynx (15%). A multidisciplinary approach is vital and normal tissue conservation and reconstructive techniques have added greatly to quality of life. Unfortunately, this patient population are ethanol and nicotine abusers and it is difficult to change their habits. Persistence of smoking and drinking contributes to their demise, often from second malignant tumors in adjacent sites (Fig. 1.7).

Remarkably, $>55\%$ of patients are alive at 5 years; the majority live to 10 years. When treatment fails, death is within 2 years in 90% of patients and is often painful and disfiguring. African Americans in particular tend to die at a higher rate (75%). Another source for assessing the gains in survival in head and neck cancers is based on the multidisciplinary approach to management in national cooperative groups. The large database accumulated by the Radiation Therapy Oncology Group allows for 5-year survival analysis by major anatomic sites and their subsites as a function of stage. Stage I patients survive at the 60% to 80% level, stage II at 40% to 60%, stage III at 30% to 60%, and stage IV at 15% to 30%. With combined modality treatment, chemoradiation and surgery yields complete response rates of 45% to 95% depending on stage (Tables 1.6 and 1.7) and often allows for preservation of normal structures (e.g., larynx).

2

Paranasal Ethmoid Sinus

The ethmoid sinuses and nasal passages are the appropriate introduction to the upper respiratory tract oncoanatomy since the malignant gradient of the ethmoid sinus is its access and communication with all of the other paranasal sinuses.

Perspective and Patterns of Spread

Ethmoid sinus cancer, although rare, is more common than cancers of the sphenoid or frontal sinus. Because of their deep-seated location, these neoplasms are even more difficult to diagnose than maxillary antral cancers. The cancer is insidious in onset, but each manifestation is explicable by the pattern of invasion of the surrounding anatomy. A deep-seated headache around or posterior to the eyes suggests invasion into the surrounding sinuses—the frontal anteriorly, the sphenoid posteriorly, or the contralateral ethmoid or the maxillary sinus inferiorly (Fig. 2.1). With lateral extension, orbital invasion and globe displacement can occur. The clinical triad of symptoms and signs of ethmoid sinus cancer are diplopia, a bloody nasal discharge, and loss of sensation in the upper lip.

These mucoperiosteum spaces have ciliated columnar epithelium that sweeps mucus to the nasal cavity. Ethmoid cancers arise from these mucosal linings of the sinus and tend to be adenocarcinomas as well as squamous cell cancers. They have been associated with the shavings and dust of furniture and cabinetmakers (Table 2.1).

TNM Staging Criteria

The ethmoid sinus is a new primary site added to the TNM staging system (Fig. 2.2). As with most sites, the cancer infiltrates the surrounding structures, depending on its site of origin; pathways of least resistance (in this instance, at its foramen or where the bone is thinnest) manifest themselves, displaying the triad of symptoms mentioned. The patterns of spread are determined by the malignant gradient, which is more favorable (T4a) with anterior and inferior spread compared with posterior

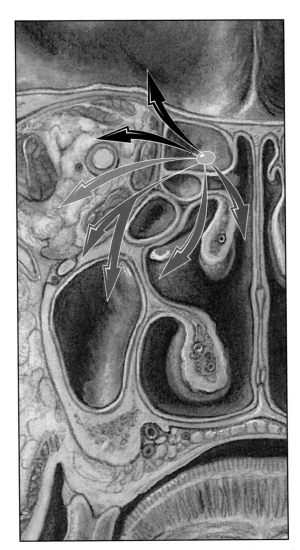

Figure 2.1 **Patterns of spread.** The primary cancer (paranasal ethmoid sinus) invades in various directions which are color-coded vectors (*arrows*) representing stage of progression: Tis, yellow; T1, green; T2, blue; T3, purple; T4a, red; T4b, black.

DEFINITION OF TNM

T1
Tumor restricted to any one subsite, with or without bony invasion

N0
No regional lymph node metastasis

T2
Tumor invading two subsites in a single region or extending to involve an adjacent region within the nasoethmoidal complex, with or without bony invasion

N0
No regional lymph node metastasis

T3
Tumor extends to invade the medial wall or floor of the orbit, maxillary sinus, palate, or cribriform plate

N1
Metastasis in a single ipsilateral lymph node, ≤3 cm in greatest dimension

T4a
Tumor invades any of the following: anterior orbital contents, skin of nose or cheek, minimal extension to anterior cranial fossa, pterygoid plates, sphenoid or frontal sinuses

N2
Metastasis in lymph nodes, none >6 cm
(N2a) Single ipsilateral, >3 cm but ≤6 cm
(N2b) Multiple ipsilateral, none >6 cm
(N2c) Bilateral or contralateral, none 6 cm

T4b
Tumor invades any of the following: orbital apex, dura, brain, middle cranial fossa, cranial nerves other than (V2), nasopharynx, or clivus

N3
Metastasis in a lymph node, >6 cm in greatest dimension

STAGE GROUPINGS

Stage I
T1 N0 M0

Stage II
T2 N0 M0

Stage III
T3 N0 M0
T1 N1 M0
T2 N1 M0
T3 N1 M0

Stage IVA
T4a N0 M0
T4a N1 M0
T1   N2 M0
T2   N2 M0
T3   N2 M0
T4a N2 M0

Stage IVB
T4b Any N M0
Any T N3   M0

Stage IVC
Any T Any N M1

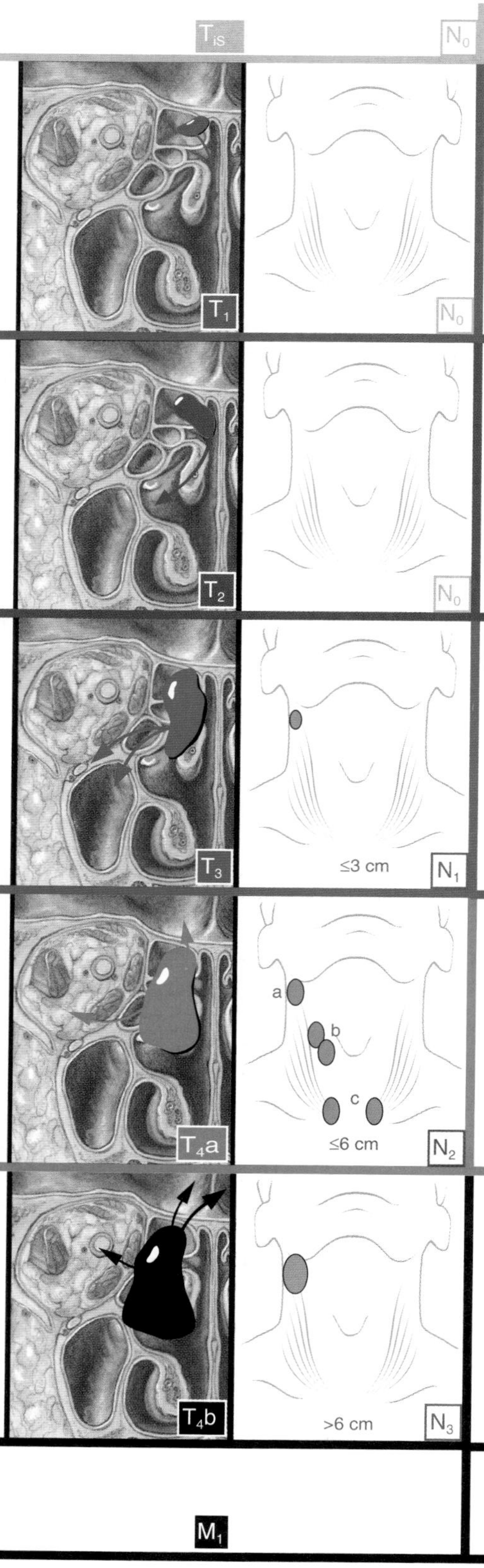

Figure 2.2 TNM stage grouping. Ethmoid cancers invade other paranasal sinuses and the orbit. Vertical presentations of stage groupings, which follow the same color code for cancer stage advancement, are organized in horizontal lanes: stage 0, yellow; I, green; II, blue; III, purple; IVA, red; IVB, black. Definitions of TN on left and stage grouping on right.

TABLE 2.1	Histopathologic Type: Common Cancers of the Paranasal Ethmoid Sinus
Squamous Cell Carcinoma Microscopic Variants	
Keratinizing; well differentiated; moderately well differentiated; poorly differentiated	
Nonkeratinizing; anaplastic squamous carcinoma	
Transitional cell carcinoma	
Spindle cell squamous carcinoma	

Adapted from Rubin P. *Clinical oncology.* 8th ed. New York: Elsevier; 2001:408.

superior vectors. The spread patterns form the basis for T4a resectable and T4b unresectable disease. With T4a, the ethmoid cancer invades the anterior orbital contents and the skin of the nose and cheek, whereas with T4b, the cancer invades posteriorly into the nasopharynx, orbital apex, and optic nerve and superiorly into the dura, brain, and middle fossa.

Summary of Changes

Nasoethmoid is new site being added with staging based on subsites and cancer extension into regional anatomy.

Orientation of Three-planar Oncoanatomy

The ethmoid sinus is the anatomic isocenter of all paranasal sinuses; the ethmoid communicates with each of the other paranasal sinuses: frontal (superoanterior), sphenoid (posterior), maxillary inferior, and lateral. The anatomic isocenter is at the level of the floor of the orbit and extends to the sphenoid at the skull base. The anterior surface bullet enters to the right or left of the midsagittal plane at or below the medial canthus of the eye (Fig. 2.3A). The lateral bullet is at or below the lateral canthus of the eye (Fig. 2.3B).

T-oncoanatomy

The ethmoid sinuses and nasal passages are the appropriate introduction to the upper respiratory tract. The eight major sinuses in the face and skull are in direct continuity. The three paired sinuses are the maxillary, ethmoid, frontal sinuses, and the sphenoid. Although the sphenoid appears as a single midline sinus, it is a paired sinus. A three-dimensional reconstruction, focusing on bony anatomy, allows for an understanding of the interrelationships. The anatomy may be divided by drawing three parallel lines across the frontal view of the skull, one line passing above and another below the orbits, the third passing through the floor of the antra or hard palate. The two vertical lines separate the ethmoid and nasal fossa from the maxillary antra. The nasal septum separates the ethmoid and nasal fossa into right

and left sides. In a comparison with anteroposterior and lateral projections or coronal and sagittal sections, three important planes become evident: (i) The floor of the anterior fossa of the skull is the roof of the nasal cavity and ethmoid; (ii) The hard palate is the floor of the maxillary antra; and (iii) An imaginary plane below the orbits divides the paranasal sinuses into a suprastructure and an infrastructure. The suprastructure contains the ethmoids, anterior to which is the apex of the nasal cavity and cribriform (olfactory region). Posterior to this are the sphenoid sinuses, medial are the orbits, and inferior are the nasal fossa and turbinates. The infrastructure contains the maxillary antra and the major portion of the nasal cavity or vestibule. These planes are helpful in relating the surface anatomy to the radiographic anatomy. The three-dimensional planar views are crucial to understanding the malignant gradient:

- *Coronal plane* (Fig. 2.4A): In the coronal view, the lateral anterior wall separates the ethmoid sinus from the orbit and inferiorly drains into the nasal cavity.
- *Sagittal plane* (Fig. 2.4B): The relationship to the maxillary antrum is readily seen as well as to the sphenoid sinus. Anterior to the ethmoid is the cribriform plate and cranial nerve I (olfactory).
- *Axial plane* (Fig. 2.4C): The orbit and its relation to the ethmoid sinus is shown and illustrates the fineness of the walls separating the two cavities. The sphenoid sinus has the most complex anatomic location in contrast to the frontal sinus, which has the simplest. To understand cranial nerve anatomy, one must relate the course of the first six nerves to the walls of the sphenoid sinuses. The various divisions and branches of the cranial nerve V and its trigeminal ganglion are in its vicinity. This is detailed when studying the nasopharynx, which is directly below the sphenoid sinuses and cavernous sinus.

N-oncoanatomy

The sentinel nodes are the high retroparapharyngeal and parapharyngeal nodes along the carotid sheath; when they are involved and extend into the retrostyloid compartment (Fig. 2.5). This leads to entrapment of the

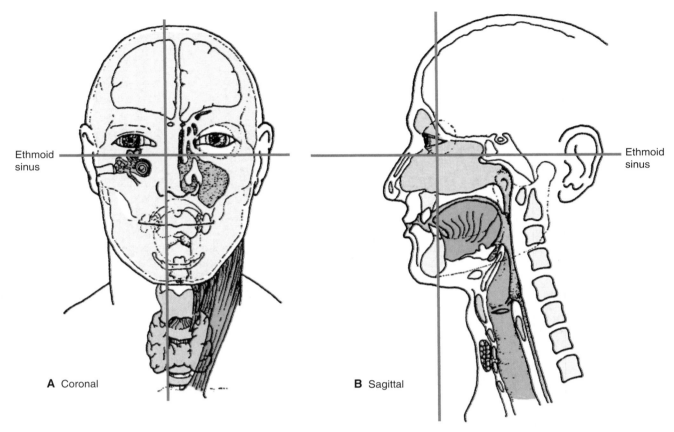

Ethmoid
sinus

Ethmoid
sinus

A Coronal

B Sagittal

Figure 2.3 Orientation of three-planar T-oncoanatomy. The anatomic isocenter is at the axial level of the sphenoid sinus. **A.** Coronal. **B.** Sagittal.

cranial nerves emerging alongside the jugular foramen. The nodes in this region are named after Rouviere, famous for his treatise on lymphoid anatomy. Again, numerous neurologic syndromes can occur. The retroparotidian syndrome, or the jugular foramen syndrome, is characterized by loss of the gag reflex (cranial nerve IX), vocal cord paralysis (cranial nerve X), atrophy of the trapezius muscle (cranial nerve XI), and deviation of the uvula (cranial nerve X) and tongue on protrusion (cranial nerve XII).

M-oncoanatomy

The lateral pterygoid buccal venous plexus drains into the jugular vein and then into the subclavan vein and right superior vena cava. Hematogenous spread, although uncommon, can include lung and bone as favored sites of involvement; distant metastases occur infrequently (Fig 2.6).

Rules of Classification and Staging

Clinical Staging and Imaging

Inspection and palpation of paranasal sinuses is limited in early localized stages. For ethmoid cancers, orbital invasion may displace the globe and trap the anterior ethmoid branch of cranial nerve V_1, leading to altered sensation in the upper lip. Maxillary antral cancers, when advanced, fill the gingival buccal gutter, loosen molar teeth, and invade the cheek and hard palate. Infection and inflammatory sinusitis obscures cancers. Both magnetic resonance imaging (MRI) and computed tomography enhancement (CT_e) are recommended to distinguish tumor from fluid. CT_e is best for determining bone erosion of the paper-thin lamina bones of sinus walls. For evaluation of retropharyngeal nodes imaging is essential (see Table 1.5).

Pathologic Staging

The gross specimen should be evaluated for margins. Unresected gross residual tumor must be included and marked with clips. All resected lymph node specimens should describe size, number, and level of involved nodes and whether there is extracapsular spread. Specimens taken after radiation or chemotherapy need to be noted as such; specimen shrinkages may occur up to 30% after resection itself. Designations pT and pN should be used after histopathologic evaluation. Perineural invasion deserves special notation.

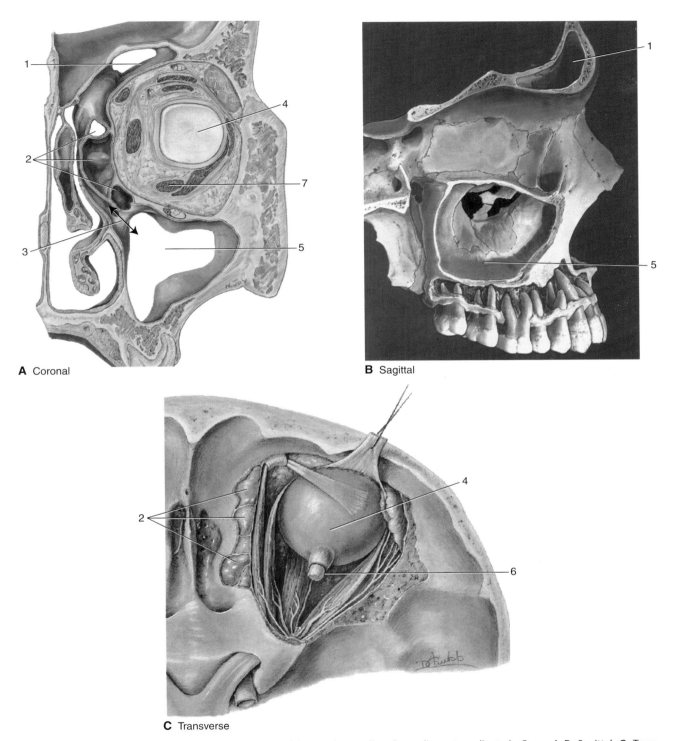

A Coronal

B Sagittal

C Transverse

Figure 2.4 **T-oncoanatomy.** Three-planar views are crucial to understanding the malignant gradient. **A.** Coronal. **B.** Sagittal. **C.** Transverse. (1) Frontal sinus. (2) Ethmoidal cells. (3) Opening of maxillary sinus. (4) Eyeball. (5) Maxillary sinus. (6) Optic nerve. (7) Orbital content.

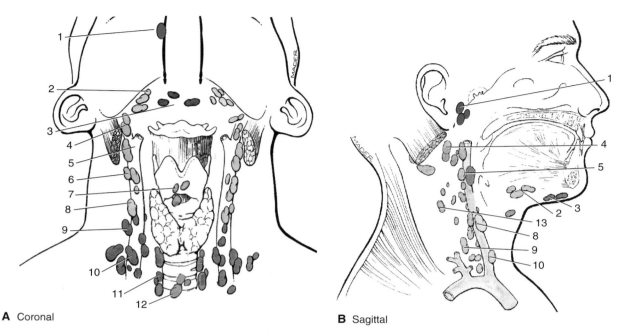

A Coronal   **B** Sagittal

Figure 2.5 N-oncoanatomy. The red node highlights the sentinel node, which is the highest retropharyngeal node. **A.** Coronal. **B.** Sagittal. Once the sentinel node is involved, all of the neck nodes are at risk for metastases. The regional nodes include: (1) retropharyngeal; (2) submandibular; (3) submental; (4) superior deep cervical; (5) jugulodigastric; and (6) midjugular. The juxtaregional nodes are: (7) prelaryngeal; (8) jugulo-omohyoid; (9) inferior deep cervical; (10) supraclavicular; (11) paratracheal; (12) pretracheal; and (13) spinal accessory.

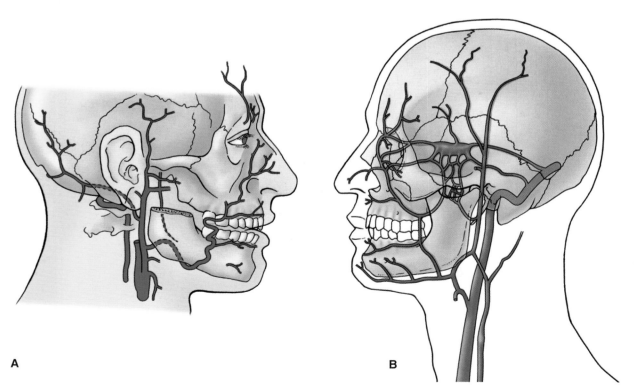

A   **B**

Figure 2.6 M-oncoanatomy. A. Carotid artery with major shown. **B.** Pterygoid plexus of veins drains most of head and neck sites into internal deep jugular. The jugular vein drains into the superior vena cava and then into the right heart, making lung the target organ.

Oncoimaging Annotations

- MRI and CT play complementary roles in the assessment and staging process for these tumors.

- MRI is best at detecting tumor extension outside the sinonasal cavity. CT is most sensitive in assessing anatomy and bone invasion with these tumors. The hallmark of sinonasal malignancy is bone destruction, seen in approximately 80% of all CT scans in these patients.

- MRI aids in separating complex sinonasal secretions/ infections from tumor. Combined T1- and T2-weighted, contrast medium-enhanced images are needed for this evaluation.

- Orbital extension is manifest on CT and MRI by bone erosion and changes in the orbital fat. MRI tends to underestimate orbital invasion.

- Sinonasal bony sclerosis caused by tumor is rare; its presence is normally related to coexistent chronic inflammatory changes.

Cancer Statistics and Survival

Generally, cancers of the oral cavity and pharynx (the upper digestive passage) account for 28,000 new cases (see Table 1.6). In addition, cancer of the larynx affects another 10,000 patients and thyroid cancers 23,600. Approximately 25% of head and neck cancer patients die annually, often owing to other causes. Long-term survival rates in patients with thyroid cancer with only 1500 deaths (5%), is the exception. The improvement in survival rates in patients with oral cavity and pharyngeal tumors from 1950 to 2000 was modest at 14% and matches that for patients with tumors of the larynx at 15%. A multidisciplinary approach is vital, and normal tissue conservation and reconstructive techniques have both added greatly to quality of life. Unfortunately, this patient population are ethanol and nicotine abusers and it is difficult to change these habits. Persistence of smoking and drinking contributes to their demise, often from second malignant tumors in adjacent sites.

Specifically, paranasal sinus cancers are detected late due to being mistaken for sinusitis. Both ethmoid and maxillary central cancers remain well below 50% 5-year survival.

3

Maxillary Sinus Antrum

The use of Ohngren's plane provides the malignant gradient of the maxillary antrum, dividing the sinus into an anterior/inferior compartment and a posterior/superior pocket.

Perspective and Patterns of Spread

Tumors arising in the paranasal sinuses can be both very destructive and deforming. Fortunately, they are uncommon. Cancers of the maxillary antrum and ethmoid are among those more frequently encountered. The unique anatomic feature at these sites is the direct juxtaposition of the mucous membrane with very thin bony walls. Unfortunately, the manifestations of localized cancers are similar to sinusitis. Consequently, most cancers masquerade as infections and go unrecognized. It is no surprise, therefore, that the first detectable clinical signs of cancer are of advanced spread, most often owing to invasion through bony walls (Fig. 3.1). To the astute clinician, a persistent unilateral sinusitis may be a clue to an underlying cancer.

Most maxillary antral cancers are squamous cell cancers (Table 3.1). Ethmoid cancers can be either squamous cell or adenocarcinomas. In contrast, tumors of the nose are highly varied, although again, they are most often squamous cell cancers. As for most sites, the cancer infiltrates the surrounding structures, which depends on its site of origin. Pathways of least resistance are at the foramena or where the bone is thinnest and are manifested by displaying a number of typical signs. The infrastructure of the maxillary sinus is the most common site of cancer origin, and the medial wall is easy to penetrate because of the normal ostia. Bloody nasal discharge appears before erosion of this paper-thin wall. As the mass extends medially into the nose, nasal obstruction can occur. The floor of the maxillary sinus is in close contact with molar dental roots and their nerves. Consequently, as the bone is destroyed with inferior spread, there is filling of the gingivobucal gutter, loosening of teeth, and finally an ulcerating lesion and loss of the alveolar bone with extension into the hard palate.

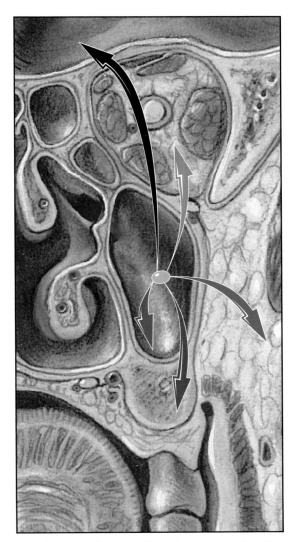

Figure 3.1 **Patterns of spread.** The primary cancer (maxillary sinus antrum) invades in various directions which are color-coded vectors (*arrows*) representing stage of progression. Tis, yellow; T1, green; T2, blue; T3, purple; T4a, red; and T4b, black.

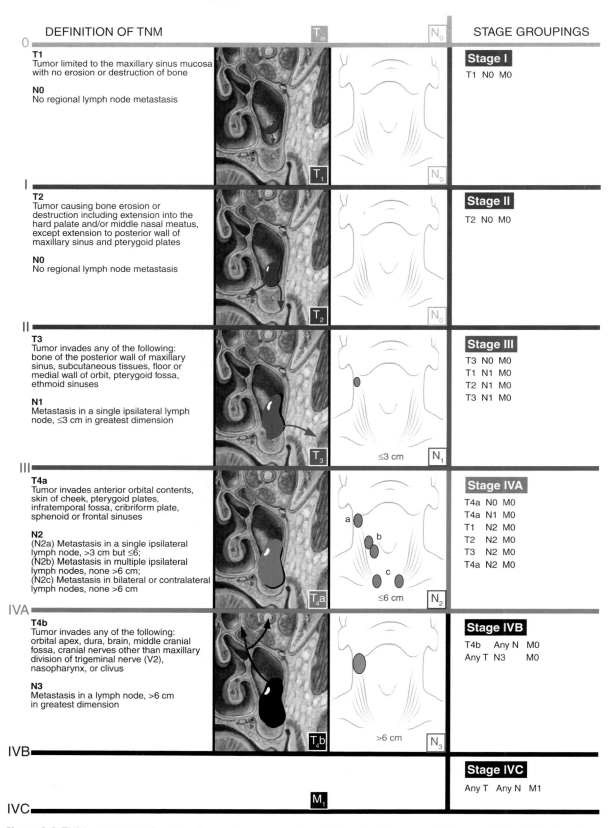

Figure 3.2 TNM stage grouping. Maxillary antrum cancers invade through their paper-thin bone walls in all six directions. Vertical presentations of stage groupings which follow same color code for cancer stage advancement are organized in horizontal lanes. Stage 0, yellow; I, green; II, blue; III, purple; IVA, red; IVB and IVC, black. Definitions of TN on left and stage grouping on right.

TABLE 3.1	Histopathologic Type: Common Cancers of the Maxillary Antrum

Squamous Cell Carcinoma Microscopic Variants

Keratinizing; well differentiated; moderately well differentiated; poorly differentiated

Nonkeratinizing; anaplastic squamous carcinoma

Transitional cell carcinoma

Spindle cell squamous carcinoma

Adapted from Rubin P. *Clinical Oncology.* 8th Ed. New York: Elsevier; 2001:408.

Cancers of the suprastructure usually occur at the summit of the sinusoidal pyramid. They extend into the malar bone and the outer half of the floor of the orbit into the temporal fossa. The skin of the cheek rapidly expands, often as a result of infection, and the zygomatic arch can be destroyed. The eye can be displaced and become proptotic when there is superior invasion. A posterior location and spread of cancer is less common, but in advanced states, the tumor, particularly when it is aggressive, can explode the sinus cavity and move in all directions via the associated infection. Under these circumstances, the cancer invades the pterygoid plates and muscles, leading to trismus.

TNM Staging Criteria

The TNM criteria for the maxillary antrum were introduced with the 4th edition of the American Joint Committee on Cancer/International Union Against Cancer (1992) and are based on patterns of spread rather than size (Fig. 3.2). The use of Ohngren's plane provides the malignant gradient of the maxillary antrum, dividing the sinus into an anterior/inferior compartment and a posterior/superior pocket. With massive invasion, cancer of the maxillary sinus can invade other paranasal sinuses, enter into the cranial fossa, and even reach the lateral pterygoid space.

Summary of Changes

As stated, TNM patterns of spread are based on an imaginary oblique plane, referred to as Ohngren's line, which divides the antrum into the anterior/inferior portion resectable T4a and a posterior/superior half unresectable T4b. T4a/b was introduced with the 6th edition (2003). The major sites invaded are as follows: T4a, cheek and zygoma (anteriorly and laterally), floor of the maxilla and mouth (inferiorly), turbinates and nasal cavity (medially); and T4b, ethmoid sinus (superiorly), floor of the orbit (superiorly), and pterygoid plates and fossa (posteriorly). Eventually, the cancer extends into the brain, middle cranial fossa, and nasopharynx. The T stages are based on patterns of spread and not size as for other head and neck sites.

Orientation of Three-planar Oncoanatomy

For the maxillary antrum the anatomic isocenter is at the level of the clivus. The anterior surface bullet is at the level of or slightly inferior to the bridge of the nose to the right and left of the midline (Fig. 3.3A). Centered inferior to the pupil of the eye (Fig 3.3B), the lateral bullet is at the level of the external auditory canal and inferior to a line connecting the lateral canthus of the eye and the external auditory canal.

T-oncoanatomy

To appreciate the manifestation of cancer of the paranasal sinus, a thorough knowledge of the three-dimensional aspects of paranasal sinus anatomy is essential. The eight major sinuses in the face and skull are in direct continuity. The three paired sinuses are the maxillary, the ethmoid, frontal sinuses, and the sphenoid. Although the sphenoid appears as a single midline sinus, it is also a paired sinus. A three-dimensional reconstruction, focusing on bony anatomy, allows for an understanding of the interrelationships. The anatomy may be divided by drawing three parallel lines across the frontal view of the skull, one line passing above and another below the orbits, the third passing through the floor of the antra or hard palate. The two vertical lines separate the ethmoid and nasal fossa from the maxillary antra. The nasal septum separates the ethmoid and nasal fossa into the right and left sides.

- *Coronal plane* (Fig. 3.4A): In a comparison of antero-posterior and lateral projections or coronal and sagittal sections, three important planes become evident: (i) The floor of the anterior fossa of the skull (in the roof of the nasal cavity and ethmoid); (ii) The hard palate, in the floor of the maxillary antra; and (iii) An imaginary plane below the orbits that divides the paranasal sinuses into a suprastructure and an infrastructure. The suprastructure contains the ethmoids,

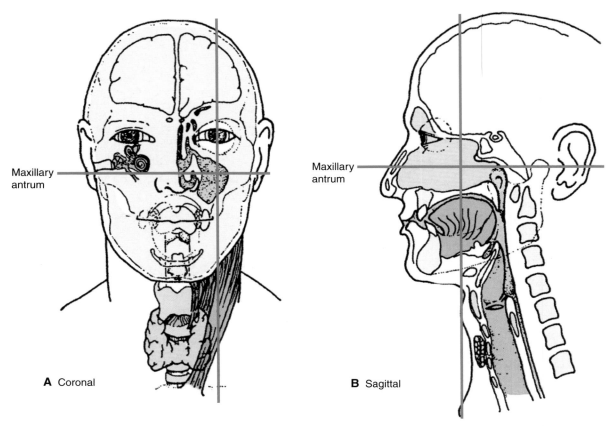

Maxillary
antrum

Maxillary
antrum

A Coronal

B Sagittal

Figure 3.3 **Orientation of three-planar T-oncoanatomy.** The anatomic isocenter is at the axial level of the clivus. **A.** Coronal **B.** Sagittal.

anterior to which is the apex of the nasal cavity and cribriform (olfactory region). The sphenoid sinus is posterior, the orbits are medial, and the nasal fossa and turbinates are inferior to the suprastructure. The infrastructure contains the maxillary antra and the major portion of the nasal cavity or vestibule. These planes are helpful in relating the external anatomy of physical diagnosis to the radiographic anatomy.

- *Sagittal plane* (Fig. 3.4B): The relationship of the teeth in the superior alveolus determines which teeth are affected as tumor invasion of the floor occurs. First, the second premolar or bicuspid, and the first and second molars are in the floor itself and become loosened. The upper canine may become involved when there is more anterior invasion. Rarely, however, are the incisors affected. The third molar can be loosened when there is posterior extension. The ethmoid sinuses are the central paranasal space in the suprastructure with communication to the frontal sphenoid sinuses and the nasal cavity. The ethmoid bone also constitutes the cribriform plate and the superior and medial concha. The important nerves in its walls are (a) the anterior ethmoidal branch of the

ophthalmic division of the cranial nerve V (anterior at the junction with the frontal sinus); (b) the olfactory nerve and bulb in and above the cribriform plate; and (c) the nasociliary nerve inside the orbit that branches into the posterior and anterior ethmoidal nerves, infratrochlear, and the internal nasal branches.

- *Transverse plane* (Fig. 3.4C): The maxillary antrum is the essential paranasal sinus to study in the infrastructure. It is pyramidal with its apex at the malar arch and base at the nasal cavity. It projects as a triangulated space from virtually every view. The bony walls consist of the maxillary bone in its entirety, laterally, anteriorly, and inferiorly. The medial wall is constituted inferiorly by the concha and palatine bone, superiorly and laterally by the zygomatic bone, and posteriorly by the pterygoid plates of the sphenoid. The important nerves to identify in these walls are those in the infraorbital branch of the maxillary division of cranial nerve V through the canal in the perpendicular plate of the palatine posteriorly. The posterior aspect and its relationship to the pterygoid plates and muscle with its access to major vessels and retropharyngeal nodes.

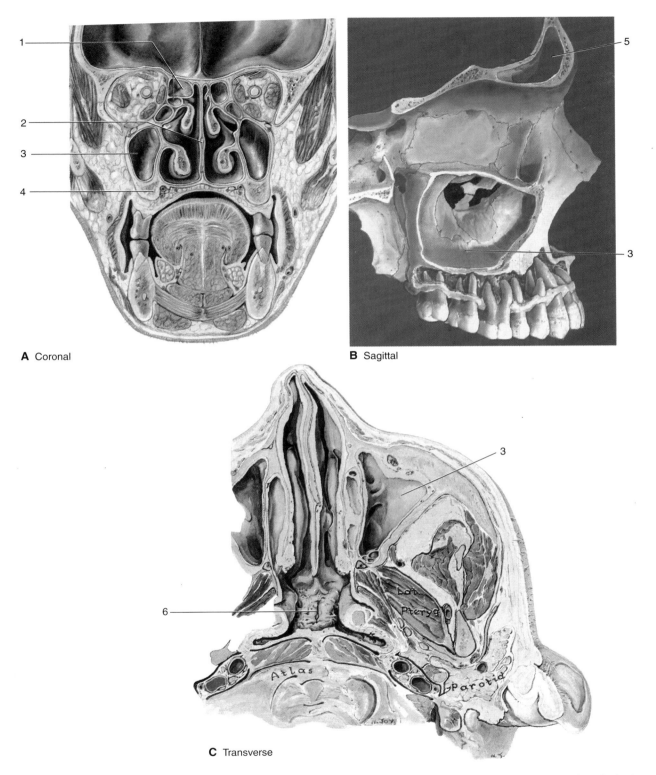

A Coronal

B Sagittal

C Transverse

Figure 3.4 **T-oncoanatomy.** The three-planar views are crucial to understanding the malignant gradient. **A.** Coronal. **B.** Sagittal. **C.** Transverse. (1) Ethmoidal cells. (2) Middle nasal meatus. (3) Maxillary sinus. (4) Hard palate. (5) Frontal sinus. (6) Pharyngeal tonsil.

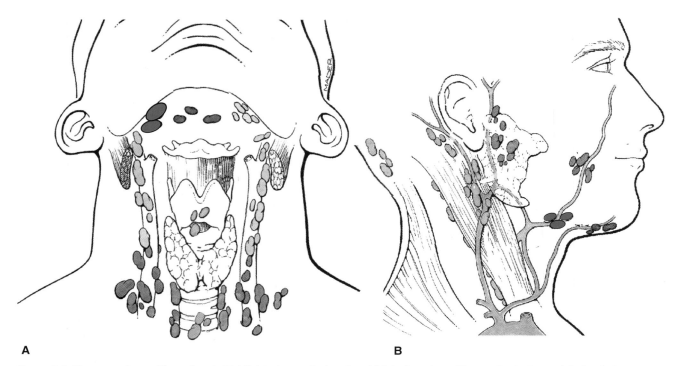

A   **B**

Figure 3.5 N-oncoanatomy. The red node highlights the sentinel node, which is the submaxillary node. **A.** Coronal. **B.** Sagittal.

N-oncoanatomy

Lymphatic involvement occurs late, despite extensive disease. The submaxillary node is usually the first (often the only) node invaded and it is the sentinel node (Fig. 3.5). The major lymphatic drainage of the maxillary antrum is through the lateral and inferior collecting trunks to the first station submaxillary, parotid, and jugulodigastric nodes, and via the superoposterior trunk to the retropharyngeal and deep cervical nodes.

M-oncoanatomy

The pterygoid plexus of veins drains the maxillary sinuses into the internal jugular vein, the subclavian and right heart. The target organ for metastases is the lung (see Fig. 2.6).

Rules of Classification and Staging

Clinical Staging and Imaging

Inspection and palpation of paranasal sinuses is limited in early localized stages. For ethmoid cancers, orbital in-

vasion may displace the globe and trap the anterior ethmoid branch of cranial nerve V_1 leading to altered sensation in the upper lip. Maxillary antral cancers when advanced fill the gingival buccal gutter, loosen molar teeth, and invade the cheek and hard palate. Infection and inflammatory sinusitis obscures cancers. Both magnetic resonance imaging (MRI) and computed tomography enhancement (CT_e) are recommended to distinguish tumor from fluid. CT_e is best for determining bone erosion of the paper-thin lamina bones of sinus walls. Imaging is essential for evaluation of submandibular and retropharyngeal nodes (see Table 1.5).

Pathologic Staging

The gross specimen should be evaluated for margins. Unresected gross residual tumor must be included and marked with clips. All resected lymph node specimens should describe size, number, and level of involved nodes and whether there is extracapsular spread. Specimens after radiation, chemotherapy, or both need to so noted, but specimen shrinkages may occur up to 30% after resection itself. Designations pT and pN should be

TABLE 3.2	Approximate Determinate 5-Year Survival by Stages at Diagnosis (1992–1998)				
	5-Year Survival by Stage Grouping (%)				
Site	All Stages	I	II	III	IV
Maxillary sinus	25	35	—	15	—

used after histopathologic evaluation. Perineural invasion deserves special notation.

Oncoimaging Annotations

- MRI and CT play complementary roles in the assessment and staging process for these tumors.

- Most minor salivary gland neoplasms arise from the palate and secondarily extend into the nasal cavity and paranasal sinuses.

- MRI is best at detecting tumor extension outside the sinonasal cavity. CT is most sensitive in assessing anatomy and bone invasion with these tumors. The hallmark of sinonasal malignancy is bone destruction, seen in approximately 80% of all CT scans in these patients.

- Enlargement of the infraorbital foramen on CT occurs with perineural invasion of the infraorbital nerve, a branch of cranial nerve V_2.

- MRI aids in separating complex sinonasal secretions/infections from tumor. Combined T1- and T2-weighted, contrast medium-enhanced images are needed for this evaluation.

- Orbital extension is manifest on CT and MRI by bone erosion and changes in the orbital fat. Unfortunately, the absence of orbital fat abnormality does not exclude invasion. MRI tends to underestimate orbital invasion.

- Sinonasal bony sclerosis caused by tumor is rare; its presence is normally related to coexistent chronic inflammatory changes.

- Carotid encasement is a relative contraindication to surgery and is suggested by MRI when the internal carotid artery is surrounded by >270 degrees with tumor.

- Mature scar after treatment can usually be distinguished from tumor by the absence of a mass effect, a hypodense appearance on T2-weighted images, and the lack of contrast medium enhancement.

Cancer Statistics and Survival

Generally, cancers of the oral cavity, pharynx, and the upper digestive passage, account for 28,000 new cases (see Table 1.6). In addition, cancer of the larynx affects another 10,000 patients and thyroid cancers, 23,600. Approximately 25% of head and neck cancer patients die annually, often owing to other causes (Table 3.2). Thyroid cancer is the exception for long-term survival, with only 1,500 deaths (5%). The improvement in oral cavity and pharyngeal tumors from 1950 to 2000 was modest at 14% and matches larynx at 15%. A multidisciplinary approach is vital and normal tissue conservation and reconstruction techniques have both added greatly to quality of life. Unfortunately, this patient population comprise ethanol and nicotine abusers and it is difficult to change these habits. Persistence of smoking and drinking contributes to their demise, often from second malignant tumors in adjacent sites.

Specifically, paranasal sinus cancers are detected late due to being mistaken for sinusitis. Both ethmoid and maxillary sinus cancers remain well below 50% for 5-year survival rates.

4

Nasopharynx

To understand the malignant gradient of the nasopharynx in terms of the oncoanatomy of the head and face, it is essential to understand both its superior aspect and its relationship to the cavernous sinus in the skull.

Perspective and Patterns of Spread

Nasopharyngeal cancer is uncommon in white populations and accounts for only 2% of all head and neck cancers in the United States. The nasopharynx can be a harbinger of malignant disease, particularly common among the Chinese population. This is true for specific provinces and subpopulations; the risk is maintained even after migrating to the United States and applies to second-generation Chinese. Its etiology is being investigated from the point of view of viral induction, immunologic response, environmental pollutants, and ingestion of nitrates in food. The Epstein-Barr virus is commonly identified in elevated antibody titers, but it also has been associated with other malignances and is not truly specific for this site.

The epithelium of the nasopharynx varies from a stratified squamous in its lower part to a pseudostratified ciliated columnar epithelium along its walls and roof. Because of Waldeyer's lymphatic ring, many different tumors can arise in this site—lymphoepitheliomas and lymphosarcomas in addition to carcinomas (Table 4.1). The most common, however, are carcinomas, which are locally invasive and destructive to the bony structures of the skull (Fig. 4.1). Lymphoepitheliomas tend to spread bilaterally to nodes in the neck and may present in this fashion. Lymphosarcomas are bulky lesions that tend to interfere with breathing but tend to be less destructive.

Cancer of the nasopharynx has two major spread patterns, depending on whether the primary tumor extends locally or metastasizes to parapharyngeal nodes. The juxtaposition of the mucosa to the base of the skull allows for immediate access to the cranial fossa. The foramen lacerum is accessible and is the only foramen medial to the pharyngeal tube and its fascia. Once the base of the skull is invaded, the tumor enters into the cavernous

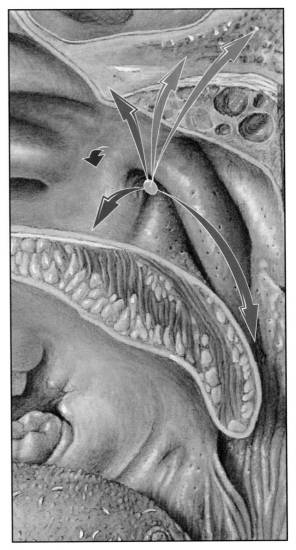

Figure 4.1 **Patterns of spread.** The primary cancer (nasopharynx) invades in various directions which are color-coded vectors (*arrows*) representing stage of progression: Tis, yellow; T1, green; T2, blue; T3, purple; T4, red; and T4, black.

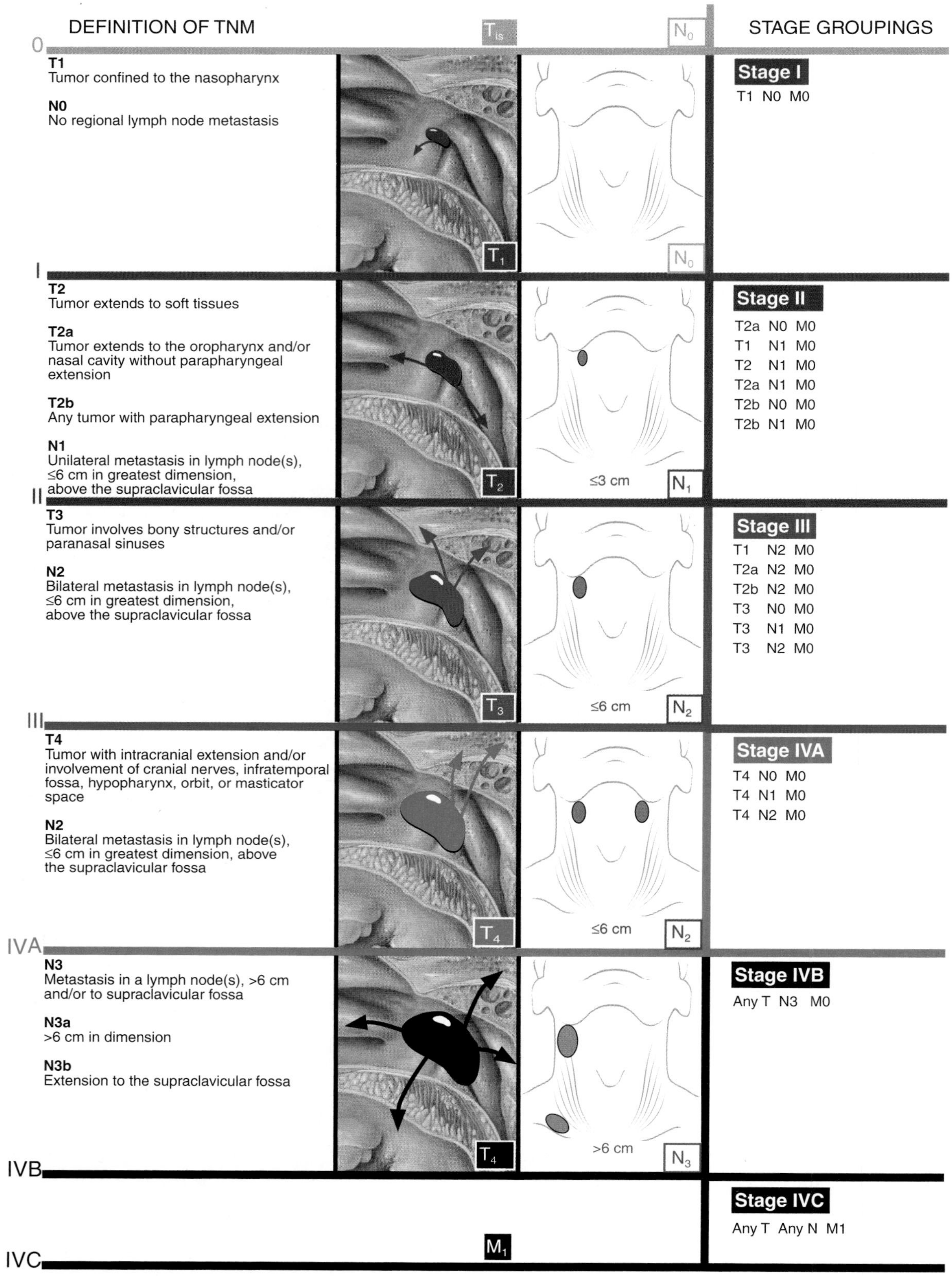

DEFINITION OF TNM T_{is} N_0 STAGE GROUPINGS

0

T1
Tumor confined to the nasopharynx

N0
No regional lymph node metastasis

T_1 N_0

Stage I
T1 N0 M0

I

T2
Tumor extends to soft tissues

T2a
Tumor extends to the oropharynx and/or
nasal cavity without parapharyngeal
extension

T2b
Any tumor with parapharyngeal extension

N1
Unilateral metastasis in lymph node(s),
≤6 cm in greatest dimension,
above the supraclavicular fossa

T_2 ≤3 cm N_1

Stage II
T2a N0 M0
T1   N1 M0
T2   N1 M0
T2a N1 M0
T2b N0 M0
T2b N1 M0

II

T3
Tumor involves bony structures and/or
paranasal sinuses

N2
Bilateral metastasis in lymph node(s),
≤6 cm in greatest dimension,
above the supraclavicular fossa

T_3 ≤6 cm N_2

Stage III
T1   N2 M0
T2a N2 M0
T2b N2 M0
T3   N0 M0
T3   N1 M0
T3   N2 M0

III

T4
Tumor with intracranial extension and/or
involvement of cranial nerves, infratemporal
fossa, hypopharynx, orbit, or masticator
space

N2
Bilateral metastasis in lymph node(s),
≤6 cm in greatest dimension, above
the supraclavicular fossa

T_4 ≤6 cm N_2

Stage IVA
T4 N0 M0
T4 N1 M0
T4 N2 M0

IVA

N3
Metastasis in a lymph node(s), >6 cm
and/or to supraclavicular fossa

N3a
>6 cm in dimension

N3b
Extension to the supraclavicular fossa

T_4 >6 cm N_3

Stage IVB
Any T N3 M0

IVB

M_1

Stage IVC
Any T Any N M1

IVC

Figure 4.2 TNM stage grouping. Nasopharyngeal cancers are not resectable and staging categories differ from other head
and neck sites as to T/N definitions. Vertical presentations of stage groupings, which follow same color code for cancer stage
advancement are organized in horizontal lanes: Stage 0, yellow; I, green; II, blue; III, purple; IVA, red; and IVB, black. Definitions
of TN on left and stage grouping on right.

TABLE 4.1	Histopathologic Type: Common Cancers of the Nasopharyngeal Carcinoma
WHO Classification	**Former Terminology**
Type 1	
Squamous cell carcinoma	Squamous cell carcinoma
Type 2	
Nonkeratinizing carcinoma Without lymphoid stroma With lymphoid stroma	Transitional cell carcinoma Intermediate cell carcinoma Lymphoepithelial carcinoma (Regaud)
Type 3	
Undifferentiated carcinoma Without lymphoid stroma With lymphoid stroma	Anaplastic carcinoma Clear cell carcinoma Lymphoepithelial carcinoma (Schminke)

From the American Joint Committee on Cancer (AJCC). *AJCC Cancer Staging Manual*. 6th ed. New York: Springer; 2002:37.

sinus and can involve a number of cranial nerves. There are numerous clinical syndromes, depending on which combination of nerves are involved. Invasion of cranial nerves, inferiorly to superiorly, are cranial nerves III, IV, and VI, which can cause diplopia or ophthalmoplegia because of the resultant partial paralysis of one eye. Deafness is caused by local obstruction of the eustachian tube leading to tympanic membrane fixation, and not caused by involvement of cranial nerve VIII. The acoustic nerve is well encased in the mastoid bone of the inner ear with its meatus in the posterior fossa. Despite the fact that the eustachian tube is open, cancer rarely invades along this pathway into the middle ear, probably because of the cartilaginous wall of the tube and the absence of a good vascular bed. Proptosis, periorbital edema, and orbital invasion are a result of extensive invasion along the base of the skull and/or thrombosis of the cavernous sinuses.

TNM Staging Criteria

The classification and staging of nasopharyngeal cancers is different from other cancers of the head and neck, but has remained relatively unchanged since its introduction in the third editions of the International Union Against Cancer and American Joint Committee on Cancer classifications (1988; Fig. 4.2). The vectors of invasion vary with the biologic behavior of these different malignancies.

Summary of Changes

Knowledge of the anatomy is essential for staging, which has been recently revised in the 6th edition (2002). Nasopharyn-

geal cancer, which spreads on the surface anteriorly into the nasal cavity or inferiorly into the oropharynx is T2a; with penetration into the parapharyngeal space, it becomes T2b; bone destruction T3 is better prognostically than perineural invasion; T4 intracranial disease, cranial nerve involvement implies a poor outcome.

Orientation of Three-planar Oncoanatomy

For the nasopharynx, the anatomic isocenter is at the level of C1, the atlas. The anterior surface bullet enters through the tip of the nose (Fig. 4.3A) and the lateral bullet is at the temporal mandibular joint, just below the level of the external auditory canal (Fig. 4.3B).

T-oncoanatomy

The nasopharynx is a small, box-like space in the center of the head, posterior to the nasal cavity and superior to the pharyngeal tube. The anterior limit of the nasopharynx is the chona, through which it is continuous with the nasal cavity. Its roof is attached to the base of the skull, and slopes downward to become continuous with the posterior pharyngeal wall. The lateral wall is composed of the torus tubarius, the eustachian tube orifice, and that posterior portion of the mucosa, the fossa of Rosenmüller extending up to its apex and junction with the roof. The inferior limit of the nasopharynx is level with the plane of the hard palate.

To understand the importance of the nasopharynx in terms of the anatomy of the head and face, it is essential to understand both its superior aspect and its relationship to the skull and lateral walls. The pharyngeal fascia is attached to the base of the skull. This can be diagrammed in relationship to those foramena,

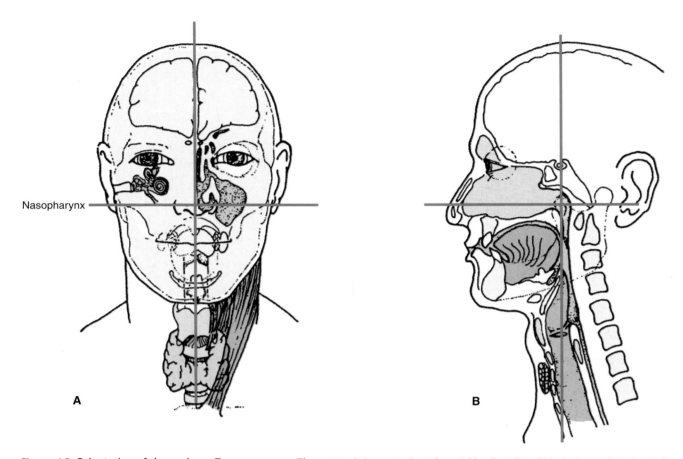

A

B

Figure 4.3 Orientation of three-planar T-oncoanatomy. The anatomic isocenter is at the axial level at clivus/C1. **A.** Coronal. **B.** Sagittal.

which may be invaded and destroyed by carcinomas. The superior attachment of the pharyngobasilar fascia starts from the midline pharyngeal tubercle on the basi-occiput, extending across the petrous portion of the temporal bone to a point in front of the carotid canal. From there, it passes posteromedially to the petrotympanic fissure in the region where the eustachian tube attaches and the levator palati originates, and then attaches to the medial pterygoid lamina. The fascia inferiorly is continuous over the superior pharyngeal constrictor muscle.

- *Coronal section* (Fig. 4.4A) provides a view from retropharyngeal space. The roof of the nasopharynx is occupied by the sphenoid sinus, alongside of which are cavernous sinuses. Within its contents are three cranial nerves responsible for extraocular motion (III, IV, and VI), laterally lies the Gasserian (trigeminal) ganglion (cranial nerve V), and its major branches as they exit through different foramena along the base of the skull into the parapharyngeal space, paranasal sinuses, and orbit.
- *Sagittal plane* (Fig. 4.4B) shows the lateral walls of the nasopharynx, which consist of the eustachian tube

and its two related muscles, the tensor veli palatini and the levator veli palati, the latter of which is more important functionally for tubal patency. The muscles are continuous with the palatopharyngeus muscles and superior constrictor, forming the pharyngeal muscular tube.

- *Transverse plane* (Fig. 4.4C) shows the parapharyngeal space divided into three compartments by the styloid process, its muscles, and the related fascial expansions from the carotid sheath and prevertebral fascia. A neoplastic process may extend into and follow these preformed spaces but, unlike an inflammatory process, also may extend through these barriers and invade nerves.

The *retropharyngeal compartment* houses Rouviere's node, which is a major focus of metastatic spread. As these parapharyngeal nodes enlarge, they compress the neurovascular bundle in the carotid sheath. The *retrostyloid compartment* contains the internal carotid artery, the last four cranial nerves, and cervical sympathetics. The *prestyloid* is formed by the tensor palatini muscle and the pterygoid muscles. It contains the maxillary artery and important nerves. Once this latter space is invaded,

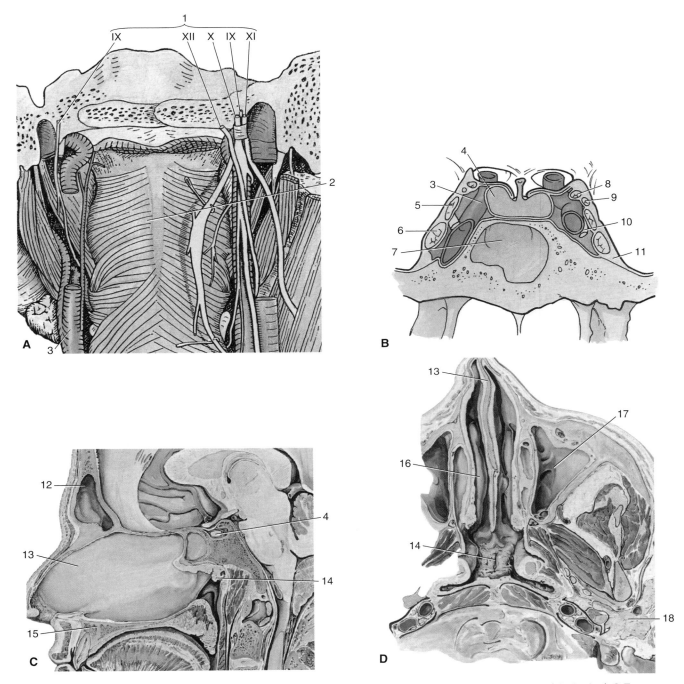

Figure 4.4 **T-oncoanatomy.** The three-planar views are crucial in understanding the malignant gradient. **A.** Coronal. **B.** Sagittal. **C.** Transverse. (1) Cranial nerves IX, X, XI, XII. (2) Superior pharyngeal constrictor. (3) Internal carotid artery. (4) Hypophysis. (5) Ophthalmic nerve (V1). (6) Maxillary nerve (V2). (7) Sphenoid sinus. (8) Oculomotor nerve (III). (9) Trochlear nerve (IV). (10) Abducent nerve (VI). (11) Dura mater. (12) Frontal sinus. (13) Nasal septum. (14) Pharyngeal tonsil. (15) Palate. (16) Inferior concha. (17) Maxillary sinus. (18) Parotid gland nodes.

access is gained laterally into the deep portion of the parotid gland and inferiorly to the submaxillary gland.

N-oncoanatomy

With nodal dissemination, the high parapharyngeal nodes along the carotid sheath are involved and ex-

tend into the retrostyloid compartment (Fig. 4.5). This leads to entrapment of the cranial nerves emerging alongside the jugular foramen. The nodes in this region are named after Rouviere–famous for his treatise on lymphoid anatomy. Again, numerous neurologic syndromes can occur. The retroparotidian syndrome, or the

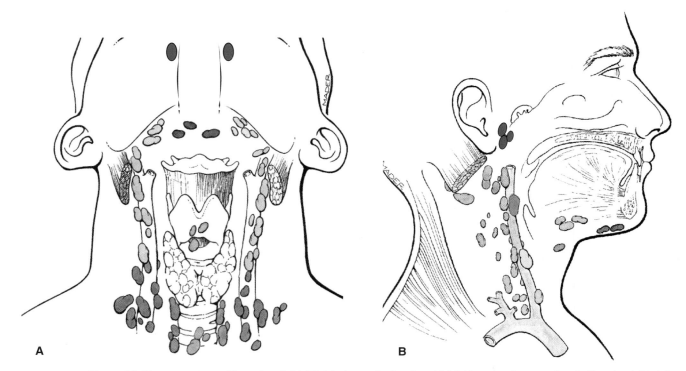

Figure 4.5 N-oncoanatomy. The red node highlights the sentinel node, which is the retropharyngeal node (Rouviere's Node). **A.** Coronal. **B.** Sagittal.

jugular foramen syndrome, is characterized by loss of the gag reflex (cranial nerve IX), vocal cord paralysis (cranial nerve X), atrophy of the trapezius muscle (cranial nerve XI), and deviation of the uvula (cranial nerve IX) and tongue on protrusion (cranial nerve XII).

In addition to retropharyngeal and parapharyngeal nodes, the main routes of lymphatic spread of the nasopharynx are into the first station nodes, that is, the jugulodigastric, jugulo-omohyoid, upper deep cervical, lower deep cervical, and submaxillary and submental lymph nodes. Bilateral node spread is common. Mediastinal lymph node metastases are considered distant metastases. Distant spread to the lungs is common in this type of cancer.

M-oncoanatomy

The cavernous sinus and lateral pterygoid buccal venous plexus drains into the jugular vein, brachiocephalic vein and then into the subclavian vein and right superior vena cava. Hematogenous spread, although uncommon, can include lung and bone as favored sites of involvement. Skeletal and other distant metastases occur infrequently (see Fig. 2.6).

Rules of Classification and Staging

Clinical Staging and Imaging

For nasopharyngeal cancers, careful history taking, and inspection and palpations of the face and neck are essen-

tial. Testing all cranial nerves is critical. Both direct and indirect endoscopy are useful. Despite patient cooperation, pharyngeal cancers are inaccessible and imaging is important. To determine the true extent of primary nasopharyngeal cancers, imaging is essential. Magnetic resonance imaging (MRI) is superior to computed tomography (CT) in demonstrating soft tissue extension, skull base bone changes, and perineural invasion (see Table 1.5).

Pathologic Staging

Histopathologic verification of primary and nodes is performed by needle aspiration or biopsy. Nasopharyngeal cancers are not resectable.

Oncoimaging Annotations

- Most nasopharyngeal tumors arise in the fossa of Rosenmüller and tend to spread deeply, often obstructing the eustachian tube.
- The vast majority (75%) of nasopharyngeal cancer patients have cervical node metastases at presentation. Bilateral involvement occurs in up to 80%.
- MRI is superior to CT in demonstrating the soft tissue extent of the tumor and skull base changes. CT often underestimates the frequency and extent of skull base involvement.
- After successful radiation therapy, there is usually complete tumor resolution on images within 3 months. A baseline, a posttreatment scan should be

obtained at approximately 6 months. Differentiating tumor recurrence from fibrosis can be a formidable task.

- Positron emission tomography (PET) with fluorine-18–labeled deoxy-D-glucose (FDG) enhancement may be useful in evaluating tumor recurrence. Both PET and thallium 201 single-photon emission computed tomography (SPECT) may be used to differentiate tumor from radiation-induced necrosis.
- CT and MRI can identify Rouviere's Node opposite C_1 transverse process.

Cancer Statistics and Survival

Generally, cancers of the oral cavity and pharynx, the upper digestive passage, account for 28,000 new cases (see Table 1.6). In addition, cancer of the larynx affects another 10,000 patients and thyroid cancers, 23,600. Approximately 25% of head and neck cancer patients die annually, often due to other causes. Long-term survival in thyroid cancer is the exception, with only 1,500 deaths (5%). The improvement in oral cavity and pharyngeal tumors from 1950 to 2000 was modest at 14% and matches larynx at 15%. A multidisciplinary approach is vital.

Specifically, nasopharyngeal cancers are difficult to detect and metastasize to bilateral neck nodes with generally poor overall survival for all stages. When encountered in early stages in high-risk Chinese populations, 5-year survival is at the 90% level. Combined chemoradiation regimens (Cisplatinum and 5-fluoracil with radiation) have dramatically improved response rates and survival.

5

Oral Cavity

In the oral cavity, the location of the cancer is a powerful prognosticator of its malignant gradient; a shift of a few centimeters alters the prognosis of the cancer significantly.

Perspective and Patterns of Spread

Each specific cancer subsite in the oral cavity has the potential to give rise to different manifestations. Each requires individualized management, dictated by local anatomy and patterns of spread (Fig. 5.1). Thus, lip cancers appear as superficial ulcerations that grow slowly. They rarely enter lymphatic channels or have metastases to lymph nodes, unless there is a deep invasion of the orbicularis oris muscle. By contrast, cancers of the tongue tend to arise along the lateral borders due to irritation of broken teeth and the microtrauma of swallowing foods, alcohol, and smoking tobacco. The underlying musculature is readily invaded and, because of its rich lymphatic network, leads to rapid infiltration and lymph node involvement.

There are a large variety of carcinomas (Table 5.1), but the most common are squamous cell cancers; adenocarcinomas are less common. Oral cavity cancers are the most common upper aerodigestive cancer and are predominantly male (88%); lip followed by tongue is the most common site. *The malignant gradient in the oral cavity increases from anterior to posterior and from lateral to medial loci.* Cancers arising in the posterior portion of the floor of the mouth tend to carry a poor prognosis because the mylohyoid muscle is shorter in its anterior–posterior diameter and is deficient in its posterior part, no longer providing a muscular floor to the oral cavity. Invasion at this particular junction allows the tumor to extend directly into a gap and enter into direct contact with the submandibular salivary gland and tissues of the neck. This leads to the retromylohyoid space and permits the easy propagation of both an infectious and/or neoplastic process directly from the mouth to the neck. The buccal mucosa gives rise to superficial lesions, much as the lip; they tend to be ulcerating, and also arise from irritation due to broken teeth. Deep invasion into the

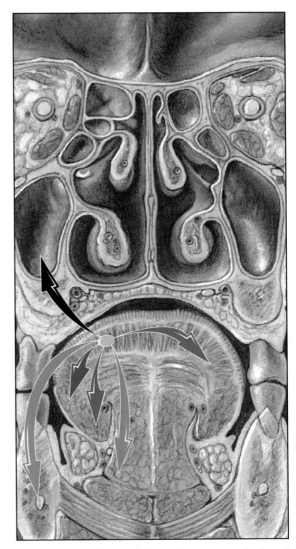

Figure 5.1 **Patterns of spread.** The primary cancer (oral cavity) invades in various directions, which are color-coded vectors (*arrows*) representing stage of progression: Tis, yellow; T1, green; T2, blue; T3, purple; T4A, red; and T4B, black.

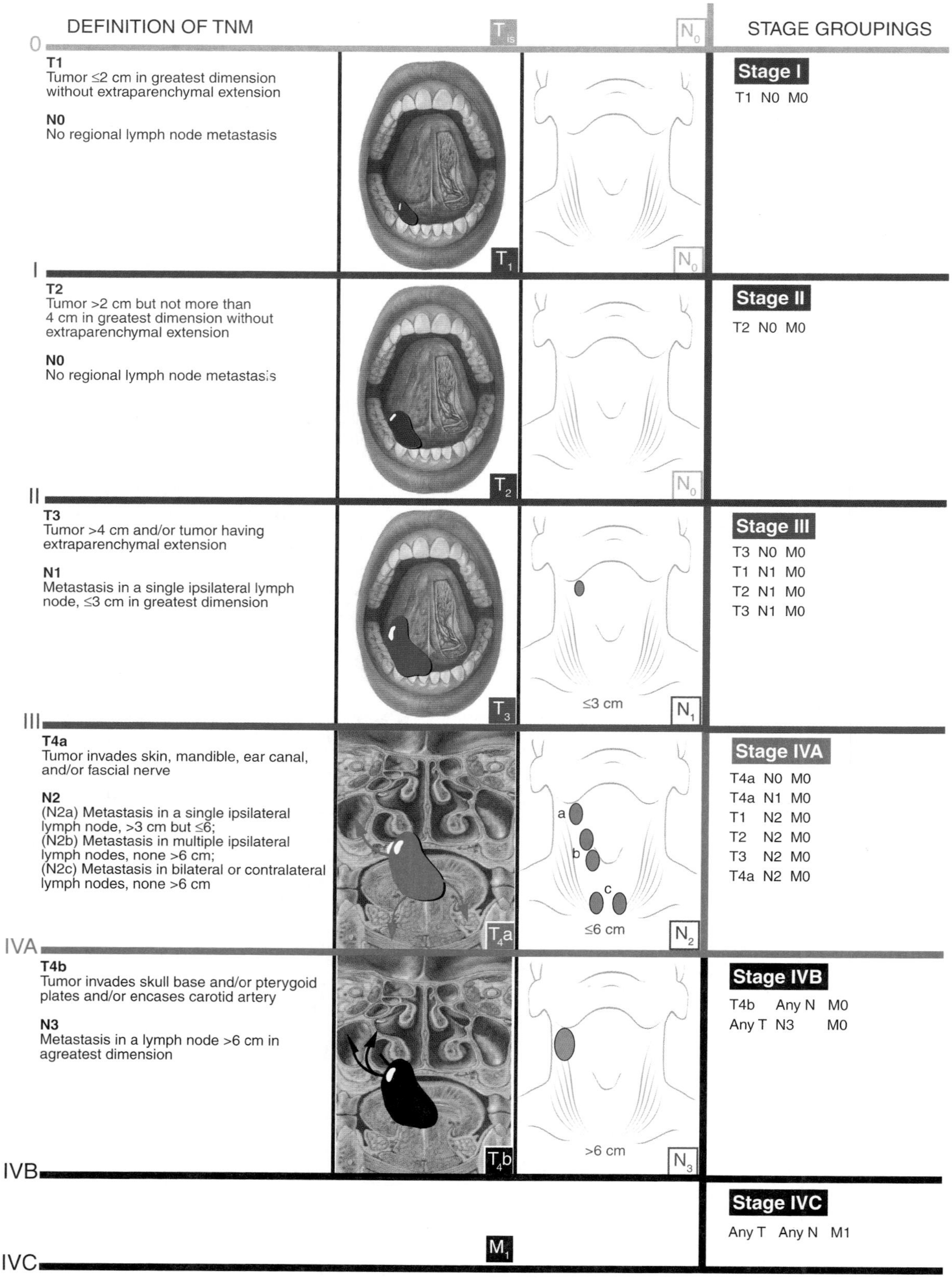

DEFINITION OF TNM

STAGE GROUPINGS

T1
Tumor ≤2 cm in greatest dimension without extraparenchymal extension

N0
No regional lymph node metastasis

Stage I
T1 N0 M0

T2
Tumor >2 cm but not more than 4 cm in greatest dimension without extraparenchymal extension

N0
No regional lymph node metastasis

Stage II
T2 N0 M0

T3
Tumor >4 cm and/or tumor having extraparenchymal extension

N1
Metastasis in a single ipsilateral lymph node, ≤3 cm in greatest dimension

Stage III
T3 N0 M0
T1 N1 M0
T2 N1 M0
T3 N1 M0

≤3 cm

T4a
Tumor invades skin, mandible, ear canal, and/or fascial nerve

N2
(N2a) Metastasis in a single ipsilateral lymph node, >3 cm but ≤6;
(N2b) Metastasis in multiple ipsilateral lymph nodes, none >6 cm;
(N2c) Metastasis in bilateral or contralateral lymph nodes, none >6 cm

Stage IVA
T4a N0 M0
T4a N1 M0
T1 N2 M0
T2 N2 M0
T3 N2 M0
T4a N2 M0

≤6 cm

T4b
Tumor invades skull base and/or pterygoid plates and/or encases carotid artery

N3
Metastasis in a lymph node >6 cm in agreatest dimension

Stage IVB
T4b Any N M0
Any T N3   M0

>6 cm

Stage IVC
Any T Any N M1

Figure 5.2 TNM stage grouping. Oral cavity cancers tend to occur in the lateral gutters. Oral tongue cancers invade floor of mouth because of interdigitation of intrinsic and extrinsic musculature. Vertical presentations of stage groupings, which follow same color code for cancer stage advancement are organized in horizontal lanes: Stage 0, yellow; I, green; II, blue; III, purple; IVA, red; and IVB, black. Definitions of TN on left and stage grouping on right.

TABLE 5.1	Histopathologic Type: Common Cancers of the Oral Cavity	
Squamous Cell Carcinoma Microscopic Variants	**Adenocarcinoma Major or Minor Salivary Gland**
Keratinizing; well differentiated; moderately well differentiated; poorly differentiated	Low-grade adenocarcinoma Adenoid cystic carcinoma
Nonkeratinizing; anaplastic squamous carcinoma	Mucoepidermoid (low or high grade)
Lymphoepithelioma	With lymphoid stroma
Transitional cell carcinoma	Carcinoma expleomorphic adenoma
Spindle cell squamous carcinoma	Poorly differentiated adenocarcinoma

Adapted from Rubin P. *Clinical Oncology*. 8th ed. New York: Elsevier; 2001:408.

buccinator muscle can lead to swelling of the cheek and access to the deep pterygoid plexus of veins. Unrecognized advancement can become rapidly debilitating, interfering with speech and swallowing, and producing a malodorous halitosis.

TNM Staging Criteria

These lesions tend to be either exophytic or endophytic, with the greatest concern being cancer of the tongue that, because of the interdigitations of its intrinsic and extrinsic muscles, leads to invasion of the floor of the mouth (Fig. 5.2). Cancers arising in the floor of the mouth tend to be shallow ulcerations, usually in the gutters, and invade into the muscles of the tongue. They can readily attach and destroy the mandible. The lateral angles of the floor are important and precise landmarks for cancer spread in the mouth, because they merge into the alveololingual sulcus of the oropharynx.

In the oral cavity, the location of the cancer is a powerful prognosticator. As noted, a shift of a few centimeters alters the prognosis of the cancer significantly. Buccal cancers, alveolar ridges, and retromolar cancers are more unilaterally localized and are likely to spread into ipsilateral lymph nodes. Structures in the midline, such as the tongue, floor of the mouth, and palate, tend to drain bilaterally and have a poorer prognosis.

Summary of Changes

The staging of cancers is size dependent; the new definitions of T4a resectable and T4b unresectable are characterized by two different patterns of spread. T4a is a lateralized cancer, which can invade the floor of mouth, oral tongue, buccal mucosa, and alveolar ridge. T4b cancers of the buccal mucosa and retromolar trigone can invade deeply into the retroparotidian space, pterygoid plates, and oropharynx, becoming unresectable.

Orientation of Three-planar Oncoanatomy

The anatomic isocenter of the oral cavity is the C2/C3 level. The anterior bullet enters in the midline at the upper lip (Fig. 5.3A) and the lateral bullet is posterior to the lateral commissure of the lips (Fig. 5.3B).

T-oncoanatomy

The oral cavity extends from the skin–vermillion junction of the lips to the junction of the hard and soft palate anteriorly and the anterior pillar (palatoglossal of the oropharynx and to the line of the circumvallate papillae inferiorly, which divides the tongue into the anterior two-thirds and posterior one third of the tongue. The various subsites of the oral cavity are noted. The major structures are the tongue, floor of the mouth, alveolar ridges, gingival, and hard palate within the oral cavity proper; the mandible separates the buccal mucosa and lips.

The deeper and more complex anatomy requires knowledge of the underlying musculature, which suspends the upper aerodigestive tract from the mandible and hyoid bone to the vertebral column and base of the skull. Swallowing, mastication, and the initiation of digestion through salivary gland secretion occur in the oral cavity. The tongue aids in food consumption and the sensation of taste is principally located here. The tongue is vital to social intercourse for verbalization, articulation, conversation, and osculation. All of these complex functions relate to the musculature, namely, the muscles of the lips and cheek, including the orbicularis oris and the deeper muscles of the face, the levator anguli oris, the mentalis, and the buccinator muscle of the cheek. The muscles of the tongue and floor of the mouth include the intrinsic muscles of the tongue (longitudinal, transverse, and vertical), the extrinsic tongue muscles (genioglossus, styloglossus, and hyoglossus), and the geniohyoid and mylohyoid muscles, which are the muscles of the floor of the mouth.

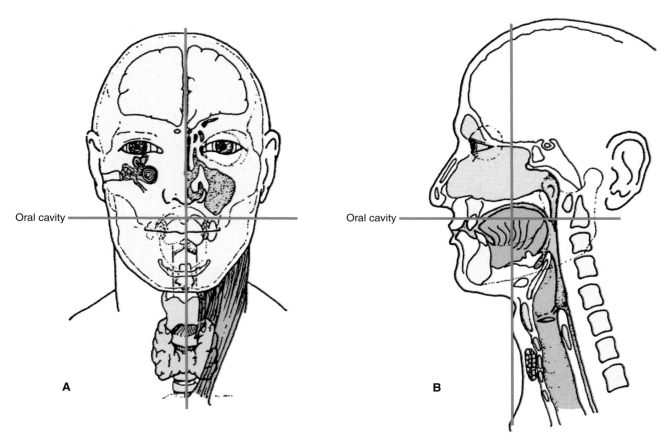

Oral cavity

A

Oral cavity

B

Figure 5.3 **Orientation of three-planar T-oncoanatomy.** The anatomic isocenter is at the axial level at C2/C3. **A.** Coronal. **B.** Sagittal.

The retromolar trigone, when viewed from its superficial mucosa to its deeper underlying structure, shows the complexity of the oral cavity particularly as it relates to the oropharynx. Beneath the retromolar trigone mucosa lies the pterygomandibular raphe, which forms the boundary between the vestibule of the oral cavity and the anterior pillar of the fauces, containing the palatoglossal muscle in it free border. The fibers of the superior pharyngeal constrictor muscle attach laterally and the buccinator anterior to the pterygomandibular raphe. When these muscles and the superior constrictor muscle are removed, the various spaces around the tonsillar fossa and the mandible are readily identified with the important underlying nerves. The lingual nerve and buccal nerve are identified, as is the glossopharyngeal nerve and the inferior alveolar nerve. The various spaces are the parapharyngeal space, which lies medial to the lateral pterygoid muscle; the pterygomandibular space, which is occupied by buccal fat and lies lateral to the medial pterygoid muscle; the buccal space, which is lateral to the mandible; and the masseter muscle.

Perhaps no area illustrates the complexity of the underlying anatomy of the oral cavity better than the retro-

molar trigone. This site is of particular interest to radiation oncologists because cancers in this area tend to be more radiosensitive and carry a better prognosis than cancers of the oropharynx. The retromolar trigone is formed by the posterior boundary of the retromolar space, posterior to the opening of Stensen's (parotid) duct, and extends posteriorly to the anterior surface of the mandible. With the mouth open, the retromolar trigone comes into prominence and assumes a triangular form with a pale mucous membrane. The base of the retromolar trigone is situated superiorly behind the third upper molar tooth and the apex lies inferiorly behind the third lower molar tooth. The stretching of the mucous membrane in this region results in the lengthening and projection of the underlying elevator muscles. The medial boundary of the trigone forms the border between the oral cavity and the oropharynx.

- *Coronal plane* (Fig. 5.4A): The coronal plane stratifies the oral tongue and floor of mouth as a set of interdigitating muscles constituted by the intrinsic and extrinsic muscles of the oral cavity.
- *Sagittal plane* (Fig. 5.4B): This view presents the tongue as a contiguous structure of both the oral

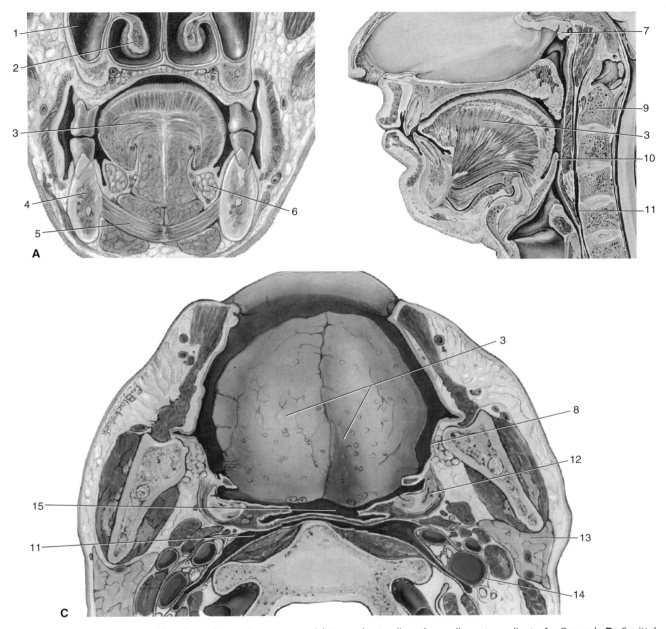

Figure 5.4 **T-oncoanatomy.** The three-planar views are crucial to understanding the malignant gradient. **A.** Coronal. **B.** Sagittal. **C.** Transverse. (1) Maxillary sinus. (2) Inferior concha. (3) Tongue. (4) Mandible. (5) Mylohyoid. (6) Sublingual gland. (7) Pharyngeal tonsil. (8) Retromolar trigone. (9) Axis (C2). (10) Epiglottis. (11) Retropharyngeal space. (12) Palatine tonsil. (13) Parotid gland. (14) Carotid sheath. (15) Cavity of pharynx.

cavity and tongue attached to the mandible and hyoid bone, respectively.

- *Transverse plane* (Fig. 5.4C): Note the pterygomandibular raphe, which defines the retromolar trigone as the buccal mucosa anterior to the anterior tonsillar pillar. The buccinator muscle and medial pterygoid meet at the raphe. The parapharyngeal space and the pterygomandibular space are avenues into lymph nodes, carotid artery encasement, and

perineural invasion of the lingual and glossal pharyngeal nerves.

N-oncoanatomy

Generally there are two patterns of lymph node involvement that depend on location (Fig. 5.5). Anterior cancer sites such as the lips, floor of mouth, and mobile oral tongue, are drained by lymph channels into the

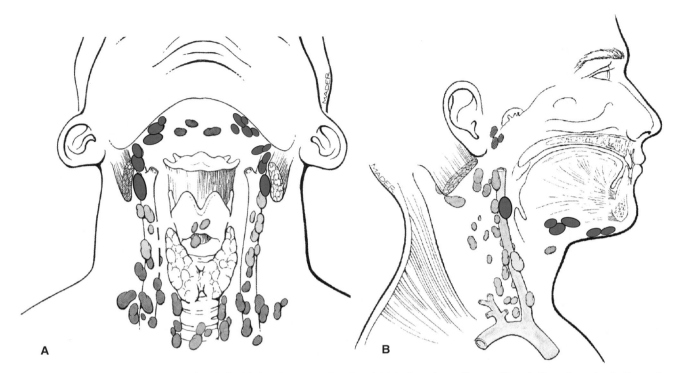

Figure 5.5 N-oncoanatomy. The red node highlights the sentinel node, which is the submaxillary and jugulodigastric node. **A**. Coronal. **B**. Sagittal.

submental and submandibular lymph nodes. The more posteriorly located cancers drain into the jugulodigastric nodes. Midline tongue cancers can drain and lead to bilateral nodal infiltrations. The gingival and buccal mucosa tend to have unilateral disease.

M-oncoanatomy

Distant metastases are also possible because of the plexus of pharyngeal veins that drain into the jugular vein, and then into the superior vena cava, the right heart, and finally the lungs. The vascular supply of the pharynx arises from the external carotid. The carotid body and sinus located at the bifurcation of the common carotid

is an arterial chemoreceptor and baroreceptor area, respectively (see Fig. 2.6).

Rules of Classification and Staging

Clinical Staging and Imaging

For all mucosal cancers, careful inspection and palpation of the primary site and all uninvolved subsites are essential. Regional nodes deserve careful evaluation, recognizing that the anterior location of tongue-type cancers can drain into submental areas or pass directly to the supraclavicular region. The mid tongue drains to the mid neck node. Posterior tongue favors the jugulodigastric nodes.

TABLE 5.2	Approximate Determinate 5-Year Survival by Stages at Diagnosis (1992–1998)				
	5-Year Survival According to Stage Grouping (%)				
Site	**All Stages**	**I**	**II**	**III**	**IV**
Oral cavity					
Mobile tongue	45	80	60	30	15
Floor of mouth	50	80	70	60	30
Buccal mucosa	45	75	65	30	15
Retromolar trigone	60	75	70	60	30
Lower gingival	65	75	60	50	30
Lip	85	90	85	70	60

Both computed tomography enhancement (CT$_e$) and magnetic resonance imaging (MRI) are recommended for soft tissue and bony involvement; preference is often based absence of artifacts (teeth fillings and crowns create streaking on CT; see Table 1.5).

Pathologic Staging

The gross specimen should be evaluated for margins. Unresected gross residual tumor must be included and marked with clips. All resected lymph node specimens should describe size, number, level of involved nodes, and whether there is extracapsular spread. Specimens taken after radiation and/or chemotherapy need to be so noted, but specimen shrinkages may occur up to 30% after resection itself. Designations pT and pN should be used after histopathologic evaluation. Perineural invasion deserves special notation.

Oncoimaging Annotations
- The tongue is richly supplied with lymphatics and a high percentage of patients (30%) have bilateral metastatic nodes at the time of initial clinical presentation. Many of these nodes are clinically silent and are detected only on imaging studies.
- With oral cavity tumors, the specific imaging issues to be addressed are those of the bone erosion and degree of submucosal extension.
- To assess perineural spread of tumor, MRI should be performed in patients with adenoid cystic carcinoma of the hard palate.

Cancer Statistics and Survival

Generally, cancers of the oral cavity, pharynx, and upper digestive passage, account for 28,000 new cases (see Table 1.6). In addition, cancer of the larynx affects another 10,000 patients and thyroid cancers 23,600. Approximately 25% of head and neck cancer patients die annually, often due to other causes (Table 5.2). Thyroid cancers are the exception; long-term survival is high, with only 1,500 deaths (5%). The improvement in oral cavity and pharyngeal tumors 1950 to 2000 was modest at 14% and matches larynx at 15%. A multidisciplinary approach is vital and normal tissue conservation and reconstructive techniques have both added greatly to quality of life. Unfortunately, this patient population abuse ethanol and nicotine; it is difficult to change these habits. Persistence of smoking and drinking contributes to their demise often from second malignant tumors in adjacent sites (see Fig. 1.7).

Specifically, oral cavity cancers encompass six subsites with a wide range of success. Lip cancers are readily recognized in local stages I/II and are successfully controlled in 85% of patients. The buccal mucosa and retromolar trigone spread to ipsilateral nodes and are intermediate; 5-year survival rates are 60% to 65%. Cancers of oral tongue and floor of both are more common; they spread rapidly and deeply due to the anatomic interdigitation of the intrinsic and extrinsic muscles of the tongue. Lymphatic drainage is bilateral from these sites. Survival rates range from 45% to 50%. Best chance for a favorable outcome is detection as stage I disease; 80% of patients are alive at 5 years.

6

Parotid Gland

The parotid gland has its malignant gradient from superficial to deep by virtue of its anatomic location and bilobed configuration, which surrounds the ramus of the mandible and houses cranial nerve VII.

Perspective and Patterns of Spread

Salivary gland tumors are uncommon, accounting for 5% to 7% of all head and neck malignancies; this constitutes 2,000 to 2,500 cases in the United States, mainly in the parotid gland (85%). Fortunately, the majority are relatively benign, and are most often mixed salivary gland tumors or pleomorphic adenomas. Tumors in the submaxillary and sublingual glands tend more toward being malignant. The histopathology can be highly varied reflecting the cellular components of the acinar glands, which tend to be serous or mucous with an elaborate ductal system. The relationship of cell type and derivative tumor is shown in Figure 6.1 and Table 6.1.

The parotid gland, by virtue of its anatomic location and bilobed configuration surrounding the ramus of the mandible, presents therapeutic challenges. Foremost is the preservation of the facial nerve (cranial nerve VII), which traverses through its isocenter. The malignant gradient is from anterior to posterior, from lateral to medial, that is, the superficial to deep lobe. The major salivary glands are branched tubuloalveolar exocrine glands whose connective tissue septa subdivide the gland into lobes and lobules. Embedded in the gland are lymph nodes and neural components that can affect survival outcomes.

Alterations in salivary gland flow can be discerned as dryness or abnormal taste in the subclinical phase of tumor growth. It is usually swelling that alerts the patient; once facial paresis appears, medical care is actively sought. Tumors arising in the superficial lobe involve skin and facial nerve and its various branches when aggressive and resection demands sacrificing the facial nerve (T4a). Of greater concern is the deep lobe, where the cancer can enter into the parapharyngeal area by way of the retroparotidian space. The carotid artery, jugular vein, and cranial nerves IX, X, XI, and XII can be involved.

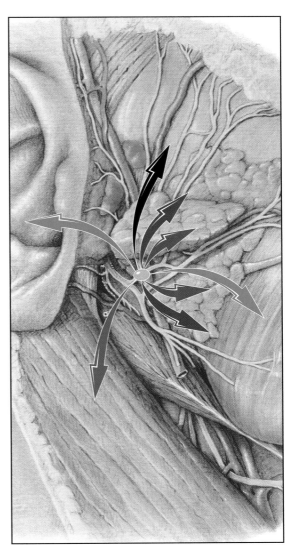

Figure 6.1 **Patterns of spread.** The primary cancer (parotid gland) invades in various directions which are color-coded vectors (*arrows*) representing stage of progression: T$_0$, yellow; T1, green; T2, blue; T3, purple; T4a, red; and T4b, black.

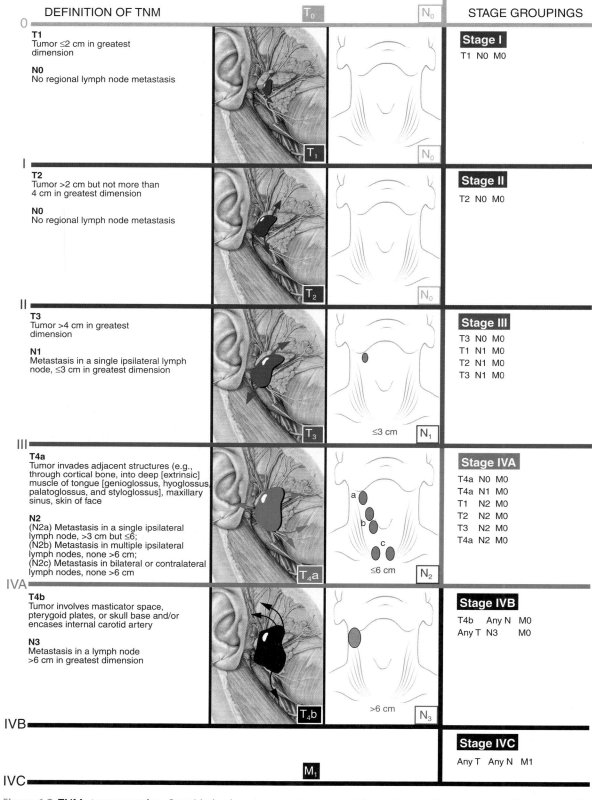

DEFINITION OF TNM

T1
Tumor ≤2 cm in greatest dimension

N0
No regional lymph node metastasis

T2
Tumor >2 cm but not more than 4 cm in greatest dimension

N0
No regional lymph node metastasis

T3
Tumor >4 cm in greatest dimension

N1
Metastasis in a single ipsilateral lymph node, ≤3 cm in greatest dimension

T4a
Tumor invades adjacent structures (e.g., through cortical bone, into deep [extrinsic] muscle of tongue [genioglossus, hyoglossus, palatoglossus, and styloglossus], maxillary sinus, skin of face

N2
(N2a) Metastasis in a single ipsilateral lymph node, >3 cm but ≤6;
(N2b) Metastasis in multiple ipsilateral lymph nodes, none >6 cm;
(N2c) Metastasis in bilateral or contralateral lymph nodes, none >6 cm

T4b
Tumor involves masticator space, pterygoid plates, or skull base and/or encases internal carotid artery

N3
Metastasis in a lymph node >6 cm in greatest dimension

STAGE GROUPINGS

Stage I
T1 N0 M0

Stage II
T2 N0 M0

Stage III
T3 N0 M0
T1 N1 M0
T2 N1 M0
T3 N1 M0

Stage IVA
T4a N0 M0
T4a N1 M0
T1 N2 M0
T2 N2 M0
T3 N2 M0
T4a N2 M0

Stage IVB
T4b Any N M0
Any T N3 M0

Stage IVC
Any T Any N M1

Figure 6.2 TNM stage grouping. Parotid gland cancers are highly varied histopathologically and perineural invasion of the VIIth and Vth cranial nerves are the major concern. Vertical presentations of stage groupings, which follow same color code for cancer stage advancement are organized in horizontal lanes: Stage 0, yellow; I, green; II, blue; III, purple; IVA, red; and IVB, black. Definitions of TN on left and stage grouping on right.

TABLE 6.1	Histopathologic Type: Common Cancers of the Parotid Proposed by the World Health Organization	
Acinic cell carcinoma		Oncocytic carcinoma
Mucoepidermoid carcinoma		Salivary duct carcinoma
Adenoid cystic carcinoma		Adenocarcinoma
Polymorphous low-grade adenocarcinoma		Myoepithelial carcinoma
Epithelial-myoepithelial carcinoma		Carcinoma in pleomorphic adenoma
Basal cell adenocarcinoma		Squamous cell carcinoma
Sebaceous carcinoma		Small cell carcinoma
Papillary cystadenocarcinoma		Other carcinomas
Mucinous adenocarcinoma		

American Joint Committee on Cancer (AJCC). *AJCC Cancer Staging Manual.* 6th ed. New York: Springer; 2002:70.

TNM Staging Criteria

The staging system for salivary glands appeared in the fourth edition of the American Joint Committee on Cancer/International Union Against Cancer guidelines (1992), and was based on an extensive retrospective study of malignant tumors of the major salivary glands collected from 11 participating American and Canadian institutions. Although statistical analysis of the data revealed that numerous factors affected patient survival, the classification proposed involved only four clinical variables: Tumor size, local extension of the tumor, palpability and suspicion of nodes, and presence or absence of distant metastasis. The anatomic configuration and location predetermines the staging features of the parotid gland. Involvement of the pterygoid plates or skull base renders tumors unresectable (T4b).

Summary of Changes

The staging of parotid gland cancers have been revised in the sixth edition (2002) to be consistent with other head and neck cancers, which are predominantly categorized by size; T1 <2 cm, T2 2–4 cm, and T3 >4 cm with T4a and T4b defining cancer resectability as previously described (Fig. 6.2).

Orientation of Three-planar Oncoanatomy

The parotid is a superficial gland above the angle of the mandible and wraps around the ramus. The anatomic isocenter is axially at the level of the bodies of C2 and C3. The anterior bullet skims the cheek at the level of the lobule of the external ear (Fig. 6.3A) and the lateral bullet is through the body of the ramus of the mandible superior to the angle of the jaw (Fig. 6.3B).

T-oncoanatomy

The parotid, submaxillary, and sublingual glands are the major salivary glands in contradistinction to the many minor salivary glands, each and all providing digestive enzymes, lubrication, or both for the lumen of the upper digestive passage. The major salivary glands are best oriented (Fig. 6.3AB) to the oral cavity because their major ducts empty into this region. Stensen's duct opens into the buccal cavity opposite the molars and Wharton's duct empties into the floor of mouth along the frenulum of the tongue. The three-dimensional planar views (Fig. 6.4ABC) are essential to appreciate the oncoanatomy.

- *Sagittal plane* (Fig. 6.4A): The sagittal view is the most informative; cranial nerve VII facial nerve enters and exits through the parotid gland between the superficial lobe and the mandible, innervating the multiple muscles of the face. Equally important are branches of cranial nerve V3 and the lingual nerve, both of which can be involved with deep lobe cancers. Perineural invasion can occur, particularly with cylindromas. Such cancers can travel retrograde along the nerve and penetrate into the middle fossa of the skull and the Gasserian ganglion of cranial nerve V.
- *Coronal plane* (Fig. 6.4B): The coronal view demonstrates the relationship of the parotid and submaxillary gland to the mandible.
- *Transverse plane* (Fig. 6.4C): This view is essential to define the retroparotidian space through which the carotid artery, jugular vein, parapharyngeal nodes, and cranial nerves IX, X, XI, and XII pass along the posterior pharyngeal wall.

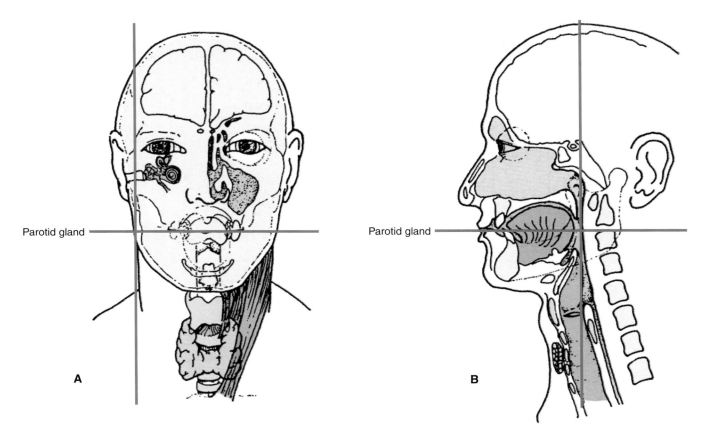

Figure 6.3 **Orientation of three-planar T-oncoanatomy.** The anatomic isocenter is at the axial level at C2/C3. **A**. Coronal. **B**. Sagittal.

N-oncoanatomy

The rich network of superficial lymphatics of the face including the scalp and eyelids drain into the preauricular and parotid lymph nodes (Fig. 6.5). The jugulodigastric lymph node is just inferior to the parotid gland. The deep lobe of the parotid drains into the retropharyngeal lymph nodes. The submaxillary gland drains into submandibular nodes.

M-oncoanatomy

The parotid gland drains to the pterygoid venous plexus, facial vein, internal jugular vein, brachiocephalic vein and superior vena cava, into the right side of the heart. The target metastatic organ is lung, but the pulmonary vascular bed acts as a sanctuary housing metastases that often do not produce any severe or life-threatening loss of pulmonary function (see Fig. 2.6).

Rules of Classification and Staging

Clinical Staging and Imaging

Careful history, physical examination, inspection, and palpation are essential. Full assessment of cranial nerves should be fully evaluated, especially for cylindromas. Computed tomography (CT) and magnetic resonance imaging (MRI) are complementary for assessing deep extraglandular tumor spread, perineural and bone invasion (see Table 1.5).

Pathologic Staging

The gross specimen should be evaluated for margins. Unresected gross residual tumor must be included and marked with clips. All resected lymph node specimens should describe size, number, and level of involved nodes and whether there is extracapsular spread. Specimens taken after radiation, chemotherapy, or both need to so noted, but specimen shrinkages may occur up to 30% after resection itself. Designations pT and pN should be used after histopathologic evaluation. Perineural invasion deserves special notation.

Oncoimaging Annotations

- Perineural invasion of cranial nerve VII is best appreciated on MRI.
- Perineural invasion of cranial nerve V3 with extension in a retrograde fashion to the middle fossa of the skull is best seen on MRI.

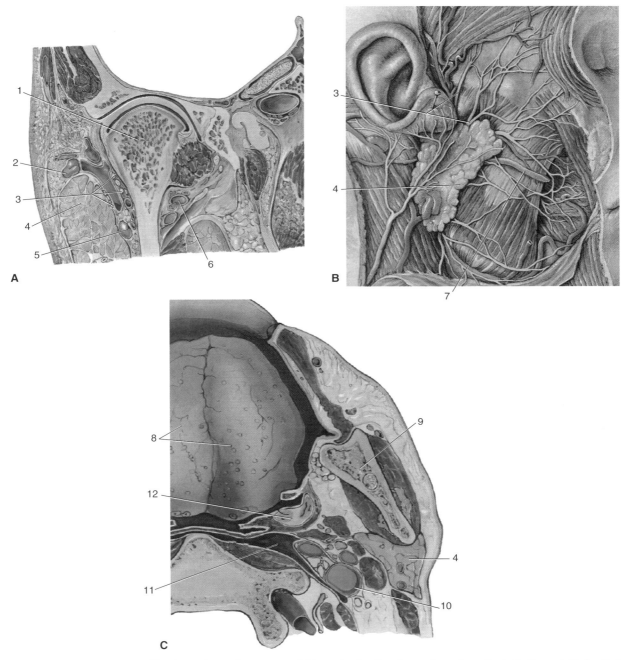

Figure 6.4 **T-oncoanatomy.** The three planar views are crucial to understanding the malignant gradient. **A.** Coronal. **B.** Sagittal. **C.** Transverse. (1) Head of mandible. (2) Superficial parotid lymph node. (3) Branches of facial nerve. (4) Parotid gland. (5) Deep parotid lymph node. (6) Maxillary artery. (7) Parotid duct. (8) Tongue. (9) Ramus of mandible. (10) Carotid sheath. (11) Retropharyngeal space. (12) Palatine tonsil.

- Lung CT should be performed in advanced stage cancer because the lung is most often the metastatic target site.

Cancer Statistics and Survival

Generally, cancers of the oral cavity, pharynx, and upper digestive passage, account for 28,000 new cases (see Table 1.6). In addition, cancer of the larynx affects another 10,000 patients and thyroid cancers 23,600. Approximately 25% of head and neck cancer patients die annually, often due to other causes. Long-term survival is exceptional in thyroid cancer (1,500 deaths [5%]). The improvement in oral cavity and pharyngeal tumors from 1950 to 2000 was modest at 14% and matches larynx at 15% (see Fig. 1.7). A multidisciplinary approach

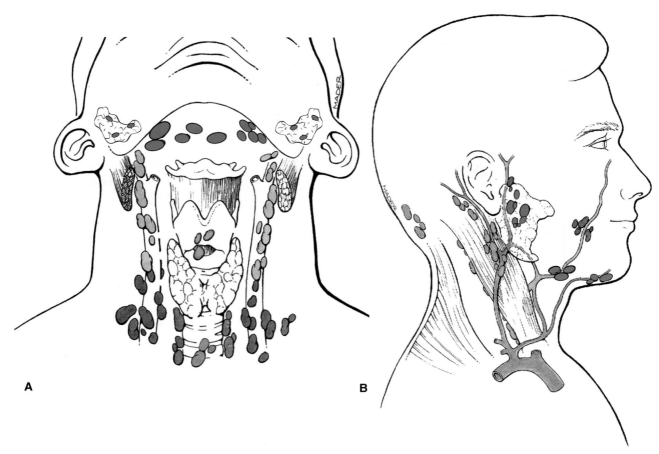

Figure 6.5 N-oncoanatomy. The red node highlights the sentinel node, which is the parotid node. **A.** Coronal. **B.** Sagittal.

is vital and normal tissue conservation and reconstructive techniques have both added greatly to quality of life.

Specifically, improvements in salivary gland tumors dramatically occurred with fast neutron therapy, in which more than 50% of advanced stages responded and were locally controlled. As surgical techniques improved, and when combined with post-operative megavoltage photon and electron therapy, 55% 5-year survival rose to 75% in the assessment of many series in the literature.

7

Oropharynx

The TNM patterns of spread and the malignant gradient are predetermined by the underlying musculature anatomy of the tonsillar pillars.

Perspective and Patterns of Spread

The oropharynx is the isocenter of the upper aerodigestive tract and is composed of a series of large sphincters, which receives the bolus of food and initiates the act of swallowing. The need for sphincteric mechanisms arises because the physiology of deglutition ensures that the contents of tubular structures move in one direction to ensure their proper digestion. Once the bolus is swallowed, a series of involuntary muscular movements of the tube propels the food onward. The chief sphincter of the upper aerodigestive tract is the muscular pharynx (Fig. 7.1).

Tumors of the oropharynx arise from the mucosal lining and are similar to those of the nasopharynx; the tonsil and base of the tongue are a continuation of Waldeyer's ring. The most common neoplasms are squamous cell cancers exhibiting varying degrees of differentiation and anaplasia; most of the discussion surrounding these neoplasms refers to their pattern of spread (Table 7.1). Lymphomas tend to be bulky exophytic lesions. They enlarge the palatine tonsils and/or lingual tonsils without deep infiltration. Although cancers can be exophytic, they invariably have a significant endophytic component. Lymphoepitheliomas have both epithelial and lymphatic cells, and behave in a fashion consistent with both of these two components. Large primaries with bilateral adenopathy are frequently present at their onset.

Cancers of the anterior pillar follow the palatoglossal muscle, which either encircle the soft palate and uvula or alternately, follow the fascial plane inferiorly and infiltrate the tongue. Cancers of the pharyngonasal sphincter (Passavant's fold) consist of palatal neoplasms that act as a nasopharyngeal neoplasm. This sphincter prevents nasal regurgitation and, in effect, ensures closure and separation of the nasal passage from the oral cavity

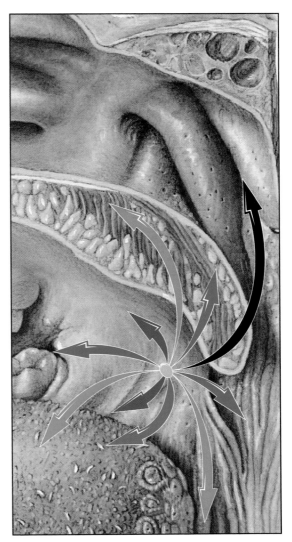

Figure 7.1 **Patterns of spread.** The primary cancer (oropharynx) invades in various directions, which are color-coded vectors (*arrows*) representing stage of progression: Tis, yellow; T1, green; T2, blue; T3, purple; T4a, red; and T4b, black.

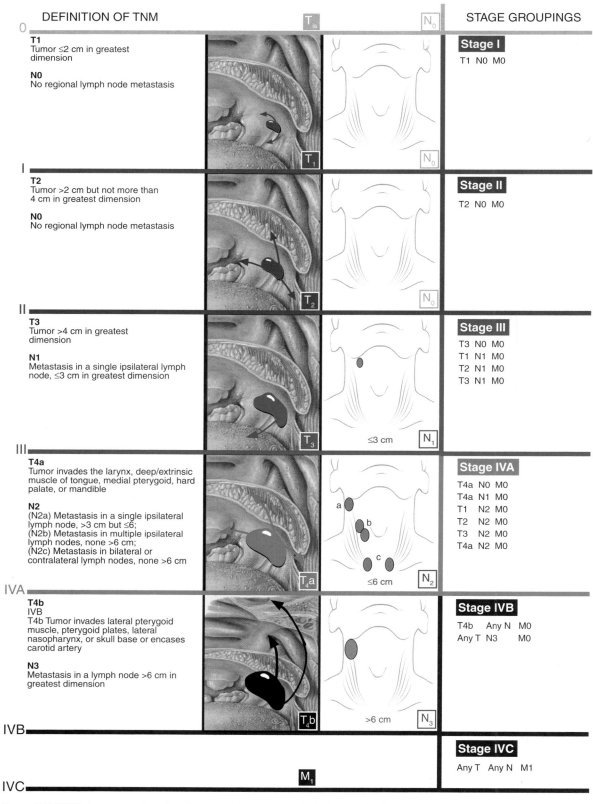

DEFINITION OF TNM

T1
Tumor ≤2 cm in greatest dimension

N0
No regional lymph node metastasis

T2
Tumor >2 cm but not more than 4 cm in greatest dimension

N0
No regional lymph node metastasis

T3
Tumor >4 cm in greatest dimension

N1
Metastasis in a single ipsilateral lymph node, ≤3 cm in greatest dimension

T4a
Tumor invades the larynx, deep/extrinsic muscle of tongue, medial pterygoid, hard palate, or mandible

N2
(N2a) Metastasis in a single ipsilateral lymph node, >3 cm but ≤6;
(N2b) Metastasis in multiple ipsilateral lymph nodes, none >6 cm;
(N2c) Metastasis in bilateral or contralateral lymph nodes, none >6 cm

T4b
IVB
T4b Tumor invades lateral pterygoid muscle, pterygoid plates, lateral nasopharynx, or skull base or encases carotid artery

N3
Metastasis in a lymph node >6 cm in greatest dimension

STAGE GROUPINGS

Stage I
T1 N0 M0

Stage II
T2 N0 M0

Stage III
T3 N0 M0
T1 N1 M0
T2 N1 M0
T3 N1 M0

Stage IVA
T4a N0 M0
T4a N1 M0
T1   N2 M0
T2   N2 M0
T3   N2 M0
T4a N2 M0

Stage IVB
T4b Any N M0
Any T N3   M0

Stage IVC
Any T Any N M1

Figure 7.2 TNM stage grouping. Oropharyngeal cancers spread via the muscle planes into tongue and pharynx from palate in a circumferential fashion. Vertical presentations of stage groupings, which follow same color code for cancer stage advancement are organized in horizontal lanes: Stage 0, yellow; I, green; II, blue; III, purple; IVA, red; and IVB, black. Definitions of TN on left and stage grouping on right.

TABLE 7.1	Histopathologic Type: Common Cancers of the Oropharynx	
Squamous Cell Carcinoma Microscopic Variants	**Adenocarcinoma Major or Minor Salivary Gland**
Keratinizing; well differentiated; moderately well differentiated; poorly differentiated	Low-grade adenocarcinoma
Nonkeratinizing; anaplastic squamous carcinoma	Adenoid cystic carcinoma
Lymphoepithelioma	Mucoepidermoid (low or high grade)
Transitional cell carcinoma	Carcinoma expleomorphic adenoma
Spindle cell squamous carcinoma	Poorly differentiated adenocarcinoma

Adapted from Rubin P. *Clinical Oncology*. 8th ed. New York: Elsevier; 2001:408.

and pharynx while swallowing. Cancers of the posterior pillar (palatopharyngeal muscle) of the tonsil invade the posterior wall of the pharynx (Fig. 7.2). The contraction of the superior constrictor muscle of the pharynx during swallowing forms a prominence known as Passavant's fold on the posterior wall of the nasopharynx which acts as a protective barrier. Cancers in this area tend to appear as irregular surface lesions, spreading circumferentially on the oral and pharyngeal surface. Odynophagia (pain on swallowing) may be ignored and attributed to the common cold. To the astute clinician, dysphagia-producing pain referred to the middle ear is attributed to the referral of pain to the nerve of Jacobsen, a branch of the glossopharyngeal nerve (cranial nerve IX).

TNM Staging Criteria

The TNM patterns of spread are predetermined by the underlying musculature anatomy (Fig. 7.2). The two pillars of the tonsillar fossa, which need to be distinguished from true tonsil remnants, are readily appreciated on surface anatomy. The two sphincters of the oropharynx are the pharyngonasal and buccopharyngeal sphincters.

Cancers can arise in the posterior pharyngeal wall in the area of the mucous membrane between the posterior pillars on the posterior pharyngeal wall over the bodies of C2 and C3. More frequently, the base of the tongue, which seals off regurgitation by pressing against the oropharyngeal bar, is a favored site for malignancy. The malignant gradient increases as the cancer arises in an anteromedial location versus a posterolateral site. Again, the intimate relationship of the tongue and tonsillar region is reflected in their anatomic structure and muscular arrangements. Deeply penetrating cancers from either site usually extend into and invade the other region. Unlike the oral tongue, the base of tongue contains some fat and lymphoid tissue in between the fibers, as well as

a less distinct midline septum, making invasion across to the opposite side a more likely clinical occurrence.

Summary of Changes

The size of the primary tumor determines the stage of the cancer with modification due to nodes. The staging system was revised to determine resectability, T4a, versus unresectability, T4b. Cancer spread anteriorly into the deep extrinsic muscle of the tongue and inferiorly into the larynx or laterally into the medial pterygoid is T4a. T4b cancers infiltrate the pterygoid plates, lateral pterygoid muscles or superiorly into the nasopharynx (Fig. 7.2).

Orientation of Three-planar Oncoanatomy

The anatomic isocenter is located at the C2/C3 level and located along the anterior border of the ramus of the mandible and medial to it. A vertical line from the center of the ramus runs through the center of the pharyngeal tube. The anterior surface bullet is at the level of the lips in the midline (Fig. 7.3A) and the lateral bullet penetrates at the angle of the mandible (Fig. 7.3B).

T-oncoanatomy

The pharynx is a fibromuscular tube extending from the base of the skull to the esophagus, regulating the flow of food and air in the upper aerodigestive passage. The pharynx is composed of three sections: (i) the nasal, (ii) the oral, and (iii) the laryngeal pharynx.

- *Coronal plane* (Fig. 7.4A): There are four major sphincters in the pharynx that regulate the passage of air and food to their ultimate destinations. The sphincters, at the point of the entry, are the buccopharyngeal sphincters guarding the communication between the mouth and the pharynx (fauces). They are

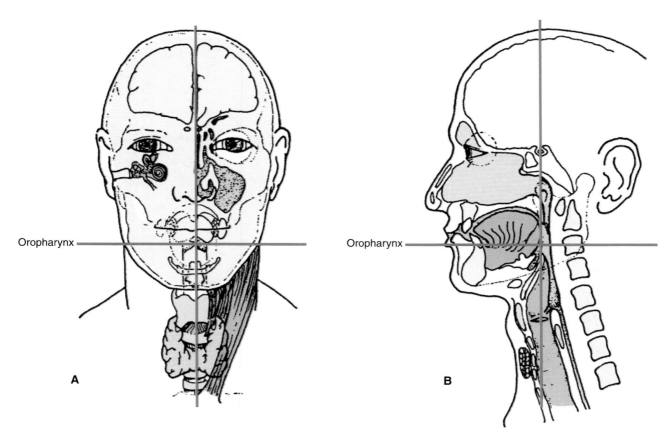

Oropharynx

A

Oropharynx

B

Figure 7.3 **Orientation of three-planar T-oncoanatomy.** The anatomic isocenter is at the axial level at C3. **A**. Coronal. **B**. Sagittal.

formed by the base of the tongue and the oropharyngeal bar, which is produced by a synchronized peristaltic contraction of the posterior oropharyngeal muscular wall. The upper or pharyngonasal opening between the nasopharynx and the oropharynx is protected by a sphincter formed by the soft palate and Passavant's fold. The lower or esophageal opening is protected by the cricopharyngeal sphincter formed by the cricopharyngeal bar and the back of the cricoid cartilage. Cancers that invade posteriorly to the pterygoid plate and superiorly into the nasopharynx to the skull base are T4b.

The fibrous coat (pharyngobasilar fascia) is strong, and anchors the pharynx to the base of the skull and the medial pterygoid plate. In a dissection of mucous membranes and tonsils from the lateral oropharyngeal wall, the following muscles may be identified: palatopharyngeus, superior constrictor, styloglossus, stylopharyngeus, and middle constrictor. As in all peristaltic activity in the digestive tract, there are constrictor muscles and longitudinal muscles. This pattern is seen in the pharyngeal wall. There are three inner constrictor muscles: (i) superior, (ii) middle, and (iii) inferior—and an outer, more longitudinal coat—the stylopharyngeus, stylohyoid,

and palatopharyngeus muscles. The constrictor muscles are strategically attached to the mandible, the hyoid bone, and the thyroid and cricoid cartilages. They provide the form and structure of the pharyngeal tube.

It is in the coronal plane that the prestyloid compartment can be identified by the fatty or areolar content from the lateral pharyngeal space with the stylopharyngeus and styloglossus muscles. The posterior belly of the digastric muscle arises posteriorly, and spreads inferiorly in this space, as does the stylohyoid. Using these same muscles and the styloid process as landmarks, the lateral pharyngeal space is better appreciated with its contents. Posterior to the styloid process is the neurovascular bundle, identified previously in the nasopharyngeal wall.

- *Sagittal plane* (Fig. 7.4B): The palatopharyngeus muscle is shown, innervation by cranial nerve IX into the base of the tongue. On deep dissection of the tonsillar fossa, the palatopharyngeal and the stylopharyngeus muscles form the longitudinal coat. The constrictor muscles, superior and mainly middle, are the circular inner coat that control swallowing. The glossopharyngeal nerve supplies one muscle, the stylopharyngeus, and provides special taste to the

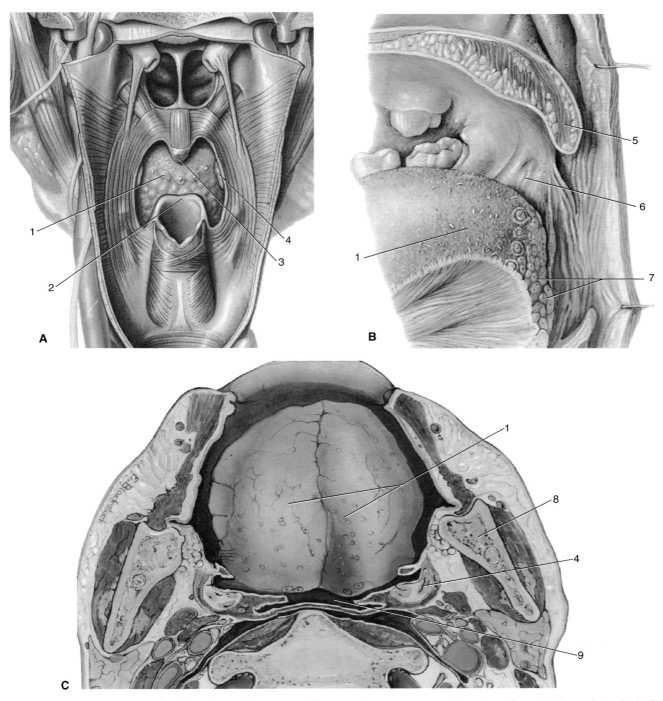

Figure 7.4 **T-oncoanatomy.** The three-planar views are crucial to understanding the malignant gradient. **A.** Coronal. **B.** Sagittal. **C.** Transverse. (1) Base of tongue. (2) Epiglottis. (3) Uvula. (4) Palatine tonsil. (5) Soft palate. (6) Tonsillar fossa. (7) Lingual follicles. (8) Ramus of mandible. (9) Cavity of pharynx.

posterior third of the tongue and sensation to an entire half of the pharyngeal wall; deviation of the uvula and absent gag reflex results when the nerve is lost.

- *Transverse view* (Fig. 7.4C): At C2, it demonstrates the medial and lateral pterygoid muscles, than posteri-

orly the retropharyngeal nodes along side the carotid and jugular vessels in the retroparotidian space laterally. Deep invasion of the posterior glossopharyngeal muscle along the posterior pillar into retropharyngeal nodes leads to neurologic loss, namely, cranial nerves IX, X, XI, and XII.

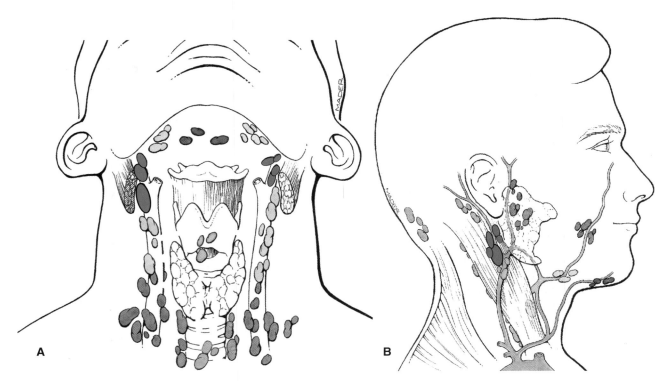

Figure 7.5 **N-oncoanatomy.** The red node highlights the sentinel node, which is the jugulodigastric node. **A.** Coronal. **B.** Sagittal.

N-oncoanatomy

There are three major collecting lymphatic trunks in the oropharynx: (i) the middle collecting, (ii) the palatine tonsil, and (iii) the posterior lingual. These drain into the parapharyngeal or retropharyngeal nodes (Fig. 7.5). The jugulodigastric and jugulo-omohyoid are the most common draining nodes, although upper and lower deep cervical nodes also are first-station nodes. Because of the location of palatine tonsillar lymphoid tissue between the anterior and posterior pillars, and the location of lingual tonsils in the base of the tongue, lymphomas commonly arise at these sites. Occasionally, all of Waldeyer's ring can be involved with lymphomatous

infiltration, obstructing the oropharynx and nasopharynx. These tumors can become large, growing rapidly and remaining submucosal. Both lymphomas and carcinomas often spread into the jugulodigastric and omodigastric nodes. Rapid spread into other cervical nodes and bilateral involvement is common, reflecting the bilateral drainage of the base of the tongue.

M-oncoanatomy

Distant metastases are also possible because of the plexus of pharyngeal veins that drain into the jugular vein, and then into the superior vena cava, the right heart, and

	5-Year Survival According to Stage Grouping (%)				
Site	All Stages	I	II	III	IV
Oropharynx					
Tonsil	45	90	60	40	15
Base of tongue	30	60	40	20	10
Pharyngeal wall	20	50	30	20	10
Soft palate	50	85	60	30	15

TABLE 7.2 | **Approximate Determinate 5-Year Survival by Stages at Diagnosis (1992–1998)**

finally the lungs. The vascular supply of the pharynx arises from the external carotid. The carotid body and sinus located at the bifurcation of the common carotid are arterial chemoreceptor and baroreceptor areas, respectively (see Fig. 2.6).

Rules of Classification and Staging

Clinical Staging and Imaging

For oropharyngeal cancers, careful history taking, inspection, and palpation of the face and neck are essential. Testing of all cranial nerves is critical. Both direct and indirect endoscopy are useful. Despite cooperation of the patient, pharyngeal cancers may be inaccessible and imaging is important. To determine the true extent of primary oropharyngeal cancers, imaging is essential. Magnetic resonance imaging (MRI) is superior to computed tomography (CT) in demonstrating soft tissue extension, skull base changes, and perineural invasion (see Table 1.5).

Pathologic Staging

The gross specimen should be evaluated for margins. Unresected gross residual tumor must be included and marked with clips. All resected lymph node specimens should describe size, number, and level of involved nodes and whether there is extracapsular spread. Specimens taken after radiation, chemotherapy, or both need to so noted; specimen shrinkages may occur up to 30% after resection itself. Designations pT and pN should be used after histopathologic evaluation. Perineural invasion deserves special notation.

Oncoimaging Annotations

* Staging systems for oropharyngeal carcinomas are based mainly on tumor size criteria and deep extensions.

* All CT studies should be performed after contrast enhancement administered by using a bolus technique.

* Thirty percent of patients with squamous cell carcinoma of the base of the tongue have bilateral metastatic nodes at the time of initial clinical presentation. Many of these nodes are clinically silent and are detected on imaging studies.

* Evaluation of tonsillar and soft palate carcinomas is best done with MRI to determine soft tissue invasion.

Cancer Statistics and Survival

Generally, cancers of the oral cavity, pharynx, and the upper digestive passage account for 28,000 new cases (see Table 1.6). In addition, cancer of the larynx affect another 10,000 patients and thyroid cancers 23,600. Approximately 25% of head and neck cancer patients die annually, often due to other causes (Table 7.2). Long-term survival for patients with thyroid cancers is an exception, with only 1,500 deaths (5%). The improvement in oral cavity and pharyngeal tumors from 1950 to 2000 was modest at 14% and matches larynx at 15% (see Fig. 1.7). A multidisciplinary approach is vital and normal tissue conservation and reconstructive techniques have both added greatly to quality of life. Unfortunately, this patient population abuse ethanol and nicotine and it is difficult to change these habits. Persistence of smoking and drinking contributes to their demise often from second malignant tumors in adjacent sites.

Specifically, oropharyngeal cancer is often advanced stage II or III when detected and overall survival is only 20% to 40%. The best outcome is with early stage I tonsillar cancers and soft palate as compared to base of tongue and pharyngeal wall, that is, 85% to 90% versus 50% to 60% respectively.

8

Hypopharynx

The malignant gradient is an oblique plane following the hypopharyngeal circle. The circle begins with the valleculae at the base of the tongue and worsens as it extends to the piriform recesses laterally. The poorest prognosis is posteriorly at the postcricoid region above the esophageal inlet with the completion of the circle.

Perspective and Patterns of Spread

Although the hypopharynx (laryngopharynx) and larynx are anatomically distinct, they require presentation together. *In hunting animals as the wolf and fox, the larynx projects into the nasopharynx providing continuity for airways.* There is no oropharynx when the epiglottis overrides the uvula and soft palate, providing a continuous air column. *With evolution the two-part pharynx arose; as in bipedal man, the food bypasses the larynx laterally in the piriform recess.* In this anatomic arrangement, food and fluids can be aspirated and is a common complaint when tumors arise in the hypopharynx. There is a malignant gradient of cancers arising in this site with anterior location as the valleculae being more favorable than the lateral piriform fossae and the least desirable are posterior pharyngeal and postcricoid in location (Fig. 8.1). The common epithelial cancer is squamous cell with other varieties occurring less often. The pharyngeal mucosa tends to be nonkeratinized stratified squamous epithelium giving rise to squamous cell cancers predominantly with varying degrees of differentiation (Table 8.1).

The major sites of malignancy in the hypopharynx occur in the zones of food traffic. The hypopharynx can be viewed as a circular gutter designed to allow the food bolus to circumvent the larynx, which is closed during deglutition. The circle, starting anteriorly, begins with the valleculae at the base of the tongue, extends to the piriform recesses laterally, and is completed posteriorly at the postcricoid region above the esophageal inlet. The epithelial cancers of the piriform recess are by far the most common. Cancers of the piriform recess are usually squamous cell carcinomas, most often undifferentiated and advanced, spreading in all directions. Superiorly, they extend into the lateral pharyngeal wall and the base of the tongue, and inferiorly into the cricopharyngeal area. Medially, they can spill into the larynx by

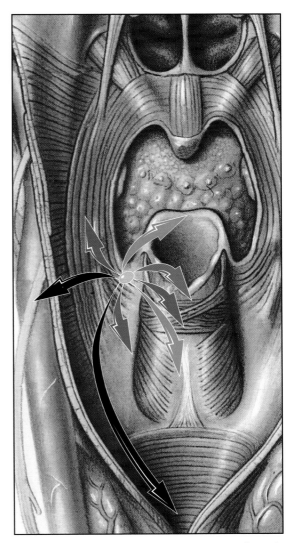

Figure 8.1 **Patterns of spread.** The primary cancer (hypopharynx) invades in various directions, which are color-coded vectors (*arrows*) representing stage of progression: Tis, yellow; T1, green; T2, blue; T3, purple; T4a, red; and T4b, black.

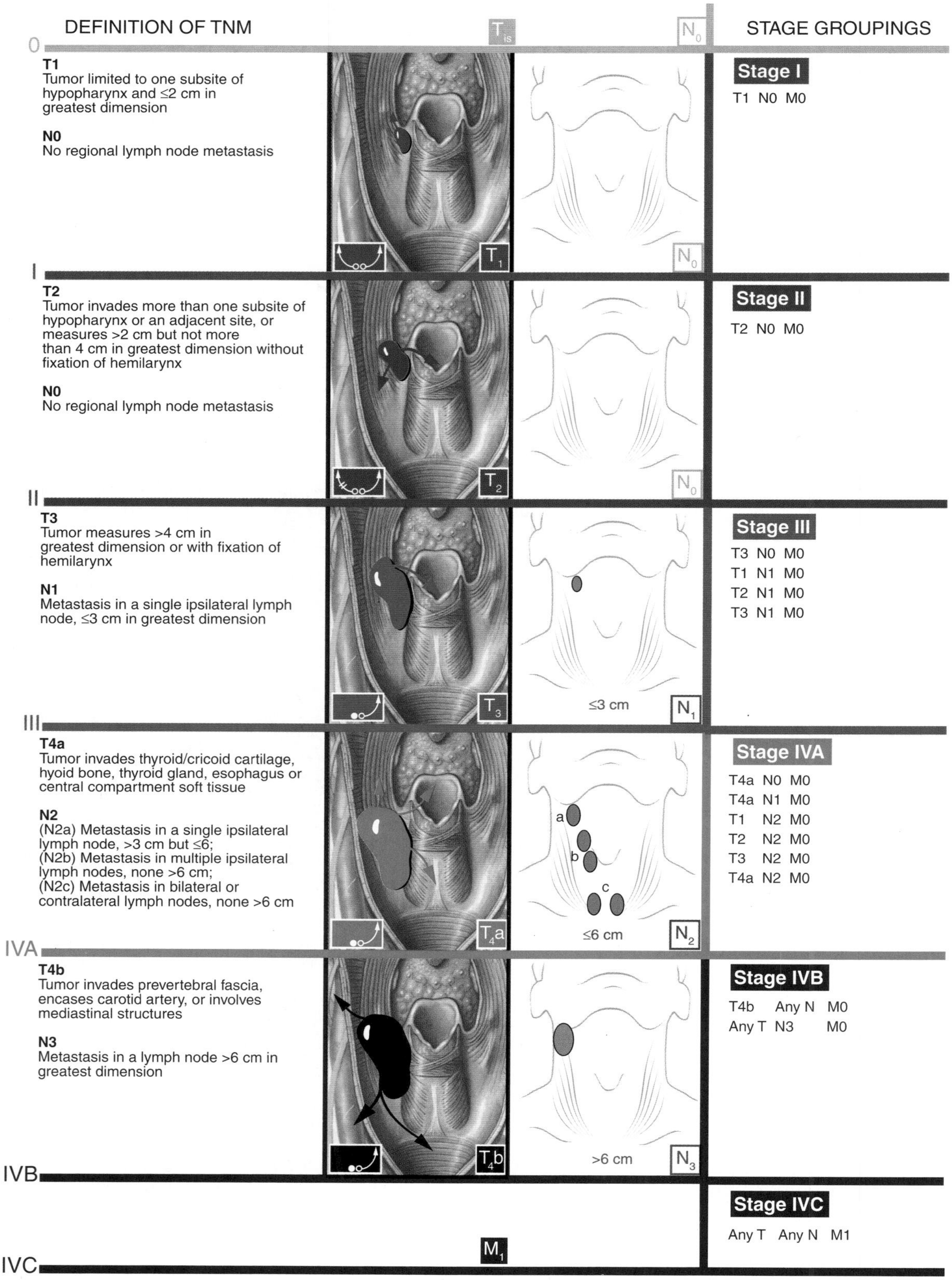

DEFINITION OF TNM

STAGE GROUPINGS

T1
Tumor limited to one subsite of hypopharynx and ≤2 cm in greatest dimension

N0
No regional lymph node metastasis

Stage I

T1 N0 M0

T2
Tumor invades more than one subsite of hypopharynx or an adjacent site, or measures >2 cm but not more than 4 cm in greatest dimension without fixation of hemilarynx

N0
No regional lymph node metastasis

Stage II

T2 N0 M0

T3
Tumor measures >4 cm in greatest dimension or with fixation of hemilarynx

N1
Metastasis in a single ipsilateral lymph node, ≤3 cm in greatest dimension

Stage III

T3 N0 M0
T1 N1 M0
T2 N1 M0
T3 N1 M0

≤3 cm

T4a
Tumor invades thyroid/cricoid cartilage, hyoid bone, thyroid gland, esophagus or central compartment soft tissue

N2
(N2a) Metastasis in a single ipsilateral lymph node, >3 cm but ≤6;
(N2b) Metastasis in multiple ipsilateral lymph nodes, none >6 cm;
(N2c) Metastasis in bilateral or contralateral lymph nodes, none >6 cm

Stage IVA

T4a N0 M0
T4a N1 M0
T1   N2 M0
T2   N2 M0
T3   N2 M0
T4a N2 M0

≤6 cm

T4b
Tumor invades prevertebral fascia, encases carotid artery, or involves mediastinal structures

N3
Metastasis in a lymph node >6 cm in greatest dimension

Stage IVB

T4b   Any N   M0
Any T N3   M0

>6 cm

Stage IVC

Any T Any N M1

Figure 8.2 TNM stage grouping. Hypopharyngeal cancers are aggressive malignancies that invade into the larynx and/or directly into cervical neck nodes. Vertical presentations of stage groupings, which follow same color code for cancer stage advancement are organized in horizontal lanes: Stage 0, yellow; I, green; II, blue; III, purple; IVA, red; IVB, black. Definitions of TN on left and stage grouping on right.

TABLE 8.1	Histopathologic Type: Common Cancers of the Hypopharynx

Squamous Cell Carcinoma Microscopic Variants	Adenocarcinoma Major or Minor Salivary Gland
Keratinizing; well differentiated; moderately well differentiated; poorly differentiated	Low-grade adenocarcinoma
Nonkeratinizing; anaplastic squamous carcinoma	Adenoid cystic carcinoma
Lymphoepithelioma	Mucoepidermoid (low or high grade)
Transitional cell carcinoma	Carcinoma expleomorphic adenoma
Spindle cell squamous carcinoma	Poorly differentiated adenocarcinoma

Adapted from Rubin P. *Clinical Oncology*. 8th ed. New York: Elsevier; 2001:408.

infiltrating over the aryepiglottic fold. Very often they invade laterally directly into the soft tissues of the neck. An obscure piriform sinus cancer can present as aspiration pneumonitis. A majority of patients complain of difficulty in swallowing with referral of pain to the external ear, which is attributed to Arnold's nerve, a branch of the vagus nerve (cranial nerve X). This neurologic sign indicates invasion of the larynx. Other signs of cancer progression are fetor oris, difficulty swallowing saliva, and dyspnea. Hoarseness also indicates laryngeal invasion.

TNM Staging Criteria

True postcricoid tumors are often difficult to distinguish from cancer of the cervical esophagus (Fig. 8.2). There are three definite groups of tumors: (i) cricopharyngeal, (ii) pharyngoesophageal, and (iii) cervical esophageal. There are certain peculiarities in these tumors. For example, they seem to be more common in women, and are associated with difficulty in swallowing. The cricopharyngeus muscle, a muscular band formed by the lower part of the inferior constrictor, usually directs the tumor in an encircling fashion, where it tends to remain with extension superiorly. Involvement of the true larynx with invasion into the arytenoids and into the glottis is possible, but much less likely than inferior spread into the esophagus or superior spread into the posterior pharyngeal wall in the direction of peristalsis.

The most difficult cancers to recognize are those in the valleculae, which tend to burrow into the base of the tongue and destroy the epiglottis. Necrosis is common, and deep sinuses may develop in the tongue. Cartilage erosion and disfiguration of the epiglottis are frequently noted. Invasion of the pre-epiglottic, fat-filled space is common; it offers no resistance to cancer spread.

As stated, the malignant gradient of the hypopharynx is less anteriorly in the valleculae where the prognosis is better than posteriorly and laterally in the piriform recess and postcricoid regions. However, direct invasion into the soft tissues of the neck and even the jugular vein often lead to distant metastases.

Summary of Changes

The major modification of the staging system is defining the resectable versus the unresectable spread of cancer. The resectable patterns of spread T4a of these cancers are typified by pyriform recess cancers, which extend medially to the aryepiglottic fold, then spilling over into the supraglottis (the laryngeal face of the epiglottis), or the arytenoids, and from there to the false and true vocal folds. The invasions of the anterior and central compartmental tissues of the neck T4a are distinguished from the more unfavorable invasion of the posterior neck compartment. Unresectable T4b refers to invasion of the prevertebral fascia. Inferiorly, cancer can extend into the postcricoid region toward the inlet of the esophagus or involves mediastinal structures beyond the esophagus.

Orientation of Three-planar Oncoanatomy

The anatomic isocenter of the hypopharynx is at the C4/C5 level. It is vertically in line with the anterior border of the ramus of the mandible and its inferior border anteriorly begins at level of the hyoid bone. The anterior bullet is the level of the hyoid bone to the left and right of midline (Fig. 8.3A) and the lateral bullet is just below the greater horns of the hyoid bone (Fig. 8.3B).

T-oncoanatomy

The hypopharynx is the lower continuation of the pharyngeal tube and is anatomically defined laterally and posteriorly by the middle and inferior constrictor muscles and anteriorly by the hyoid bone, thyroid, and cricoid cartilage (Fig. 8.4). If the larynx were postnasal, anatomy would be less complex and the oropharynx

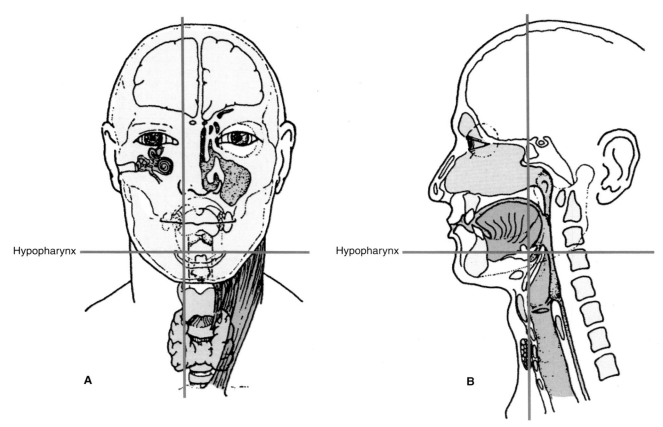

Figure 8.3 **Orientation of three-planar T-oncoanatomy.** The anatomic isocenter is at the axial level at C5. **A.** Coronal. **B.** Sagittal.

and hypopharynx functionally and structurally would be one. The descent of the larynx transforms the tube into a series of symmetrical gutters surrounding the larynx (Fig. 8.4).

- *Coronal view*: The hypopharynx is best understood anatomically from a posterior coronal view (Fig. 8.4A), obtained by separating the inferior constrictor muscles at the midline. The hypopharyngeal sphincters and the piriform recesses circumvent the larynx to lead food into the esophagus. The recurrent laryngeal nerve enters the larynx and can be trapped by piriform sinus cancers.
- *Sagittal plane* (Fig. 8.4B) allows identification of the postcricoid region and establishes the relationship to the larynx of the beginning of the trachea and the beginning of the esophagus.
- *Transverse plane* and a cross-section at C4/5 (Fig. 8.4C) basically identifies the intimate relationship of the pharyngeal tube to the cartilages, bones, and muscles in the neck. The carotid artery and its branches, and the jugular vein in the retropharyngeal space, has only cranial nerve X and the cervical sympathetics. Most of the neck volume is posterior to the pre-

vertebral fascia, which contains the spinal cord and nerve trunks to form the brachial plexus.

N-oncoanatomy

The major lymph node drainage is into the jugular chain of nodes (Fig. 8.5). The deep cervical node and posterior triangle nodes are also readily related to the hypopharynx. The vagus nerve (cranial nerve X) plays an important role in sensation and muscular innervation of the hypopharynx and larynx. Note that only the vagus nerve is left in the lower neck as the other cranial nerves terminate in the head with the exception of the spinal accessory XI nerve. The jugulo-omohyoid node is often the sentinel node for hypopharyngeal cancers. There is a high degree of lymph node involvement including the parapharyngeal and retropharyngeal nodes, as well as the jugulodigastric and jugulo-omohyoid nodes.

M-oncoanatomy

Distant metastases are also possible because of the plexus of pharyngeal veins that drain into the jugular vein, and then into the superior vena cava, the right heart, and finally the lungs. The vascular supply of the pharynx

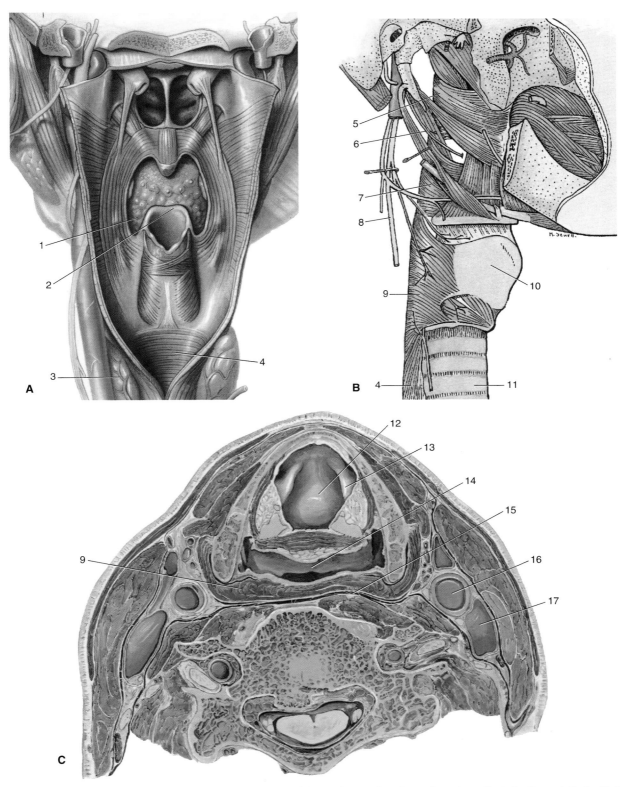

Figure 8.4 **T-oncoanatomy.** The three planar views are crucial to understanding the malignant gradient. **A.** Coronal. **B.** Sagittal. **C.** Transverse. (1) Root of tongue. (2) Epiglottis. (3) Thyroid gland. (4) Esophagus. (5) Superior pharyngeal constrictor. (6) Glossopharyngeal nerve. (7) Middle pharyngeal constrictor. (8) Vagus nerve. (9) Inferior pharyngeal constrictor. (10) Thyroid lamina. (11) Trachea. (12) Larynx. (13) Vestibular fold. (14) Pharynx. (15) Retropharyngeal space. (16) Common carotid artery. (17) Internal jugular vein.

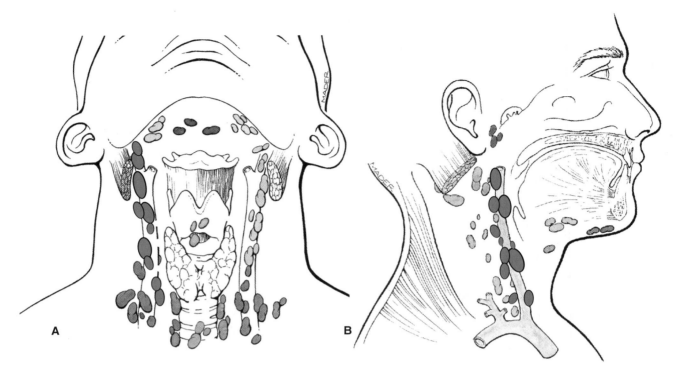

Figure 8.5 **N-oncoanatomy.** The red node highlights the sentinel node, which is the jugulo-omohyoid node. **A.** Coronal. **B.** Sagittal.

arises from the external carotid. The carotid body and sinus located at the bifurcation of the common carotid is an arterial chemoreceptor and baroreceptor area, respectively (see Fig. 2.6).

Rules of Classification and Staging

Clinical Staging and Imaging

For hypopharyngeal cancers, careful history taking, inspection, and palpations of the face and neck are essential. Testing all cranial nerves is critical. Both direct and indirect endoscopy are useful. Despite patient cooperation, pharyngeal cancers are inaccessible and imaging is important. To determine the true extent of primary

hypopharyngeal cancers, imaging is essential. Magnetic resonance imaging (MRI) is superior to computed tomography (CT) in demonstrating soft tissue extension, skull base changes, and perineural invasion (see Table 1.5).

Pathologic Staging

The gross specimen should be evaluated for margins. Unresected gross residual tumor must be included and marked with clips. All resected lymph node specimens should describe size, number, and level of involved nodes and whether there is extracapsular spread. Specimens taken after radiation, chemotherapy, or both need to so noted, but specimen shrinkages may occur up to 30% after resection itself. Designations pT and pN

TABLE 8.2	Approximate Determinate 5-Year Survival by Stages at Diagnosis (1992–1998)				
	5-Year Survival According to Stage Grouping (%)				
Site	All Stages	I	II	III	IV
Hypopharynx					
Piriform sinus	25	30	20	15	5
Postcricoid	20	ID	ID	ID	ID
ID, insufficient data.					

should be used after histopathologic evaluation. Perineural invasion deserves special notation.

Oncoimaging Annotations

- With hypopharyngeal carcinomas, cartilage invasion is often clinically occult and is therefore best detected by imaging. Submucosal extension is also better detected with imaging.
- All CT studies should be performed after contrast enhancement administered by using a bolus technique.
- A collapsed (paralyzed) piriform sinus may mimic a tumor on both CT and MRI studies.

Cancer Statistics and Survival

Generally, cancers of the oral cavity, pharynx, and upper digestive passage account for 28,000 new cases (see Table 1.6). In addition, cancer of the larynx affect another 10,000 patients and thyroid cancers 23,600. Approximately 25% of head and neck cancer patients die annually, often due to other causes (Table 8.2). Long-term survival is exceptional in thyroid cancers, with only 1,500 deaths (5%). The improvement in oral cavity and pharyngeal tumors from 1950 to 2000 was modest at 14% and matches larynx at 15% (see Fig. 1.7). A multidisciplinary approach is vital, and normal tissue conservation and reconstructive techniques have both added greatly to quality of life. Unfortunately, this patient population abuses ethanol and nicotine, and it is difficult to change these habits. Persistence of smoking and drinking contributes to their demise, often from second malignant tumors in adjacent sites.

Specifically, hypopharyngeal cancers are found in advanced stages, particularly pyriform sinus and postcricoid cancers, with the poorest survival in head and neck sites at 20% to 25% at 5 years. Localized early cancers have a 5-year survival rate of 75%, whereas advanced malignancies hover in the 25% range.

9

Supraglottic Larynx

The malignant gradient is in reference to the horizontal midplane through the true glottis. Cancers above have a better outcome and below have a poorer prognosis.

Perspective and Patterns of Spread

Cancers of the larynx are among the commonly occurring cancers in the upper respiratory passage and present the challenge of preservation of phonation. The larynx is a critical structure in the respiratory tract and is the major sphincter through which air enters and exits from the lung. It performs the essential function of closure to the airway entrance during deglutition. Once involved, laryngeal cancer can be an isolated nodule, but is often part of a field cancerization process due to habitual smoking. The likelihood of a recurrence or second primary in lung is inevitable if the host is either unwilling or unable to give up tobacco. Persistent hoarseness demands an otologic examination. The larynx is lined by pseudostratified ciliated columnar epithelium except on the superior surface of the epiglottis and vocal cords, which are covered by stratified squamous non keratinized epithelium (Fig. 9.1). Most cancers are squamous cell cancers, but a variety of malignancies can occur (Table 9.1). Vocal cord cancers tend to be well differentiated and supraglottic and subglottic cancers tend to be more undifferentiated. The malignant gradient is greater from anterior to posterior, from superior to inferior, and from medial to lateral. Most important is sparing of the vocal cords and voice preservation. A number of randomized studies have confirmed that chemoradiation regimens are able to yield comparable survival with laryngeal preservation versus radical laryngectomy.

Cancers arising in the different subsites of the larynx have patterns of spread that reflect the anatomy of a larynx in its development and function. The malignant gradient is in reference to the horizontal midplane through the true glottis. Cancers above have a less favorable outcome and below have a poorer prognosis for readily apparent reasons relating to the ease of detection of supraglottic compared with subglottic cancers obscured

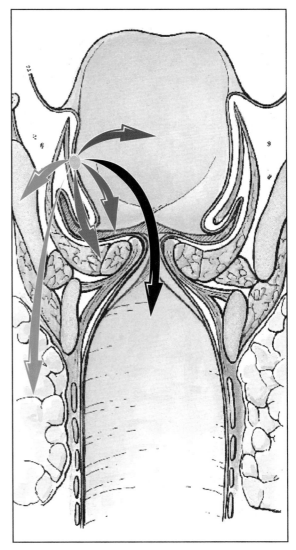

Figure 9.1 **Patterns of spread.** The primary cancer (supraglottic larynx) invades in various directions, which are color-coded vectors (*arrows*) representing stage of progression: Tis, yellow; T1, green; T2, blue; T3, purple; T4a, red; and T4b, black.

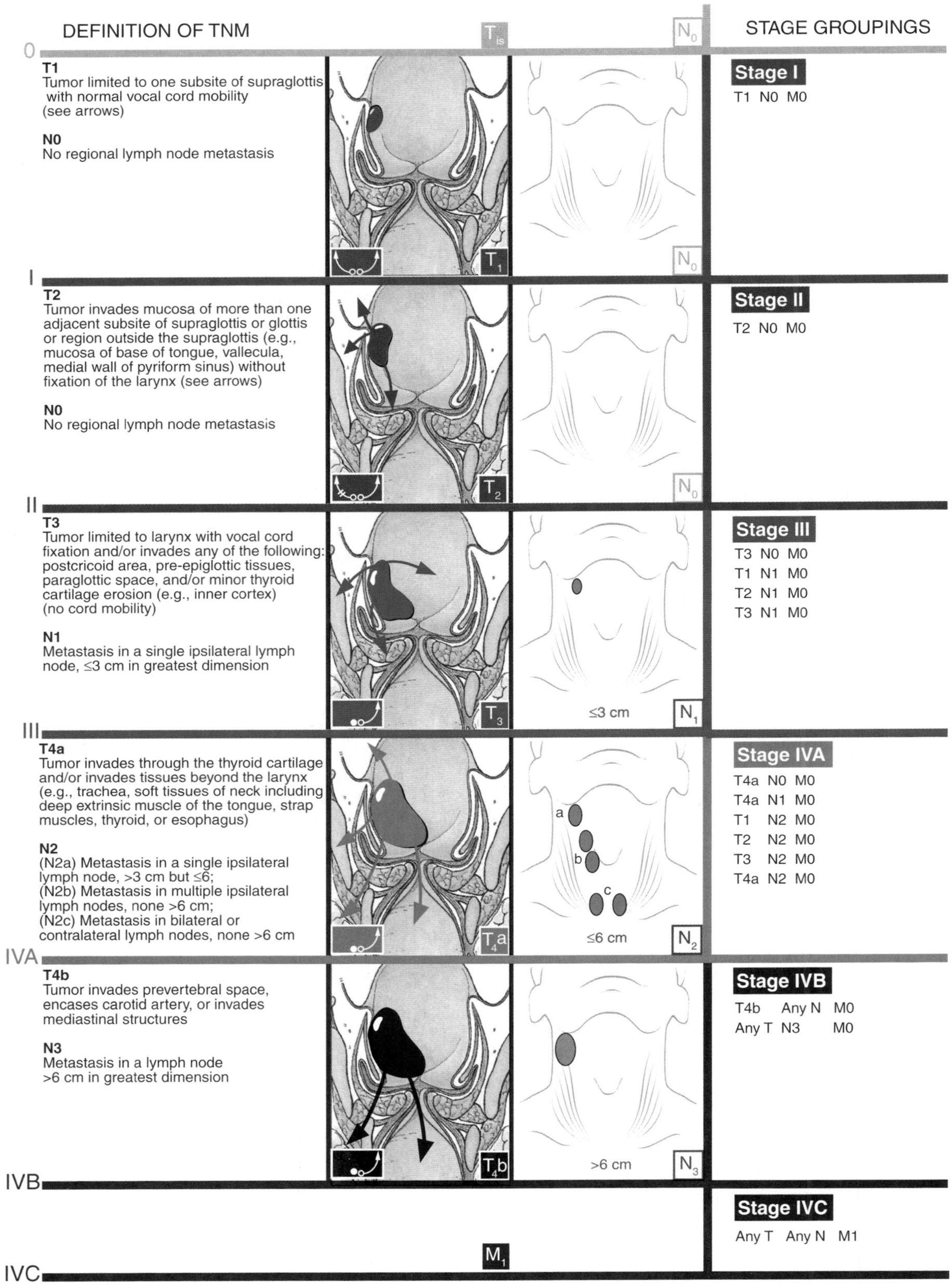

DEFINITION OF TNM T_{is} N_0 STAGE GROUPINGS

0

T1
Tumor limited to one subsite of supraglottis
with normal vocal cord mobility
(see arrows)

N0
No regional lymph node metastasis

Stage I
T1 N0 M0

I

T2
Tumor invades mucosa of more than one
adjacent subsite of supraglottis or glottis
or region outside the supraglottis (e.g.,
mucosa of base of tongue, vallecula,
medial wall of pyriform sinus) without
fixation of the larynx (see arrows)

N0
No regional lymph node metastasis

Stage II
T2 N0 M0

II

T3
Tumor limited to larynx with vocal cord
fixation and/or invades any of the following:
postcricoid area, pre-epiglottic tissues,
paraglottic space, and/or minor thyroid
cartilage erosion (e.g., inner cortex)
(no cord mobility)

N1
Metastasis in a single ipsilateral lymph
node, ≤3 cm in greatest dimension

Stage III
T3 N0 M0
T1 N1 M0
T2 N1 M0
T3 N1 M0

III

T4a
Tumor invades through the thyroid cartilage
and/or invades tissues beyond the larynx
(e.g., trachea, soft tissues of neck including
deep extrinsic muscle of the tongue, strap
muscles, thyroid, or esophagus)

N2
(N2a) Metastasis in a single ipsilateral
lymph node, >3 cm but ≤6;
(N2b) Metastasis in multiple ipsilateral
lymph nodes, none >6 cm;
(N2c) Metastasis in bilateral or
contralateral lymph nodes, none >6 cm

Stage IVA
T4a N0 M0
T4a N1 M0
T1 N2 M0
T2 N2 M0
T3 N2 M0
T4a N2 M0

IVA

T4b
Tumor invades prevertebral space,
encases carotid artery, or invades
mediastinal structures

N3
Metastasis in a lymph node
>6 cm in greatest dimension

Stage IVB
T4b Any N M0
Any T N3   M0

IVB

M_1

Stage IVC
Any T Any N M1

IVC

Figure 9.2 TNM stage grouping. Supraglottic cancers spread insidiously and may not be detected until surrounding structures are invaded as vocal cords or spill into piriform fossa. Vertical presentations of stage groupings, which follow same color code for cancer stage advancement are organized in horizontal lanes: Stage 0, yellow; I, green; II, blue; III, purple; IVA, red; and IVB, black. Definitions of TN on left and stage grouping on right. Note inferior box on T-oncoanatomy provides a key to vocal cord mobility.

TABLE 9.1	Histopathologic Type: Common Cancers of the Glottic Larynx
Squamous Cell Carcinoma Microscopic Variants	
Keratinizing; well differentiated; moderately well differentiated; poorly differentiated	
Nonkeratinizing; anaplastic squamous carcinoma	
Transitional cell carcinoma	
Spindle cell squamous carcinoma	
Adapted from Rubin P. *Clinical Oncology.* 8th ed. New York: Elsevier; 2001:408.	

by the vocal cords. Cancers of the true vocal cord are detected early because they alter voice quality and lead to hoarseness. They tend to arise from the free margin, but frequently cross to the opposite cord via the anterior commissure. The vocal cords are relatively avascular and are poor in lymphatics. Consequently, lymph node involvement and distant metastases are rare.

TNM Staging Criteria

Supraglottic cancers can arise from a variety of different locations, and tend to cause few symptoms until advanced (Fig. 9.2). The free surface of the epiglottis, false cords, and ventricles can all be involved. Transglottic cancers are usually advanced cancers that extend from the supraglottic area, invade the vocal cords, and impair their function. These tumors spread rapidly because of the rich lymphatic network of this region. Bilateral neck nodes are often encountered. Another favored area of spread is the pre-epiglottic fat space.

Epilaryngeal cancers arise from the free border of the larynx where they come into contact with the pharynx. Cancers of the tip of the epiglottis can spill into the valleculae and can appear like a golf ball on a tee. Another common point of origin is the aryepiglottic fold, from which the cancer can spread into the supraglottic larynx or into the piriform sinus. Arytenoids cancers are unusual and obscure the normal double-beaded appearance of the posterior cartilages of the larynx.

Subglottic cancers, in terms of prognosis, are worse than other types. This is probably due to their tendency to invade the trachea, and to reach a more advanced state before detection.

The larynx was initially staged with the development of the TNM system and appeared in the joint first edition of the American Joint Committee on Cancer/International Union Against Cancer guidelines (1978). The basis of progression of laryngeal cancers is related to their spread patterns to subsites (T2) as well as advancement from any one major site: Glottic, supraglottic, subglottic to another, T2 if cord mobility is preserved. Loss of cord mobility indicates T3.

Summary of Changes

In the sixth edition (2002), a revision of stage 4 into resectable T4a and unresectable T4b invasion in emphasized. If the involvement is limited to the central and anterior neck compartment it is T4a and resectable; if the prevertebral space and fascia are penetrated by posterior spread, the stage is T4b. Extension from the neck to mediastinal structures also constitutes a very advanced stage T4b.

Orientation of Three-planar Oncoanatomy

The anatomic isocenter of the supraglottic larynx is at the C4 level. The anterior surface bullet is at the level of the thyroid cartilage notch (Fig. 9.3A) and the lateral surface bullet is at the same level anterior to the greater horn of the thyroid cartilage (Fig. 9.3B).

T-oncoanatomy

The introduction to three-dimensional planar view of the larynx is best appreciated from the posterior coronal view with the constrictor musculature split.

- *Coronal plane* (Fig. 9.4A): The larynx is divided into three parts: (i) supraglottis, (ii) glottis, and (iii) subglottis; these three parts are known as the vestibule, ventricle (glottis), and infraglottic cavity. The epiglottis is readily visualized at its vestibule. The opening of the larynx, referred to as the *aditus larynges* or the *superior laryngeal aperture*, can be traced from the epiglottis to the arytenoids. The aryepiglottic folds start at the free edge of the epiglottis and terminates at the corniculate and arytenoids cartilages. The false cords and the true cords are separated by the ventricle. The true cords act as a sphincter that closes off the airway.

- *Sagittal plane* (Fig. 9.4B): The cartilaginous skeleton of the larynx consists of the epiglottis, thyroid, cricoid, arytenoids, and corniculate cartilages and hyoid bone. A set of fine membranes and muscles hold this cartilage together forming a rigid structure that is not easily destroyed by cancer invasion. The cricoid

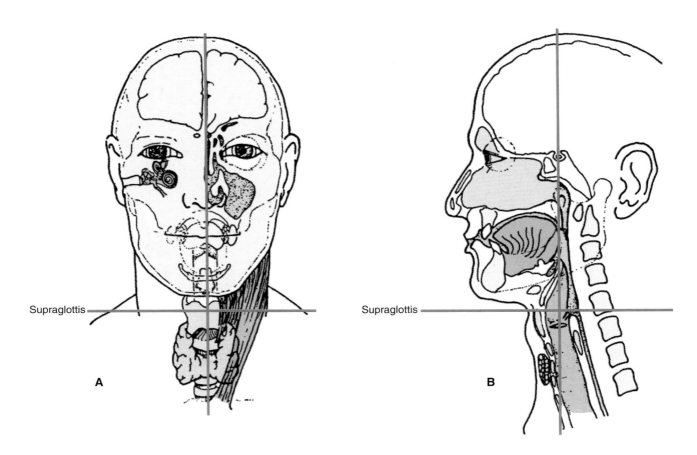

Figure 9.3 **Orientation of three-planar T-oncoanatomy.** The anatomic isocenter is at the axial level at C5. **A.** Coronal. **B.** Sagittal.

muscle tenses the vocal cords. The intrinsic muscles include the posterior cricoarytenoid, thyroarytenoids, vocalis, thyroepiglottis, and aryepiglottis. The essential function of these muscles is to open and close the glottis during breathing and to regulate cord tension during speaking. The true cords and the false cords are separated by a ventricle. The pre-epiglottic fat-filled space can be readily infiltrated from a cancer in the supraglottic region at its base because the epiglottic cartilage sits as an upside-down paddle. These features are best appreciated in the coronal and sagittal views.

- *Transverse view* (Fig. 9.4C): The axial view illustrates the paralaryngeal space between the thyroid and epiglottal cartilage and the position of the larynx to the pharynx. The prevertebral space is separated from the larynx by the hypopharynx and the prevertebral fascia is rarely invaded by true laryngeal malignancies.

N-oncoanatomy

Each segment of the larynx drains to a different sentinel node (Fig. 9.5). The glottis or true vocal cords are not rich in lymphatics and drain to pretracheal or paralaryngeal lymph nodes. The supraglottis is richer in lymphatics and vascularization, with drainage favoring midjugular and jugulodigastric nodes. Subglottic cancers drain to deeper cervical nodes, the jugulo-omohyoid, and even the scalene nodes.

M-oncoanatomy

The venous drainage of the larynx is by way of laryngeal veins into the internal jugular vein and then into the superior vena cava. Metastases are most likely to target the lung (see Fig. 1.6).

Rules of Classification and Staging

Clinical Staging and Imaging

Assessment of the larynx in its three compartments—supraglottis, glottis, and subglottis—is optimally performed with fiberoptic laryngoscope and often requires general anesthesia, which is advised often after completion of diagnostic imaging studies. Determining vocal cord motion, either partial or complete paralysis, is difficult; the normal cord can cross over to meet the involved cord. Imaging studies do not supplant

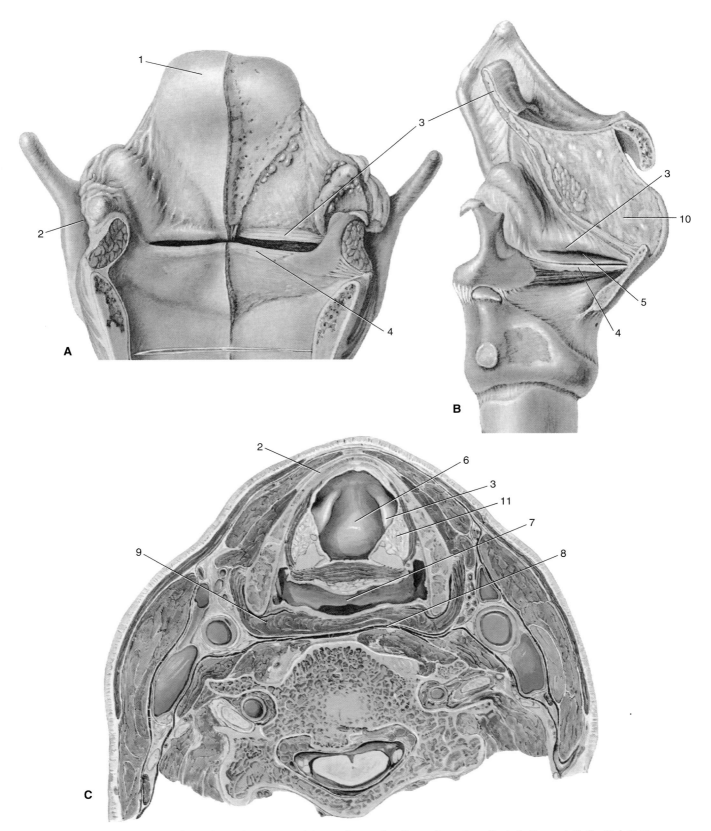

Figure 9.4 **T-oncoanatomy.** The three planar views are crucial to understanding the malignant gradient. **A.** Coronal. **B.** Sagittal. **C.** Transverse. (1) Epiglottis. (2) Thyroid cartilage. (3) Vestibular fold. (4) Vocal fold. (5) Ventricle of larynx. (6) Vestibule of larynx. (7) Pharynx. (8) Retropharyngeal space. (9) Inferior pharyngeal constrictor. (10) Pre-epiglottic space. (11) Para-epiglottic space.

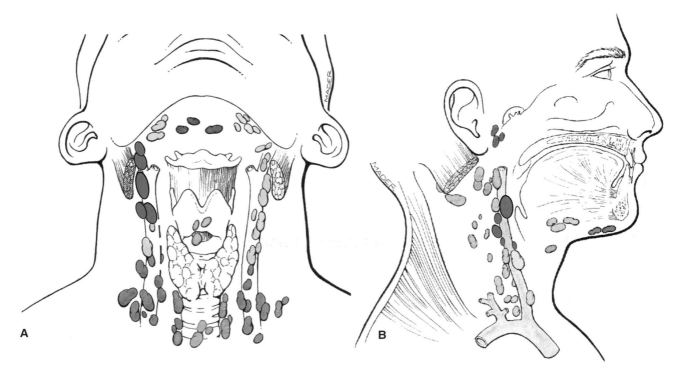

Figure 9.5 **N-oncoanatomy.** The red node highlights the sentinel node, which is the jugulodigastric node. **A.** Coronal. **B.** Sagittal.

endoscopy and are viewed as complimentary. Distinction between the three compartments is essential to staging. Computed tomography (CT) and magnetic resonance imaging (MRI) are often complimentary (see Table 1.5).

Pathologic Staging

The gross specimen should be evaluated for margins. Unresected gross residual tumor must be included and marked with clips. All resected lymph node specimens should describe size, number, and level of involved nodes and whether there is extracapsular spread. Specimens taken after radiation, chemotherapy, or both need

to so noted; specimen shrinkages may occur up to 30% after resection itself. Designations pT and pN should be used after histopathologic evaluation. Perineural invasion deserves special notation.

Oncoimaging Annotations

- After contrast administration, cross-section CT studies of the larynx should be performed, extending from C1 to the thoracic inlet.
- MRI should be performed before and after gadolinium enhancement.
- Extralaryngeal tumor spread can cause cartilage sclerosis, erosion, and lysis, suggestive of cartilaginous cancer invasion on CT.

TABLE 9.2	Cancer Curability by Stages at Diagnosis (1992–1998)			
	5-Year Survival Rate (%)			
Site	All Stages	Local	Regional	Distant
Oral cavity and pharynx	56	95	81	31
Larynx	64	82	51	38
Thyroid	96	99	95	44

From Ries LAG, Eisner MP, Kosary CL, et al, eds. *SEER Cancer Statistics Review, 1975–2001* [Tables XII-4 and XIX-4]. Bethesda, MD: National Cancer Institute. Available at: http://seer.cancer.gov/csr/1975_2001/.

- A positive diagnosis of cartilage invasion on MRI should be made with caution because the positive predictive value of the altered signal behavior as a sign of invasion is low.

- Pretreatment CT imaging is predictive of local tumor control in patients treated with definitive radiation therapy. Tumor diameters of less than 2 cm have a high likelihood of local control, whereas tumor diameters greater than 2 cm have only a 50% chance of control.

- Both positron emission tomography with fluorine-18-labeled-deoxy-glucose and thallium-201 single photon emission computed tomography have useful potential in differentiating post-treatment radiation changes from recurrent tumor.

Cancer Statistics and Survival

Generally, cancers of the oral cavity, pharynx, and upper digestive passage accounts for 28,000 new cases (see Table 1.6). In addition, cancer of the larynx affects another 10,000 patients and thyroid cancers 23,600. Approximately 25% of head and neck cancer patients die annually, often due to other causes (Table 9.2). Long-term survival in thyroid cancers is exceptional, with only 1,500 deaths (5%). The improvement in oral cavity and pharyngeal tumors from 1950 to 2000 was modest at 14% and matches larynx at 15% (see Fig. 1.7). A multi-disciplinary approach is vital and normal tissue conservation and reconstructive techniques have both added greatly to quality of life. Unfortunately, this patient population abuse ethanol and nicotine and it is difficult to change these habits. Persistence of smoking and drinking contributes to their demise often from second malignant tumors in adjacent sites.

Specifically, laryngeal cancers are a more favorable site in head and neck cancers because hoarseness allows for early detection. With early detection, stage I glottic cancers have 95% survival at 5 years and overall stages at 85%. Success in advanced stages in both survival and preservation of voice is due to chemoradiation regimens, which yield high complete response rates.

10

Glottic Larynx

The malignant gradient is a vertical in reference to the horizontal midplane through the true glottis; it is greater above and below the vocal cords.

Perspective and Patterns of Spread

Cancers of the larynx are among the most commonly occurring cancers in the upper respiratory passage and present the challenge of preservation of phonation. The larynx is a critical structure in the respiratory tract and is the major sphincter through which air enters and exits from the lung. It performs the essential function of closure to the airway entrance during deglutition. Once involved the laryngeal cancer can be an isolated nodule, but is often part of a field cancerization process due to habitual smoking. The likelihood of a recurrence or second primary in lung is inevitable if the host is either unwilling or unable to give up tobacco. Persistent hoarseness demands an otologic examination.

The larynx is lined by pseudostratified ciliated columnar epithelium except on the superior surface of the epiglottis and vocal cords, which are covered by stratified squamous, nonkeratinized, epithelium (Fig. 10.1). Most cancers are squamous cell cancers but a variety of malignancies can occur (Table 10.1). Vocal cord cancers tend to be well differentiated and supraglottic; subglottic cancers tend to be more undifferentiated. The malignant gradient is from anterior to posterior, from superior to inferior, and from medial to lateral. Most important is sparing of the vocal cords and voice preservation. A number of randomized studies have confirmed that chemoradiation regimens are able to yield comparable survival with laryngeal preservation versus radical laryngectomy.

Cancers arising in the different subsites of the larynx have patterns of spread that reflect the anatomy of a larynx in its development and function. The malignant gradient is in reference to the horizontal midplane through the true glottis. Cancers above have a better outcome and below have a poorer prognosis for readily apparent reasons relating to the ease of detection of supraglottic compared to subglottic cancers that are obscured

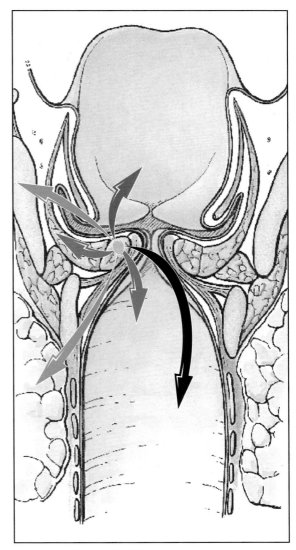

Figure 10.1 **Patterns of spread.** The primary cancer (glottic larynx) invades in various directions which are color-coded vectors (*arrows*) representing stage of progression: Tis, yellow; T1, green; T2, blue; T3, purple; T4a, red; and T4b, black.

DEFINITION OF TNM   T$_{is}$ N$_0$ STAGE GROUPINGS

0

T1
Tumor limited to the vocal cord(s) (may involve anterior or posterior commissure) with normal mobility (see arrows)

N0
No regional lymph node metastasis

Stage I
T1 N0 M0

I

T2
Tumor extends to supraglottis and/or subglottis, or with impaired vocal cord mobility (see arrows)

N0
No regional lymph node metastasis

Stage II
T2 N0 M0

II

T3
Tumor limited to the larynx with vocal cord fixation, and/or invades paraglottic space, and/or minor thyroid cartilage erosion (e.g., inner cortex; no cord mobility)

N1
Metastasis in a single ipsilateral lymph node, ≤3 cm in greatest dimension

Stage III
T3 N0 M0
T1 N1 M0
T2 N1 M0
T3 N1 M0

III

T4a
Tumor invades through the thyroid cartilag and/or invades tissues beyond the larynx (e.g., trachea, soft tissues of neck including deep extrinsic muscles of the tongue, strap muscles, thyroid, or esophagus)

N2
(N2a) Metastasis in a single ipsilateral lymph node, >3 cm but ≤6 cm
(N2b) Metastasis in multiple ipsilateral lymph nodes, none >6 cm
(N2c) Metastasis in bilateral or contralateral lymph nodes, none >6 cm

Stage IVA
T4a N0 M0
T4a N1 M0
T1   N2 M0
T2   N2 M0
T3   N2 M0
T4a N2 M0

IVA

T4b
Tumor invades prevertebral space, encases carotid artery, or invades mediastinal structures

N3
Metastasis in a lymph node >6 cm in greatest dimension

Stage IVB
T4b Any N M0
Any T N3   M0

IVB

Stage IVC
Any T Any N M1

M$_1$

IVC

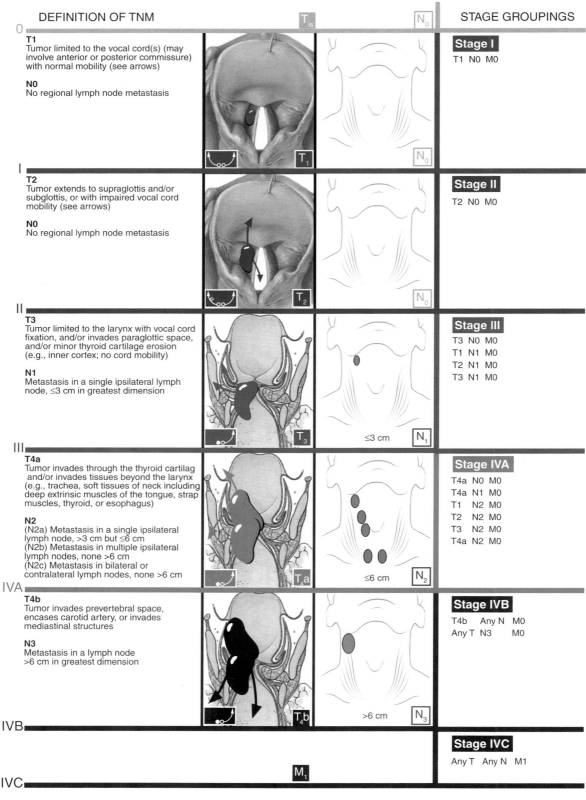

Figure 10.2 TNM stage grouping. Glottic cancers are commonly confined to vocal cords producing hoarseness early which leads to their detection. Vertical presentations of stage groupings, which follow same color code for cancer stage advancement are organized in horizontal lanes: Stage 0, yellow; I, green; II, blue; III, purple; IVA, red; and IVB, black. Definitions of TN on left and stage grouping on right. Note inferior box on T-oncoanatomy provides a key to vocal cord mobility.

TABLE 10.1	Histopathologic Type: Common Cancers of the Glottic Larynx
Squamous Cell Carcinoma Microscopic Variants	
Keratinizing; well differentiated; moderately well differentiated; poorly differentiated	
Nonkeratinizing; anaplastic squamous carcinoma	
Transitional cell carcinoma	
Spindle cell squamous carcinoma	
Adapted from Rubin P. *Clinical Oncology.* 8th ed. New York: Elsevier; 2001:408.	

by the vocal cords. Cancers of the true vocal cord are detected early because they alter voice quality and lead to hoarseness. They tend to arise from the free margin, but frequently cross to the opposite cord via the anterior commissure. The vocal cords are relatively avascular and are poor in lymphatics. Consequently, lymph node involvement and distant metastases are rare.

TNM Staging Criteria

Glottic cancers are the most common laryngeal cancers and are three times more common than others. Glottic cancers are most often confined to the true cords along its anterior free border (Fig. 10.2). However, the cancerous nodule usually is part of a field cancerization and is an alert signal to stop smoking. To halt future cancers from developing elsewhere in the respiratory and upper digestive passage, it is essential to abstain from smoking. Cancers of the true cord tend to be confined to one cord, but one third of the cases involve both cords, most often spreading across the anterior commissure where it may extend along anterior attachment (Broyles ligament) to the thyroid cartilage. Invasion of thyroid cartilage can follow with destruction of its calcified body. Posterior involvement of arytenoid cartilage is uncommon and obscures their normal double-beaded appearance.

Supraglottic cancers can arise from a variety of different locations, and tend to cause few symptoms until advanced. The free surface of the epiglottis, the false cords, and the ventricles can all be involved. Transglottic cancers are usually advanced and extend from the supraglottic area, invade the vocal cords, and impair their function. These tumors spread rapidly because of the rich lymphatic network in this region. Bilateral neck nodes are often encountered. Another favored area of spread is the pre-epiglottic fat space.

Subglottic cancers, in terms of prognosis, are worse than other types. This is probably due to their tendency to invade the trachea, and to reach a more advanced state before detection.

Subglottic cancers are often vocal cord lesions beginning on the inferior surface of the true cords but growing unrecognized. True subglottic cancers are really tracheal cancers and begin 1 cm below the vocal cords. Such cancers are rare and tend to involve the cricoid cartilage early because there is no muscle layer beneath the mucous membrane. Difficulty in breathing rather than hoarseness may be the critical complaint.

The larynx was initially staged with the development of the TNM system and appeared in the joint first edition of American Joint Committee on Cancer/International Union Against Cancer (1978). The basis of progression of laryngeal cancers is related to their spread patterns to subsites (T2) as well as advancement from any one major site: Glottic, supraglottic, subglottic to another, and (T2) if cord mobility is preserved. Loss of cord mobility indicates T3.

Summary of Changes

In the latest edition (2002), a revision of stage 4 into resectable T4a and unresectable T4b invasion is emphasized. If the involvement is limited to the central and anterior neck compartment, it is T4a and resectable; if the prevertebral space and fascia are penetrated by posterior spread, the stage is T4b. Extension from the neck to mediastinal structures also constitutes a very advanced stage T4b.

Orientation of Three-planar Oncoanatomy

The anatomic isocenter of the true glottis is at the C5 level. The anterior surface bullet enters midway below the anterior notch of the thyroid cartilage and its inferior border (Fig. 10.3A) and the lateral bullet enters through the body of the thyroid cartilage (Fig. 10.3B).

T-oncoanatomy

The introduction to three-dimensional planar view of the larynx is best appreciated from the posterior coronal view with the constrictor musculature split.

- *Coronal plane* (Fig. 10.4A): The larynx is divided into three parts: (i) the supraglottis, (ii) the glottis, and (iii) the subglottis; these three parts are known as

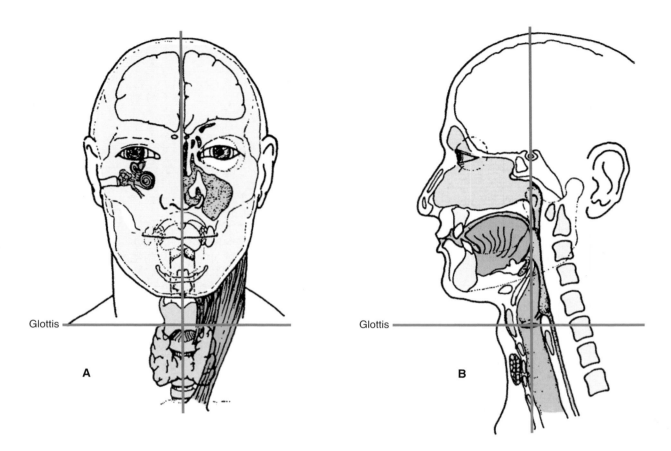

Glottis

A

Glottis

B

Figure 10.3 **Orientation of three-planar T-oncoanatomy.** The anatomic isocenter is at the axial level at C5. **A.** Coronal. **B.** Sagittal.

the vestibule, ventricle (glottis), and infraglottic cavity. The epiglottis is readily visualized at its vestibule. The opening of the larynx, referred to as the *aditus larynges* or the *superior laryngeal aperture*, can be traced from the epiglottis to the arytenoids. The aryepiglottic folds start at the free edge of the epiglottis and terminate at the corniculate and arytenoids cartilages. The false cords and true cords are separated by the ventricle. Each acts as a sphincter that closes off the airway.

- *Sagittal plane* (Fig. 10.4B): The cartilaginous skeleton of the larynx consists of the epiglottis, thyroid, cricoid, arytenoids, coniculate cartilages, and hyoid bone. A set of fine membranes and muscles hold this cartilage together forming a rigid structure, which is not easily destroyed by cancer invasion. The cricothyroid muscle tenses the vocal cords. The intrinsic muscles include the posterior cricoarytenoid, thyroarytenoids, vocalis, thyroepiglottis, and aryepiglottis. The essential function of these muscles is to open and close the glottis during breathing and to regulate cord tension during speaking. The true cords and false cords are separated by a ventricle. The pre-epiglottic fat-filled space can be readily infiltrated from a cancer in the supraglottic region at its

base because the epiglottic cartilage sits as an upside-down paddle. These features are best appreciated in the sagittal view.

- *Transverse view* (Fig. 10.4C): The axial view illustrates the paralaryngeal space between the thyroid and epiglottal cartilage and the position of the larynx to the pharynx. The prevertebral space is separated from the larynx by the hypopharynx and the prevertebral fascia is rarely invaded by true laryngeal malignancies.

N-oncoanatomy

Each segment of the larynx drains to a different sentinel node (Fig. 10.5). The glottis or true vocal cords are not rich in lymphatics and drain to pretracheal or paralaryngeal lymph nodes. The supraglottis is richer in lymphatics and vascularization, with drainage favoring midjugular and jugulodigastric nodes. Subglottic cancers drain to deeper cervical nodes, the jugulo-omohyoid, and even the scalene nodes.

M-oncoanatomy

The venous drainage of the larynx is by way of laryngeal veins into the internal jugular vein brachiocephalic

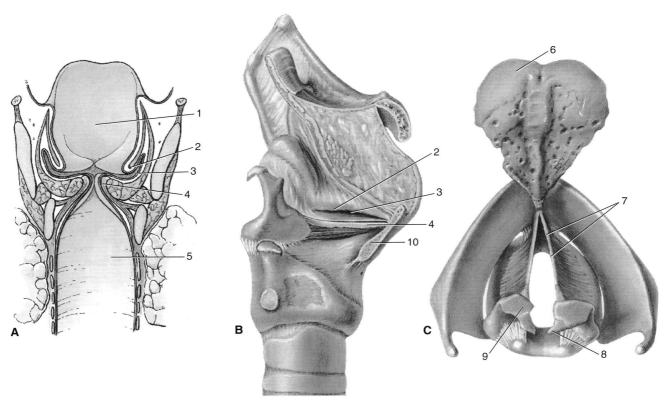

Figure 10.4 **T-oncoanatomy.** The three planar views are crucial to understanding the malignant gradient. **A.** Coronal. **B.** Sagittal. **C.** Transverse. (1) Vestibule. (2) Vestibular fold. (3) Ventricle. (4) Vocal fold. (5) Trachea. (6) Epiglottic cartilage. (7) Vocal ligament. (8) Corniculate cartilage. (9) Arytenoid cartilage. (10) Thyroid cartilage.

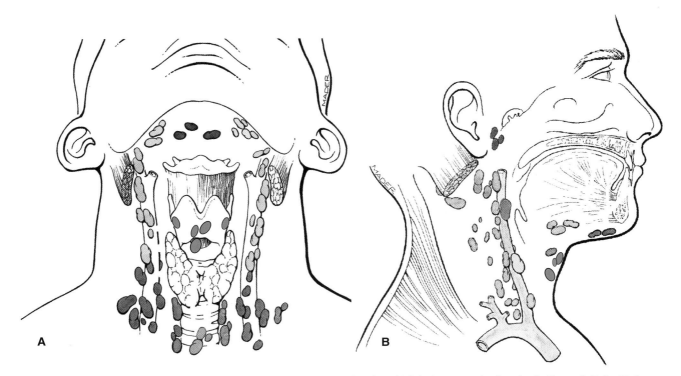

Figure 10.5 **N-oncoanatomy.** The red node highlights the sentinel node, which is the pretracheal node. **A.** Coronal. **B.** Sagittal.

TABLE 10.2	Approximate Determinate 5-Year Survival by Stages at Diagnosis (1992–1998)				
	5-Year Survival According to Stage Grouping (%)				
Site	All Stages	I	II	III	IV
Glottic larynx	85	95	85	60	35

vein and then into the superior vena cava. Metastases are most likely to target the lung (see Fig. 1.6).

Rules of Classification and Staging

Clinical Staging and Imaging

Assessment of the larynx in its three compartments—supraglottis, glottis, and subglottis—is optimally performed with a fiberoptic laryngoscope and often requires general anesthesia, which is advised often after completion of diagnostic imaging studies. Determining vocal cord motion, namely, partial or complete paralysis, is difficult because the normal cord can cross over to meet the involved cord. Imaging studies do not supplant endoscopy and are viewed as complimentary. Distinction between the three compartments is essential to staging. Computed tomography (CT) and magnetic resonance imaging (MRI) are often complimentary (see Table 1.5).

Pathologic Staging

The gross specimen should be evaluated for margins. Unresected gross residual tumor must be included and marked with clips. All resected lymph node specimens should describe size, number, and level of involved nodes and whether there is extracapsular spread. Specimens taken after radiation, chemotherapy, or both need to so noted; specimen shrinkages may occur up to 30% after resection itself. Designations pT and pN should be used after histopathologic evaluation. Perineural invasion deserves special notation.

Oncoimaging Annotations

- After contrast administration, cross-sectional CT studies of the larynx should be performed, extending from C1 to the thoracic inlet.
- MRI should be performed before and after gadolinium enhancement.
- Extralaryngeal tumor spread, sclerosis, erosion, and lysis suggest cartilaginous cancer invasion. The negative predictive value of this combination of findings is high, but the specificity is low.

- A positive diagnosis of cartilage invasion on MRI should be made with caution because the positive predictive value of the altered signal behavior as a sign of invasion is low.
- Pretreatment CT imaging is predictive of local tumor control in patients treated with definitive radiation therapy. Tumor diameters less than 2 cm have a high likelihood of local control, whereas tumors with diameters greater than 2 cm have only a 50% chance of control.
- Both positron emission tomography with fluorine-18-labeled-deoxy-glucose (FDG) and thallium-201 single photon emission computed tomography have useful potential in differentiating post-treatment radiation changes from recurrent tumor.

Cancer Statistics and Survival

Generally, cancers of the oral cavity and pharynx, the upper digestive passage, account for 28,000 new cases (see Table 1.5). In addition, cancer of the larynx affects another 10,000 patients and thyroid cancers 23,600. Approximately 25% of head and neck cancer patients die annually, often due to other causes (Table 10.2). Long-term survival in thyroid cancers is exceptional, with only 1,500 deaths (5%). The improvement in oral cavity and pharyngeal tumors from 1950 to 2000 was modest at 14% and matches larynx at 15% (see Fig. 1.7). A multidisciplinary approach is vital; normal tissue conservation and reconstructive techniques have both added greatly to quality of life. Unfortunately, this patient population abuse ethanol and nicotine, and it is difficult to change these habits. Persistence of smoking and drinking contributes to their demise often from second malignant tumors in adjacent sites.

Specifically, laryngeal cancers are a more favorable site in head and neck cancers because hoarseness allows for early detection. With early detection, stage I glottic cancers have a 95% 5-year survival level; overall stages survive at 85%. Success in advanced stages in both survival and preservation of voice is due to chemoradiation regimens, which yield high complete response rates. Cessation of smoking is essential to cure and prevention of cancer recurrence.

11

Subglottic Larynx

The malignant gradient is in reference to the horizontal midplane through the true glottis; cancers below have the poorest prognosis.

Perspective and Patterns of Spread

Cancers of the larynx are among the commonly occurring cancers in the upper respiratory passage and present the challenge of preservation of phonation. The larynx is a critical structure in the respiratory tract and is the major sphincter through which air enters and exits from the lung. It performs the essential function of closure to the airway entrance during deglutition. Once involved the laryngeal cancer can be an isolated nodule, but is often part of a field cancerization process due to habitual smoking. The likelihood of a recurrence or second primary in lung is inevitable if the host is either unwilling or unable to give up tobacco. Persistent hoarseness demands an otologic examination.

Subglottic cancers are often vocal cord lesions beginning on the inferior surface of the true cords but growing unrecognized. True subglottic cancers are really tracheal cancers and begin 1 cm below the vocal cords. Such cancers are rare and tend to involve the cricoid cartilage early because there is no muscle layer beneath the mucous membrane. Difficulty in breathing rather than hoarseness is often the critical initial complaint.

The larynx is lined by pseudostratified ciliated columnar epithelium except on the superior surface of the epiglottis and vocal cords, which are covered by stratified squamous, not keratinized, epithelium (Fig. 11.1). Most cancers are squamous cell cancers, but a variety of malignancies can occur (Table 11.1). Vocal cord cancers tend to be well differentiated and supraglottic; subglottic cancers tend to be more undifferentiated. Most important is sparing of the vocal cords and voice preservation. A number of randomized studies have confirmed that chemoradiation regimens are able to yield comparable survival with laryngeal preservation versus radical laryngectomy.

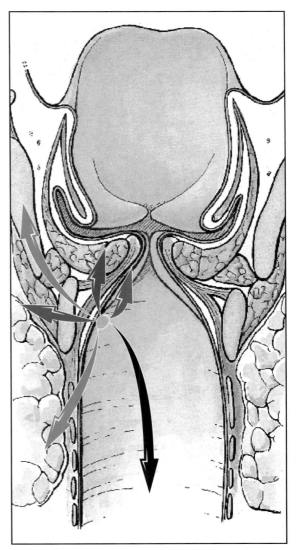

Figure 11.1 **Patterns of spread.** The primary cancer (subglottic larynx) invades in various directions which are color-coded vectors (*arrows*) representing stage of progression: Tis, yellow; T1, green; T2, blue; T3, purple; T4a, red; and T4b, black.

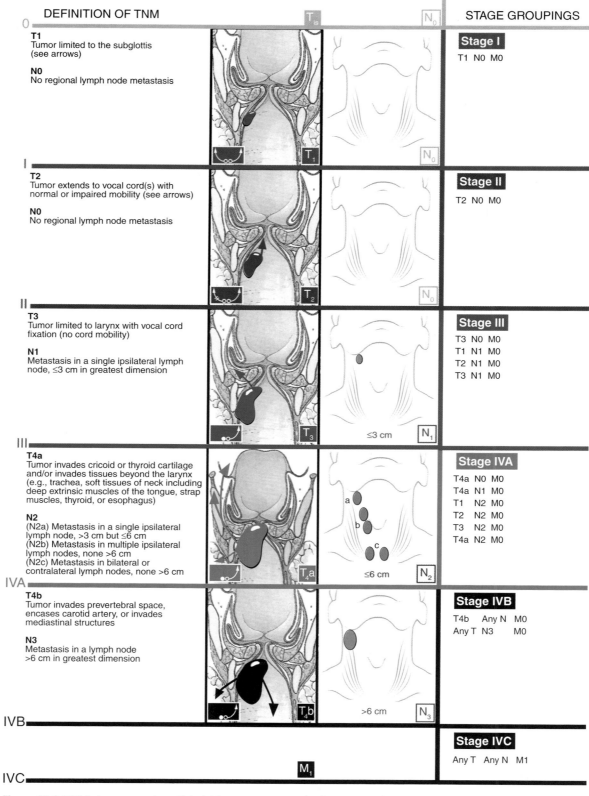

DEFINITION OF TNM

T1
Tumor limited to the subglottis (see arrows)

N0
No regional lymph node metastasis

T2
Tumor extends to vocal cord(s) with normal or impaired mobility (see arrows)

N0
No regional lymph node metastasis

T3
Tumor limited to larynx with vocal cord fixation (no cord mobility)

N1
Metastasis in a single ipsilateral lymph node, ≤3 cm in greatest dimension

T4a
Tumor invades cricoid or thyroid cartilage and/or invades tissues beyond the larynx (e.g., trachea, soft tissues of neck including deep extrinsic muscles of the tongue, strap muscles, thyroid, or esophagus)

N2
(N2a) Metastasis in a single ipsilateral lymph node, >3 cm but ≤6 cm
(N2b) Metastasis in multiple ipsilateral lymph nodes, none >6 cm
(N2c) Metastasis in bilateral or contralateral lymph nodes, none >6 cm

T4b
Tumor invades prevertebral space, encases carotid artery, or invades mediastinal structures

N3
Metastasis in a lymph node >6 cm in greatest dimension

STAGE GROUPINGS

Stage I
T1 N0 M0

Stage II
T2 N0 M0

Stage III
T3 N0 M0
T1 N1 M0
T2 N1 M0
T3 N1 M0

Stage IVA
T4a N0 M0
T4a N1 M0
T1 N2 M0
T2 N2 M0
T3 N2 M0
T4a N2 M0

Stage IVB
T4b Any N M0
Any T N3 M0

Stage IVC
Any T Any N M1

Figure 11.2 TNM stage grouping. Subglottic cancers are tracheal tumors and are often life threatening because of their vital location and present as advanced cancers. Vertical presentations of stage groupings, which follow same color code for cancer stage advancement are organized in horizontal lanes: Stage 0, yellow; I, green; II, blue; III, purple; IVA, red; and IVB, black. Definitions of TN on left and stage grouping on right. Note inferior box on T-oncoanatomy provides a key to vocal cord mobility.

TABLE 11.1	Histopathologic Type: Common Cancers of the Subglottic Larynx
Squamous Cell Carcinoma Microscopic Variants	
Keratinizing; well differentiated; moderately well differentiated; poorly differentiated	
Nonkeratinizing; anaplastic squamous carcinoma	
Transitional cell carcinoma	
Spindle cell squamous carcinoma	
Adapted from Rubin P. *Clinical Oncology.* 8th ed. New York: Elsevier; 2001:408	

TNM Staging Criteria

Cancers arising in the different subsites of the larynx have patterns of spread that reflect the anatomy of a larynx in its development and function (Fig. 11.2). The malignant gradient is in reference to the horizontal midplane through the true glottis. Cancers above have a better outcome and below have a poorer prognosis for readily apparent reasons relating to the ease of detection of supraglottic compared with subglottic cancers that are obscured by the vocal cords. Cancers of the true vocal cord are detected early, because they alter voice quality and lead to hoarseness. They tend to arise from the free margin, but frequently cross to the opposite cord via the anterior commissure. The vocal cords are relatively avascular and are poor in lymphatics. Consequently, lymph node involvement and distant metastases are rare.

Subglottic cancers, in terms of prognosis, are worse than other types. This is probably due to their tendency to invade the trachea, and to reach a more advanced stage before detection.

The larynx was initially staged with the development of the TNM system and appeared in the joint first edition of American Joint Committee on Cancer/International Union Against Cancer (1978). The basis of progression of laryngeal cancers is related to their spread patterns to subsites as well as advancement from any one major site: glottic, supraglottic, and subglottic to another; (T2) if cord mobility is preserved. Loss of cord mobility indicates T3.

Summary of Changes

In the latest edition (2002), a revision of stage 4 into resectable T4a and unresectable T4b invasion is emphasized. If the involvement is limited to the central and anterior neck compartment, it is T4a and resectable; if the prevertebral space and fascia are penetrated by posterior spread, the stage is T4b. Extension from the neck to mediastinal structures also constitutes a very advanced stage T4b.

Orientation of Three-planar Oncoanatomy

The anatomic isocenter of the subglottic larynx is at C6/C7 level and superior to the cricoid cartilage and within its grasp. The anterior bullet enters in the midline at the cricoid cartilage (Fig. 11.3A) and the lateral bullet is at the inferior horn of the thyroid cartilage (Fig. 11.3B).

T-oncoanatomy

The introduction to three-dimensional planar view of the larynx is best appreciated from the posterior coronal view with the constrictor musculature split.

• *Coronal plane* (Fig. 11.4A): The larynx is divided into three parts: (i) the supraglottis, (ii) the glottis, and (iii) the subglottis; these three parts are known as the vestibule, ventricle (glottis), and infraglottic cavity. The epiglottis is readily visualized at its vestibule. The opening of the larynx, referred to as the *aditus larynges* or the *superior laryngeal aperture*, can be traced from the epiglottis to the arytenoids. The aryepiglottic folds start at the free edge of the epiglottis and terminate at the corniculate and arytenoids cartilages. The false cords and true cords are separated by the ventricle. Each acts as a sphincter that closes off the airway.

• *Sagittal plane* (Fig. 11.4B): The cartilaginous skeleton of the larynx consists of the epiglottis, thyroid, cricoid, arytenoids, coniculate cartilages, and hyoid bone. A set of fine membranes and muscles hold this cartilage together forming a rigid structure that is not easily destroyed by cancer invasion. The cricoid muscle tenses the vocal cords. The intrinsic muscles include the cricoarytenoid, thyroarytenoids, vocalis, thyroepiglottis, and aryepiglottis. The essential function of these muscles is to open and close the glottis during breath and to regulate core tension during speaking. The true cords and false cords are separated by a ventricle. The pre-epiglottic fat-filled space can be readily infiltrated from a cancer in the supraglottic region at its base because the epiglottic cartilage

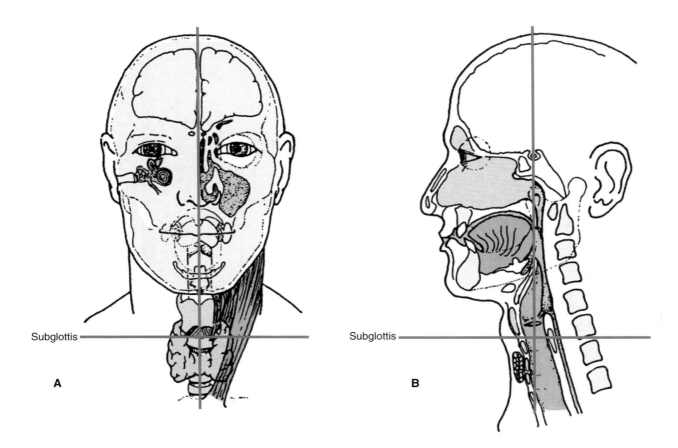

Subglottis ——————————

A

Subglottis ——————————

B

Figure 11.3 **Orientation of three-planar T-oncoanatomy.** The anatomic isocenter is at the axial level at C6. **A.** Coronal. **B.** Sagittal.

sits as an upside-down paddle. These features are best appreciated in the sagittal view.

- *Transverse view* (Fig. 11.4C): The axial view illustrates the paralaryngeal space between the thyroid and epiglottal cartilage and the position of the larynx to the pharynx. The prevertebral space is separated from the larynx by the hypopharynx and the prevertebral fascia is rarely invaded by true laryngeal malignancies.

N-oncoanatomy

Each segment of the larynx drains to a different sentinel node (Fig. 11.5). Subglottic cancers drain to deeper cervical nodes, the jugulo-omohyoid, and even the scalene nodes. The glottis or true vocal cords are not rich in lymphatics and drain to pretracheal or paralaryngeal lymph nodes. The supraglottis is richer in lymphatics and vascularization, with drainage favoring midjugular and jugulodigastric nodes.

M-oncoanatomy

Venous drainage of the larynx is by way of laryngeal veins into the internal jugular vein and then into the

superior vena cava. Metastases are most likely to target the lung (see Fig. 1.6).

Rules of Classification and Staging

Clinical Staging and Imaging

Assessment of the larynx in its three compartments—supraglottis, glottis, and subglottis—is optimally performed with a fiberoptic laryngoscope and often requires general anesthesia, which is advised often after completion of diagnostic imaging studies. Determining vocal cord motion, either partial or complete paralysis, is difficult because the normal cord can cross over to meet the involved cord. Imaging studies do not supplant endoscopy and are viewed as complimentary. Distinction between the three compartments is essential to staging. Computed tomography (CT) and magnetic resonance imaging (MRI) are often complimentary (see Table 1.5).

Pathologic Staging

The gross specimen should be evaluated for margins. Unresected gross residual tumor must be included and marked with clips. All resected lymph node specimens

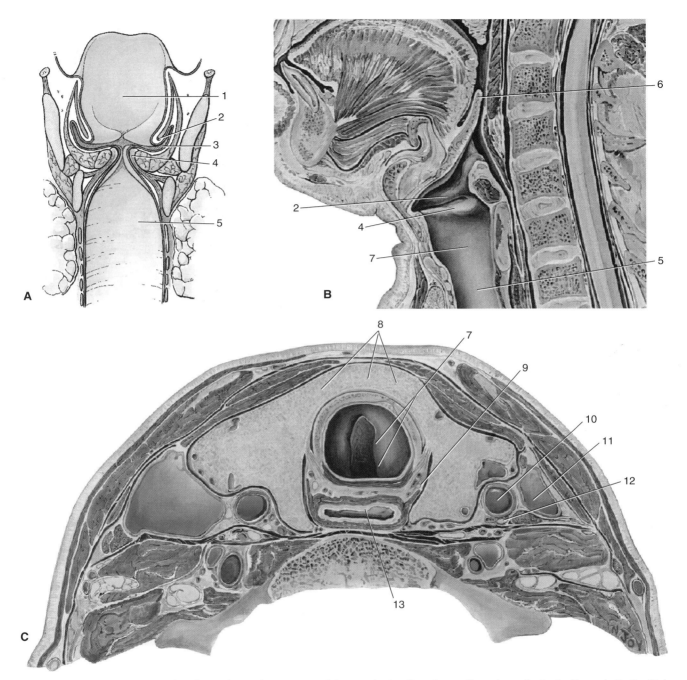

Figure 11.4 **T-oncoanatomy.** The three planar views are crucial to understanding the malignant gradient. **A.** Coronal. **B.** Sagittal. **C.** Transverse. (1) Vestibule. (2) Vestibular fold. (3) Ventricle. (4) Vocal fold. (5) Trachea. (6) Epiglottis. (7) Larynx. (8) Thyroid gland. (9) Recurrent laryngeal nerve. (10) Common carotid artery. (11) Internal jugular vein. (12) Vagus nerve. (13) Esophagus.

should describe size, number, and level of involved nodes and whether there is extracapsular spread. Specimens taken after radiation, chemotherapy, or both need to be noted; specimen shrinkages may occur up to 30% after resection itself. Designations pT and pN should be used after histopathologic evaluation. Perineural invasion deserves special notation.

Oncoimaging Annotations

- After contrast administration, cross-sectional CT studies of the larynx should be performed, extending from C1 to the thoracic inlet.
- MRI should be performed before and after gadolinium enhancement.

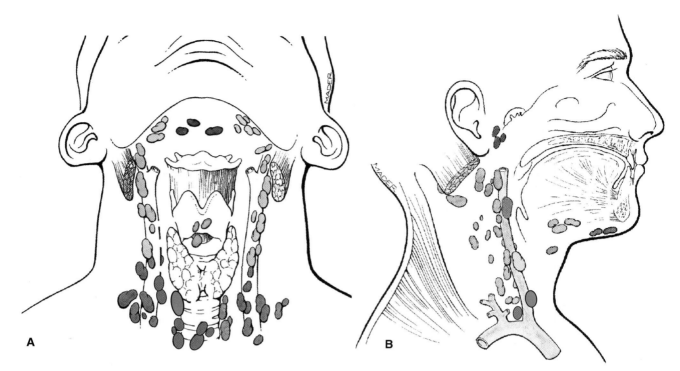

Figure 11.5 **N-oncoanatomy.** The red node highlights the sentinel node, which is the jugulo-omohyoid node. **A.** Coronal. **B.** Sagittal.

- Extralaryngeal tumor spread, sclerosis, erosion, and lysis on CT suggest cartilaginous invasion. The negative predictive value of this combination of findings is high, but specificity is low.

- A positive diagnosis of cartilage invasion on MRI should be made with caution because the positive predictive value of the altered signal behavior as a sign of invasion is low.

- Both positron emission tomography with fluorine-18-labeled-deoxy-glucose and thallium-201 single photon emission computed tomography have useful potential in differentiating post-treatment radiation changes from recurrent tumor.

Cancer Statistics and Survival

Generally, cancers of the oral cavity and pharynx, the upper digestive passage, account for 28,000 new cases (see Table 1.6). In addition, cancer of the larynx affects another 10,000 patients and thyroid cancers 23,600. Ap-

proximately 25% of head and neck cancer patients die annually, often due to other causes. Long-term survival in thyroid cancers is exceptional, with only 1,500 deaths (5%). The improvement in oral cavity and pharyngeal tumors from 1950 to 2000 was modest at 14% and matches larynx at 15%. A multidisciplinary approach is vital and normal tissue conservation and reconstructive techniques have both added greatly to quality of life. Unfortunately, this patient population abuse ethanol and nicotine, and it is difficult to change these habits. Persistence of smoking and drinking contributes to their demise often from second malignant tumors in adjacent sites.

Specifically, laryngeal cancers are a more favorable site in head and neck cancers because hoarseness allows for early detection. With early detection, stage I glottic cancers have a 95% 5-year survival level and overall stages are at 85%. Success in advanced stages in both survival and preservation of voice is due to chemoradiation regimens, which yield high complete response rates. Unfortunately, subglottic cancers are really tracheal cancers and are inevitably advanced lethal cancers when detected.

Histogenesis rather than anatomic extent determines the malignant gradient in thyroid cancer staging because it determines behavior clinically and pathologically.

Perspective and Patterns of Spread

The thyroid nodule is a common occurrence in clinical medicine and most often nodular glands are benign and functioning. The concern as to the possibility of a malignancy is heightened with a history of irradiation as an infant for an "enlarged thymus" or for acne as a teenager. The thyroid scinitiscan of concern is nonfunctioning (cold) compared with a hyperfunctioning (hot) nodule in thyrotoxic patients. Thyroid cancer is two to four times more common among women than men. Median age is 45 to 50 years with a wide range of young to older patients afflicted annually in the United States. There are 14,000 new cases and 1,100 deaths every year. The disparity between incidence and deaths represents their "benign" course as well as improvements in detection, diagnosis, and treatment.

The histopathology as well as the surrounding anatomy determines the spread patterns. There are five distinct different cancers, each with different management features (Table 12.1). The vectors of the more common differentiated variety tend to be local regional, although hematogenous and lymphatic dissemination occur (Fig. 12.1).

TNM Staging Criteria

Histogenesis is the major factor in thyroid cancer staging because it determines behavior clinically and pathologically (Fig. 12.2). Thyroid adenomas are by far the most common tumors of this endocrine gland. They are, for the most part, low-grade carcinomas, which invade into the gland substance and are considered multicentric in origin, although intraglandular spread may seem to be similar. Nodules of the thyroid are much more common than parathyroid adenomas and malignant degeneration similarly is a much more likely event in the thyroid. Depending on the type of thyroid malignancy,

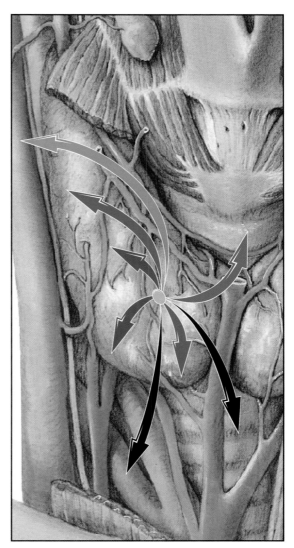

Figure 12.1 **Patterns of spread.** Patterns of spread. The primary cancer (thyroid) invades in various directions which are color-coded vectors (*arrows*) representing stage of progression: T_0, yellow; T_1, green; T_2, blue; T_3, purple; T_{4a}, red; and T_{4b}, black.

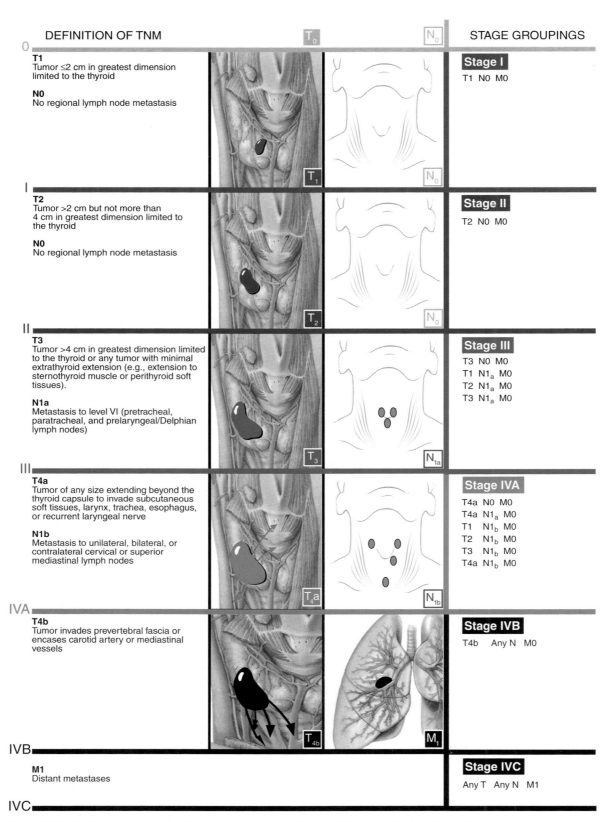

DEFINITION OF TNM

T1
Tumor ≤2 cm in greatest dimension
limited to the thyroid

N0
No regional lymph node metastasis

T2
Tumor >2 cm but not more than
4 cm in greatest dimension limited to
the thyroid

N0
No regional lymph node metastasis

T3
Tumor >4 cm in greatest dimension limited
to the thyroid or any tumor with minimal
extrathyroid extension (e.g., extension to
sternothyroid muscle or perithyroid soft
tissues).

N1a
Metastasis to level VI (pretracheal,
paratracheal, and prelaryngeal/Delphian
lymph nodes)

T4a
Tumor of any size extending beyond the
thyroid capsule to invade subcutaneous
soft tissues, larynx, trachea, esophagus,
or recurrent laryngeal nerve

N1b
Metastasis to unilateral, bilateral, or
contralateral cervical or superior
mediastinal lymph nodes

T4b
Tumor invades prevertebral fascia or
encases carotid artery or mediastinal
vessels

M1
Distant metastases

STAGE GROUPINGS

Stage I
T1 N0 M0

Stage II
T2 N0 M0

Stage III
T3 N0 M0
T1 N1$_a$ M0
T2 N1$_a$ M0
T3 N1$_a$ M0

Stage IVA
T4a N0 M0
T4a N1$_a$ M0
T1   N1$_b$ M0
T2   N1$_b$ M0
T3   N1$_b$ M0
T4a N1$_b$ M0

Stage IVB
T4b   Any N M0

Stage IVC
Any T Any N M1

Figure 12.2 TNM stage grouping. Thyroid cancers are highly varied histologically and their cellular phenotype determines their biologic behavior which ranges from a benign course to highly malignant. Vertical presentations of stage groupings, which follow same color code for cancer stage advancement are organized in horizontal lanes: Stage 0, yellow; I, green; II, blue; III, purple; IVA, red; and IVB, and IVC, black. Definitions of TN on left and stage grouping on right.

TABLE 12.1	Histopathologic Type: Common Cancers of the Thyroid

There are four major histopathologic types:

Papillary carcinoma (including follicular variant of the papillary carcinoma)

Follicular carcinoma (including Hurthle cell carcinoma)

Medullary carcinoma

Undifferentiated (anaplastic) carcinoma

American Joint Committee on Cancer (AJCC). *AJCC Cancer Staging Manual.* 6th ed. New York: Springer; 2002:79.

different spread patterns occur. Common types can be divided into the follicular adenocarcinoma, papillary adenocarcinoma, medullary, and anaplastic tumors, which are either small or large cell carcinomas.

Follicular carcinoma tends to be nodular and encapsulated and is more likely to displace than invade into the gland substance and its surrounding structures. Its major spread pattern is via the venous system into the systemic circulation, leading to lung and bone metastases.

Papillary adenocarcinomas are the most common tumor of the thyroid and tend to be more invasive locally, breaking through and invading through the thyroid capsule into surrounding tissues. They rarely tend to be locally recurrent after their resection, indicating only low-grade local aggressiveness. Distant hematogenous spread is uncommon; these cancers tend to invade into regional lymph nodes, which can be involved bilaterally. Occasionally, the oncologic presentations can be as metastatic cervical lymph nodes of unknown origin. Neck node dissections can be effective treatments rather than radical neck node resections.

Medullary thyroid cancers account for 10% of all thyroid cancers, can be familial, and are transmitted as an autosomal-dominant trait with high penetrance. Multiple endocrine tumors can be present as pheochromocytomas, parathyroid adenomas, or ganglioneuromatosis. These medullary thyroid cancers tend to localize between the upper third and lower two thirds of the lobe and appear on cut section as a red hard lesion consisting of C-cells, physiologically producing calcitonin. They can be locally invasive, spreading into regional nodes, or form distant metastases in liver, lung, and bones. Fortunately, these lesions tend to be slow growing.

Anaplastic small and large cell carcinomas can be very rapidly growing tumors, very invasive, and aggressive locally, leading to tracheal and/or esophageal invasion and compression. If they extend into the superior mediastinum, they can lead to compression of the superior vena cava. The recurrent laryngeal nerves are very intimately involved posterior to the thyroid gland and can be invaded; these tumors aggressively infiltrate through the capsule of the thyroid gland.

All anaplastic cancers are considered as T4. Their staging has been modified into T4a and T4b as to resectability. The size of the tumor as in other head and neck sites does not apply; and T3. T4a is a cancer nodule with anterior extrathyroid extension involving the sternohyoid muscle surrounding soft tissues larynx, trachea, esophagus, recurrent laryngeal nerve. T4b is for posterior extension and invasion into the prevertebral space.

In summary, the major spread patterns are intraglandular spread; T4a, extraglandular spread into the sternocleidomastoid muscle and skin; into surrounding structures such as the trachea and esophagus; and into the recurrent laryngeal nerves, particularly on the right side. T4b is spread posteriorly into the prevertebral muscle and or inferiorly deep into the mediastinum, carotid artery.

Summary of Changes

- *Tumor staging (T) has been revised and the categories redefined.*
- *T4 is now divided into T4a and T4b.*
- *Nodal staging (N) has been revised.*
- *All anaplastic carcinomas are considered T4. The T4 category for anaplastic carcinomas is divided into T4a (intrathyroidal anaplastic carcinoma—surgically resectable) and T4b (extrathyroidal anaplastic carcinoma—surgically unresectable).*
- *For papillary and follicular carcinomas, the stage grouping for patients older than 45 has been revised. Stage III includes tumors with minimal extrathyroid extension. Stage IVA includes tumors of any size extending beyond the thyroid capsule to invade subcutaneous soft tissues, larynx, trachea, esophagus OR recurrent laryngeal nerve. Stage IVB includes tumors that invade prevertebral fascia, carotid artery, or mediastinal vessels. Stage IVC includes advanced tumors with distant metastasis.*

Orientation of Three-planar Oncoanatomy

The anatomic isocenter for thyroid gland is at C7 level and inferior to the cricoid cartilage, readily palpable on swallowing when the gland moves vertically. The

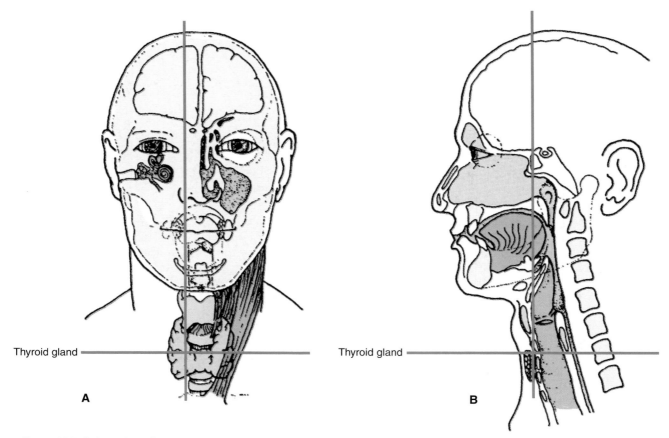

Figure 12.3 **Orientation of three-planar T-oncoanatomy.** The anatomic isocenter is at the axial level at C7. **A.** Coronal. **B.** Sagittal.

anterior bullet enters below the cricoid cartilage (Fig. 12.3A) and the lateral bullet through the anterior surface of the trachea (Fig. 12.3B).

T-oncoanatomy

The thyroid gland is a bilobed structure, symmetrical in size and connected by an isthmus. It is approximately 2 to 3 cm long and wide, and is shaped like a horseshoe.

- *Coronal plane* (Fig. 12.4A): From the anterior view, the gland is in close proximity to the cervical portion of the trachea, below the thyroid cartilage. It is located deep to the strap muscles of the neck, which include the sternocleidomastoid, sternohyoid, and sternothyroid muscles.
- *Sagittal plane* (Fig. 12.4B): Deep to the thyroid gland are the jugular vein and the carotid artery. The recurrent laryngeal nerve lies posterior to the thyroid gland, particularly on the left side where it courses along the gland's entire length into the thorax; the right recurrent laryngeal is more lateral in its location as it hooks around the subclavian artery.
- *Transverse plane* (Fig. 12.4C): Deep to the left lobe of the thyroid is also the thoracic duct, which rises into

the neck and extends anteriorly, inserting into the junction of the jugular and subclavian vein.

N-oncoanatomy

The nodal drainage of the thyroid is into the anterior and deep cervical lymph nodes (Fig. 12.5). There is a small Delphic node, which sits in the midline at the superior margin of the isthmus.

M-oncoanatomy

The thyroid gland is supplied by branches from the external carotid artery, superior thyroid and subclavian artery with the inferior thyroid artery, which arises directly from the carotid artery. The venous pattern follows the arterial blood supply and drains into the internal jugular vein via superior, middle and inferior veins (see Fig. 1.6).

Rules of Classification and Staging

Clinical Staging and Imaging

Assessment of thyroid tumor depends on inspection and palpation of the thyroid gland and regional neck nodes. Indirect laryngoscopy is essential to determine if vocal cord paresis or paralysis is present because of the

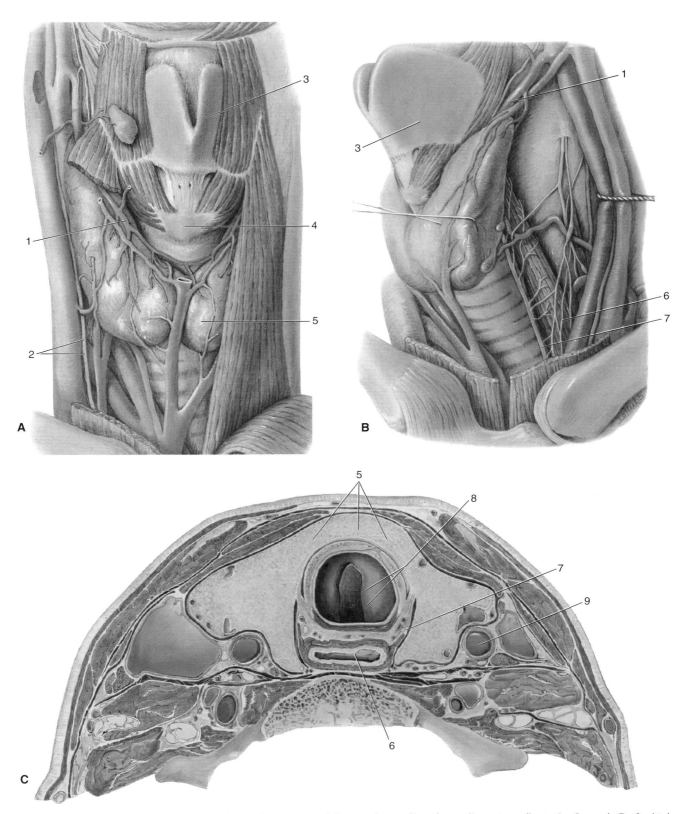

Figure 12.4 **T-oncoanatomy.** The three planar views are crucial to understanding the malignant gradient. **A.** Coronal. **B.** Sagittal. **C.** Transverse. (1) Superior thyroid artery. (2) Vagus nerve. (3) Thyroid cartilage. (4) Cricoid cartilage. (5) Thyroid gland. (6) Esophagus. (7) Recurrent laryngeal nerve. (8) Larynx. (9) Common carotid artery.

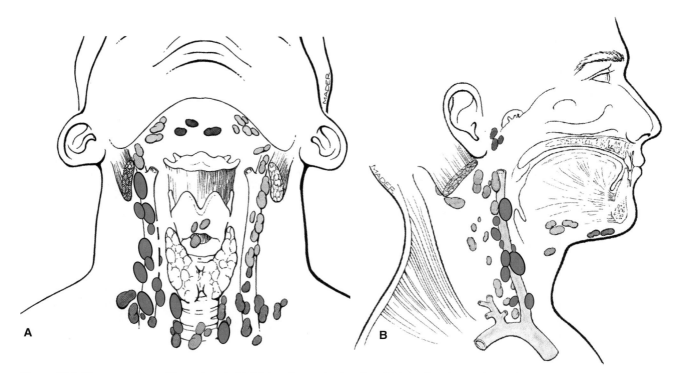

Figure 12.5 N-oncoanatomy. The red node highlights the sentinel node, which is after the jugulo-omohyoid node (J.O.) but all deep cervical jugular nodes are at risk on ipsilateral side. **A.** Coronal. **B.** Sagittal.

proximity of recurrent laryngeal nerves. A large variety of imaging procedures are available, particularly the I^{131} scintiscan and uptake, which requires no iodine contrast be used before this test is done. Technetium 99M protechnetate is currently the most widely used thyroid imaging agent. Ultrasound is the most sensitive technique for detecting focal pathology and is used for screening persons at risk. Radionuclide SPECT utilizing a variety of agents are recommended in Table 1.5.

Pathologic Staging

The gross specimen should be evaluated for margins. Unresected gross residual tumor must be included and marked with clips. All resected lymph node specimens should describe size, number, and level of involved nodes and whether there is extracapsular spread. Specimens taken after radiation and/or chemotherapy need to so noted; specimen shrinkages may occur up to 30% after resection itself. Designations pT and pN should be used after histopathologic evaluation. Perineural invasion deserves special notation.

Oncoimaging Annotations

- Microcalcifications are almost exclusively found in malignancies, mainly papillary and medullary carcinomas.

- Ultrasound is the most sensitive technique for detecting focal pathology and plays an important role in screening those at risk of developing thyroid malignancy.

TABLE 12.2	Cancer Curability by Stages at Diagnosis (1992–1998)			
	5-Year Survival Rate (%)			
Site	All Stages	Local	Regional	Distant
Oral cavity and pharynx	56	**95**	81	31
Larynx	64	**82**	51	38
Thyroid	96	**99**	95	44

From Ries LAG, Eisner MP, Kosary CL, Hankey BF, Miller BA, Clegg L, Mariotto A, Feuer EJ, Edwards BK, eds. *SEER Cancer Statistics Review, 1975–2001*. National Cancer Institute. Bethesda, MD. Available at: http://seer.cancer.gov/csr/1975_2001/, 2004. Tables XII-4, XIX-4, and XXV-4.

- Ultrasound-guided fine-needle aspiration remains the most accurate means of distinguishing between benign and malignant lesions.
- Cystic papillary carcinoma are anechoic, with solid nodules protruding into the cyst and calcification in intracystic nodules.
- Tc-99m pertechnetate is the most widely used thyroid imaging agent; a solitary cold nodule is associated with malignancy in 10% to 20% of cases.
- Tc(99m) DMSA and In-111 pentreotide are the imaging agents of choice for medullary carcinoma.
- Computed tomography or magnetic resonance imaging of the thyroid demonstrating surrounding structures (strap muscles) and encasement of the great vessels and recurrent laryngeal nerve is pathognomonic for cancer.
- Enlarged cervical nodes, especially ipsilaterally, are common findings. Size per se is nonspecific, but the presence of microcalcifacation or complete cystic degeneration are characteristic of cancer.
- Total body I^{131} scan is utilized in searching for functioning follicular and/or papillary metastatic pulmonary and osseous foci post total thyroidectomy.

Cancer Statistics and Survival

Generally, cancers of the oral cavity, pharynx, and upper digestive passage account for 28,000 new cases (see Table 1.6). In addition, cancer of the larynx affects another 10,000 patients and thyroid cancers 23,600. Approximately 25% of head and neck cancer patients die annually, often due to other causes (Table 12.2). Long-term survival in thyroid cancers is exceptional, with only 1,500 deaths (5%). The improvement in oral cavity and pharyngeal tumors from 1950 to 2000 was modest at 14% and matches larynx at 15%. The multidisciplinary approach is vital and normal tissue conservation and reconstructive techniques have both added greatly to quality of life. Unfortunately, this patient population abuse ethanol and nicotine and it is difficult to change these habits. Persistence of smoking and drinking contributes to their demise, often from second malignant tumors in adjacent sites.

Specifically, the success in treating thyroid cancer is reflected in the large population of patients who are long-term survivors. The dominant papillary and follicular carcinomas yield 80% to 95% 10-year survival. Anaplastic cancers both small and large cell varieties are highly lethal.

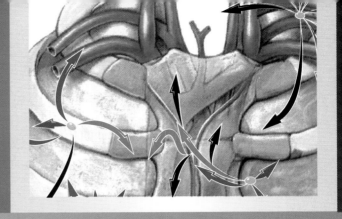

SECTION 2

THORAX PRIMARY SITES

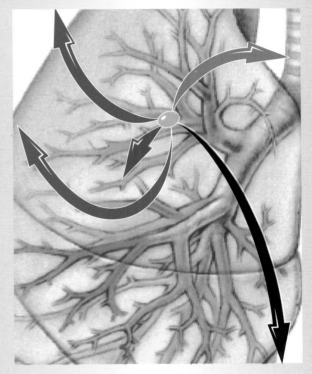

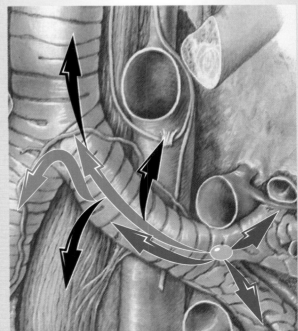

13

Introduction and Orientation

The TNM lung cancer staging system reflects the oncoanatomy of the bronchial tree and its numerous divisions into pulmonary segments and functioning respiratory units, with variations in lining epithelial cell phenotypes.

The thorax is associated with two major malignancies: pulmonary and breast cancers. To paraphrase Dickens as to the survival outcomes of these two highly prevalent cancers: one is the worst of our time and the other among the best of our time. Both organs consist of an elaborate branching ductile systems ending in a vaster fine network of functioning acini. In the lung, its extensive bronchial labyrinth terminates in a huge alveolar micromesh for aeration. In the breast, its more pliable, but fine ductwork terminate in a myriad of compound tubuloalveolar acini that, under the stimulus of pregnancy and elevated levels of estrogens and progesterones, can expand rapidly for lactation.

Lung cancer, one of the most malignant cancers, generally strikes active men and women in the prime of their lives, and is associated consistently with a 20- to 30-year history of smoking. Even the earliest signs, unfortunately, are indicative of advanced spread. A patient who presents with unresolved and recurrent pneumonia or persistent cough leading to mild or severe chest pain often has unresectable disease. Cancers of the lung are highly invasive, rapidly metastasizing tumors. *Lung cancer* is used in reference to many different histopathologic types (Table 13.1), which can masquerade in the form of a large number of benign pulmonary conditions. A collage of patterns of cancer spread presents the basis for the large diversification on clinical presentations (Fig. 13.1).

Cancers of the bronchi and lung are highly lethal tumors. More than 90% of lung cancer patients do not survive this disease, and more than 50% have distant metastases at the time of diagnosis. In women, the death rate associated with lung cancer began to exceed that of breast cancer by 1987. Two million people in the United States died from lung cancer by 2000 before better diagnostic and therapeutic methods were developed. Breast cancer strikes one out of every seven women in the United States, and accounts for more than 25% of all cancers in women. With advances in diagnosis and treatment, survival rates have improved by 25% over the past five decades ranging as high as 97% 5-year survival for early stage node-negative disease.

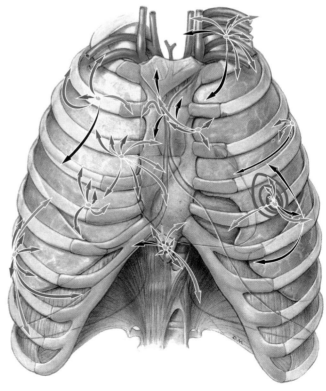

Figure 13.1 **Cancer spread patterns.** Lung cancer can arise in many different sites in the bronchial tree and therefore presenting symptoms and signs are highly variable depending on its anatomic location. The cancer crabs are color-coded for T stage: Tis, yellow; T1, green; T2, blue; T3, purple; T4, red; and metastatic, black.

DEFINITION OF TNM

T1
Tumor ≤3 cm, surrounded by lung or visceral pleura, without bronchoscopic evidence of invasion more proximal than the lobar bronchus

T2
Tumor with any of the following features of size or extent: >3 cm; involves main bronchus, ≥2 cm distal to the carina; invades the visceral pleura; associated with the atelectasis or obstructive pneumonitis that extends to the hilar region but does not involve the entire lung

N0
No regional lymph node metastasis

T1
Tumor ≤3 cm, surrounded by lung or visceral pleura, without bronchoscopic evidence of invasion more proximal than the lobar bronchus

T2
Tumor with any of the following features of size or extent: >3 cm; involves main bronchus, ≥2 cm distal to the carina; invades the visceral pleura; associated with the atelectasis or obstructive pneumonitis that extends to the hilar region but does not involve the entire lung

N1
Metastasis to ipsilateral peribronchial and/or ipsilateral hilar lymph nodes, and intrapulmonary nodes including involvement by direct extension of the primary tumor

T3
Tumor of any size that directly invades any of the following: chest wall (including superior sulcus tumors), diaphragm, mediastinal pleura, parietal pericardium; or tumor in the main bronchus <2 cm distal to the carina, but without involvement of the carina; or associated atelectasis or obstructive pneumonitis of the entire lung

N2
Metastasis to ipsilateral mediastinal, and/or subcarinal lymph node(s)

T4
Tumor of any size that invades any of the following: mediastinum, heart, great vessels, trachea, esophagus, vertebral body, carina; or separate tumor nodules in the same lobe; or tumor with malignant pleural effusion

N3
Metastasis to contralateral mediastinal, contralateral hilar, ipsilateral or contralateral scalene, or supraclavicular lymph node(s)

Nm
Juxtaregional, cervical nodes

M1
Distant metastases

STAGE GROUPINGS

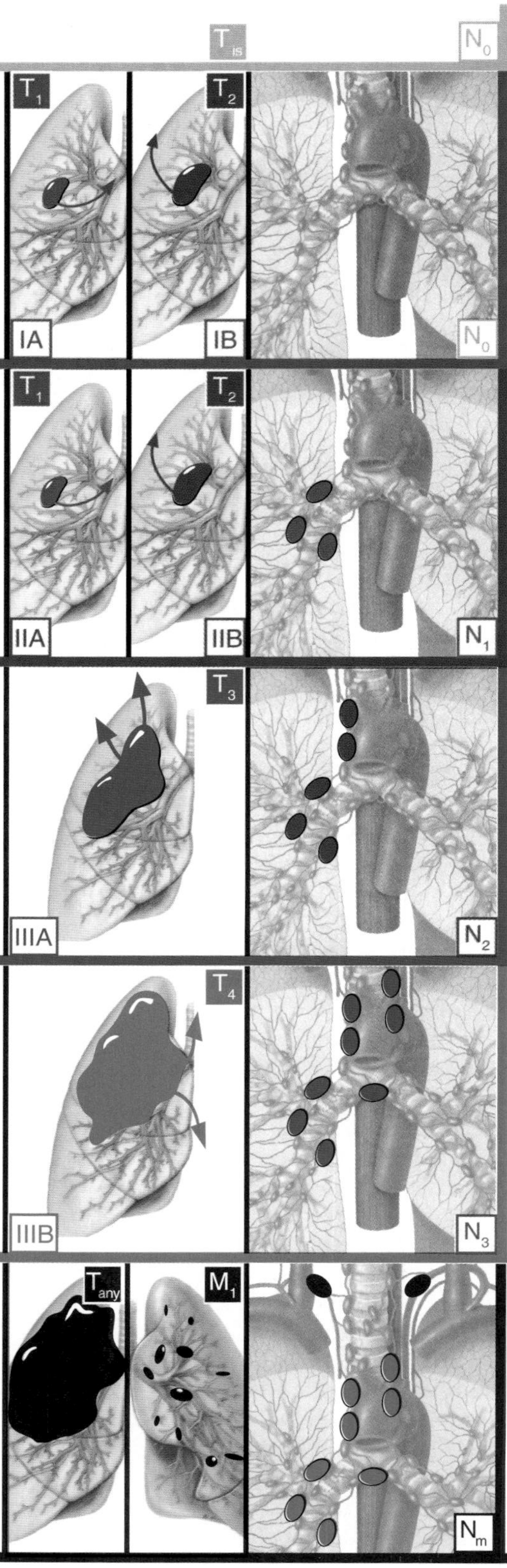

Stage IA
T1 N0 M0

Stage IB
T2 N0 M0

Stage IIA
T1 N1 M0

Stage IIB
T2 N1 M0
T3 N0 M0

Stage IIIA
T1 N2 M0
T2 N2 M0
T3 N1 M0
T3 N2 M0

Stage IIIB
Any T N3 M0
T4 Any N M0

Stage IV
Any T Any N M1

Figure 13.2 TNM staging diagram. The vertical arrangement with color bars encompassing TN combinations shows progression: Stage 0, yellow, Stage I green, Stage II blue, Stage IIIA purple, Stage IIIB Red, Stage IV black. Definitions of T are on left and Stage Groupings Right Read Stage/Color Code Bar on left which encompasses T and N categories which are diagramed and color coded numerically as shown in figure 1. Stage groupings are in right side clustered.

TABLE 13.1	Histopathologic Type
Main Pathologic Cell Type Variant	

Adenocarcinoma
  Acinar
  Papillary
	SCC
	  Combined SCC Squamous cell carcinoma
	  Papillary
	  Clear cell
	  Small cell
	  Basaloid

Bronchoalveolar carcinoma
  Nonmucinous
  Mucinous
  Mixed mucinous and non-mucinous or indeterminate
  Solid adenocarcinoma with mucin formation
	Large cell carcinoma
	  Large cell neuroendocrine carcinoma
	  Combined large cell neuroendocrine carcinoma
	  Basaloid carcinoma
	  Lymphepithelioma-like carcinoma
	  Clear cell carcinoma
	  Large cell carcinoma with rhabdoid phenotype

Adenocarcinoma with mixed subtypes
  Well differentiated fetal adenocarcinoma
  Mucinous ("colloid" adenocarcinoma)
  Mucinous cystadenocarcinoma
  Signet ring adenocarcinoma
  Clear cell adenocarcinoma	

SQCC, squamous cell cancer.

If one views normal lung and lung cancers as derived from a pluripotential stem cell, then it is possible to understand its capability of expressing different features of the complex pulmonary anatomy as well as a variety of malignant phenotypes. The highly varied characteristics of each lung cancer's biologic behavior reflect their normal cell histiogenic counter part. These cells include pseudostratified epithelial reserve cells, type II pneumocytes, ciliated goblet columnar cells, and neuroendocrine cells, each giving rise to a specific type of cancer. Utilizing this construct, the microscopic and macroscopic behavior of the various lung cancers and their spread patterns provides a logical basis for understanding the various staging notations and clarifications that have gradually evolved over time while maintaining a consistently defined set of criteria for its staging. The current classification and staging was agreed to by the American Joint Committee on Cancer (AJCC)/International Union Against Cancer (UICC) in the third edition (1978); however, in subsequent editions annotations have been added to provide detailed explanations as modifications of the basic staging system, again recognizing that lung cancer is more than one disease.

Lung cancer spreads in different patterns depending on its inherent biopathology and anatomic location in the bronchial tree. Briefly, centrally located bronchial tumors tend to be squamous cell cancers (SQCC), whereas tumors arising in peripheral bronchioles and alveoli more often are adenocarcinomas. Bronchioalveolar cancers appear in a peripheral scar or as a patchy, diffuse pneumonitis and can be bilateral in distribution. Adenocarcinomas tend

to arise in the segmental bronchi and are associated with lobar pneumonitis and atelectasis. SQCCs are true bronchogenic cancers arising in the major bronchi. Small cell anaplastic cancers tend to be central masses, whereas large cell anaplastic carcinomas are more peripheral and extensively infiltrating. No structure in the thorax or mediastinum is spared. Compression of mediastinal structures is associated invariably with advanced lymph node involvement, which can lead either to esophageal compression and difficulty in swallowing, venous compression, and congestion associated with collateral circulation, or tracheal compression. Signs of metastatic disease involving such remote sites as the liver, brain, or bone are seen before any knowledge of a primary lung lesion.

TNM Staging Criteria

Lung cancer classification and staging has been stable since the first AJCC edition 1977 (Fig. 13.2). A major change in T categories occurred in the third edition (1988), when T3 resectable advanced disease was distinguished from T4 unresectable advanced disease. Also, N2 mediastinal nodes was divided into N2 ipsilateral and N3 contralateral nodes. Specific clarifications as to special presentations and histopathologic types were added in subsequent editions. In the third edition (1988), the AJCC introduced an elaborate numbering system for intrapulmonary and mediastinal nodes. The nodal status determines the stage grouping rather than the primary

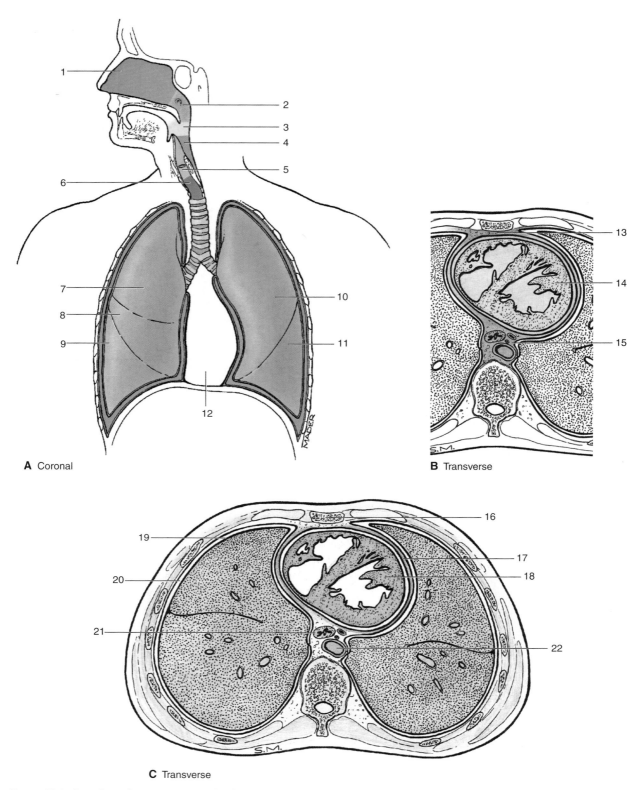

A Coronal

B Transverse

C Transverse

Figure 13.3 **Overview of oncoanatomy.** The three sectors of thorax are shown in three views. **A.** Coronal. **B.** Transverse. **C.** Axial. These sectors are: Lungs and bronchi (purple), mediastinum (green) including the heart (blue), and the breast and chest wall (orange). **A.** (1) Nasal cavity. (2) Nasopharynx. (3) Oropharynx. (4) Laryngopharynx (hypopharynx). (5) Larynx. (6) Trachea. (7) Superior lobe, right lung. (8) Middle lobe, right lung. (9) Inferior lobe, right lung. (10) Superior lobe, right lung. (11) Inferior lobe, right lung. (12) Mediastinum. **B.** (13) Anterior mediastinum. (14) Middle mediastinum (heart). (15) Posterior mediastinum. **C.** (16) Sternum. (17) Pericardium. (18) Heart. (19) Visceral pleura. (20) Parietal pleura. (21) Esophagus. (22) Aorta. (*continued*)

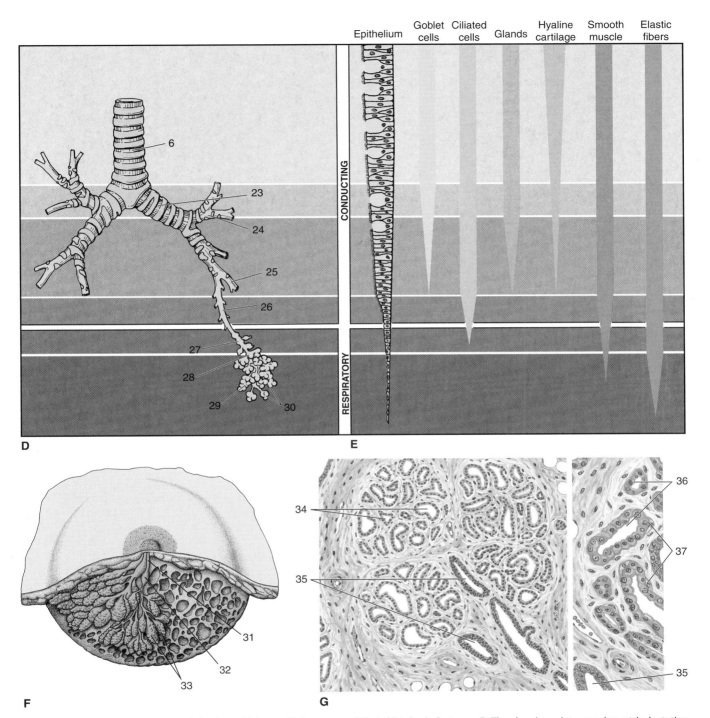

Figure 13.3 (*Continued*) **D.** Divisions of the bronchial tree. **E.** Summary of their histologic features. **F.** The drawing pictures a breast in lactation to emphasize the morphology. **G.** The terminal portion of the tubuloalveolar glands shows several lobules with numerous branching ducts lined by epithelial cells. The epithelial cells of the ducts (ductal carcinoma) exceed the epithelial cells of the lobules (lobular carcinoma) in undergoing carcinogenesis. With lactation, there is a marked proliferation of ducts, giving rise to secretory acini. The duct lining epithelia are secretory, making them difficult to distinguish from epithelium of acini. **D.** (6) Trachea. (23) Main bronchus. (24) Lobar bronchus. (25) Segmental bronchus. (26) Terminal bronchiole. (27) Respiratory bronchiole. (28) Alveolar duct. (29) Alveolar sac. (30) Alveoli. **E** and **F.** (31) Lactiferous duct. (32) Lactiferous sinus. (33) Lobules of tubuloalveolar glands. (34) Alveoli. (35) Interlobular excretory ducts. (36) Alveolus. (37) Myoepithelial cell.

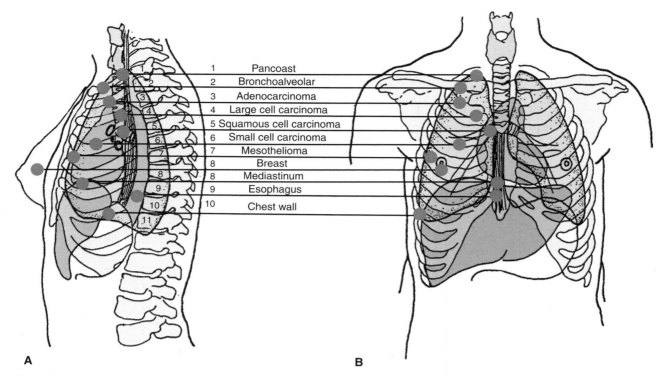

1	Pancoast
2	Bronchoalveolar
3	Adenocarcinoma
4	Large cell carcinoma
5	Squamous cell carcinoma
6	Small cell carcinoma
7	Mesothelioma
8	Breast
8	Mediastinum
9	Esophagus
10	Chest wall

A   **B**

Figure 13.4 **Orientation of three-planar T-oncoanatomy of nine primary sites in the thorax. A.** Anterior coronal. **B.** Lateral sagittal. Because of the angulation of the vertebrae to the convex curvature of the thoracic spine, the reference levels are between the vertebrae.

cancer status. Stage I is N0; stage II is N1; and stages IIIA and IIIB are determined by anatomic node location in the mediastinum, namely, ipsilateral or contralateral. In the fifth edition (1997), T3 N0 was downstaged to stage IIB due to better survival for node-negative advanced disease patients. Then, nodal status is unresectable and assignment to stage IV would have been just as logical. Prognostic factors including molecular, biologic, and genetic markers are noted, but are considered investigational and have not been incorporated into the staging system.

The origin of breast cancer is mainly within its glandular or ductal structure infiltrating the lobule of its origin, then its quadrant invading in one of two directions, toward skin or chest wall. The chest wall, for both breast and lung cancer, when involved is a sign of advancement. It is essential to understand the oncologic anatomy of the mammary gland to appreciate breast cancer's clinical manifestations and patterns of spread. Detection requires knowledge of the cancer's pathologic behavior, the surrounding structures that are commonly invaded, the location of the regional lymph nodes, and how the cancer can spread to remote sites through the breast's rich vascular network. Knowing this anatomy is a fundamental step toward the diagnosis and staging of this cancer.

The basic T and N categories for breast cancer have been modified over the decades with integration of clin-ical and pathologic criteria. The impact of screening mammography has gradually transformed breast cancer into noninvasive and early microinvasive cancers with numerous subcategories. The impact of sentinel nodes detected by lymphoscintography has redefined early stage lymph node involvement. Numerous putative prognostic variables continue to be analyzed, but have not led to any modifications of stage grouping. The T language alphabet has been extended to incorporate three orders of subcategories based on surgical pathologic findings. T stage determines stage grouping with stage subgrouping into A, B, and C being assigned by nodal status.

Overview of Oncoanatomy

In the thorax, there are three major sectors (Fig. 13.3A–C) and four major cancer sites that are staged. The first sector is the lung, major bronchi, and its visceral pleura. The second sector is the chest wall, which includes the parietal pleura and breast. The third sector is anatomically the most diverse, namely, the mediastinum and its contents: the heart and great vessels, thymus gland, major intrathoracic lymph node chains, thoracic duct, and esophagus. A cancer arising in one of the sectors tends to remain localized within that sector until it spreads into regional nodes or invades hematogenously. The boney

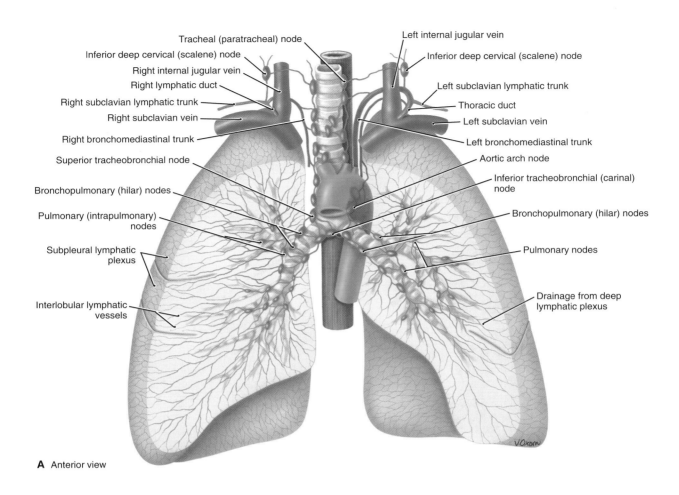

A Anterior view

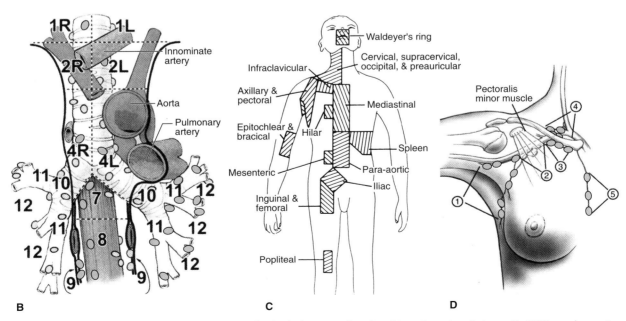

B

C

D

Figure 13.5 **Orientation of N-oncoanatomy: Lymphatic drainage and regional lymph nodes. A.** Lung. **B.** AJCC number system of lung and mediastinal nodes (see Table 13.4). **C.** Anatomic definition of separate lymph nodes regions. **D.** Schematic diagram of the breast and regional lymph nodes. (1) Low axillary, level I. (2) Midaxillary, level II. (3) High axillary, apical, level III. (4) Supraclavicular. (5) Internal mammary nodes (parasternal).

TABLE 13.2	Orientation of Histogenesis of Primary Cancer Sites		
Primary Site Normal Anatomic Structures	Derivative Normal Cell	Cancer Histopathologic Type Primary Site	Thorax Axial Level Assigned*
Terminal bronchiole	Simple cuboidal	Pancoast cancer (adenocarcinoma)	T1/T2
Respiratory bronchiole, acini, alveoli	Type II pneumocyte	Bronchiolalveolar cancer	T2/T3
Segmental bronchi	Goblet cell ciliated columnar	Adenocarcinoma with mixed subtypes	T3/T4
Bronchial neuroendocrine cells	Transdifferentiated neuroendocrine	Large cell anaplastic cancer	T4/T5
Main bronchi	Metaplasia of pseudostratified columnar cells	SQCC	T5/T6
Lobar bronchi	Dedifferentiated stem cell ~Lung bud	Small cell cancer	T6/T7
Visceral parietal pleura and space	Mesothelial cell	Mesothelioma	T7/T8
Breast (chest wall)	Breast duct and lobule cells	Adenocarcinoma	T8/T9
Esophagus (mediastinum and diaphragm)	Stratified squamous cell	SQCC	T9/T10

SQCC, squamous cell cancer.
*Assigned thoracic axial level is designed to encompass and illustrate the different thoracic anatomic sectors and planes.

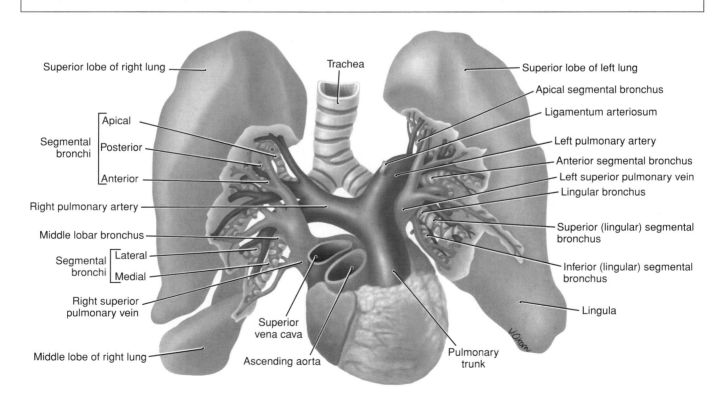

Anterior View

Figure 13.6 **Orientation of M-oncoanatomy.** Pulmonary anterior views are related to metastatic spread to and from lung, respectively.

thorax and intercostal musculature are anatomic structures that surround the lung and mediastinum.

- The bronchial tree (Fig. 13.3D) originates at the tracheal carina starting with the *main bronchi*; then divide within the visceral pleura into the pulmonary parenchyma as *lobar bronchi* (secondary bronchi). The left lung is divided into two lobes and further divides into 10 bronchopulmonary segments. The right lung divides into three lobes and also into 10 bronchopulmonary segments. The segmental bronchus and its associated lung parenchyma constitute a bronchopulmonary segment. Each segment of each lobe has its own blood supply, (bronchial, pulmonary arteries, and veins) and can be resected along their connective tissue septa. The bronchi undergo another five to six orders of divisions downsizing into *terminal bronchioles* that finally end in *respiratory bronchioles*. The smallest functional unit of pulmonary structure consists of a single respiratory bronchiole, which allows for gas exchange via its acini and their multiple alveolar sacs.

- *The subdivisions of the bronchial tree and summary of its histologic features are shown in Figure 13.3E. An anatomic relationship is postulated between lining epithelial cells and specific pulmonary cancers.* Relating these different anatomic divisions of the bronchi to the origin of each histopathologic cancer types provides a rationale for many of the notations and clarifications for specific lung cancers and their staging features. The mesothelial pleural surfaces are barriers to cancer penetration. The lungs are encased in membranes called *visceral pleura*; the chest cavity is lined with a similar, although more fibrous, membrane called the *parietal pleura*. The potential space between these two membranes is the pleural cavity that allows for the smooth movement of lungs with respiration. Pleural mesotheliomas represent a new category that has been staged and classified for the first time in the sixth edition of the AJCC/UICC.

- The mammary gland consists of 15 to 20 lobes of glandular tissue with varying amounts of fat, in a dense fibroareolar stroma, and is attached to the anterior chest wall. In cross-sections starting from the nipple, there are openings of the lactiferous ducts and their lactiferous sinuses, which are the conduits for the secretions of the hormonally stimulated breast glands. These ducts are distinct and individual for each lobule; they first run dorsally from the nipple and then spread radially into the glandular tissue. The breast can be viewed three-dimensionally in terms of its anatomic relationship to other structures. As a superficial gland, it is covered by skin. Posteriorly, it is bounded by the underlying muscles of the chest. Deep to the glandular tissue there is usually a small amount of fat, which, along with the breast proper, is bounded by a deeper layer of superficial

fascia. This layer can usually be dissected free from the deep fascia investing the pectoralis major muscle. Connective tissue septa called the *suspensory ligaments* (of Cooper) form subdivisions of the breast, dividing the breast into lobes. The pectoralis major, the muscle underlying the breast, consists of two heads that arise from the clavicle, sternum, cartilages of the true ribs, and the sixth rib. The schematic of the breast dramatizes the largely ductal branched tubuloalveolar glands contained within a dense connective tissue stroma and variable amounts of adipose tissue. Each of the 15 to 20 lobes of the breast radiates from the mammary papilla (nipple), and each is connected by a specific lactiferous duct with its own lacuna or dilated sinus (Fig. 13.3F, G).

- The esophagus consists of three principle regions (cervical, thoracic, cardiac) and bridges the head and neck, thoracic, and abdominal oncoanatomies. Its mediastinal course allows for a rapid overview of the various organs and structures in the mediastinum, especially those contained in the posterior compartment, which includes the sympathetic and parasympathetic nerves and ganglia, the spinal cord and thoracic vertebrae, the thoracic duct and the aorta, which has the longest contact with the esophagus as both of these structures descend in the chest and exit via their own diaphragmatic stoma into the abdomen. In summary, the thorax oncoanatomy is presented to encompass all the potential primary sites and their malignant gradient.

- The lung oncoanatomy rests on its bronchial tree and its order of 10 subdivisions, lung lobes, and segments and the variation in cell lining phenotypes. The malignant gradient tends to worsen as cancers in the periphery arise in more central locations.

- The breast oncoanatomy rests on its more pliable 15 to 20 lobules, their extensive ductal arrays with the malignant gradient tends to worsen as cancers arise in the periphery and invade into the chest wall and more rapidly into lymphatics.

- The esophagus is a thin-walled structure that courses through the mediastinum with a high malignant gradient throughout; cancers penetrate vital structures and viscera in the different mediastinal compartments.

Orientation of Three-planar T-oncoanatomy of Primary Sites

The three-planar anatomy to overcome the physiologic changes with respiratory and cardiac motion are correlated with anatomic views in dissection atlases, highlighting selected coronal and sagittal planes. The transverse planes are assigned to different lung cancers to provide a basis to encompass the complexities of

TABLE 13.3	Anatomic Isocenters of Primary Cancer Sites		
Normal Structure (Cancer Type)	**Relevant Anatomy**	**Thorax Axial Level Assigned***	
Terminal bronchi (superior sulcus cancer)	Supraclavicular, brachial plexus, stellate ganglion	T1/T2	L/R subclavian, carotid artery
Respiratory bronchi (bronchioalveolar)	Surface anatomy of lung periphery, segmental/lobar arrangements	T3/T4	L/R subclavian, carotid brachiocephalic trunk
Segmental bronchi (adenocarcinoma)	Bronchial tree in situ emphasis on lobar divisions	T3/T4	Arch of aorta Azygos vein
Lobar bronchi (large cell anaplastic)	Large arteries, aorta, and innervations	T4/T5	Ascending and descending aorta
Main bronchi (SQCC)	Trachea, carina, bifurcation of bronchi	T5/T6	Pulmonary arteries
Lung bud, roots (small cell anaplastic)	Large veins, SVC, and azygos and collateral hemiazygos	T6/T7	Pulmonary veins
Pleural space (mesothelioma)	Pleural space extends from neck into abdomen	T7/T8	R/L auricle heart
Mammary glands (breast cancer)	Chest wall construct: intercostal muscle, nerves, vessels	T8/T9	R/L ventricle Apex of heart
Mediastinum (esophagus)	Paraesophageal, neck through posterior mediastinum to abdomen	T9/T10	Base of heart

*Assigned thoracic axial level is designed to encompass and illustrate the different thoracic anatomic sectors and planes.
SQCC, squamous cell cancer.

thoracic anatomy. The assigned axial level is provided at 10 different levels to act as a scaffold for correlative computed tomography (CT) and cross-sectional magnetic resonance imaging (MRI).

The multiplanar diagrams in anterior (Fig. 13.4A) and lateral (Fig. 13.4B) views present the different thoracic malignancies, as variations of lung cancer histopathology and its intrinsic anatomy. Again, the biologic behavior and invasions of pulmonary cancer are determined in large part by the anatomy. To encompass the thoracic and pulmonary anatomy the presentation of the 10 different primary site isocenters is utilized. Therefore, in Table 13.2 *a specific anatomic aspect of the normal lung will be correlated with each cancer type reinforcing concepts as to classification, staging, primary anatomy, lymph node drainage and vascular drainage.* A cephalad to caudad odyssey follows (Table 13.3).

1. Pancoast *cancers arise in the neck rather than the chest emphasizing the apex of the lung which extends above and behind the clavicle.* The symptom complex or syndrome caused by the apical cancer is readily apparent clinically since the superior sulcus of the lung is in direct contact with the inferior portion of the brachial plexus (C7 and T1). Also the stellate ganglion of the sympathetic chain is often compressed against the T1 transverse process as the cancer invades perineurally.

2. Bronchoalveolar cancers (BACs) *arise from the peripheral and most terminal part of the bronchoalveolar segment at which point respiratory bronchioles (without cartilage) branch into an acinus consisting of alveolar sacs.* BACs typically consist of large, mucus-containing cells, reminiscent of the type II pneumocytes and appear as parenchymal nodules. With their lipedic, scale-like growth pattern, they often appear in association with peripheral scars. BACs account for 5% to 9% of all lung cancers but in recent studies have increased to 20% to 24% of all lung cancers.

3. Adenocarcinomas *are the most common histopathology type of lung cancer and arise from the intrapulmonary bronchi that branch like limbs of a tree in each lung then dividing into segmental and subsegmental bronchi, characterized by cartilage in their walls.* They tend to

be intrapulmonary in location, arising from glandular forming epithelial lining cells of bronchi. Four subtypes or variants exist and range from abundant mucus production in well-differentiated cancers and to a cancer that becomes more undifferentiated, losing the glandular arrangement. The lobar anatomy is stressed because atelectasis and obstructive pneumonitis are common and extend to the hilar area.

4. Small cell carcinoma (SCC) are the most dedifferentiated cancers and tend to be more central in location close to the mediastinum. Such cancers arise from or *revert to anlage pluripotential epithelial stem cells and one may draw an appropriate analogy to the endoderm forming cells at the time in embryogenesis when the epithelia of the future lung airways, appearing as right and left lung buds* giving rise to lobar and segmental airways. SCCs are extremely aggressive cancers and in the majority of presentations (80%) are central mediastinal tumors, disseminating rapidly into submucosal lymphatic vessels and regional lymph nodes are almost always present without bronchial invasion. This pattern of spread is to hilar and mediastinal nodes with no evident primary bronchial lesion.

5. Squamous cell cancers (SQCC) *are true bronchogenic cancers arising in major bronchi which are often extrapleural in location with a different blood supply,* namely, bronchial arteries instead of pulmonary arteries. SQCCs are a common cancer although they are less than 50% incidence, more in the 30% to 35% range. Smoking is invariably part of the history and, when hemoptysis is associated with a coarse hilar rhonchial wheeze, this triad is diagnostic of bronchogenic carcinoma.

6. *Large cell anaplastic cancers* are a histologic diagnosis of exclusion and behave similarly to small cell anaplastic cancers. *They, the large cell anaplastic cancers, are more proximal in location and locally tend to invade the mediastinum and its structures early.* Pericardial effusion is currently categorized as T4 if malignant cells are present. The most common cardiac involvement is a pericardial malignancy secondary to pulmonary cancer or to a lesser degree breast cancer. If pericardial cytology is negative, an incidental viral pericarditis needs to be ruled out. Although metastatic hematogenous spread places malignant cells in direct contact with the endocardial surface of the heart, metastatic myocardial nodules are a terminal event and are most often found at post mortem. Large cell anaplastic cancers behave similarly to small cell cancers and are known for their rapid fatal spread.

7. Mesotheliomas *are pleural-based malignancies derived from the cell lining the pleuroperitoneal membranes of the diaphragm* that separates the pleural and peri-

toneal cavities from each other during their embryonal development. The mesenchyme lining these cavities differentiates into a simple single layer of squamous epithelium or mesothelium. *The mesothelium of the lung is the visceral pleura.* In contrast, the *parietal pleura lines the diaphragm, thoracic wall, and mediastinum.* Pleural-based malignancies are designated as mesotheliomas and most often are due to asbestosis exposure years earlier.

8. Breast cancers arise in the mammary glands, an appendage on the chest wall. Cancers of the *mammary gland predominate amongst tumors of the chest wall,* which are both *benign and malignant.* Breast cancers can invade their rich lymphatic plexus and drain to the axillary and internal mammary nodes (parasternal), which are essential features of its anatomic spread. As the most common female cancer, it has been thoroughly studied and analyzed. The anatomic origin is most often either intraductal or the terminal lobule. It gradually invades the lobar segments and their suspensory ligaments with dimpling of the skin owing to the loss of their elasticity. Extensive invasion of dermal lymphatics leads to a *peau d'orange* pitting, which is caused by the pull of multiple Cooper ligament insertions in the edematous dermal layer. Invasion into the pectoral muscle and chest wall leads to fixation of the cancer.

9. *Mediastinal tumors* can arise from any structure, encompassed between the anterior manubrial sternal boney plate and the posterior spine, which are invested in the mediastinal pleura. *A multitude of malignancies arise in the different compartments of the mediastinum, which is divided into superior, anterior, middle, and posterior segments.* The superior mediastinum is defined by a plane intersecting T4 with the manubriosternal junction, and the other compartments are located below with the heart in the middle mediastinum separating the anterior and posterior compartments. A tabulation of malignant mediastinal tumors and the compartments they typically arise in and reflect the key anatomic structures are presented.

10. *Esophageal cancers* arise in different anatomic regions ranging from its cervical origin to the longer longitudinal intrathoracic portion terminating at the cardia of the stomach. *Although the esophagus is thought of as a thoracic organ, esophageal cancers can present in the neck and abdomen as well as the chest.* The TNM staging for esophageal cancer is presented as an introduction to gastrointestinal malignancies. Its thin muscular walls once invaded rapidly disseminate epithelial cancers mistaking them for a bolus of food. The peristaltic milking activity allows for its rapid dissemination through its submucosal lymphatics and its drainage into regional lymph nodes.

TABLE 13.4	Orientation of Sentinel Lymph Nodes (see Fig. 13.5B)	
Primary Site Structure	**Sentinel Node(s) (Fig. 13.5D)**	**AJCC Thorax Number Assigned (Fig. 13.5B)**
Pancoast	Scalene	IR/IL
Bronchiolalveolar	Intrapulmonary, hilar	12, 10
Adenocarcinoma	Interlobar, hilar	11, 10
Large cell anaplastic	Hilar	10
SQCC	Carinal	4R/4L/7
Small cell cancer	Mediastinal	3, 4, 5, 6
Mesothelioma	Intercostal (posterior, mediastinal, hilar)	3p, 8, 9
Breast	Axillary, internal mammary	1, 2, 5
Mediastinum	Paratracheal, pericardial	2, 3, 4, 5, 6
Esophagus	Paraesophageal	2, 3, 4, 5, 6

AJCC, American Joint Committee on Cancer; SQCC, squamous cell cancer.

N-oncoanatomy of Regional Nodes

The lymph node anatomy of the thorax follows the orientation of the three sectors of primary site anatomy and its complexity is a result of their interconnectivity.

- The lung and its bronchial tree reflects the pulmonary lobar and segmental anatomy, which drains into hilar and mediastinal nodes.
- The breast or mammary gland is a chest wall appendage that drains into axillary, interpectoral, and internal mammary (parasternal) lymph nodes.
- The esophagus has paraesophageal lymph nodes that drain into the posterior mediastinal nodes.

Another important aspect that needs to be appreciated is that as cancer infiltrates and replaces a node, lymph flow alters its prograde direction into collateral or retrograde channels reaching lymph nodes that are not normally at risk of becoming involved.

For the lung, the first stations of lymph nodes are the intrapulmonary and bronchopulmonary lymph nodes that lie within the visceral pleura. *Their designation follows the bronchial divisions: hilar, interlobar, lobar bronchi, segmental, and subsegmental (Fig. 13.5A).* These drain into second station carinal and mediastinal nodes. The entire right lung drains to the right hilar nodes and ipsilateral superior mediastinal nodes. The left lower lobe lymphatics cross over from the carinal region to the contralateral right side of the superior mediastinum. The left upper lobe and lingula drain to the ipsilateral left superior mediastinal nodes. A right scalene node biopsy is often favored because its drainage encompasses both right and left lungs. The lymph nodes of the lower posterior mediastinum do not appear to drain the lower lobes unless lower lobe cancers invade the pleural surfaces.

For the mediastinum, lymph nodes range from the thoracic inlet to the diaphragm and the major structures as the thymus and esophagus intermingle their paraortic lymph nodes with those from lung. The heart has pericardial nodes at its apex and base along the diaphragm. Mediastinal lymph nodes are within the right and left parietal pleura. Most important is the thoracic duct, which runs the vertical length of the thorax, crossing from right to left at the T6 to T4 levels. When the thoracic duct is compressed and invaded, a right-sided chylothorax can result. The AJCC utilizes a numbering system from 1 to 14 to locate thoracic lymph nodes, which is helpful to thoracic surgeons resecting and labeling mediastinal nodes (Fig. 13.5B; Table 13.4). For lymphomas, again in contrast is the concept of a lymph node–bearing region wherein the entire mediastinum is one node-bearing region with each hilar region designated separately (Fig. 13.5C).

For breast, its drainage encompasses much of the axilla and chest wall via four major routes: axillary, transpectoral, internal thoracic, and parasternal or internal mammary. Depending on which quadrant the breast cancer arises in, first station nodes include axillary (low, middle), axillary apex, supraclavicular, internal thoracic, parasternal nodes, interpectoral, and subclavicular nodes. Other pathways include crossover lymphatic channels to the opposite breast and inferior drainage into diaphragmatic and subdiaphragmatic channels. Disease involvement in all other nodes—cervical, contralateral supraclavicular and contralateral internal thoracic mammary—is equivalent to distant

TABLE 13.5	Anatomic Distribution of Distant Metastases of Lung			
Site of Metastasis	Squamous	Small Cell	Anaplastic	Adenocarcinoma
Lymph nodes	137 (54%)	163 (85%)	135 (76%)	42 (75%)
Liver	58 (23%)	122 (54%)	67 (38%)	26 (47%)
Adrenals	54 (21%)	84 (44%)	69 (39%)	17 (30%)
Bones	59 (21%)	75 (39%)	53 (30%)	23 (41%)
Brain	26 (17%)	45 (42%)	30 (24%)	13 (39%)
Kidney	39 (15%)	28 (14.5%)	24 (13.5%)	11 (20%)
Pancreas	9 (3.5%)	46 (24%)	25 (14%)	3 (5%)
Lung	31 (12%)	13 (7%)	15 (8%)	8 (14%)
Pleura	18 (7%)	21 (11%)	9 (%)	3 (5%)
Total	255	191	179	56

Used with permission from Line DH, Deeley TJ. The necropsy findings in carcinoma of the bronchus. *Br J Dis Chest* 1971;65:238–242.

metastases. The AJCC divides the axilla into three levels: (i) low axillary, (ii) mid axillary, beneath the pectoralis minor muscle insertion, and (iii) high axillary and apical (Fig. 13.5D).

M-oncoanatomy of Regional Veins and Neurovascular Bundle

The major vessels of the thorax are great vessels of the mediastinum, the aorta, and its divisions into innominate and subclavian arteries (Fig. 13.6). The great veins consist of the anterior located, superior vena cava and brachiocephalic vein, the midthoracic pulmonary veins, and the posterior azygos and hemiazygos venous complex. The major neurovascular bundle is the autonomic nervous system of parasympathetic and sympathetic ganglions and nerves located in posterior mediastinum. Metastatic spread to distant organs according to the histopathologic type of lung cancer is listed in Table 13.5. The anatomic distribution of distant metastases is presented as a function of histopathologic type of lung cancer.

Rules of Classification and Staging

Clinical Staging and Imaging

Lung cancer masquerades as many different pulmonary diseases and their clinical presentations are radiologically shown in Figure 13.7. The most commonly used procedure for staging lung, mediastinal, and breast cancers is the spiral CT. This is utilized to define the extent

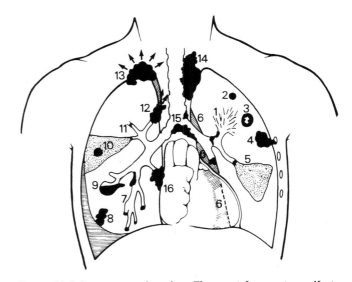

Figure 13.7 Lung cancer imaging: The most frequent manifestation or masquerades of bronchial cancers (1) to (16). (1) Hilar lung cancer with endobronchial growth (relatively early elicitation of the cough reflex). (2) Typical round focus. (3) Tumor cavern (note the thick irregular walls). (4) Subpleural focus infiltrating the chest wall. (5) Obstructive segmental discontinuation with retention in pneumonia, (10) already with abscess formation. (6) Atelectasis, which is hidden behind the cardiac shadow (lateral radiograph). (7) Secondary bronchiectasis due to partial stenosis. (8) Focus near to the pleura, with effusion. (9) Necrotizing tumor with draining bronchus (abscess symptom). (11) Obstruction emphysema due to valve occlusion. (12) and (13) Outbreak of carcinoma into the mediastinum, for example, in the direction of the vena cava (upper inflow congestion) or as Pancoast tumor. (14) Lymph node involvement in the upper mediastinum and paratracheally, extending to the upper clavicular fossa. Detection by lymph node biopsy according to Daniels or by mediastinoscopy: (15) and (16) carcinoma spreading to the trachea and pericardium, respectively. *Note:* A bronchial carcinoma can be masked even in a normal radiograph.

Method	Capability	Recommended
TABLE 13.6	**Imaging Modalities for Diagnosis and Staging**	
Primary tumor and regional nodes workup		
Chest films	Baseline image	Yes
CT/spiral CT	Most useful of all modalities for determining characteristics of T and N in the thorax and M in the brain and liver	Yes
MRI	Not as good as CT	No
Percutaneous needle biopsy	Guided by fluoroscopy or CT, accurate in establishing cytologic diagnosis from T (particularly peripheral lung lesions); M(especially liver or bone); less experience with N	Yes
Mediastinoscopy/thoracoscopy	Confirmation of nodal involvement	Yes
Metastatic work-up for clinically suspected metastases		
CT/echography	For liver, adrenals	Yes
CT/MRI	For brain	Yes
Bone scan	For the bone	Yes
PET scan/MRI spectroscopy	Diagnosis of peripheral lesions, staging; can differentiate between cystic and solid lesions	Yes, if clinically indicated

CT, computed tomography; M, metastasis; MRI, magnetic resonance imaging; N, node; PET, positron emission tomography; T, tumor.

of both lung and breast cancer when they are invasive and advanced. MRI is useful for assessing the mediastinal malignancies or adenopathy related to pulmonary and breast lymphatic invasion. Metastatic spread workup, which is common to lung and breast cancer, includes bone scans when osseous metastases are suspected. MRI is often utilized for brain and CT liver metastases. The workup for metastatic disease is based on symptoms being present rather than electively (Table 13.6).

Pathologic Staging

Pathologic staging is described in each chapter in more detail.

Oncoimaging Annotations

- Chest radiographs seldom detect primary lung cancers in their early stages.
- Spiral CT is useful in high-risk patients to detect nodule and infiltrates.
- Positron emission tomography PET imaging with [18]FDG appears to be of value in discriminating malignant versus benign nodules.
- CT can detect and mediastinal adenopathy but histologic verification is essential to ascertain if it is malignant.
- Determining N2 versus N3 mediastinal nodes is important; it establishes resectability.
- MRI can be of value in assessing mediastinal invasion, chest wall and rib erosion, and compromised large vein involvement.

Cancer Statistics and Survival

The 5-year survival rates for thoracic cancer over five decades presents the best and worst achievements in controlling cancer deaths. Because breast cancer is slowly increasing in incidence and prevalence, it is anticipated that there will be more than 200,000 new diagnoses of invasive breast cancers annually in this country alone. In addition, there are 60,000 cases of highly curable preinvasive cancers. Breast cancer is currently found with mammography, mainly in noninvasive or early stage I cancers where survival rates are at the 95% mark. The improvement in breast cancer survival over the past five decades has been dramatic, with a doubling in the survival rate from 45% to 90%, also reflecting the advances in multimodal management. Breast cancer is the most common cancer in women (215,990), which translates to one third of all neoplasms. Fortunately, most patients with breast cancer survive and only 40,110 deaths (15%) can be attributed to the malignancy.

Lung and bronchus cancers are the second most common cancers at almost 95,000 new male patients and a comparable 80,000 female patients, accounting for 13% and 12%, respectively, of cancer patients. However, lung and bronchus cancer is public enemy number one and is the leading cause of death for men 92,000 (32%) and 68,500 (25%) women. An estimated 175,000 new cases of lung cancer annually will be diagnosed by 2005, with a predicted 160,000 deaths in the same year (Tables 13.7 and 13.8). This is one of the most dismal cancer survival rates at 15% 5-year survival. Despite the progress of research, the causes of this disease and mortality rates have not been reduced.

TABLE 13.7	Cancer Statistics for Thorax		
Site	New Diagnoses	Deaths	5-Year Survival Rates (%) 1950–2000, % Gain
Lung and bronchus	172,570	163,510	15
Breast	212,930	40,870	88
Esophagus	14,520	13,570	14

TABLE 13.8	Cancer Curability by Stages at Diagnosis (1992–1998)			
	5-Year Survival Rate (%)			
Site	All Stages	Local	Regional	Advanced
Lung and bronchus	15.2	48.4	16.1	2.1
Breast	87.7	97.5	80.4	25.5
Esophagus	14.3	29.3	13.3	3.1

TABLE 13.9	Clinical and Pathologic Surgical Survival Results by Stage of Non-Small Cell Lung Cancer				
		Clinical		Surgical	
Stage	TNM	5-Year Survival (%)	1-Year Survival (%)	5-Year Survival (%)	1-Year Survival (%)
IA	T1, N0, M0	91	61	94	67
IB	T2, N0, M0	72	38	87	57
IIA	T1, N1, M0	79	34	89	55
IIB	T2, N1, M0	61	24	78	39
	T3, N0, M0	55	22	76	38
IIIA	T3, N1, M0	56	9	65	25
	T1-2-3, N2, M0	50	13	64	23
IIIB/IV	T4, N0-1-2, M0	37	7		
	Any T, N3, M0	32	3		
	Any T, Any N, M1	20	5		

T, tumor; N, node; M, metastasis.
Modified with permission from Mountain CF: Revisions in the international system for staging lung cancer. *Chest* 1997;111:1710–1717.

Curability concepts can only be applied to breast cancer with 86% of all stages surviving 5 years, and with excellent results for all stages: 88% 5-year and an impressive 97% 5-year for localized disease and even 78% for regional nodes. For lung and esophageal cancers, most patients are in advanced stages with only 2% to 3% lasting 5 years. Although there have been improvements in multimodal approaches, only about 10% of such patients survive.

Whereas the 10% gain in lung cancer survival over five decades also represents a doubling in survival rates, it remains one of the most lethal of all cancers despite gains in knowledge. To end on a positive note, early stage I lung cancer can result in a better than 50% survival (Table 13.9). Although routine spiral CT scans of the thorax in high-risk patients have yielded a high number of early stage lung cancers, this procedure is too costly to apply routinely. However, it is recommended for the habitual heavy smoker on an annual basis. Large cohorts of patients have been screened and early detection of small lung cancers have been found with an increase in their survival rate.

14

Pancoast Cancer

The designation of Pancoast refers to a tumor arising in the apex of lung in the neck that involves the brachial plexus and the stellate ganglion.

Perspective and Patterns of Spread

The apex of the lung is in the base of the neck. The anatomy between the neck and thorax is a transitional zone because the thoracic vertebrae T1 and T2 are in the neck above the suprasternal notch. The "Pancoast" tumor refers to a symptom complex or syndrome caused by a tumor arising in the superior sulcus of the lung, which is juxtaposed and therefore involves the inferior branches of the brachial plexus (C8 and T1) and traps the stellate ganglion of the cervical sympathetic chain which resides on the transverse process of T1 resulting in a Horner's syndrome (shoulder and arm pain with ptosis, myosis, unilateral flushing, and anhydrosis).

A variety of histopathologic tumor types are possible (Table 14.1). The cells of tumor origin are in the terminal bronchioles ranging from ciliated simple columnar to simple cuboidal cells. Cancers vary from 25% to 40% squamous cell, 25% to 60% adenocarcinoma, 5% to 15% large cell, and 2% to 5% small cell. The apical location and superior sulcus cancers in the lung apex do not present in a typical fashion with a productive cough, hemoptysis, or blood-streaked sputum, but as a progressive neuralgia with referred shoulder pain to the ulnar side of the arm. Horner's syndrome is usually subtle in onset and misleading; symptoms are related to a neurologic syndrome rather than a neoplastic process in lung. The intimate anatomic relationship of lung apex to brachial plexus and the stellate ganglion explains the onset of symptoms once the cancer spread is into the soft tissues of the neck (Fig. 14.1).

TNM Staging Criteria

The designation of Pancoast tumors refers to the symptom complex or syndrome caused by a tumor arising in the superior sulcus of the lung that involves the inferior branches

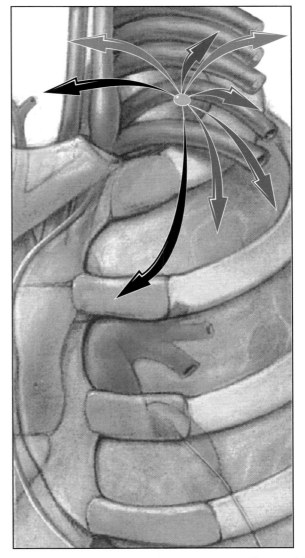

Figure 14.1 **Patterns of spread.** The primary cancer (Pancoast) invades in various directions, which are color-coded vectors (*arrows*) representing stage of progression: Tis, yellow; T1, green; T2, blue; T3, purple; T4, red; and when metastatic, black.

DEFINITION OF TNM

T_{is} N_0

STAGE GROUPINGS

0

T1
Tumor ≤3 cm, surrounded by lung or visceral pleura, without bronchoscopic evidence of invasion more proximal than the lobar bronchus

T2
Tumor with any of the following features of size or extent: >3 cm; invades the visceral pleura; associated with the atelectasis or obstructive pneumonitis that extends to the hilar region

N0
No regional lymph node metastasis

T_1 T_2

IA   IB N_0

Stage IA
T1 N0 M0

Stage IB
T2 N0 M0

I

T1
Tumor ≤3 cm, surrounded by lung or visceral pleura, without bronchoscopic evidence of invasion more proximal than the lobar bronchus

T2
Tumor with any of the following features of size or extent: >3 cm; invades the visceral pleura; associated with the atelectasis or obstructive pneumonitis that extends to the hilar region.

N1
Metastasis to ipsilateral peribronchial and/or ipsilateral hilar lymph nodes, and intrapulmonary nodes including involvement by direct extension of the primary tumor

T_1 T_3

IIA   IIB N_1

Stage IIA
T1 N1 M0

Stage IIB
T2 N1 M0
T3 N0 M0

II

T3
Tumor of any size that directly invades any of the following: chest wall (including superior sulcus tumors), mediastinal pleura. Tumor involves the inferior branches of the brachial plexus (C8 and/or T1) and the sympathetic nerve trunks, including the stellate ganglion.

N2
Metastasis to ipsilateral mediastinal, and/or subcarinal lymph node(s)

T_3

IIIA N_2

Stage IIIA
T1 N2 M0*
T2 N2 M0*
T3 N1 M0*
T3 N2 M0

*not illustrated

IIIA

T4
Tumor of any size that invades any of the following: mediastinum, great vessels, trachea, esophagus; or separate tumor nodules in the same lobe; or tumor with malignant pleural effusion; evidence of invasion of the vertebral body or spinal canal, encasement of the subclavian vessels, or unequivocal involvement of the superior branches of the brachial plexus (C8 or above).

N3
Metastasis to contralateral mediastinal, contralateral hilar, ipsilateral or contralateral scalene, or supraclavicular lymph node(s)

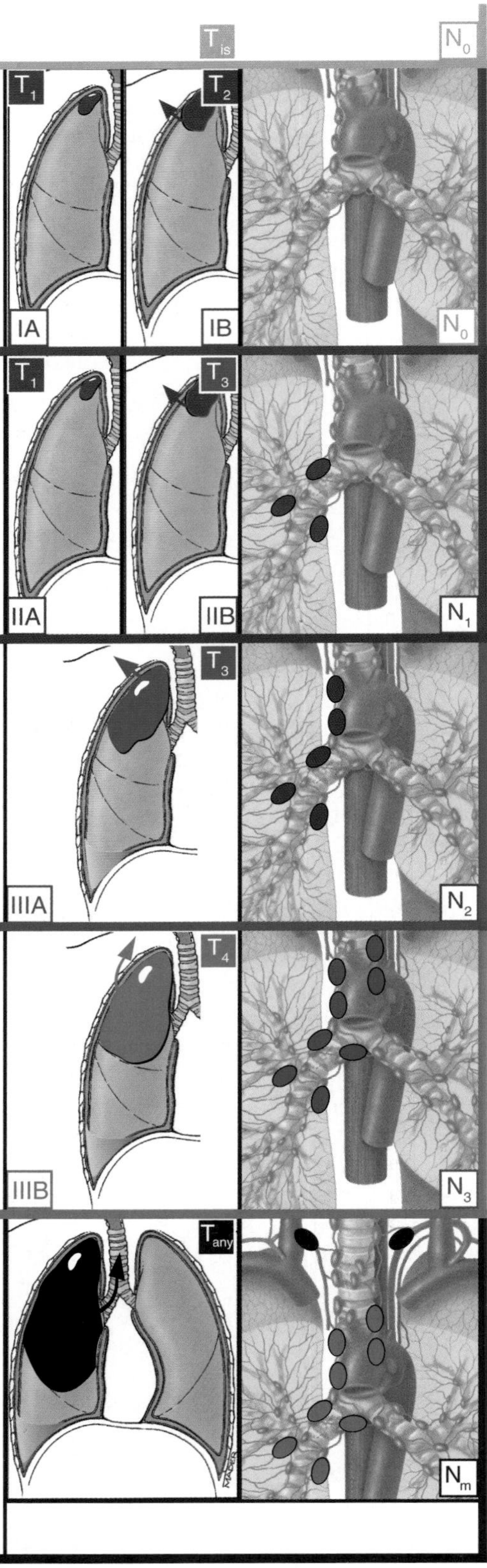

T_4

IIIB N_3

Stage IIIB
Any T   N3   M0
T4   Any N M0

IIIB

M1
Distant metastases

Nm
Node metastatic
Juxtaregional, Cervical nodes

T_{any}

N_m

Stage IV
Any T   Any N   M1

IV

Figure 14.2 TNM staging diagram. Pancoast cancers originate in cupula of lungs and are located in the base of the neck and spread into supraclavicular and cervical nodes. Vertical presentations of stage groupings, which follow same color code for cancer stage advancement are organized in horizontal lanes: Stage 0, yellow; I, green; IIIA, purple; IIIB, red; and metastatic stage IV, black. Definitions of TN on left and stage grouping on right.

TABLE 14.1	Histopathologic Type	
Main Pathologic Cell Type	**Variant**
Adenocarcinoma with mixed subtypes	Well differentiated fetal adenocarcinoma
	Mucinous ("colloid" adenocarcinoma)
	Mucinous cystadenocarcinoma
	Signet ring adenocarcinoma
	Clear cell adenocarcinoma

of the brachial plexus (C8 and/or T1) and the sympathetic nerve trunks, including the stellate ganglion. Some superior sulcus tumors are more anteriorly located and may cause fewer neurologic symptoms even when they are very locally advanced and encase the subclavian vessels. If there is evidence of invasion of the vertebral body or spinal canal, encasement of the subclavian vessels or unequivocal involvement of the superior branches of the brachial plexus (C8 or above), then the tumor is classified as T4. If no criteria for T4 disease pertain, the tumor is classified as T3.

Although the usual TNM criteria apply, because of the anatomic location, some exceptional findings need to be appreciated. T1 and T2 lesions <3 cm or >3 cm are difficult to detect on routine chest films owing to overlay of ribs and clavicle, which obscures small opacities in the lung. Diagnosis is most often made when the cancer reaches stage T3 because of persistent shoulder pain, which leads to discovering chest wall invasion and posterior rib erosion on film before extensive perineural invasion, while resection is possible. Patterns of neurologic involvement vary according to which surface the cancer invades first. Thus, with superior invasion of the brachial plexus trunks of TI, C8, and C7, ribs are eroded laterally, vertebrae are invaded posteriorly, and major vessels (subclavian artery and vein) are involved anteriorly at the thoracic inlet. The difference between stages T3 and T4 is that the latter can be due to invasion of the vertebral body, and unequivocal involvement of spinal cord at C8 with disastrous paraplegia or complete cord transection and quadriplegia before death. Invasion of the chest wall, pleura, and ribs imply resection is possible and therefore is considered to be T3 (Fig. 14.2).

Summary of Changes

There have been no changes from the fifth edition of the AJCC CSM.

Orientation of Three-planar Oncoanatomy

The isocenter of the pulmonary apex is in the neck, around which the three-planar anatomy is presented,

especially as it relates to the brachial plexus and sympathetic chain of cervical ganglion. It is important to note that T1 and T2 are above the thoracic inlet and form a transitional zone between the neck and the chest, that is, the thoracic inlet (Fig. 14.3).

T-oncoanatomy

Designated at the T1/T2 level, *the Pancoast tumor is fitting to introduce lung cancer as a disease with many different presentations, which masquerade the underlying cancer.* The misleading signs and symptoms in the presentation of a Pancoast cancer stem from the anatomic location of the superior sulcus of the lung in the neck and not the thorax. Grave signs are direct vertebral invasion, which can result in spinal cord encroachment and transection leading to paraplegia or entrapment of major vessels, namely, the subclavian artery and vein. The coronal and sagittal views are more revealing of the critical anatomy of the superior sulcus (Fig. 14.4).

- *Coronal:* The juxtaposition of the brachial plexus superior and posterior to the lung apex is readily seen.
- *Sagittal:* The brachial plexus and subclavian artery are appreciated as to their proximity to the lung apex posteriorly and anteriorly, respectively.
- *Transverse:* The medial location of the stellate ganglion anterior to the transverse process of T1. The spinal cord is accessible once the vertebral foramen are eroded. This is a striking view of the roof of the thoracic cavity from a diaphragmatic vantage point. The thoracic inlet is the zone that allows cancers to trap nerves, arteries, and veins and compress them against boney ribs and vertebrae; they are between the proverbial rock and a hard place.

N-oncoanatomy

Once the pleural surface is invaded, the cancer drains into scalene or cervical nodes by way of the superior intercostal lymphatics. These lymph nodes often are the ones involved and do not deter the resectability of Pancoast cancers. Intrapulmonary nodes and hilar nodes are possibly, albeit uncommonly, involved (Fig. 14.5; Table 14.2). Ironically, sentinel nodes are metastatic cervical nodes.

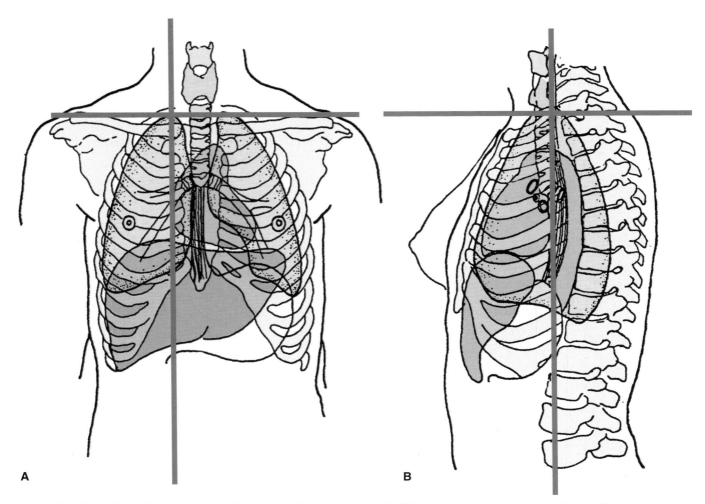

A   **B**

Figure 14.3 **Orientation of T-oncoanatomy.** The anatomic isocenter is at the T1/T2 level at the base of the neck in its transition to the thoracic inlet. **A.** Coronal. **B.** Sagittal.

M-oncoanatomy

Cancer invasion of chest wall drains into intercostal veins, then the azygos vein, and then the superior vena cava, which leads to lung dissemination (Fig. 14.6; see also Table 13.5).

Rules for Classification and Staging

Clinical Staging and Imaging

The TNM classification system is primarily for staging non–small cell lung cancers. The most important change dates back to the fourthedition of the American Joint Committee on Cancer (AJCC), where T3, resectable disease, was distinguished from T4 unresectable disease. Simultaneously, a greater reliance on more sophisticated imaging has occurred. It is with the sixthedition that computed tomography (CT) and positron emission to-

pography (PET) are allowed. The imaging modalities for detection and diagnosis apply to staging (Table 14.3). Chest films and CT (preferably spiral) are essential steps in both diagnosis and staging. PET combined with CT helps to overcome motion artifacts. Magnetic resonance imaging (MRI) is useful for mediastinal evaluation. Another advantage of CT over MRI for staging is that it allows for metastatic workup of lung, liver, adrenal and for ribs, and vertebrae, especially for Pancoast cancers.

Pathologic Staging

All pathologic specimens from clinical invasive procedures—bronchoscopy, mediastinoscopy, mediastinotomy, thoracentesis and thoracoscopy—are applicable to pathologic stage. Thoracotomy and resection of primary and lymph nodes are the mainstay of pathologic

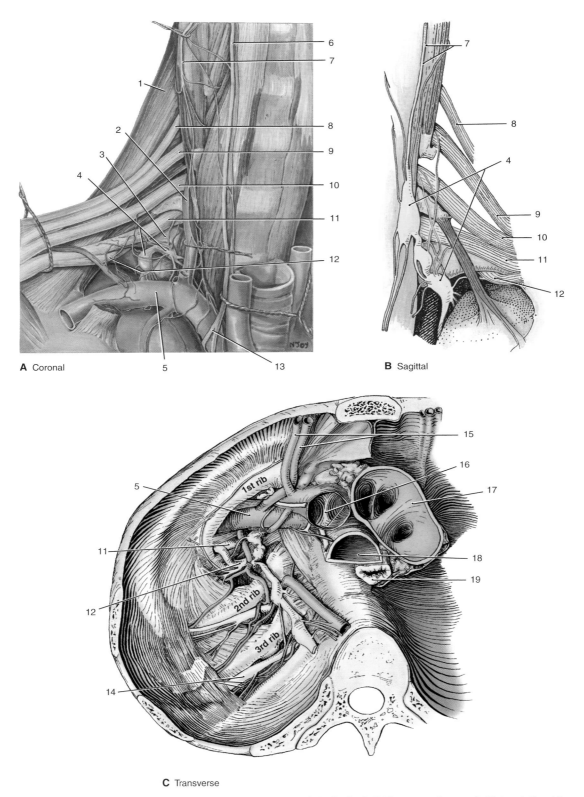

A Coronal

B Sagittal

C Transverse

Figure 14.4 **T-oncoanatomy three-planar views. A.** Coronal. **B.** Sagittal. **C.** Transverse (see text). Note relationship of brachial plexus to apex of lung. **A.** (1) Middle scalene muscle. (2) Vertebral artery. (3) First rib. (4) Stellate ganglion. (5) Subclavian artery. (6) Vagus nerve. (7) Sympathetic trunk. (8) C5. (9) C6. (10) C7. (11) C8. (12) T1. (13) Right recurrent laryngeal nerve. **B.** and **C.** (14) Intercostal nerve and vessels. (15) Internal thoracic vein and artery. (16) Superior vena cava. (17) Arch of aorta. (18) Trachea. (19) Esophagus.

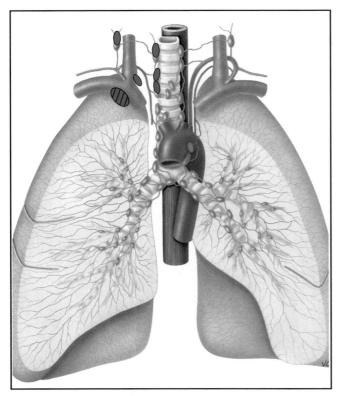

Figure 14.5 N-oncoanatomy. Sentinel nodes are scalene and supra-clavicular.

staging. Margin status and any residual cancer need to be noted. Preferably, six nodes should be examined.

Surgical resection of primary and regional nodes needs to be carefully evaluated at bronchial stump for adequate margins. All resected nodes should be numbered according to AJCC system and assessed for tumor.

Oncoimaging Annotations

- Chest radiographs seldom detect primary lung cancers in their early stages.
- Spiral CT is useful in high-risk patients to detect nodule and infiltrates.
- PET imaging with [18]FDG appears to be of value in discriminating malignant versus benign nodules.
- CT can detect and mediastinal adenopathy, but histologic verification is essential to ascertain if it is malignant.
- Determining N2 versus N3 mediastinal nodes is important; it establishes resectability.
- MRI can be of value in assessing mediastinal invasion, chest wall and rib erosion, and compromised large vein involvement.
- Pancoast cancers are difficult to diagnose on routine chest films.
- CT scan using bone windows detects invasion of ribs and vertebrae.
- MRI is useful for detecting invasion of vertebrae and tumor compressing spinal cord.

TABLE 14.2	Lymph Nodes of the Lung

Sentinel nodes are scalene and supraclavicular nodes and lower deep cervical nodes.

N1 nodes: All N1 nodes lie distal to the mediastinal pleural reflection and *within the visceral pleura.*

Hilar nodes
Interlobar nodes
Lobar nodes bronchi
Segmental nodes
Subsegmental nodes

N2 nodes: All N2 nodes lie within the mediastinal pleural envelope on the ipsilateral side.

Highest mediastinal nodes
Upper paratracheal nodes
Prevascular and retrotracheal nodes
Lower paratracheal nodes
Subaortic nodes (aortopulmonary window)
Para-aortic nodes (ascending aorta or phrenic)
Subcarinal nodes
Paraesophageal nodes (below carina)
Pulmonary ligament nodes

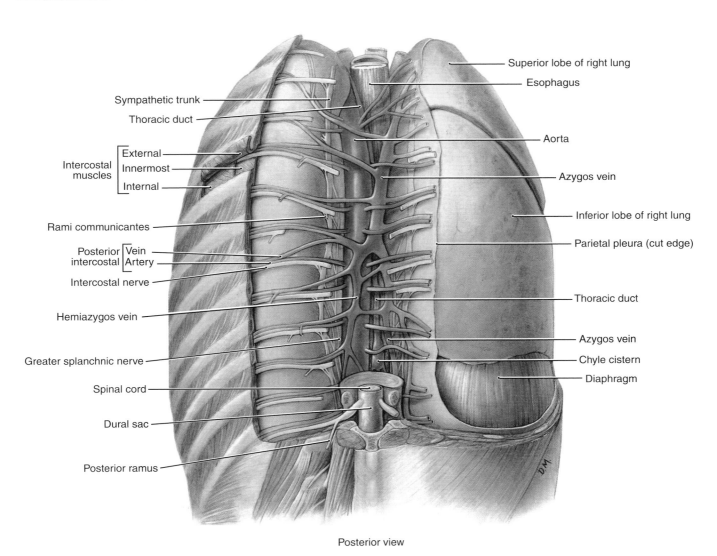

Posterior view

Figure 14.6 M-oncoanatomy. The intercostal arteries and veins drain into the azygos, then the superior vena cava to the right heart. Circulating cancer cells exit via the pulmonary artery to the lung bed.

Cancer Statistics and Survival

Generally, according to Surveillance Epidemiology and End Results data based on 16,000 patients, the relative 5-year survival is 8% to 10% and 10-year survival 5% to 7%. Surprisingly, there is a small attrition for 5-year survivors with the majority 70% remaining alive at 10 years. Female gender, good Karnofsky performance status, and cessation of smoking contribute to longer survival.

Staging is a major factor in survival and the data analyzed by Mountain present the findings in Figure 14.7 (see Table 13.9). For stage IA cancers, the 90% T1 N0 M0 patient decreases to 61% at 5 years and stage IB 70% at 1 year is almost halved at 5 years at 38%. The 50% 5-year survival for stage I decreases to 30% indicating that once hilar nodes are positive, metastatic disease is highly likely. Stage IIIA represents the most favorable advanced

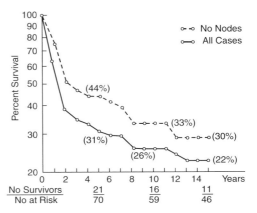

Figure 14.7 Five-, 10-, and 15-year actuarial survival curves after combined preoperative radiation, followed by en bloc surgical resection (1956–83) in patients with no lymph nodes involved and including those with nodal involvement.

TABLE 14.3	Imaging Modalities for Diagnosis and Staging	
Method	**Capability**	**Recommended**
Primary tumor and regional nodes workup		
Chest films	Baseline image	Yes
CT/spiral CT	Most useful of all modalities for determining characteristics of T and N in the thorax and M in the brain and liver	Yes
MRI	Superior to CT in superior sulcus tumors to determine involvement of lower branches of brachial plexus and subclavian vessels in coronal and sagittal planes.	Yes
Percutaneous needle biopsy	Guided by fluoroscopy or CT, accurate in establishing cytologic diagnosis from T (particularly peripheral lung lesions); M (especially liver or bone); less experience with N	Yes
Mediastinoscopy/thoracoscopy	Confirmation of nodal involvement	Yes
Metastatic workup for clinically suspected metastases		
CT/echography	For liver, adrenals	Yes
CT/MRI	For brain	Yes
Bone scan	For the bone	Yes
PET scan/MRI spectroscopy	Diagnosis of peripheral lesions, staging. Can differentiate between cystic and solid lesions.	Yes, if clinically indicated

CT, computed tomography; M, metastasis; MRI, magnetic resonance imaging; N, node; PET, positron emission tomography; T, tumor.

disease patients with 50% 1-year survival and, despite vigorous chemoradiation, only decreases to 10%. Surgically staged IIIA patients do better (as expected) with 25% alive at 5 years.

Specifically, Pancoast cancers were thought to be incurable until a fortuitous long-term survivor (27 years) was reported following preoperative radiation and resection. Nodal status is important because scalene and supraclavicular nodes maybe the first involved but are not considered contraindications to surgical resection.

The ability to resect superior sulcus cancers following preoperative radiation was pioneered by Paulson, who posted a 30% 5-year survival rate with a low 3% mortality rate (Fig. 14.7). This has been reproduced by other surgical teams.

15

Bronchioloalveolar Cancer

The BACs arise from the most peripheral respiratory bronchi branching into an acinus and alveolar sacs allowing for its lepidic spread.

Perspective and Patterns of Spread

The essential cell in the evolutionary process that enabled aquatic animals to leave the sea to become air breathers is the type II pneumocyte. The cry of the newborn recapitulates that stage in our ontogeny; it ensures that air has replaced the amniotic fluid in the alveolar acini. The malignant transformation of the type II pneumocyte provides the histogenesis into a bronchioloalveolar carcinoma (BAC; Table 15.1). BACs have three distinct patterns of presentation that have been described as clinical pathologic entities: (i) Cancers in peripheral pulmonary scars; (ii) Multiple primary nodules; and (iii) Diffuse and extensive pneumonitis. BACs account for 5% to 10% of all lung cancers, but its incidence has doubled in more recent series as its cellular characteristics are increasingly appreciated.

The crucial point in understanding the concept of *"lepidic" spread (scale like) is the pre-existence of a fine microcirculatory web in the alveoli walls of the terminal intrapulmonary airways or the alveolar acini and sacs (Fig. 15.1).* The alveolar wall is lined by type I pneumocytes, which are singular, flat surface cells generated by the type II pneumocyte, which stores, manufactures, and secretes surfactant molecules. BACs arising in the terminal respiratory bronchial appear to arise in a peripheral pulmonary scar that extends to the pleural surface because a small subsegment of air sacs or alveoli collapse or become infiltrated by lepidic spread. Their histogenic features suggest they arise from the type II pneumocyte.

TNM Staging Criteria

Lepidic spread refers to the noninvasive nature of BACs, which is an oxymoron. This is possible because of a *special feature of terminal acini. Their clusters of alveolar sacs enable surface infiltration of the pre-existing*

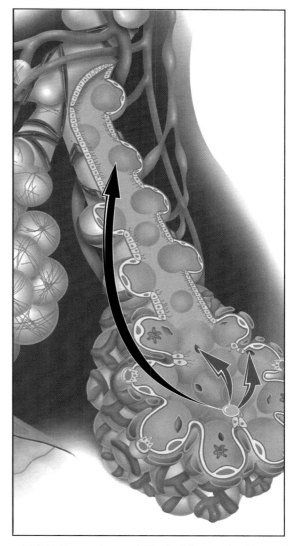

Figure 15.1 **Patterns of spread.** The lepidic spread pattern of bronchioloalveolar cancer is a scale-like peripheral infiltration of acini and alveoli through alveolar wall pores without invasion of lymphatics or microcirculation. Color code simplified: T1, peripheral nodule (green); cancer in a peripheral scar (green); and T3, dissemination.

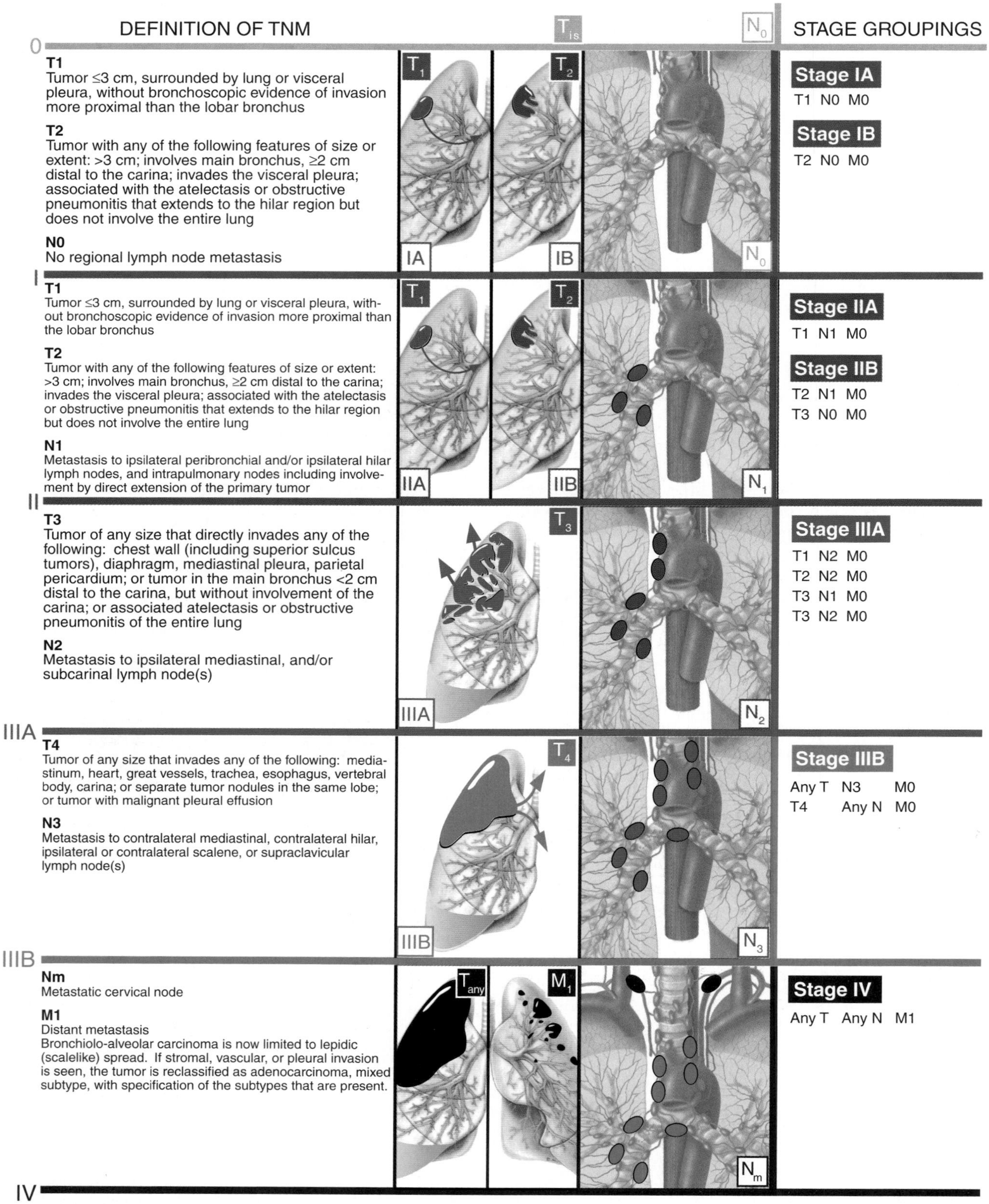

DEFINITION OF TNM

T_{is} N_0

STAGE GROUPINGS

0

T1
Tumor ≤3 cm, surrounded by lung or visceral pleura, without bronchoscopic evidence of invasion more proximal than the lobar bronchus

T2
Tumor with any of the following features of size or extent: >3 cm; involves main bronchus, ≥2 cm distal to the carina; invades the visceral pleura; associated with the atelectasis or obstructive pneumonitis that extends to the hilar region but does not involve the entire lung

N0
No regional lymph node metastasis

Stage IA
T1 N0 M0

Stage IB
T2 N0 M0

I

T1
Tumor ≤3 cm, surrounded by lung or visceral pleura, without bronchoscopic evidence of invasion more proximal than the lobar bronchus

T2
Tumor with any of the following features of size or extent: >3 cm; involves main bronchus, ≥2 cm distal to the carina; invades the visceral pleura; associated with the atelectasis or obstructive pneumonitis that extends to the hilar region but does not involve the entire lung

N1
Metastasis to ipsilateral peribronchial and/or ipsilateral hilar lymph nodes, and intrapulmonary nodes including involvement by direct extension of the primary tumor

Stage IIA
T1 N1 M0

Stage IIB
T2 N1 M0
T3 N0 M0

II

T3
Tumor of any size that directly invades any of the following: chest wall (including superior sulcus tumors), diaphragm, mediastinal pleura, parietal pericardium; or tumor in the main bronchus <2 cm distal to the carina, but without involvement of the carina; or associated atelectasis or obstructive pneumonitis of the entire lung

N2
Metastasis to ipsilateral mediastinal, and/or subcarinal lymph node(s)

Stage IIIA
T1 N2 M0
T2 N2 M0
T3 N1 M0
T3 N2 M0

IIIA

T4
Tumor of any size that invades any of the following: mediastinum, heart, great vessels, trachea, esophagus, vertebral body, carina; or separate tumor nodules in the same lobe; or tumor with malignant pleural effusion

N3
Metastasis to contralateral mediastinal, contralateral hilar, ipsilateral or contralateral scalene, or supraclavicular lymph node(s)

Stage IIIB

Any T   N3   M0
T4   Any N   M0

IIIB

Nm
Metastatic cervical node

M1
Distant metastasis
Bronchiolo-alveolar carcinoma is now limited to lepidic (scalelike) spread. If stromal, vascular, or pleural invasion is seen, the tumor is reclassified as adenocarcinoma, mixed subtype, with specification of the subtypes that are present.

Stage IV

Any T Any N M1

IV

Figure 15.2 TNM staging diagram. Bronchioloalveolar cancers are usually detected as peripheral cancers with scarring and subsegmental collapse. They are considered non-invasive but multicentric as in T3 and Tany. When invasion occurs as in T4, it is considered to be an adenocarcinoma or mixed type. Color coding: Stage 0, yellow; I, green; II, blue; IIIA, purple; IIIB, red; IV, black (metastatic). Definitions of TN on left and stage grouping on right. Although shown, stromal, vascular and pleural invasion require reclassification as adenocarcinoma.

TABLE 15.1	Histopathologic Type
Main Pathologic Cell Type	**Variant**
Bronchoalveolar carcinoma	Nonmucinous
	Mucinous
	Mixed mucinous and nonmucinous or indeterminate
	Solid adenocarcinoma with mucin formation

pulmonary capillary bed, namely the acini that communicate through the "pores of Kohn" between their alveolar walls. This allows bronchioloalveolar cancers to spread without the need for generating their own tumor neovascular bed and blood supply. If these lepidic features are not evident—that is, stromal, vascular, or pleural invasion is seen—then the cancer needs to be reclassified as adenocarcinoma (Fig. 15.2). Mixed subtypes require that each subtype present be specified.

True solitary BACs carry an excellent prognosis, with a 70% 5-year survival. Another feature is its presentation as *multiple primaries that are metachronous or synchronous.* According to the American Joint Committee on Cancer (AJCC)/International Union Against Cancer criteria as originally proposed by Martini and Melamed: *The two tumors need to be the same histologic type but in separate lobes without evidence of nodal metastasis within a common nodal drainage, that is, interlobar nodes common to upper and lower lobes.* The third scenario is the pneumonitic presentation, which can be multifocal and rapidly fills intrapulmonary acinar airways resulting in an "air bronchogram." Multiple nodules in the same lobe as the primary are considered to be metastatic and staged as T4. Survival for this multifocal disseminated form of cancer is nil.

Summary of Changes

There have been no changes from the fifth edition of the AJCC CSM.

Orientation of Three-planar Oncoanatomy

The respiratory bronchioles and their acini and alveoli constitute the breeding ground for BACs. Although the axial orientation is at the T3/T4 level, a microscopic/macroscopic view of the intrapulmonary airways is required to appreciate the very fine bronchiole divisions as they become subsegmental, intrasegmental, and lose the cartilage in their walls, and terminate as respiratory bronchioles. *These respiratory bronchioles end in acini with alveolar sacs and alveoli.* The intrapulmonary fine capillary meshwork is optimally designed for a lepidic cancer spread pattern owing to the preconfigured mi-

crovasculature of the alveoli which BACs adopt as they extend through the pores of Kohn (Fig. 15.3).

T-oncoanatomy

The peripheral pleural anatomy of the lung is the geographic zones for the BACs. The presentation of the bronchopulmonary segmental anatomy follows (Fig. 15.4):

- *Coronal:* Anterior and posterior views demonstrate the lobar and segmental anatomy of the lungs. Note the asymmetry of right and left lung with middle lobe on right being equivalent to the lingula except the middle lobe bronchus arises from the lower lobe bronchus and the lingual from the upper lobe.

- *Sagittal:* Note superior segment of lower lobes appears in upper part of the lung fields. Both the middle lobe and lingual are anterior and medial and can be obscured by the cardiac silhouette if partially collapsed.

- *Axial transverse:* At T3/4 level and sternoclavicular joints, this shows great vessels, trachea, esophagus, upper lobe segments. Midline structures are bronchiocephalic arterial trunk, trachea, esophagus with thoracic duct and nodes to left.

N-oncoanatomy

The parallelism of the branching intrapulmonary bronchiole tree and the intrapulmonary nodes are presented according to the International Anatomical Terminology designation and contrasted with AJCC numbering of lymph node stations. The interstitial pulmonary lymphatics are usually visible under certain abnormal pathophysiologic circumstances. The most peripheral lymph nodes are intrapulmonary segmental or subsegmental lymph nodes (Fig. 15.5; Table 15.2).

M-oncoanatomy

By definition, BACs can only invade the lung by so-called lepidic spread, wherein local segmental collapse occurs or an extensive pneumonitic invasion appears. This unique obliteration of intrapulmonary airways is lethal when extensive, multifocal, and mimics bronchiolitis obliterans. The destruction of multiple separate

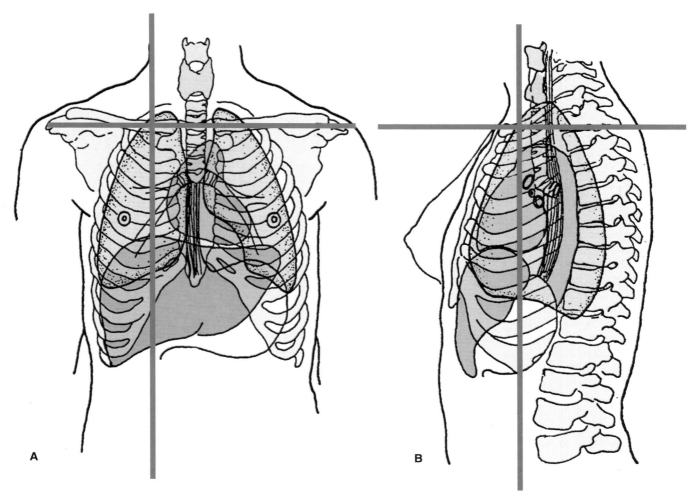

Figure 15.3 Orientation of T-oncoanatomy. A. Coronal. The anatomic isocenter is in the peripheral region of the lung. **B.** Sagittal. The anatomic isocenter is at transverse thoracic vertebral level T3/T4 at thoracic inlet.

synchronous primaries versus metastatic spread is often applied to BACs. The key anatomic fact is the two lesions cannot share the same lymph node drainage and no lymph nodes be involved (see Fig. 13.6 and Table 13.5).

- *Coronal view:* The segmental bronchi are illustrated with their pulmonary segment. The right side has 10 and the left 8. Each bronchopulmonary segment has a tertiary bronchus, the portion of lung it ventilates an artery, a vein, and bronchopulmonary nodes.

- *Sagittal view:* Note the apical segment of lower lobes are in the superior half of the lung. The middle lobe on the right corresponds to diaphragm except the apical segment.

Rules for Classification and Staging

Clinical Staging and Imaging

The TNM classification system is primarily for staging non–small cell lung cancers. The most important change

dates back to the fourth edition of the AJCC where T3, resectable disease, was distinguished from T4, unresectable disease. Simultaneously, a greater reliance on more sophisticated imaging has occurred. It is with the sixth edition that computed tomography (CT) and positron emission topography (PET) are allowed. The imaging modalities for detection and diagnosis apply to staging (see Fig. 13.6). Chest films and CT (preferably spiral) are essential steps in both the diagnosis and staging. PET combined with CT is utilized to overcome motion artifacts. Magnetic resonance imaging (MRI) is useful for mediastinal evaluation. Another advantage of CT over MRI for staging is that it allows for metastatic workup of lung, liver, adrenal, ribs, and vertebrae, especially for Pancoast cancers.

Pathologic Staging

All pathologic specimens from clinical invasive procedures—bronchoscopy, mediastinoscopy, mediastinotomy, thoracentesis, and thorascopy—are applicable.

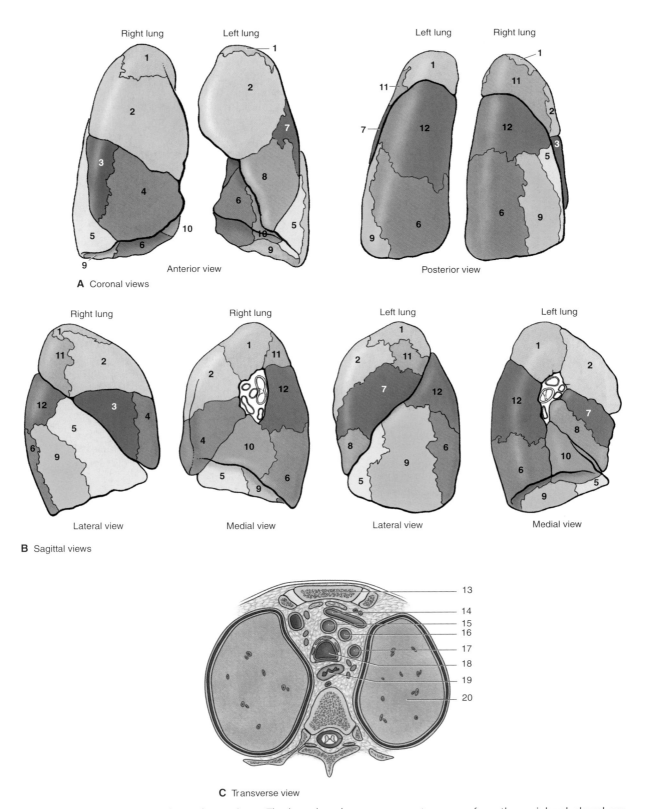

C Transverse view

Figure 15.4 **T-oncoanatomy three-planar views.** The bronchopulmonary segments as seen from the peripheral pleural sur-face of the lung (see text). **A.** Coronal anterior and posterior views. **B.** Sagittal medial and lateral views. **C.** Transverse: T3/T4 level and sternoclavicular joints. (1) Apical. (2) Anterior. (3) Lateral. (4) Medial. (5) Anterior basal. (6) Posterior basal. (7) Supe-rior lingular. (8) Inferior lingular. (9) Lateral basal. (10) Medial basal. (11) Posterior. (12) Superior. (13) Manubrium of sternum. (14) Left brachiocephalic vein. (15) Brachiocephalic trunk. (16) Left common carotid. (17) Left subclavian artery. (18) Trachea. (19) Esophagus. (20) Lung.

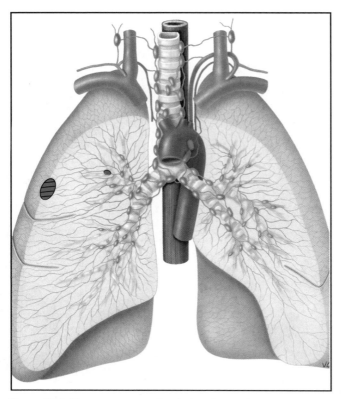

Figure 15.5 N-oncoanatomy. Sentinel nodes can be intrapulmonary nodes or interlobar bronchial nodes but are uncommon.

The thoracotomy and resection of primary and lymph nodes are the mainstay of pathologic staging. Preferably, six nodes should be examined. Surgical resection of primary and regional nodes needs to be carefully evaluated at bronchial stump for adequate margins. All resected nodes should be numbered according to AJCC system and assessed for tumor.

Cancer Statistics and Survival

According to Surveillance Epidemiology and End Results data based on 16,000 patients, the relative 5-year survival is 8% to 10% and 10-year survival 5% to 7%. Surprisingly, there is a small attrition for 5-year survivors; 70% are alive at 10 years. Females, good Karnofsky performance status, and cessation of smoking contribute to longer survival.

Staging is a major factor in survival and the data present the findings in Table 15.3 and Table 15.4. For stage IA cancers, the 90% T1 N0 M0 patient decreases to 61% at 5 years and stage IB 70% at 1 year is almost halved at 5 years at 38%. The 50% 5-year survival for stage I decreases to 30%, indicating metastatic disease is highly likely. Stage IIIA represents the most favorable advanced disease patients, with 50% 1-year survival and, despite vigorous chemoradiation, only decreases to 10%. For surgically staged IIIA patients do better as expected, with 25% alive at 5 years.

BACs have the best 5-year survival rates (65%) as compared to other histologics (Tables 15.3 and 15.4).

TABLE 15.2	Lymph Nodes of the Lung

Sentinel nodes are intrapulmonary nodes and interlobar bronchial nodes.

N1 nodes: All N1 nodes lie distal to the mediastinal pleural reflection and *within the visceral pleura.*

Hilar nodes
Interlobar nodes
Lobar nodes bronchi
Segmental nodes
Subsegmental nodes

N2 nodes: All N2 nodes lie within the mediastinal pleural envelope on the ipsilateral side.

Highest mediastinal nodes
Upper paratracheal nodes
Prevascular and retrotracheal nodes
Lower paratracheal nodes
Subaortic nodes (aortopulmonary window)
Para-aortic nodes (ascending aorta or phrenic)
Subcarinal nodes
Paraesophageal nodes (below carina)
Pulmonary ligament nodes

TABLE 15.3	Clinical and Pathological Surgical Survival Results by Stage of Non–Small Cell Lung Cancer				
		Clinical		Surgical	
Stage	TNM	1-Year Survival (%)	5-Year Survival (%)	1-Year Survival (%)	5-Year Survival (%)
IA	T1, N0, M0	91	61	94	67
IB	T2, N0, M0	72	38	87	57
IIA	T1, N1, M0	79	34	89	55
IIB	T2, N1, M0	61	25	78	39
	T3, NO, M0	55	22	76	38
IIIA	T3, N1, M0	56	9	65	25
	T1-2-3, N2, M0	50	13	64	23
IIIB/IV	T4, N0-1-2, M0	37	7		
	Any T, N3, M0	32	3		
	Any T, Any N, M1	20	5		

T, tumor; N, node; M, metastasis.
Modified from Mountain CF: Revisions in the international system for staging lung cancer. *Chest* 1997;111:1710–1717.

TABLE 15.4	Five-Year Relative Survival Rates for Non–Small Cell Lung Cancer by Histology				
		5-Year Survival (%)			
Histologic Type	No. of Cases	All Stages	Local	Regional	Distant
All carcinomas	87,128	13.9	39.6	14.4	1.5
Squamous cell carcinoma	26,407	16.5	34.3	14.9	1.5
Adenocarcinoma, NOS	20,991	46.6	49.9	16.1	1.5
Bronchioalveolar carcinoma	2,382	42.1	65.1	31.8	4.2
Papillary adenocarcinoma	568	23.7	57.4*	25.8	5.4
Adenosquamous carcinoma	1,056	21.6	49.6	19.1	2.2
Small cell carcinoma	10,656	4.6	12.3	7.5	1.4
Large cell carcinoma	7,592	11.4	34.8	13.2	1.6

NOS, not otherwise specified.
*Standard error >5% and ≤10%.
Modified from Travis WD, Travis LB, DeVessa SS: Lung cancer. *Cancer* 1995;75(1 suppl):191–198. Reproduced by permission of Wiley-Liss, Inc., a subsidiary of John Wiley & Sons, Inc.

16

Adenocarcinoma

The adenocarcinomas (ADCs) arise from the intrapul-monary bronchi that branch like limbs of a tree in each lung dividing into segmental and subsegmental bronchi.

Perspective and Patterns of Spread

Adenocarcinomas (ADC) are the most common histopathologic type of lung cancer, and have gradually exceeded squamous cell cancers in the past two decades. *The mucosal lining of the respiratory epithelium of the major bronchi is a pseudostratified ciliated columnar epithelium with goblet cells, which constitute 30% of the total cell population.* They produce the mucinogen secretions and provide the mucin lubrication when released in an aqueous environment. These gland-forming ADC cells tend to give rise to four subtypes or variants ranging from well-differentiated ADCs with abundant mucous production to undifferentiated varieties that tend to lose their glandular arrangement (Table 16.1).

These cancers tend to be pulmonary in the more pe-ripheral regions, arising in the lobar bronchi (Fig. 16.1), which is also a major factor in determining their clini-cal presentation. They are the predominant female lung cancer (69%) and constitute 45% of male lung cancers. ADCs arise in lobar bronchi, which is the key determi-nant in their clinical presentation and pattern of spread. *Because the lobar and segmental bronchi are the scaffolding for the lung, such cancers trigger segmental or lobar collapse or obstructive pneumonitis, which are more peripheral in lo-cation and do not extend beyond the lung hilus.*

The precursor lesion for pulmonary adenocarcinoma is believed to be atypical alveolar hyperplasia (ALH), typ-ically a coincidental finding in resected lung lobes. AAH is composed of proliferating Type II pneumocytes and associated with bronchioloalveolar cancer. Genetic and cytologic features often overlap making histologic dis-tinction difficult between bronchioloalveolar cancer and adenocarcinoma. Only 1–5% of AAH progress to adeno-carcinoma over a period of years.

TNM Staging Criteria

In their earliest stages, ADCs can be detected as pul-monary lesions T1 (<3 cm) or T2 (>3 cm) that are

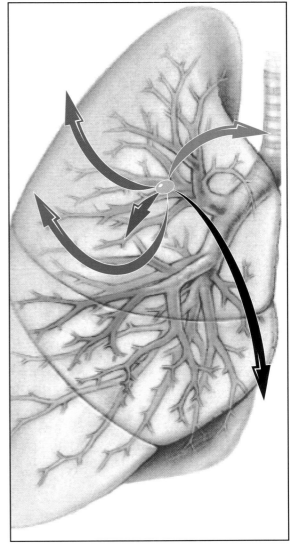

Figure 16.1 **Patterns of spread.** The primary cancer (ADC) invades in various directions, which are color coded for T stage: Tis, yellow; T1, green; T2, blue; T3, purple; T4, red; and metastatic, black.

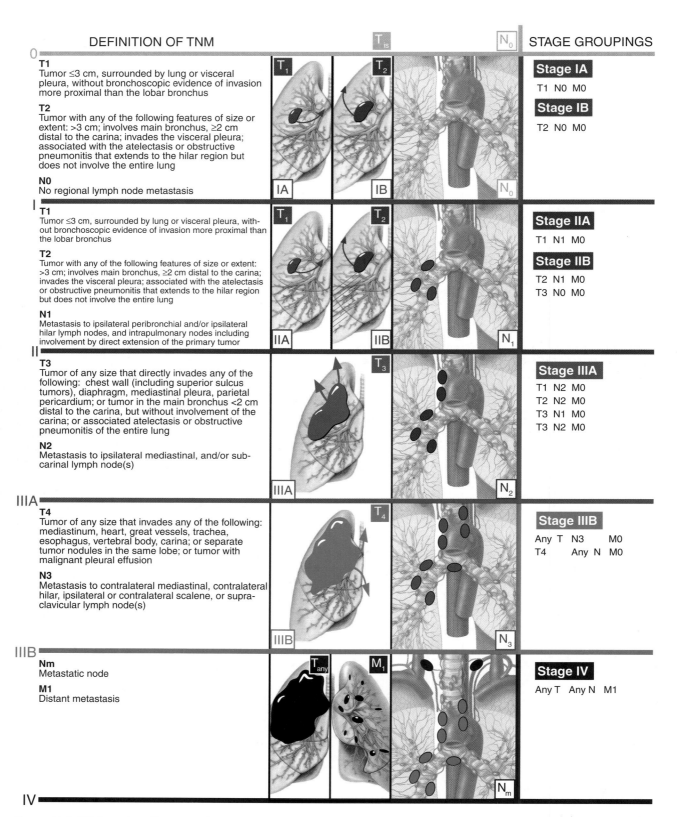

Figure 16.2 TNM staging diagram. Adenocarcinomas are peripheral arising in segmental bronchi and tend to be associated with atelectasis or obstructive pneumonitis. Vertical presentation of stage groupings, which follow same color code for cancer advancement are organized in horizontal lanes: Stage 0, yellow; I, green; II, blue; IIIA, purple; IIIB, red and metastatic stage IV, black. Definitions of TN on left and stage grouping on right.

TABLE 16.1	Histopathologic Type
Main Pathologic Cell Type	**Variant**
ADC	Acinar
ADC with mixed subtypes	Papillary Well differentiated fetal ADC Mucinous ("colloid") ADC Mucinous cystadenocarcinoma Signet ring ADC Clear cell ADC
ADC, adenocarcinoma.	

intrapulmonary. The lung segments that collapse or consolidate do not extend beyond the hilar region medially. *Such cancers lead to persistence or recurrence of symptoms and signs, namely, obstructive pneumonitis.* The pathology does not extend beyond the visceral pleura laterally. Their stage categories have been consistent over the past decade and their associated findings are highlighted in Figure 16.2. The color code corresponds to basic key, but T4 lesions are noted in red and black, with the malignant gradient being highest with mediastinal visceral invasions. The distinction between T3 and T4 occurred in the fourth edition (1992). T3 cancers do not extend to the chest wall parietal pleura and are limited in extent to the visceral pleura. The stigmata of T4, unresectable cancer, are due to invasion of mediastinal viscera as heart, esophagus, and vital structures as great vessels, aorta, and vena cava.

Summary of Changes

There have been no changes from the fifth edition of the AJCC CSM.

Orientation of Three-planar Oncoanatomy

The isocenter chosen relates to the branching lobar and segmental bronchi. The three-planar levels are chosen at thorax T4/T5 level. The plane at this level divides the superior and inferior mediastinum. It is central to understanding the thoracic anatomy (Fig. 16.3).

T-oncoanatomy

The bronchial tree in which ADCs arise branches throughout the pulmonary parenchyma undergoing 10 orders of division. The trachea, which lies in the superior mediastinum, divides into right and left main stem bronchi that extend into the right and left lungs. At that point, they divide into lobar bronchi for the upper, middle, and lower lobes on the right, and the upper and lower lobes on the left. Each lobar bronchus divides in to segmental bronchi (Fig. 16.4).

The lobes of the lung are divided into bronchopulmonary segments (10 per lung) and are defined by the branching of the segmental bronchi. The mucosa lining the bronchus is the usual site of origin for cancer of the lung, although cancer also may arise in the more peripheral areas of the bronchiolar tree.

Of particular interest are both the symmetry and asymmetry that exists between various portions of the left and right lung and the bronchial trees. The projection of the lower lobe lesions in the upper half of the lung emphasizes the need to understand this complex anatomy. It is important to be familiar with the lung lobes in different projections when viewed anteriorly and posteriorly as well as their lateral and medial faces to recognize obstructive pneumonitis on chest films.

The right lung has three lobes and the left lung has two lobes. The middle lobe in the right side arises from the lower lobe bronchus, whereas the lingula or the left side, which corresponds to the middle lobe, arises from the upper lobe bronchus. Major and segmental bronchi are presented in Figure 16.4.

- *Coronal:* Anterior view demonstrates the lobar and segmental anatomy of the bronchial tree. Note the asymmetry of right and left lung with middle lobe on right being equivalent to the lingula except the middle lobe bronchus arises from the lower lobe bronchus and the lingual from the upper lobe.

- *Transverse* (Fig. 16.4): This T4/T5 level is at the plane dividing the mediastinum. Note broadening of the trachea at the carina, the azygos vein arching into the superior vena cava on the left and the arch of the aorta, and the entry of its three major arteries—the brachiocephalic, common carotid, and subclavian. The thoracic duct is in the left.

N-oncoanatomy

The intrapulmonary lymph nodes are designated by their relationship to the bronchial tree and are referred to as lobar nodes bronchi on interlobar lymph nodes, which then drain to hilar nodes (Fig. 16.5). The AJCC

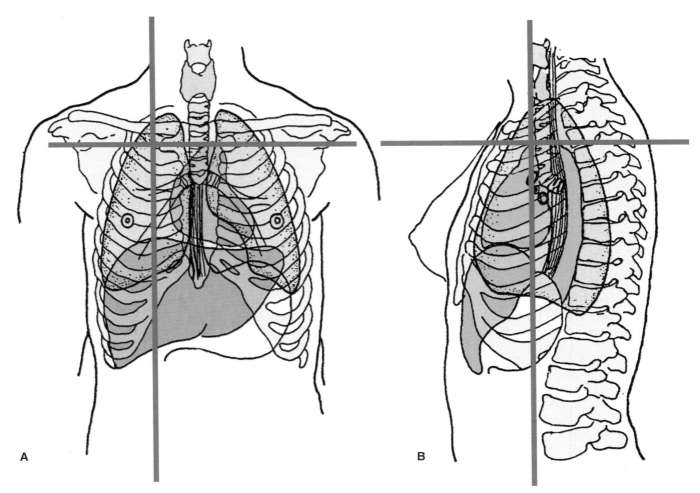

Figure 16.3 Orientation of T-oncoanatomy. A. Coronal. **B.** Sagittal. The anatomic isocenter for three-planar oncoanatomy is placed at the thoracic vertebral level T4/T5.

diagram (Fig. 13.5B) emphasizes the pleural encasement line that separates the aforementioned lymph nodes: (N1) intrapleural (visceral pleura) and intrapulmonary lymph nodes in contrast to the (N2) extrapleural mediastinal lymph nodes that lie within the mediastinal pleura (parietal pleura). N1 hilar nodes are readily resected, whereas ipsilateral (N2A) mediastinal nodes are more marginal and when they are contralateral (N2B) are inaccessible and not worth resecting. The tabulation of regional nodes is noted in Table 16.2.

M-oncoanatomy

The M-oncoanatomy emphasizes the pulmonary venous drainage, which is oxygenated, drains the pulmonary parenchymal cancers and disseminates cells to many remote anatomic states by way of the left side of the heart. Virtually every remote organ site can be involved and include liver, adrenal, bones, and brain (see Fig. 13.5). The distribution of distant metastases is noted in Table 13.5.

Rules for Classification and Staging

Clinical Staging and Imaging

The TNM classification system is primarily for staging non–small cell lung cancers. The most important change dates back to the fourth edition of the American Joint Committee on Cancer (AJCC), where T3, resectable disease, was distinguished from T4, unresectable disease. Simultaneously, a greater reliance on more sophisticated imaging has occurred. It is with the sixth edition that computed tomography (CT) and positron emission topography (PET) are allowed. The imaging modalities for detection and diagnosis apply to staging (see Table 13.6). Chest films and CT (preferably spiral) are essential steps in both the diagnosis and staging. PET combined with CT is utilized to overcome motion artifacts. Magnetic resonance imaging (MRI) is useful for mediastinal evaluation. Another advantage of CT over MRI for staging is that it allows for metastatic workup of lung, liver, adrenal, ribs, and vertebrae, especially for Pancoast cancers.

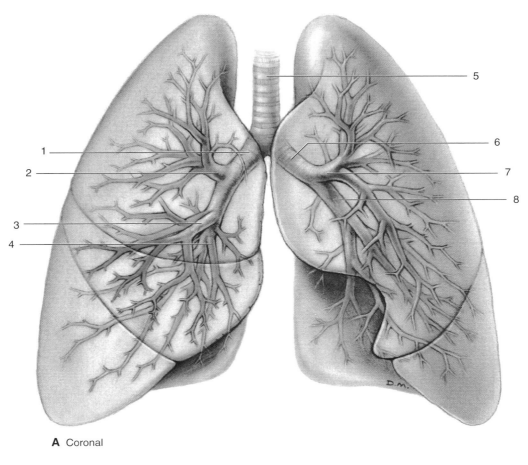

A Coronal

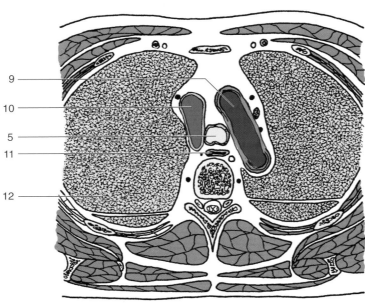

B Transverse

Figure 16.4 **T-oncoanatomy three-planar views.** The bronchopulmonary segments are shown as seen from the peripheral pleural surface of the lung (see text). **A.** Coronal. **B.** Transverse. (1) Right main bronchus. (2) Right superior lobar bronchus. (3) Right middle lobar bronchus. (4) Right lower lobar bronchus. (5) Trachea. (6) Left main bronchus. (7) Left superior lobar bronchus. (8) Left inferior lobar bronchus. B. (9) Aortic arch. (10) Superior vena cava. (11) Esophagus. (12) Right lung.

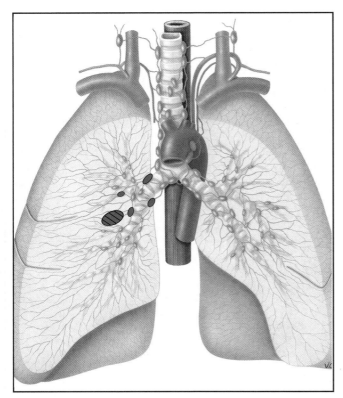

Figure 16.5 N-oncoanatomy. Interlobar bronchial nodes and hilar nodes are sentinel nodes within visceral pleura.

Pathologic Staging

All pathologic specimens from clinical invasive procedures—bronchoscopy, mediastinoscopy, mediastinotomy, thoracentesis, and thorascopy—are applicable to pathologic stage. Thoracotomy and resection of primary

and lymph nodes are the mainstay of pathologic staging. Margin status and any residual cancer need to be noted. Preferably, six nodes should be examined.

Surgical resection of primary and regional nodes needs to be carefully evaluated at bronchial stump for adequate margins. All resected nodes should be numbered according to AJCC system and assessed for tumor.

Oncoimaging Annotations

- Chest radiographs seldom detect primary lung cancers in their early stages.
- Spiral CT is useful in high-risk patients to detect nodule and infiltrates.
- PET imaging with ^{18}FDG appears to be of value in discriminating malignant versus benign nodules.
- CT can detect and mediastinal adenopathy, but histologic verification is essential to ascertain if it is malignant.
- Determining N2 versus N3 mediastinal nodes is important; it establishes resectability.
- MRI can be of value in assessing mediastinal invasion, chest wall and rib erosion, and compromised large vein involvement.
- ADCs are the most common lung cancers and often involve lobar bronchi with associated atelectasis extending to hilus.
- CT cannot distinguish mass from associated lobar collapse or pneumonitis.
- Irregular cavitation of abscess wall suggests cancer and is more frequently associated with squamous cell cancer.

TABLE 16.2	Lymph Nodes of Lung

Interlobar bronchial nodes and hilar nodes are sentinel nodes within visceral pleura.

N1 nodes: All N1 nodes lie distal to the mediastinal pleural reflection and *within the visceral pleura.*

Hilar nodes
Interlobar nodes
Lobar nodes bronchi
Segmental nodes
Subsegmental nodes

N2 nodes: All N2 nodes lie within the mediastinal pleural envelope on the ipsilateral side.

Highest mediastinal nodes
Upper paratracheal nodes
Prevascular and retrotracheal nodes
Lower paratracheal nodes
Subaortic nodes (aortopulmonary window)
Para-aortic nodes (ascending aorta or phrenic)
Subcarinal nodes
Paraesophageal nodes (below carina)
Pulmonary ligament nodes

Cancer Statistics and Survival

According to Surveillance Epidemiology and End Results data based on 16,000 patients, the relative 5-year survival is 8% to 10% and 10-year survival 5% to 7%. Surprisingly, there is a small attrition for 5-year survivors, with the majority 70% alive at 10 years. Females, good Karnofsky performance status, and cessation of smoking contribute to longer survival.

Staging is a major factor in survival and the data analyzed by Mountain present the findings in Figure 13.6 and Table 15.3. For stage IA cancers, the 90% survival rate for the T1 N0 M0 patient decreases to 61% at 5 years; for stage IB, survival is 70% at 1 year and almost halved at 5 years, to 38%. The 50% 5-year survival for stage I decreases to 30%, indicating that once hilar nodes are positive, metastatic disease is highly likely. Stage IIIA represents the most favorable advanced disease patients with 50% 1-year survival and, despite vigorous chemoradiation, only decreases to 10%. Surgically staged IIIA patients do better as expected, with 25% alive at 5 years.

Specifically, when 5-year relative survival rates for lung cancer by histology are considered (see Table 15.4), the average is 13.9% for all stages. The most favorable bronchioloalveolar is 42%, but when localized is as high as 65%. For the common non–small cell cancers, squamous cell cancer and ADCs are close to overall average at 15.4% and 16.6%, respectively. As expected, anaplastic dedifferentiated cancers do extremely poorly, that is, large cell and small cell anaplastic yield 11.6% and 4.6%, respectively.

17

Large Cell Anaplastic Cancer

Large cell anaplastic cancers arise in more proximal bronchi and have a proclivity to invade mediastinal structures early.

Perspective and Patterns of Spread

Large cell anaplastic (LCA) cancers are those cancers that are distinguished from small cell anaplastic cancers by numerous morphologic variants: Large cell neuroendocrine, basaloid carcinoma, lymphoepithelioma-like, and clear cell or large cell with rhabdoid phenotype (Table 17.1). It is not a common cancer type, accounting for 5% to 10% of lung cancers, *distinguished by its propensity to invade the mediastinum pleura and pericardium.* A paradox to ponder is the resistance of the heart to direct invasion despite circulating cancer cells, especially from lung cancers, recognizing that the endocardium is never seeded and that myocardial nodulation is more often recognized and found only at post mortem. Because most LCAs are undifferentiated, vascular infiltration occurs with rapid systemic dissemination to remote sites (Fig. 17.1; Table 17.1).

TNM Staging Criteria

As thoracic surgery improved, the need for defining criteria of unresectability became evident. The distinction between T3 and T4 entered the American Joint Committee on Cancer (AJCC)/International Union Against Cancer staging in its fourth edition (1982), as did more researched biologic and molecular markers to distinguish small cell anaplastic cancers from its variants. T4 stage applies to any tumor regardless of size that invaded any of the following: Mediastinum, heart, great vessels, trachea, esophagus, vertebral body, or malignant effusion with positive cells identified after both pleural and pericardial taps (Fig. 17.2).

Summary of Changes

There have been no changes from the fifth edition of the AJCC CSM.

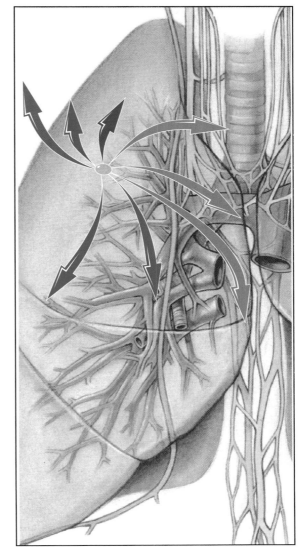

Figure 17.1 **Patterns of spread.** The primary cancer invades in various directions, which are color-coded for T stage: Tis, yellow; T1, green; T2, blue; T3, purple; T4, red; and when metastatic, black.

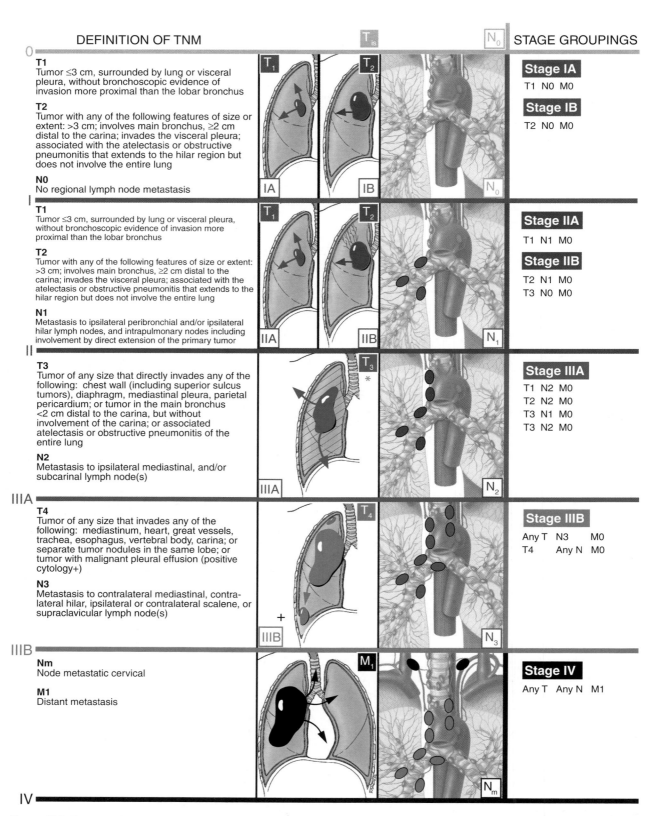

Figure 17.2 TNM staging diagram. Large cell anaplastic cancers are variants and aggressive cancers with invasive qualities often with neuroendocrine effects. Vertical presentation of stage groupings, which follow same color code for cancer advancement are organized in horizontal lanes: Stage 0, yellow; I, green; II, blue; IIIA, purple; IIIB, red and metastatic stage IV, black. Definitions of TN on left and stage grouping on right.

TABLE 17.1	Histopathologic Type
Main Pathologic Cell Type	**Variant**
Large cell carcinoma	Large cell neuroendocrine carcinoma
	Combined large cell neuroendocrine carcinoma
	Basaloid carcinoma
	Lymphepithelioma-like carcinoma
	Clear cell carcinoma
	Large cell carcinoma with rhabdoid phenotype

Orientation of Three-planar Oncoanatomy

Large cell anaplastic cancers can arise throughout the bronchial tree and its isocenter has been assigned to thoracic T6/T7 level posteriorly and to the fourth rib articulation with the sternum at the level of the horizontal fissure on the right and the cardiac contour on the left (Fig. 17.3).

T-oncoanatomy

T-oncoanatomy focuses on the left side of the mediastinum featuring the ascending aorta and descending aorta. The major nerves coursing into the thorax are the focus of the three-planar views indicating where they are vulnerable to compression or invasion (Fig. 17.4).

- *Coronal:* At the thoracic inlet the vagus nerve (cranial nerve X) enters the chest, but the recurrent laryngeal loops around the right subclavian whereas on the left it loops around the aortic arch. Compression on the right is anticipated with metastatic right supraclavicular and scalene nodes. On the left, the more common event is for mediastinal nodes to invade the recurrent laryngeal at the aortic pulmonary window. The anterior and posterior pulmonary plexus receiving sympathetic contributions from the right and left sympathetic trunks (second to fifth thoracic ganglia), and parasympathetic contributions from the right and left vagus nerves. The right and left vagus nerves passing inferiorly from the posterior pulmonary plexus to contribute fibers to the esophageal plexus. Branches from the pulmonary plexuses continuing along the bronchi and pulmonary vasculature to the lungs. The phrenic nerve passes anterior to the root of the lung to the diaphragm.
- *Sagittal:* The left side of the mediastinum is the "red side," dominated by the arch and descending portion of the aorta and the left common carotid and subclavian arteries, which obscures the trachea from view. The left vagus nerve passes posterior to the root of the lung, sending its recurrent laryngeal branch around the ligamentum arteriosum inferior, then medial to

the aortic arch. The phrenic nerve passes anterior to the root of the lung and penetrates the diaphragm more anteriorly than on the right side.

- *Transverse:* Note the juxtaposition of the ascending and descending aorta with the carina at the T5 level.

N-oncoanatomy

The first station lymph nodes are the intrapulmonary, pulmonary, and bronchopulmonary lymph nodes, which are contained within the visceral pleural reflection. There are three major collecting trunks; the superior, middle, and inferior trunks. These drain into 10 to 15 peribronchial nodes and then to hilar nodes. Second station lymph nodes are those in the mediastinum and may be paraesophageal, subcarinal, or paratracheal; and pretracheal or retrotracheal in location. Involvement of scalene, cervical, supraclavicular, and axillary nodes is considered distant metastases (Fig. 17.5, Table 17.2).

M-oncoanatomy

The vasculature of the lung is rich. The microcirculation is intimately organized into the alveolar matrix and originates from two separate circulations—the bronchial arteries and the pulmonary arteries. However, all the blood is gathered and returned by the pulmonary veins (Fig. 17.6). The anatomic distribution of distant metastases is shown in Table 13.5.

There is a major difference between the bronchial and pulmonary arteries. The pulmonary arteries are essentially venous blood carrying the right heart output into the lungs for aeration. Similarly, the pulmonary vein, unlike other veins in the body, has well-oxygenated blood carrying blood from the lungs to the left heart for injection into the general circulation. The bronchial arteries rise from the aorta and, therefore, carry oxygenated blood. An important feature of staging is the difference between T3 and T4 cancers. Once cancers penetrate both visceral and parietal pleura, respectively, they infiltrate into the costal hemiazygos veins, then caval veins and reenter the pulmonary circulation. The

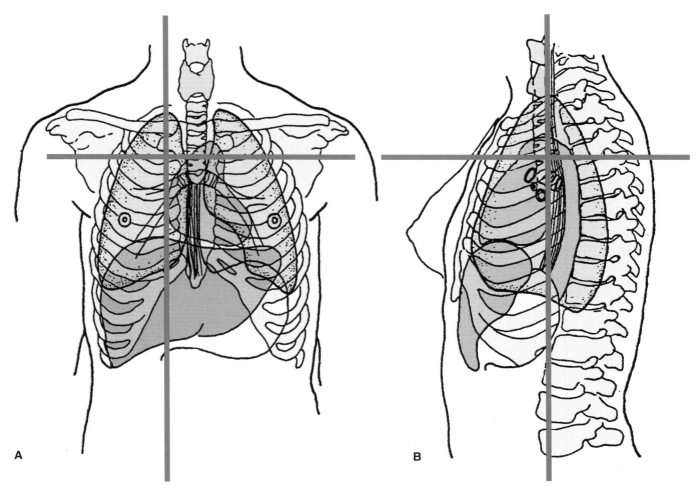

Figure 17.3 Orientation of T-oncoanatomy. The isocenter is shifted to the left lung and is at the T6/T7 level to focus on the nerves entering the thorax and their course. **A.** Coronal. **B.** Sagittal.

lungs become the target organ for their own metastatic spread.

Rules for Classification and Staging

Clinical Staging and Imaging

The TNM Classification system is primarily for staging non–small cell lung cancers. The most important change dates back to the fourth edition of the AJCC, where T3, resectable disease, was distinguished from T4, unresectable disease. Simultaneously, a greater reliance on more sophisticated imaging has occurred. It is with the sixth edition that computed tomography (CT) and positron emission topography (PET) are allowed. The imaging modalities for detection and diagnosis apply to staging (see Table 17.6). Chest films and CT (preferably spiral) are essential steps in both diagnosis and staging. PET combined with CT is utilized to overcome motion artifacts. Magnetic resonance imaging (MRI) is useful for mediastinal evaluation. Another advantage of CT over

MRI for staging is that it allows for metastatic workup of lung, liver, adrenal, ribs, and vertebrae, especially for Pancoast cancers.

Pathologic Staging

All pathologic specimens from clinical invasive procedures—bronchoscopy, mediastinoscopy, mediastinotomy, thoracentesis, and thorascopy—are applicable to pathologic stage. Thoracotomy and resection of primary and lymph nodes are the mainstay of pathologic staging. Margin status and any residual cancer needs to be noted. Preferably, six nodes should be examined.

Oncoimaging Annotations

- Chest radiographs seldom detect primary lung cancers in their early stages.
- Spiral CT is useful in high-risk patients to detect nodule and infiltrates.
- PET imaging with [18]FDG appears to be of value in discriminating malignant versus benign nodules.

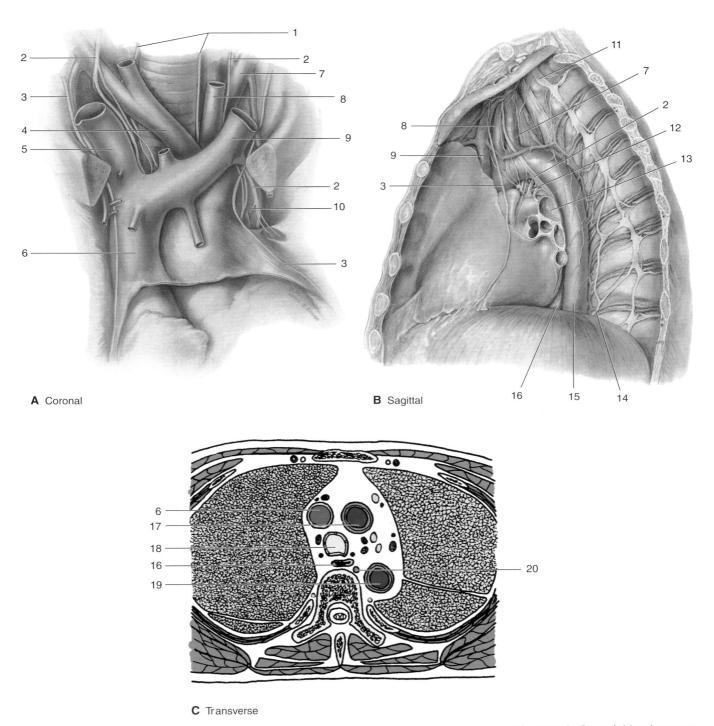

A Coronal

B Sagittal

C Transverse

Figure 17.4 **T-oncoanatomy three-planar views.** At the thoracic inlet a number of important nerves gain entry. **A.** Coronal. Most important is the vagus (cranial nerve X), which enters in the carotid sheath on the right side, the recurrent laryngeal nerve courses beneath and around the subclavian artery. The left recurrent laryngeal on left descends and circles the aortic arch. **B.** Sagittal. The phrenic nerve is most anterior, passing in front of the lung root and the sympathetic chain of ganglion are posterior paralleling the descending aorta. Note the juxtaposition of the pericardial and pleural space with lower lobe invasion of mediastinal pleura. **C.** Transverse. (1) Recurrent laryngeal nerves. (2) Vagus nerve. (3) Phrenic nerve. (4) Brachiocephalic artery. (5) Right brachiocephalic vein. (6) Superior vena cava. (7) Left subclavian artery. (8) Left common carotid artery. (9) Left brachiocephalic vein. (10) Left recurrent laryngeal nerve. (11) Sympathetic trunk. (12) Ligamentum arteriosum. (13) Left pulmonary artery. (14) Greater splanchnic nerve. (15) Aorta. (16) Esophagus. (17) Ascending aorta. (18) Trachea. (19) Descending aorta. (20) Thoracic (lymphatic) duct.

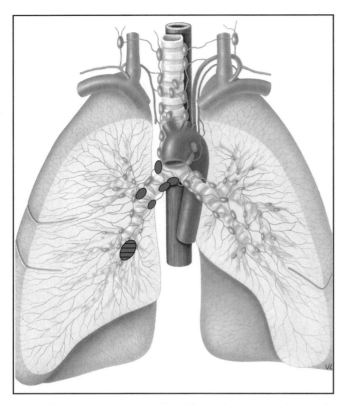

Figure 17.5 N-oncoanatomy. The hilar and coronal nodes are the sentinel nodes. However, if lower lobe cancers invade the mediastinum directly, the posterior mediastinal nodes are at risk. If the diaphragm is invaded directly, posterior and inferior mediastinal nodes are the sentinel nodes.

- CT can detect mediastinal adenopathy, but histologic verification is essential to ascertain if it is malignant.
- Determining N2 versus N3 mediastinal nodes is important; it establishes resectability.
- MRI can be of value in assessing mediastinal invasion, chest wall and rib erosion, and compromised large vein involvement.
- CT staging should include liver and adrenal glands by extending chest examinations. Most adrenal enlargements are benign and require biopsy or MRI to establish metastatic cancer.

Cancer Statistics and Survival

According to Surveillance Epidemiology and End Results data based on 16,000 patients, the relative 5-year survival is 8% to 10% and 10-year survival 5% to 7%. Surprisingly, there is a small attrition for 5-year survivors, with the majority 70% alive at 10 years. Females, good Karnofsky performance status, and cessation of smoking contribute to longer survival.

Staging is a major factor in survival and the data analyzed by Mountain present the findings in Figure 13.6 and Table 15.3. For stage IA cancers, the 90% survival rate for the T1 N0 M0 patient decreases to 61% at 5 years and for the stage IB patient, 70% survival at 1 year is almost halved at 5 years at 38%. The 50% 5-year survival for stage I decreases to 30%, indicating that once hilar nodes

TABLE 17.2	Lymph Nodes of Lung

The hilar and coronal nodes are the sentinel nodes. However, if lower lobe cancers invade the mediastinum directly, the posterior mediastinal nodes are at risk.

N1 nodes: All N1 nodes lie distal to the mediastinal pleural reflection and *within the visceral pleura.*

Hilar nodes
Interlobar nodes
Lobar nodes bronchi
Segmental nodes
Subsegmental nodes

N2 nodes: All N2 nodes lie within the mediastinal pleural envelope on the ipsilateral side.

Highest mediastinal nodes
Upper paratracheal nodes
Prevascular and retrotracheal nodes
Lower paratracheal nodes
Subaortic nodes (aortopulmonary window)
Para-aortic nodes (ascending aorta or phrenic)
Subcarinal nodes
Paraesophageal nodes (below carina)
Pulmonary ligament nodes

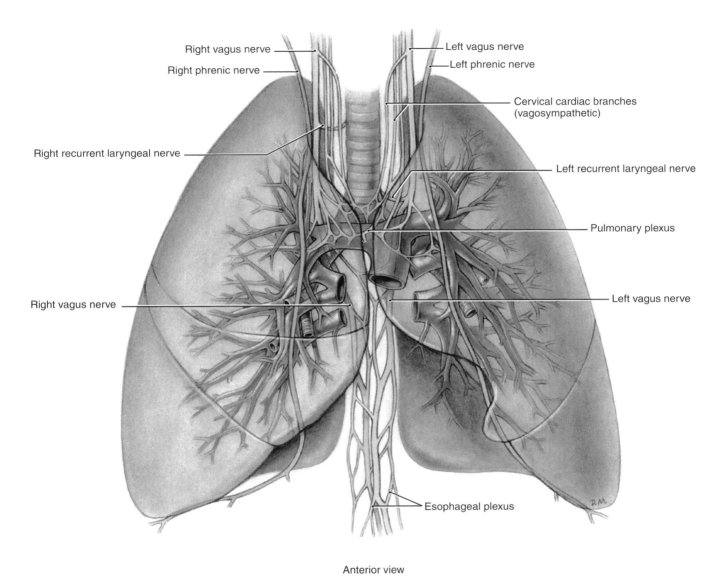

Right vagus nerve

Right phrenic nerve

Left vagus nerve

Left phrenic nerve

Cervical cardiac branches
(vagosympathetic)

Right recurrent laryngeal nerve

Left recurrent laryngeal nerve

Pulmonary plexus

Right vagus nerve

Left vagus nerve

Esophageal plexus

Anterior view

Figure 17.6 **M-oncoanatomy.** The pulmonary veins and arteries are shown with the phrenic nerve descending laterally to the diaphragm. The vagus nerve forms the esophageal plexus and the cervical sympathetics innervate the heart.

are positive, metastatic disease is highly likely. Stage IIIA represents the most favorable advanced disease patients with 50% 1-year survival and, despite vigorous chemoradiation, only decreases to 10%. Surgically staged IIIA patients do better, as expected, with 25% alive at 5 years.

Specifically, when 5-year relative survival rates for lung cancer by histology is considered in Table 15.4,

the average is 13.9% for all stages. The most favorable bronchioloalveolar is at 42%, but when localized is as high as 65%. For the common non–small cell cancers, squamous cell cancer and adenocarcinomas are close to overall average at 15.4% and 16.6%, respectively. As expected, anaplastic dedifferentiated cancers do extremely poorly, that is, large cell and small cell anaplastic yield 11.6% and 4.6%, respectively.

18

Squamous Cell Cancer

Squamous cell cancers are true bronchogenic carcinomas arising in major bronchi, which are extrapleural in location with an oxygenated arterial blood supply.

Perspective and Patterns of Spread

Squamous cell lung cancers (SQC) are often extrapulmonary cancers arising in the major bronchi—located in the mediastinum rather than lung parenchyma. The normal pseudostratified ciliated columnar epithelium with its different cell types undergoes metaplastic changes, losing its ciliation, secretory goblets, brush cells, and serous cells owing to smoking and its pollutants leading to a dry hacking "smoker's cough." As the patient's mucous thickens, his lungs and cough produce plugs of phlegm. The metaplastic changes in the columnar and cuboidal basal cells lead to stratified squamous dysplasia and, over time, to squamous cell neoplasia with malignant transformation. The epithelial surface breaks down with fine ulcerations and then rust-streaked sputum appears. The triad of coarse rhonchial breathing over a major bronchus, hemoptysis, and a long history of smoking virtually ensure a diagnosis of SQC, which can be readily confirmed with a chest film. Although SQCs at one time were the most common lung cancers (50%), they have been surpassed by adenocarcinomas, which now constitute the majority of histopathologic types (Table 18.1). The patterns of cancer invasion in major bronchi can result in dramatic obstruction, that is, complete atelectasis and collapse of one lung (Fig. 18.1).

TNM Staging Criteria

SQCs arise from metaplastic bronchial epithelium in major bronchi, which is specifically addressed, in the staging system in relationship to the carina (Fig. 18.2). T1 is an early intraluminal lesion <3 cm in diameter and >2 cm from carina. T2 is of larger size (>3 cm in diameter) and is <2 cm from carina without bronchial obstruction. Cavitation may occur due to the necrosis and is most often

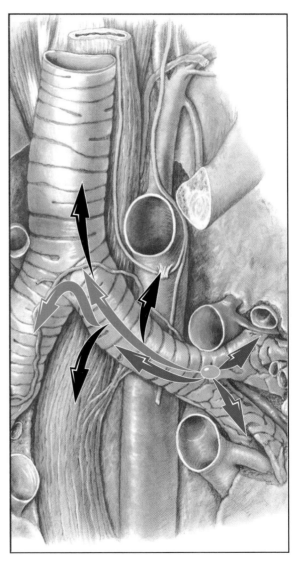

Figure 18.1 Patterns of spread. SQCs that arise in the major bronchi of lung are color coded for primary tumor spread to carina: Tis, yellow; T1, green (>2 cm); T2, blue (>2 cm) without obstruction of bronchus; T3, purple (<2 cm of carina with obstruction leading to complete lung collapse); T4, red (invading carina); M1, black (invading mediastinal structures).

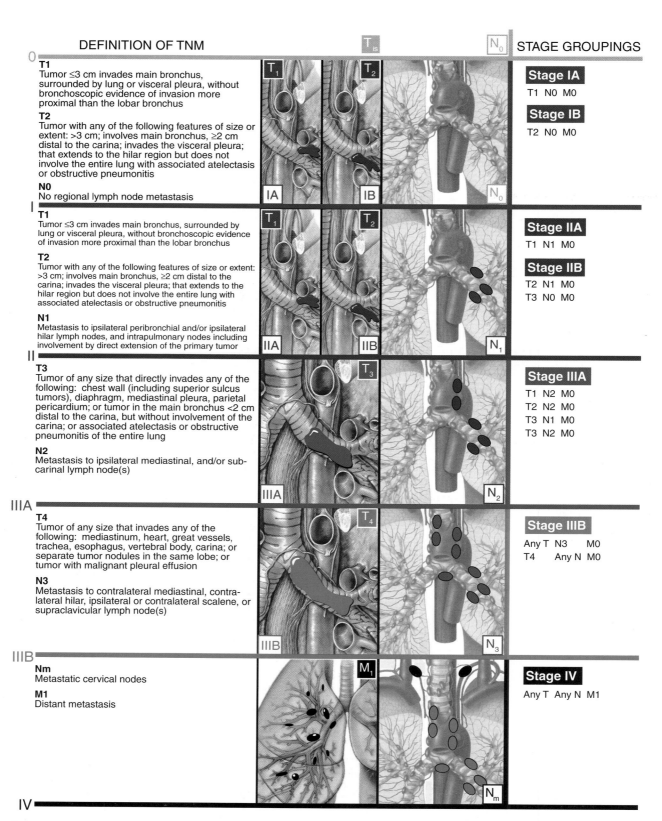

DEFINITION OF TNM

T1
Tumor ≤3 cm invades main bronchus, surrounded by lung or visceral pleura, without bronchoscopic evidence of invasion more proximal than the lobar bronchus

T2
Tumor with any of the following features of size or extent: >3 cm; involves main bronchus, ≥2 cm distal to the carina; invades the visceral pleura; that extends to the hilar region but does not involve the entire lung with associated atelectasis or obstructive pneumonitis

N0
No regional lymph node metastasis

T1
Tumor ≤3 cm invades main bronchus, surrounded by lung or visceral pleura, without bronchoscopic evidence of invasion more proximal than the lobar bronchus

T2
Tumor with any of the following features of size or extent: >3 cm; involves main bronchus, ≥2 cm distal to the carina; invades the visceral pleura; that extends to the hilar region but does not involve the entire lung with associated atelectasis or obstructive pneumonitis

N1
Metastasis to ipsilateral peribronchial and/or ipsilateral hilar lymph nodes, and intrapulmonary nodes including involvement by direct extension of the primary tumor

T3
Tumor of any size that directly invades any of the following: chest wall (including superior sulcus tumors), diaphragm, mediastinal pleura, parietal pericardium; or tumor in the main bronchus <2 cm distal to the carina, but without involvement of the carina; or associated atelectasis or obstructive pneumonitis of the entire lung

N2
Metastasis to ipsilateral mediastinal, and/or sub-carinal lymph node(s)

T4
Tumor of any size that invades any of the following: mediastinum, heart, great vessels, trachea, esophagus, vertebral body, carina; or separate tumor nodules in the same lobe; or tumor with malignant pleural effusion

N3
Metastasis to contralateral mediastinal, contra-lateral hilar, ipsilateral or contralateral scalene, or supraclavicular lymph node(s)

Nm
Metastatic cervical nodes

M1
Distant metastasis

STAGE GROUPINGS

Stage IA
T1 N0 M0

Stage IB
T2 N0 M0

Stage IIA
T1 N1 M0

Stage IIB
T2 N1 M0
T3 N0 M0

Stage IIIA
T1 N2 M0
T2 N2 M0
T3 N1 M0
T3 N2 M0

Stage IIIB
Any T   N3   M0
T4   Any N   M0

Stage IV
Any T Any N M1

Figure 18.2 TNM staging diagram. Squamous cell cancers arise in main and lobar bronchi in dysplastic epithelia that becomes neoplastic. Vertical presentation of stage groupings, which follow same color code for cancer advancement are organized in horizontal lanes: Stage 0, yellow; I, green; II, blue; IIIA, purple; IIIB, red; metastatic stage IV, black. Definitions of TN on left and stage grouping on right.

TABLE 18.1	Histopathologic Type	
Main Pathologic Cell Type		**Variant**
Squamous cell carcinoma		Papillary
		Clear cell
		Small cell
		Basaloid

occurs in SQC. T3 tumors either may occlude major stem bronchi, which may cause unilateral atelectasis and/or pneumonitis with complete collapse of an entire lung. When the cancer involves the carina or trachea, it becomes T4 and invariably invades paracarinal mediastinal nodes directly, Subcarinal, and/or contralateral nodes. The resectability of an entire lung depends on producing a well-healed stump and also providing a reasonable margin when SQC of the major bronchi approach the carina. A challenge indeed.

Summary of Changes

There have been no changes from the fifth edition of the AJCC CSM.

Orientation of Three-planar Oncoanatomy

The isocenter of the respiratory system is at the carina of the trachea and the origin of the main stem bronchi. *The isocenter of the main stem bronchi is inferior to the manubriosternal angle anteriorly and posteriorly the plane is at the thoracic vertebral level T5/T6.* The carina and 2 cm of the major bronchi are within the mediastinal pleural. The relationships of the bifurcation of the trachea built up segmentally from deep to superficial (Fig. 18.3).

T-oncoanatomy

SQC are often bronchogenic cancers involving the major bronchi, which are at the T5 level positioned inferior to the manubriosternal angle. A unique feature of this location is that the SQC are unlike other lung cancers, because they are supplied by oxygenated blood. The blood supply for SQCs is derived from the bronchial artery directly arising from the thoracic aorta. Cavitation may be more common in SQCs because its vascular attenuation may lead to severe hypoxia and necrosis. Other lung cancers, such as adenocarcinoma, are supplied with unoxygenated pulmonary arterial blood and may be more accustomed to hypoxic conditions (Fig. 18.4).

- *Coronal view:* The extrapulmonary portion of the bronchial tree is seen arising from the trachea at the carina. The left major bronchi is longer than the right, which immediately divides into right middle lobe, the bronchus intermedine, and right lower lobe with its own bronchi.

- *Sagittal view:* The hilus is a highly trafficked with pulmonary vessels anterior to the bronchi.

- *Axial view:* Pulmonary arteries dominate the middle mediastinum at the T5/T6 level along with the ascending aorta in the midline and the thoracic duct in the midline. The azygos vein enters the superior vena cava posteriorly. The descending aorta is the most posterior structure and on the left side in mediastinum.

N-oncoanatomy

Mediastinal supracarinal and subcarinal nodes rather than hilar nodes may be the first sentinel nodes because these cancers tend to be extrapulmonary and mediastinal in location. The three-planar views depict the mediastinal lymph nodes in the region of the major bronchi and carina (Fig. 18.5, Table 18.2).

M-oncoanatomy

The venous drainage is into the azygos system by bronchial veins with entry of circulating metastatic cells to the lung (see Fig. 13.5). The anatomic distribution of distant metastases is shown in Table 13.5.

Rules for Classification and Staging

Clinical Staging and Imaging

The TNM classification system is primarily for staging non–small cell lung cancers. The most important change dates back to the fourth edition of the American Joint Committee on Cancer where T3, resectable disease, was distinguished from T4, unresectable disease. Simultaneously, a greater reliance on more sophisticated imaging has occurred. It is with the sixth edition that computed tomography (CT) and positron emission topography (PET) are allowed. The imaging modalities for detection and diagnosis apply to staging (see Table 13.6). Chest films and CT (preferably spiral) are essential steps in both the diagnosis and staging. PET combined with CT is utilized to overcome motion artifacts. Magnetic resonance imaging (MRI) is useful for mediastinal

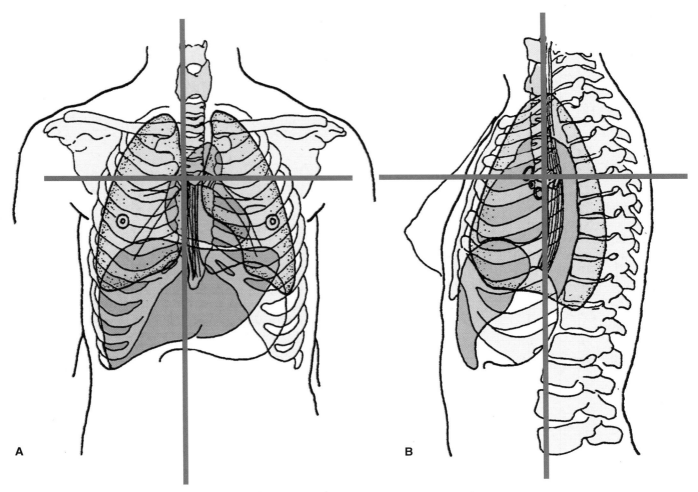

A   **B**

Figure 18.3 **Orientation of T-oncoanatomy.** The isocenter of the major bronchi are mid mediastinum and at the T5/T6 thoracic level. **A.** Coronal. **B.** Sagittal.

evaluation. Another advantage of CT over MRI for staging is that it allows for metastatic workup of lung, liver, adrenal, ribs, and vertebrae, especially for Pancoast cancers.

Pathologic Staging

All pathologic specimens from clinical invasive procedures—bronchoscopy, mediastinoscopy, mediastinotomy, thoracentesis, and thorascopy—are applicable to pathologic stage. Thoracotomy and resection of primary and lymph nodes are the mainstay of pathologic staging. Margin status and any residual cancer needs to be noted. Preferably, six nodes should be examined.

Oncoimaging Annotations

- Chest radiographs seldom detect primary lung cancers in their early stages.
- Spiral CT is useful in high-risk patients to detect nodules and infiltrates.

- PET imaging with [18]FDG appears to be of value in discriminating malignant versus benign nodules.
- CT can detect and mediastinal adenopathy, but histologic verification is essential to ascertain if it is malignant.
- Determining N2 versus N3 mediastinal nodes is important; it establishes resectability.
- MRI can be of value in assessing mediastinal invasion, chest wall and rib erosion, and compromised large vein involvement.
- Coronal cuts on CT or MRI can be useful in determining distance from major bronchi cancer's edge to carina.

Cancer Statistics and Survival

According to Surveillance Epidemiology and End Results data based on 16,000 patients, the relative 5-year survival is 8% to 10% and 10-year survival 5% to 7%. Surprisingly, there is a small attrition for 5-year survivors

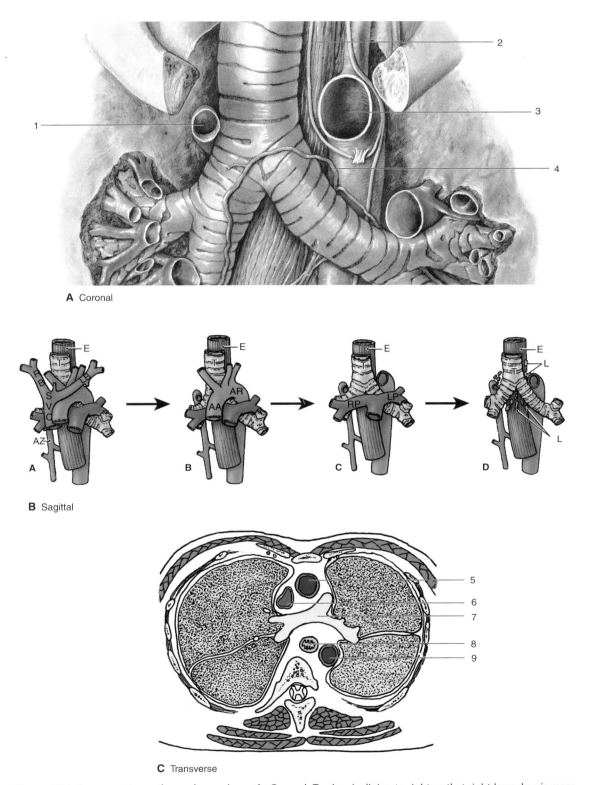

A Coronal

B Sagittal

C Transverse

Figure 18.4 **T-oncoanatomy three-planar views. A.** Coronal. Trachea inclining to right so that right bronchus is more vertical than left. **B.** Sagittal replaced with relations of bifurcation of trachea built up from deep to superficial. A. Lymph nodes at the tracheal bifurcation. B. Pulmonary arteries. C. Ascending aorta and arch of the aorta. D. Brachiocephalic veins forming the superior vena cava and the arch of the azygos vein entering it posteriorly. **C.** Axial view demonstrates bifurcation of major bronchi and location of subcarinal nodes. (1) Arch of azygos vein. (2) Left recurrent laryngeal nerve. (3) Arch of aorta. (4) Bronchial artery. (5) Ascending aorta. (6) Superior vena cava. (7) Carina bifurcation into major bronchi. (8) Esophagus. (9) Descending aorta.

TABLE 18.2	Lymph Nodes of Lung

Paracarinal and subcarinal nodes as well as hilar nodes are sentinel nodes.

N1 nodes: All N1 nodes lie distal to the mediastinal pleural reflection and *within the visceral pleura.*

Hilar nodes
Interlobar nodes
Lobar nodes bronchi
Segmental nodes
Subsegmental nodes

N2 nodes: All N2 nodes lie within the mediastinal pleural envelope on the ipsilateral side.

Highest mediastinal nodes
Upper paratracheal nodes
Prevascular and retrotracheal nodes
Lower paratracheal nodes
Subaortic nodes (aortopulmonary window)
Para-aortic nodes (ascending aorta or phrenic)
Subcarinal nodes
Paraesophageal nodes (below carina)
Pulmonary ligament nodes

with the majority (70%) alive at 10 years. Female gender, good Karnofsky performance status, and cessation of smoking contribute to longer survival.

Staging is a major factor in survival and the data analyzed by Mountain present the findings in Figure 13.6

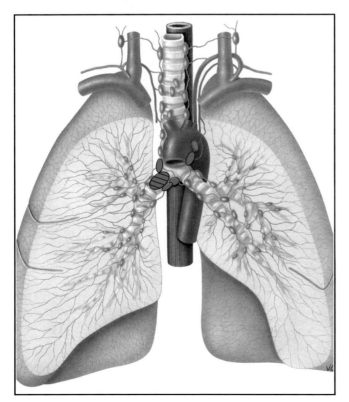

Figure 18.5 N-oncoanatomy. Paracarinal and subcarinal nodes as well as hilar nodes are sentinel nodes.

and Table 15.3. For stage IA cancers, the 90% survival rate for a T1 N0 M0 patient decreases to 61% at 5 years and for a stage IB patient, survival is 70% at 1 year, and is almost halved at 5 years at 38%. The 50% 5-year survival for stage I decreases to 30%, indicating that once hilar nodes are positive, metastatic disease is highly likely. Stage IIIA represents the most favorable advanced disease patients with 50% 1-year survival and, despite vigorous chemoradiation, only decreases to 10%. Surgically staged IIIA patients do better, as expected, with 25% alive at 5 years.

Specifically, when 5-year relative survival rates for lung cancer by histology are considered in Table 15.4, the average is 13.9% for all stages. The most favorable bronchioloalveolar is at 42%, but when localized is as high as 65%. For the common non–small cell cancers, SQC and adenocarcinomas are close to overall average at 15.4% and 16.6%, respectively. As expected, anaplastic dedifferentiated cancers do extremely poorly, that is, large cell and small cell anaplastic yield 11.6% and 4.6%, respectively.

Bronchioloalveolar cancer is characterized by the nuclear anaplasia and pleomorphism of Type II pneumocytes or clara cells. The spread pattern is in a monolayer over acinar alveoli and can when extensive (T3, T4) interfere with gas exchange and result in a right to left intrapulmonary shunt. Five subtypes have been described. Types A and B have a 100% survival and are non-invasive. Type C is transitional into an adenocarcinoma and has an 80% survival rate. Types D, E have angiolymphatic invasion to lymph nodes and beyond with higher mortality rates similar to adenocarcinomas with regional nodal invasion survival of 25–30% and with distant metastases of 5%.

19

Small Cell Anaplastic Cancer

Small cell anaplastic cancer's favored site is mostly central or proximal lung root, reminiscent of the embryonic origin of the multipotential cells of lung buds, which form the anlage of lung endoderm.

Perspective and Patterns of Spread

Small cell anaplastic cancers (SCA) are the most undifferentiated cancers. Their origin is mostly in central airways juxtaposed to the mediastinum. It is the most dedifferentiated and highly invasive lung cancer entering into lymphatics and commonly presents as a large mediastinal nodal mass. Superior vena caval obstruction as a low-pressure thin wall is more vulnerable to compression than other mediastinal structures, such as the aorta, esophagus, and trachea. These cancers are notorious for being metastatic on presentation. Of the many *solid cancers, SCAs have been genetically classified as classic versus variants depending on their biologic characteristics.* Frequently expressed mutations in tumor suppressor genes include 3P, RB, and TP_{53} (Table 19.1). The derepression of chromosomes leads to a variety of neuroendocrine and paraneoplastic syndromes including Cushing disease, severe lymphedema owing to antidiuretic hormone excess, and neuromyopathic conditions. Their favored site is mostly central or proximal lung root, reminiscent of the embryonal origin of the multipotential cells of lung buds, which form the anlage of lung endoderm. Unlike most lung cancers, SCA tends to infiltrate submucosally and distort the bronchus by extrinsic and submucosal compression. Their pattern of spread tends to create mediastinal masses (Fig. 19.1).

Research advances in genetic and molecular biology have uncovered new markers that were recognized in the fifth edition with their tabulation. However, the results were insufficient to recommend their incorporation into the staging system. In fact, in the sixth edition (2004), only brief mention and little emphasis has been made of molecular markers except to note "the marker needs to bear a strong relationship to patient prognosis" to be included.

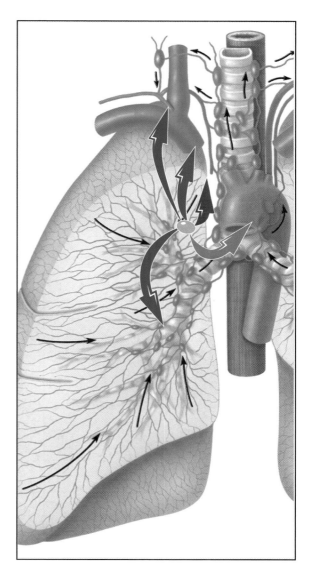

Figure 19.1 **Patterns of spread.** The proximal location of the small cell cancer and its rapid dissemination via lymphatics is stressed. Although color-coded, all T and N stages are referred to as "limited" if they are confined to the thorax.

DEFINITION OF TNM

T$_{is}$ N$_0$ STAGE GROUPINGS

0

T1
Tumor ≤3 cm, surrounded by lung or visceral pleura, without bronchoscopic evidence of invasion more proximal than the lobar bronchus

T2
Tumor with any of the following features of size or extent: >3 cm; involves main bronchus, ≥2 cm distal to the carina; invades the visceral pleura; associated with the atelectasis or obstructive pneumonitis that extends to the hilar region but does not involve the entire lung

N0
No regional lymph node metastasis

Stage IA
T1 N0 M0

Stage IB
T2 N0 M0

I

T1
Tumor ≤3 cm, surrounded by lung or visceral pleura, without bronchoscopic evidence of invasion more proximal than the lobar bronchus

T2
Tumor with any of the following features of size or extent: >3 cm; involves main bronchus, ≥2 cm distal to the carina; invades the visceral pleura; associated with the atelectasis or obstructive pneumonitis that extends to the hilar region but does not involve the entire lung

N1
Metastasis to ipsilateral peribronchial and/or ipsilateral hilar lymph nodes, and intrapulmonary nodes including involvement by direct extension of the primary tumor

Stage IIA
T1 N1 M0

Stage IIB
T2 N1 M0
T3 N0 M0

II

T3
Tumor of any size that directly invades any of the following: chest wall (including superior sulcus tumors), diaphragm, mediastinal pleura, parietal pericardium; or tumor in the main bronchus <2 cm distal to the carina, but without involvement of the carina; or associated atelectasis or obstructive pneumonitis of the entire lung

N2
Metastasis to ipsilateral mediastinal, and/or subcarinal lymph node(s)

Stage IIIA
T1 N2 M0
T2 N2 M0
T3 N1 M0
T3 N2 M0

IIIA

T4
Tumor of any size that invades any of the following: mediastinum, heart, great vessels, trachea, esophagus, vertebral body, carina; or separate tumor nodules in the same lobe; or tumor with malignant pleural effusion

N3
Metastasis to contralateral mediastinal, contralateral hilar, ipsilateral or contralateral scalene, or supraclavicular lymph node(s)

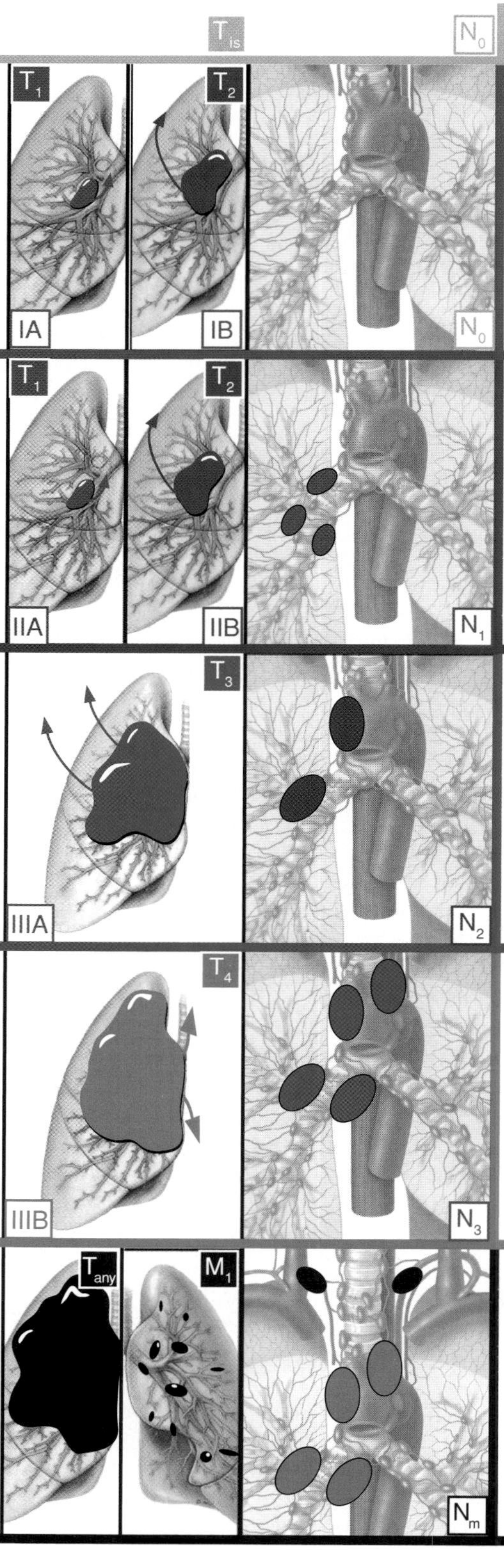

Stage IIIB
Any T   N3   M0
T4   Any N   M0

IIIB

Nm
Node metastasis

M1
Distant metastasis

Stage IV
Any T   Any N   M1

IV

Figure 19.2 TNM staging diagram. Small cell cancers have a tendency to metastasize early. They arise in central hilar locations with mediastinal invasion they often present as large masses causing suerior venous obstruction. Although shown in stages similar to other lung cancers the typical stages are clustered as LIMITED (M0) which includes all stages from IA, IB, to IIIA,B. EXTENSIVE applies to overt metastases M1 Stage IV. Small cell cancer stage I/II/IIIA/B are color-coded green/blue/red but are lumped together as **M0** ''limited'' **to thorax. Stage IV is metastatic black and referred to as ''extensive.''**

TABLE 19.1	Histopathologic Type	
Main Pathologic Cell Type	**Small Cell Variant**	
Small cell carcinoma	Oat cell carcinoma	
	Intermediate cell type	
	Fusiform cell type	
	Combined cell types	

TNM Staging Criteria

The common criteria of size in staging lung cancer do not apply to SCA. *Pragmatically, all intrathoracic T stages and N categories are lumped together into "limited" stage intrathoracic disease.* The "extensive" stage is applied to metastatic dissemination, which is all too common and, until shown otherwise, bone marrow invasion, liver, bone, and brain foci need to be excluded. For practical purposes, the staging is based on M0 versus M1 and the mainstay of treatment is systemic first because of high likelihood of occult micrometastases (Fig. 19.2).

Summary of Changes

There have been no changes from the fifth edition of the AJCC CSM.

Orientation of Three-planar Oncoanatomy

The orientation diagrams are at the T7/T8 level and the *key anatomic feature is their central locations as their point of origin akin to lung bud anlage.* The isocenter for SCA is at the hilar area, which is at the thoracic T7/T8 level (Fig. 19.3). The three main branches of each major bronchus are within the visceral pleura. The orientation diagrams C/D/E show the many varieties of epithelial cells increase as one approaches the hilar area of the bronchial tree.

T-oncoanatomy

The rich lymphatic submucosal network ensures the cancers rapid spread to the visceral pleura and cross the mediastinal pleura. The three-planar views (Fig. 19.4) emphasize the R pulmonary mediastinal surfaces and the juxtaposed R mediastinum because mediastinal mass formation and invasion are common presentations.

- *Sagittal plane:* The lung bud anlage is superior imposed on the bronchial tree. The *mediastinal structures that are commonly compressed include the low-pressure, thin-walled superior vena cava* or brachiocephalic vein and their entrapment between metastatic matted mediastinal masses of nodes and arteries. *Plugs of tumor, when entering the thoracic duct or metastatic lymph nodes, can also compress and block the lymphatic flow,* which can lead to chylous or pseudochylous effusions. Similarly, pulmonary venous compression result in serous pleural effusions. It is critical in staging to send cytospins of pleural effusions to determine if they are positive for cancer cells or whether they are cytologically negative.

- *Coronal view:* The medial aspects of the lung reflect the structures into the superior and inferior mediastinum by virtue of anatomic position. A rapidly growing neoplasm penetrates the mediastinal pleura and invades mediastinal lymphatics and nodes directly.

- *Transverse view:* The T7/T8 level is at the border between the superior and inferior mediastinum and is a critical level to appreciate. The arch of the aorta is defined, the trachea is bifurcating, and the branches of the sympathetics and parasympathetics, particularly the cardiac branches, are streaming alongside the trachea to form the cardiac plexuses that, when invaded, can lead to cardiac arrhythmias.

N-oncoanatomy

The mediastinal lymph nodes are the main focus of small cell cancers, which can and do spread into all sectors of the mediastinum. Each sector of the mediastinum has a vulnerable structure that can be invaded or compressed. Because of the central and proximal origin of SCA, they present with rapid extension to mediastinal surfaces. Small cell cancers arising in the upper and lower lobes involve mediastinal structures by juxtaposition. *The right-sided posterior nodal masses can trap the thoracic duct as it enters the chest from the abdomen. True chylous effusions tend to be right sided.* The right superior mediastinum mass can lead to superior vena caval obstruction. On the left side, the recurrent laryngeal nerve is most often compressed by nodes in the pulmonary aortic window and leads to hoarseness. Phrenic nerve invasion can lead to refractory hiccoughing due to spasmatic contractions of the diaphragm (Fig. 19.5; Table 19.2).

M-oncoanatomy

The rapid entry into the arterial system allows for widespread remote and venous dissemination and leads to multiorgan metastases. The development of superior

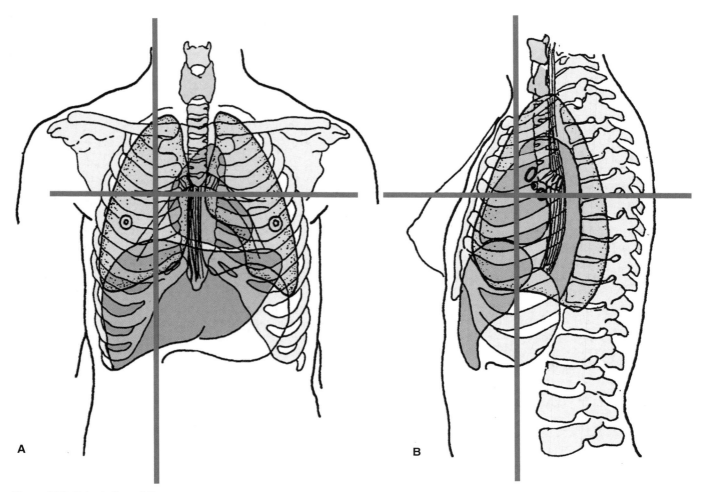

Figure 19.3 Orientation of T-oncoanatomy. A. Anterior. **B.** Lateral. The isocenter for three-planar oncoanatomy is placed centrally at the lung root and transversely at the thoracic vertebral level T7/T8.

vena cava obstruction (SVCO) emphasizes collateral venous channels or caput medusa presentations on the chest wall, shoulders, and abdomen, depending on whether the azygos vein is at or below the level of obstruction. If azygos vein is patent inferior to the SVCO, then blood flows through the hemiazygos system to the collateral channels around the shoulder. If both azygos and superior vena cava are obstructed, however, blood takes the circuitous route of intervertebral venous plexus to the femoral, iliac veins, or hemiazygos vein to the lumbar veins and inferior vena cava then anterior abdominal veins or the inferior vena cava to the right heart (see Fig. 14.6). The anatomic distribution of distant metastases is shown in Table 13.5.

Rules for Classification and Staging

Clinical Staging and Imaging

The TNM classification system is primarily for staging non–small cell lung cancers. The most important

change dates back to the fourth edition of the American Joint Committee on Cancer (AJCC) where T3, resectable disease, was distinguished from T4, unresectable disease. Simultaneously, a greater reliance on more sophisticated imaging has occurred. It is with the sixth edition that computed tomography (CT) and positron emission topography (PET) are allowed. The imaging modalities for detection and diagnosis apply to staging (Table 19.3). Chest films and CT, preferably spiral CT is an essential step in both the diagnosis and staging. PET combined with CT is utilized to overcome due to motion artifacts. Magnetic resonance imaging (MRI) is useful for mediastinal evaluation. Another advantage of CT over MRI for staging is that it allows for metastatic workup of lung, liver, adrenal, ribs, and vertebrae, especially for Pancoast cancers.

Pathologic Staging

All pathologic specimens from clinical invasive procedures—bronchoscopy, mediastinoscopy, mediastinotomy, thoracentesis, and thorascopy—are applicable to

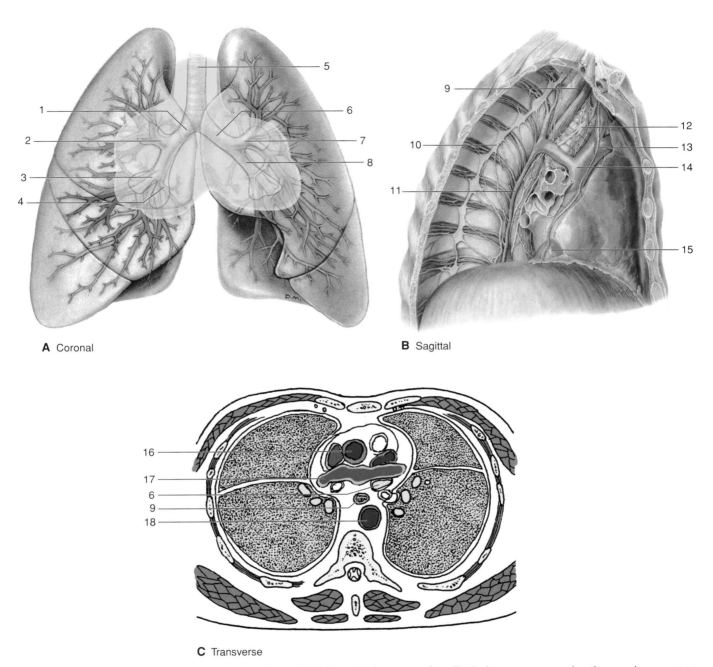

A Coronal

B Sagittal

C Transverse

Figure 19.4 **T-oncoanatomy three-planar views.** The emphasis is on the frequency of mediastinal masses compressing the superior vena cava and azygos vein. **A.** Coronal. **Superimposition of bronchi and lung anlage (yellow)** at 5 to 6 weeks on the mature bronchial tree to emphasize pluripotent cell origin of small cell cancer and their preference for a central location at lung root. **B.** Sagittal. Medial surface of right lobe is presented to emphasize proximity to superior vena cava and azygos vein since mediastinal mass presentations can lead to superior vena caval compression and collaterization. **C.** Transverse. Right and left branching of main bronchi within visceral pleura at lung roots. (1) Right main bronchus. (2) Right superior lobar bronchus. (3) Right middle lobar bronchus. (4) Right lower lobar bronchus. (5) Trachea. (6) Left main bronchus. (7) Left superior lobar bronchus. (8) Left inferior lobar bronchus. (9) Esophagus. (10) Sympathetic trunk. (11) Azygos vein. (12) Vagus nerve. (13) Phrenic nerve. (14) Superior vena cava. (15) Inferior vena cava. (16) Ascending aorta. (17) Pulmonary trunk. (18) Descending aorta.

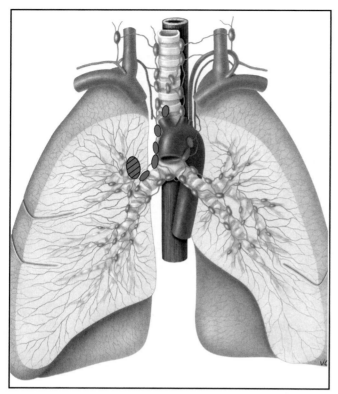

Figure 19.5 N-oncoanatomy. Hilar and ipsilateral mediastinal nodes are the sentinel nodes that are often bulky and fused with the primary mass in lung.

pathologic stage. Thoracotomy and resection of primary and lymph nodes are the mainstay of pathologic staging. Margin status and any residual cancer needs to be noted. Preferably, six nodes should be examined.

Surgical resection of primary and regional nodes needs to be carefully evaluated at bronchial stump for adequate margins. All resected nodes should be numbered according to AJCC system and assessed for tumor.

Oncoimaging Annotations

- Chest radiographs seldom detect primary lung cancers in their early stages.
- Spiral CT is useful in high-risk patients to detect nodule and infiltrates.
- PET imaging with [18]FDG appears to be of value in discriminating malignant versus benign nodules.
- CT can detect mediastinal adenopathy, but histologic verification is essential to ascertain if it is malignant.
- Determining N2 versus N3 mediastinal nodes is important; it establishes resectability.
- MRI can be of value in assessing mediastinal invasion, chest wall and rib erosion, and compromised large vein involvement.
- MRI of vertebrae may show bone marrow replacement by cancerous infiltrates of disseminated metastases.
- CT may often be unable to discriminate the primary from its mediastinal adenopathy.
- SVCO can be determined as cancer invasion versus compression by MRI rather than CT.

Cancer Statistics and Survival

According to Surveillance Epidemiology and End Results (SEER) data based on 16,000 patients, the relative 5-year survival is 8% to 10% and 10-year survival 5% to 7%.

TABLE 19.2	Lymph Nodes of Lung

Hilar and ipsilateral mediastinal nodes are the sentinel nodes that are often bulky and fused with the primary mass in lung.

N1 nodes: All N1 nodes lie distal to the mediastinal pleural reflection and *within the visceral pleura.*

Hilar nodes
Interlobar nodes
Lobar nodes bronchi
Segmental nodes
Subsegmental nodes

N2 nodes: All N2 nodes lie within the mediastinal pleural envelope on the ipsilateral side.

Highest mediastinal nodes
Upper paratracheal nodes
Prevascular and retrotracheal nodes
Lower paratracheal nodes
Subaortic nodes (aortopulmonary window)
Para-aortic nodes (ascending aorta or phrenic)
Subcarinal nodes
Paraesophageal nodes (below carina)
Pulmonary ligament nodes

TABLE 19.3	Imaging Modalities for Diagnosis and Staging	
Method	**Capability**	**Recommended**
Primary tumor and regional nodes workup		
Chest films	Baseline image	Yes
CT/spiral CT	Most useful of all modalities for determining characteristics of T and N in the thorax and M in the brain and liver	Yes
MRI	Beneficial if there are large mediastinal nodes fused with primary tumor; MRI may detect bone marrow invasion	Yes
Percutaneous needle biopsy	Guided by fluoroscopy or CT, accurate in establishing cytologic diagnosis from T (particularly peripheral lung lesions); M (especially liver or bone); less experience with N	Yes
Mediastinoscopy/thoracoscopy	Confirmation of nodal involvement	Yes
Metastatic workup for clinically suspected metastases		
MRI	For bone marrow involvement if suspected	Yes
CT/echography	For liver, adrenals	Yes
CT/MRI	For brain	Yes
Bone scan	For the bone	Yes
PET scan/MRI spectroscopy	Diagnosis of peripheral lesions, staging; can differentiate between cystic and solid lesions	Yes, if clinically indicated

CT, computed tomography; M, metastasis; MRI, Magnetic resonance imaging; N, node; PET, positron emission tomography; T, tumor.

Surprisingly, there is a small attrition for 5-year survivors with the majority (70%) alive at 10 years. Female gender, good Karnofsky performance status, and cessation of smoking contribute to longer survival.

Staging is a major factor in survival. There is a dramatic difference in survival rates for non–small cell cancers when one compares clinical versus surgical staging. There is a similar striking difference between similar stage groupings for non–small cell versus small cell cancers. For stages I and II, the 5-year results are halved; that is, stage I 46% versus 20.3%, stage II 26.1% versus 14.7%; whereas stage III and IV are identical, at 8% and 15%, respectively.

Specifically, when 5-year relative survival rates for lung cancer by histology is considered in Table 13.5, the average is 13.9% for all stages. The most favorable bronchioloalveolar is at 42%, but when localized is as high as 65%. For the common non–small cell cancers, squamous cell cancer and adenocarcinomas are close to overall average at 15.4% and 16.6%, respectively. As expected, anaplastic dedifferentiated cancers do extremely poorly; that is, large cell and SCA yield 11.6% and 4.6%, respectively (see Table 13.5).

Despite effective chemotherapy, survival results are frustratingly poor due to recurrence, relapse, or second primaries in lung. According to SEER data, 2-, 3-, and 5-year results are 11.6%, 7.1%, and 4.6%, respectively, and late morbidity from multimodal treatment includes neurologic impairment in 13%, pulmonary fibrosis in 18%, and cardiac disorders in 10%.

20

Mesothelioma

Mesotheliomas render the invisible pleural space visible by developing nodular lesions on its visceral and parietal surfaces, extending in a corkscrew fashion into fissure surfaces.

Perspective and Patterns of Spread

Malignant mesotheliomas are extremely aggressive, but uncommon thoracic neoplasms, accounting for 2% of chest tumors. The bioassociation with asbestos exposure is well recognized, with long latency periods of 20 to 25 years. Routine chest radiographs are inadequate to detect fibers, the amphiboles, particularly crocidolite, which gradually wiggles into the pulmonary lymphatics reaching the visceral pleura and irritating the smooth surface lining of mesothelial cells. With time, nodular lesions develop on visceral and parietal surfaces, extending in a corkscrew fashion into fissure surfaces. Although slow growing, their insidious onset obscures early detection. Recent data suggest early stage diagnosis and multimodal treatment can yield long-term survival (Fig. 20.1).

Pathologically, these tumors are divided into four types: Epithelioid, mesenchymal (sarcomatous), desmoplastic, and mixed or by basic (at least 10% of both epithelioid and sarcomatoid) elements. Pure epithelioid carry a better prognosis than the sarcomatous and, although desmoplastic reactions appear benign, these tumors have the poorest survival (Table 20.1).

TNM Staging Criteria

The American Joint Committee on Cancer (AJCC) has adopted the staging system of the International Mesothelioma Interest Group (IMIG) and is based on patterns of spread of this aggressive thoracic malignancy (Fig. 20.2). The pleura is like the peritoneum; although it consists of only a single layer of cells, they act as a barrier to cancer spread. Thus, T1 tumors are focal nodular lesions of parietal pleura; T2 indicates spread to visceral pleura and lung; and T3 is deeper invasion of the chest wall and mediastinum, but potentially resectable. The

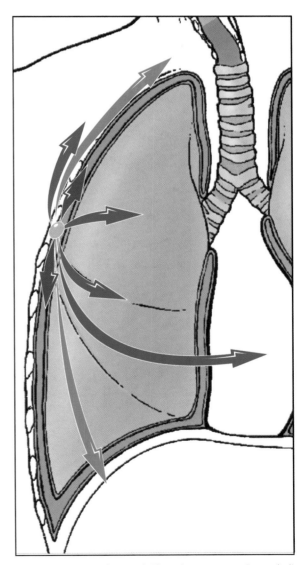

Figure 20.1 **Patterns of spread.** The primary cancer (mesothelioma) invades in various directions, which are color-coded vectors (*arrows*) representing stage of progression: T_0, yellow; T1, green; T2, blue; T3, purple; T4, red; and when metastatic, black.

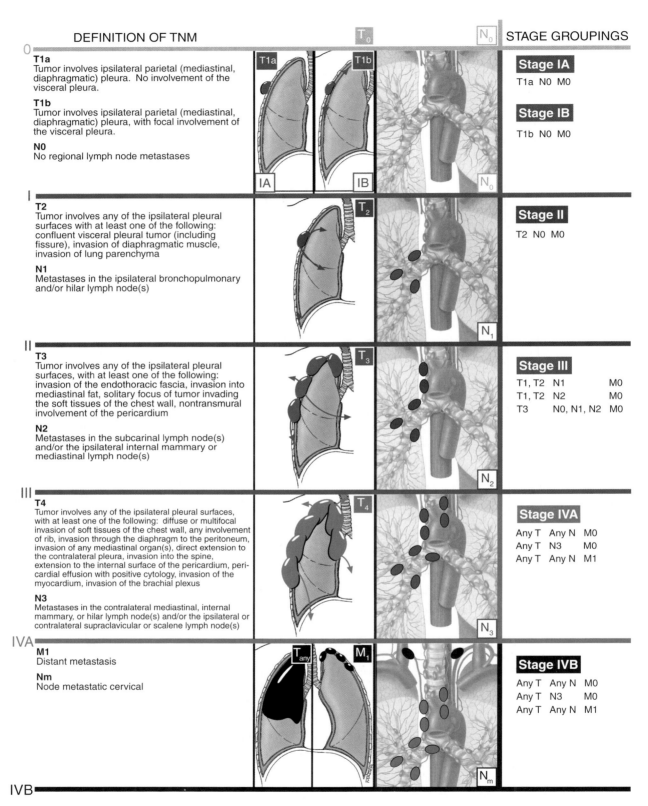

DEFINITION OF TNM

T1a
Tumor involves ipsilateral parietal (mediastinal, diaphragmatic) pleura. No involvement of the visceral pleura.

T1b
Tumor involves ipsilateral parietal (mediastinal, diaphragmatic) pleura, with focal involvement of the visceral pleura.

N0
No regional lymph node metastases

T2
Tumor involves any of the ipsilateral pleural surfaces with at least one of the following: confluent visceral pleural tumor (including fissure), invasion of diaphragmatic muscle, invasion of lung parenchyma

N1
Metastases in the ipsilateral bronchopulmonary and/or hilar lymph node(s)

T3
Tumor involves any of the ipsilateral pleural surfaces, with at least one of the following: invasion of the endothoracic fascia, invasion into mediastinal fat, solitary focus of tumor invading the soft tissues of the chest wall, nontransmural involvement of the pericardium

N2
Metastases in the subcarinal lymph node(s) and/or the ipsilateral internal mammary or mediastinal lymph node(s)

T4
Tumor involves any of the ipsilateral pleural surfaces, with at least one of the following: diffuse or multifocal invasion of soft tissues of the chest wall, any involvement of rib, invasion through the diaphragm to the peritoneum, invasion of any mediastinal organ(s), direct extension to the contralateral pleura, invasion into the spine, extension to the internal surface of the pericardium, pericardial effusion with positive cytology, invasion of the myocardium, invasion of the brachial plexus

N3
Metastases in the contralateral mediastinal, internal mammary, or hilar lymph node(s) and/or the ipsilateral or contralateral supraclavicular or scalene lymph node(s)

M1
Distant metastasis

Nm
Node metastatic cervical

STAGE GROUPINGS

Stage IA
T1a N0 M0

Stage IB
T1b N0 M0

Stage II
T2 N0 M0

Stage III

T1, T2	N1	M0
T1, T2	N2	M0
T3	N0, N1, N2	M0

Stage IVA

Any T	Any N	M0
Any T	N3	M0
Any T	Any N	M1

Stage IVB

Any T	Any N	M0
Any T	N3	M0
Any T	Any N	M1

Figure 20.2 TNM staging diagram. Mesotheliomas arise in the pleural spaces, first on the parietal, visceral pleura and continue invading into fissures. Then the aggressive malignancy spreads into the parietal pleura, chest wall and mediastinal pleura and mediastinal structures. Unlike lung cancers, Stage IVA is T4N3M0 and Stage IVB M1 is metastatic. Vertical presentations of stage groupings, which follow same color code for cancer stage advancement are organized in horizontal lanes: Stage 0, yellow; I, green; II, blue; III, purple; IVA, red; and metastatic stage IVB, black. Definitions of TN on left and stage grouping on right.

TABLE 20.1	Histopathologic Type: Common Cancers of the Pleural Mesothelioma
Type[a]
Epithelioid
Biphasic (at least 10% of both epithelioid and sarcomatoid components)
Sarcomatoid
Desmoplastic

[a]Listed here in descending order of frequency.
From Greene FL, Page DL, Fleming ID, et al. (eds): *AJCC Cancer Staging Manual.* 6th ed. New York: Springer; 2002. Used with the permission of the American Joint Committee on Cancer (AJCC), Chicago, Illinois.

major feature of unresectability are T4 criteria and include destruction of the chest wall ribs or vertebra or mediastinal, visceral infiltration and extension through the diaphragm into the peritoneal cavity or into the contralateral pleural space or the brachial plexus in the neck.

Summary of Changes

- *The AJCC has adopted the staging system proposed by the IMIG in 1995. It is based on updated information about the relationships between tumor T and N status and overall survival. This staging system applies only to tumors arising in the pleura.*

- *T categories have been redefined.*

- *T1 lesions have been divided into T1a and T1b, leading to a division of stage I into stage IA and stage IB.*

- *T3 is defined as locally advanced but potentially resectable tumor.*

- *T4 is defined as locally advanced, technically unresectable tumor.*

- *Stage II no longer involves tumors with nodal metastasis; all nodal metastasis is categorized in stage III or IV.*

Orientation of Three-planar Oncoanatomy

The pleural space is coated by the visceral and parietal pleura of the chest wall and mediastinal pleura. This is presented at the thoracic T7/T8 level (Fig. 20.3).

T-oncoanatomy

The pleural space is readily recognized during pathologic states as a pleural effusion or pneumothorax; in its nor-

mal state, it is invisible but shown in reference to the lung in expiration (Fig. 20.4).

- *Coronal:* Anterior and posterior views, the pleura extends into the neck and enters the costadiaphragmatic recess. The visceral pulmonary pleura faces the parietal pleura on the chest wall and medially the mediastinal pleura. The horizontal and oblique fissures are due to visceral pleural invagination on the right side and, similarly, the oblique fissure of the left lung as constituted by visceral pleura.

- *Sagittal:* The pleura invaginates its layers to form fissures. In the lateral view, pleural recesses are more shallow.

- *Transverse:* The diaphragmatic surface can be viewed as separating the pleural and peritoneal cavities.

N-oncoanatomy

The regional lymph nodes are dependent on invasion patterns. Generally, they are mediastinal nodes, but with lung invasion, pulmonary and hilar nodes are at risk, and with chest wall invasion, costal nodes and internal thoracic nodes are at risk. The AJCC notes regional nodes are similar to lymph node map, nomenclature and numbering on for lung cancers (Fig. 20.5; Table 20.2).

M-oncoanatomy

The chest wall has a rich venous network of intercostals veins, azygos and hemiazygos veins interdigitating with intervertebral veins. Metastases to spinal cord and brain; contralateral spread to opposite chest and lung can occur. Most common metastatic sites are on the mesothelial surfaces as opposed to pleura, pericardial, and peritoneal cavity. With dissemination, uncommon sites as thyroid and prostate have been noted (see Fig. 14.6).

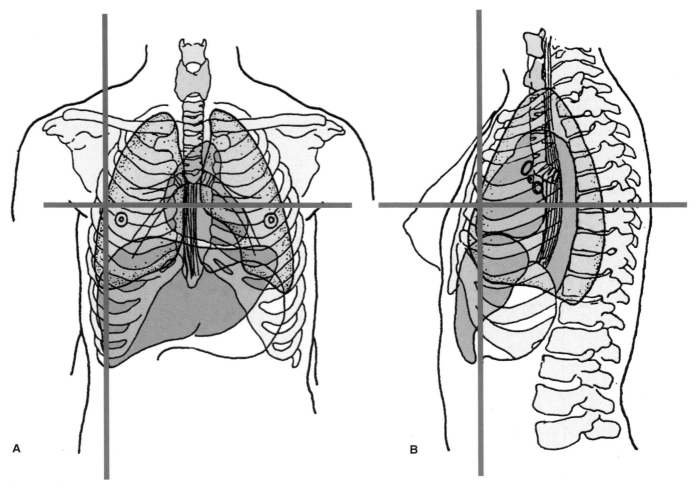

A

B

Figure 20.3 **Orientation of T-oncoanatomy.** The isocenter for three-planar oncoanatomy in the coronal view is at the T7/T8 level. **A.** Coronal. **B.** Sagittal.

Rules for Classification and Staging

Clinical Staging and Imaging

The TNM classification system is primarily for staging non–small cell lung cancers. The most important change dates back to the fourth edition of the AJCC where T3, resectable disease, was distinguished from T4, unresectable disease. Simultaneously, a greater reliance on more sophisticated imaging has occurred. It is with the sixth edition that computed tomography (CT) and positron emission topography (PET) are allowed. The imaging modalities for detection and diagnosis apply to staging (see Table 13.6). Chest films and CT (preferably spiral) are essential steps in both diagnosis and staging. PET combined with CT is utilized to overcome motion artifacts. Magnetic resonance imaging (MRI) is useful for mediastinal evaluation. Another advantage of CT over MRI for staging is that it allows for metastatic workup

of lung, liver, adrenal, ribs, and vertebrae, especially for Pancoast cancers (see Table 13.6).

Pathologic Staging

All pathologic specimens from clinical invasive procedures—bronchoscopy, mediastinoscopy, mediastinotomy, thoracentesis, and thorascopy—are applicable to pathologic stage. Thoracotomy and resection of primary and lymph nodes are the mainstay of pathologic staging. Margin status and any residual cancer need to be noted. Preferably, six nodes are examined.

Oncoimaging Annotations

- Chest radiographs seldom detect primary mesotheliomas in their early stages.

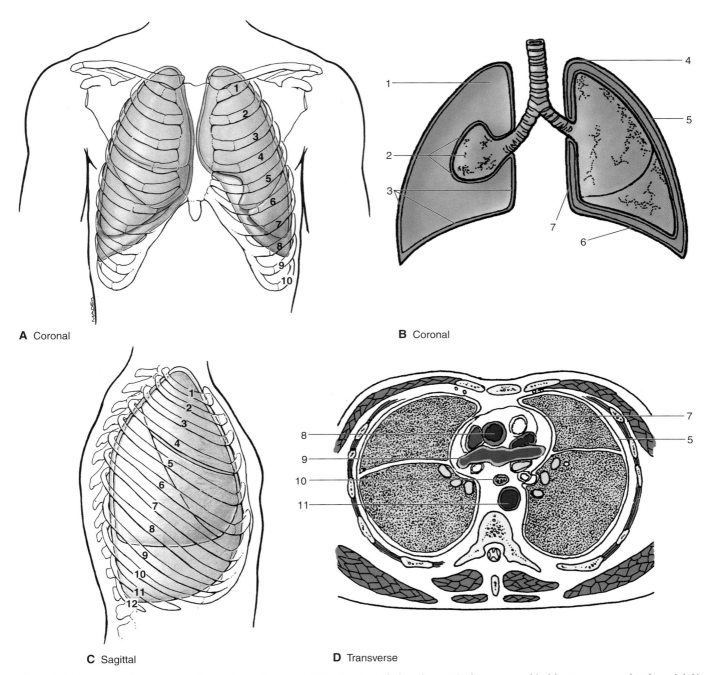

A Coronal

B Coronal

C Sagittal

D Transverse

Figure 20.4 **T-oncoanatomy three-planar views. A.** Coronal anterior view of pleural space is demonstrated in blue as compared to lung (pink) extending to the eighth rib anteriorly. **B.** Coronal. (1) Pleural cavity. (2) Visceral pleura. (3) Parietal pleura. (4) Cervical pleura. (5) Costal pleura. (6) Diaphragmatic pleura. (7) Mediastinal pleura. With lung collapsed as with a pneumothorax, the pleural space is definitely shown. **C.** Sagittal and lateral view demonstrates the excursion of the pleural space from eighth to twelfth rib, anterior to posterior. **D.** Transverse axial presentation at T7/T8 shows the subdivisions of the inferior mediastinum: anterior, middle (heart), and posterior. Note the juxtaposition of parietal mediastinal pleura fused with pericardial parietal surface. (8) Ascending aorta. (9) Pulmonary trunk. (10) Esophagus. (11) Descending aorta.

TABLE 20.2	Lymph Nodes of Lung

With pulmonary invasion, intrapulmonary and interbronchial nodes are involved. With extension to mediastinal pleura, the mediastinal nodes are at risk.

N1 nodes: All N1 nodes lie distal to the mediastinal pleural reflection and *within the visceral pleura.*

Hilar nodes
Interlobar nodes
Lobar nodes bronchi
Segmental nodes
Subsegmental nodes

N2 nodes: All N2 nodes lie within the mediastinal pleural envelope on the ipsilateral side.

Highest mediastinal nodes
Upper paratracheal nodes
Prevascular and retrotracheal nodes
Lower paratracheal nodes
Subaortic nodes (aortopulmonary window)
Para-aortic nodes (ascending aorta or phrenic)
Subcarinal nodes
Paraesophageal nodes (below carina)
Pulmonary ligament nodes

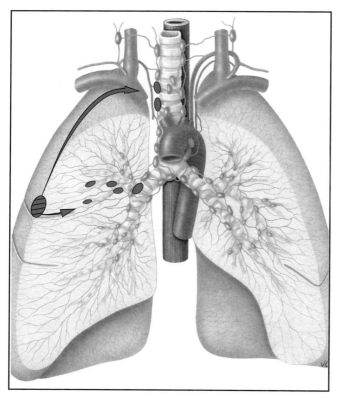

Figure 20.5 N-oncoanatomy. With pulmonary invasion, intrapulmonary and interbronchial nodes are involved. With extension to mediastinal pleura, the mediastinal nodes are at risk.

- Spiral CT is useful in high-risk patients to detect nodule and infiltrates.
- PET imaging with ^{18}FDG appears to be of value in discriminating malignant versus benign nodules.
- CT can detect and mediastinal adenopathy, but histologic verification is essential to ascertain if it is malignant.
- Determining N2 versus N3 mediastinal nodes is important; it establishes resectability.
- MRI can be of value in assessing mediastinal invasion, chest wall and rib erosion, and compromised large vein involvement.

Cancer Statistics and Survival

It is difficult to find a malignancy more lethal than lung cancer, especially small cell cancers, which are overall about 5%. However, mesotheliomas have virtually no 5-year survivors. Most reports with radical extrapleural pneumonectomy with chemoradiation are yielding median survival of less than 1 year (9 months) with high complication rates with mortality rates down to 10% or less. Elegant radiation using three-dimensional conformal techniques with intensity modulation has not been able to alter the dismal course of events.

21

Cancers of the mammary gland predominate among tumors of the chest wall and their oncoanatomy emphasizes their rich lymphatics and microvasculature.

Perspective and Patterns of Spread

Breast cancer is the most prevalent female malignancy and exceeds the incidence of the next two common cancers of lung and colorectal areas combined. At an annual rate of 215,000 new patients and death rate of 40,000, virtually everyone has a family or friend who has encountered or experienced breast cancer. With the widespread use of mammography, most cancers are detected in early stages and are most often not palpable. Especially important is the ability to identify preinvasive carcinomas in situ. The majority (85%) are ductal carcinomas in situ and the rest are lobular cancer in situ, which run a more benign course. The histopathologic varieties of breast cancer are tabulated in Table 21.1. It is recommended that all invasive breast cancers be graded utilizing the Nottingham system, in which point scores based on specific features are equated with grades 1 to 3. A comprehensive review of the literature of histologic grade and outcome in early stage breast cancer in the current American Joint Committee on Cancer (AJCC) sixth edition indicates its robustness as a prognostic factor. It seems certain that emerging data will support its incorporation into staging in the next edition, similar to the Gleason grade for prostate cancer staging.

The patterns of spread account for the physical signs associated with breast cancer. Most commonly, a small palpable nodule, often without tenderness, appears to be a thickening or swelling, which is freely movable. If the lesion causes skin wrinkling with positional changes, Cooper's suspensory ligaments are involved. Lactiferous ductal invasion can result in expression of a bloody secretion from the nipple or even nipple inversion. Loss of mobility strongly suggests invasion of the pectoralis major or chest wall. When loss of mobility occurs with muscle flexion, it is due to muscle invasion; chest wall infiltration leads to a permanent loss of mobility (Fig. 21.1).

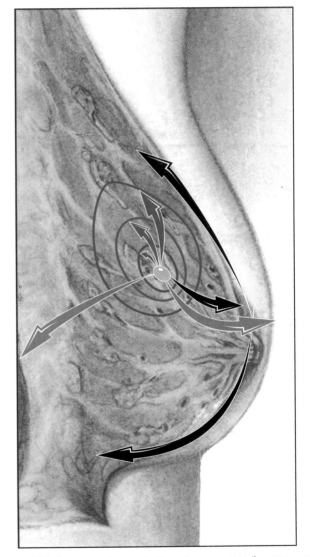

Figure 21.1 **Patterns of spread.** The primary cancer (breast cancer) invades in various directions, which are color-coded vectors (*arrows*) representing stage of progression: Tis, yellow; T1, green; T2, blue; T3, purple; T4, red; and metastatic, black.

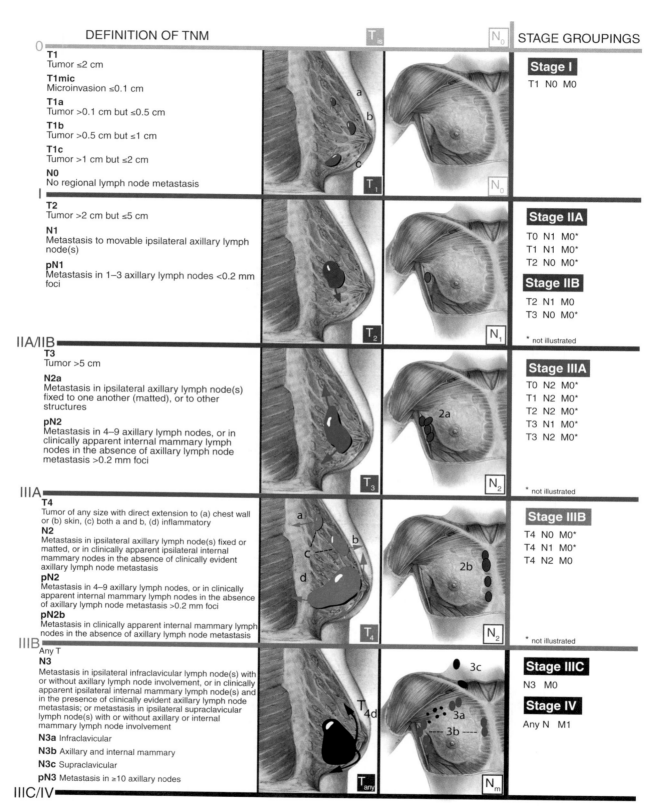

DEFINITION OF TNM

T$_{is}$ N$_0$ STAGE GROUPINGS

T1
Tumor ≤2 cm

T1mic
Microinvasion ≤0.1 cm

T1a
Tumor >0.1 cm but ≤0.5 cm

T1b
Tumor >0.5 cm but ≤1 cm

T1c
Tumor >1 cm but ≤2 cm

N0
No regional lymph node metastasis

Stage I
T1 N0 M0

T2
Tumor >2 cm but ≤5 cm

N1
Metastasis to movable ipsilateral axillary lymph node(s)

pN1
Metastasis in 1–3 axillary lymph nodes <0.2 mm foci

Stage IIA
T0 N1 M0*
T1 N1 M0*
T2 N0 M0*

Stage IIB
T2 N1 M0
T3 N0 M0*

* not illustrated

T3
Tumor >5 cm

N2a
Metastasis in ipsilateral axillary lymph node(s) fixed to one another (matted), or to other structures

pN2
Metastasis in 4–9 axillary lymph nodes, or in clinically apparent internal mammary lymph nodes in the absence of axillary lymph node metastasis >0.2 mm foci

Stage IIIA
T0 N2 M0*
T1 N2 M0*
T2 N2 M0*
T3 N1 M0*
T3 N2 M0*

* not illustrated

T4
Tumor of any size with direct extension to (a) chest wall or (b) skin, (c) both a and b, (d) inflammatory

N2
Metastasis in ipsilateral axillary lymph node(s) fixed or matted, or in clinically apparent ipsilateral internal mammary nodes in the absence of clinically evident axillary lymph node metastasis

pN2
Metastasis in 4–9 axillary lymph nodes, or in clinically apparent internal mammary lymph nodes in the absence of axillary lymph node metastasis >0.2 mm foci

pN2b
Metastasis in clinically apparent internal mammary lymph nodes in the absence of axillary lymph node metastasis

Stage IIIB
T4 N0 M0*
T4 N1 M0*
T4 N2 M0

* not illustrated

Any T

N3
Metastasis in ipsilateral infraclavicular lymph node(s) with or without axillary lymph node involvement, or in clinically apparent ipsilateral internal mammary lymph node(s) and in the presence of clinically evident axillary lymph node metastasis; or metastasis in ipsilateral supraclavicular lymph node(s) with or without axillary or internal mammary lymph node involvement

N3a Infraclavicular

N3b Axillary and internal mammary

N3c Supraclavicular

pN3 Metastasis in ≥10 axillary nodes

Stage IIIC
N3 M0

Stage IV
Any N M1

Figure 21.2 TNM staging diagram. Breast cancers are mammary gland cancers and because of the effectiveness of mammography screening the classification has become more of a pathologic staging system for both primary and lymph nodes. Note Stage III is divided into A/B/C as distinct from Stage IV. Vertical presentation of stage groupings, which follow same color code for cancer advancement are organized in horizontal lanes: Stage 0, yellow; I, green; II, blue; IIIA, purple; IIIB, red; and metastatic stage IIIC and IV, black. Definitions of TN on left and stage grouping on right.

TABLE 21.1	Histopathologic Type: Common Cancers of the Breast

Type[a]

In situ carcinomas

NOS
Intraductal
Paget disease and intraductal

Invasive carcinomas

NOS
Ductal
Inflammatory
Medullary, NOS
Medullary with lymphoid stroma
Mucinous
Papillary (predominantly micropapillary pattern)
Tubular
Lobular
Paget disease and infiltrating
Undifferentiated
Squamous cell
Adenoid cyst
Secretory
Cribriform

[a]NOS, not otherwise specified.
From Greene FL, Page DL, Fleming ID, et al. (eds): *AJCC Cancer Staging Manual*. 6th ed. New York: Springer; 2002. Used with the permission of the American Joint Committee on Cancer (AJCC) Chicago, Illinois.

TNM Staging Criteria

Breast cancer has been among the earliest cancers staged utilizing the TNM system and was proposed in 1954 by the International Union Against Cancer (UICC). Agreement by both UICC/AJCC (the first joint publication in 1968) has enabled the staging criteria to remain constant over the past three decades. The modifications relate to the frequent use of surgical findings and their histopathologic examination. The clinical basis for primary breast cancer staging is size: T1, <2 cm; T2, 2 to 5 cm; and T3, >5 cm in any dimension. Evidence of fixation to the chest wall appeared as a modifier in each stage, that is, A or B. The lymph node staging applied to axillary nodes mainly.

In the fourth edition (1992), the impact of mammography was acknowledged and tumor size was so noted and used to create subcategories for stage I: T1A, 0.5 cm; T1B, 0.5 to 1 cm; T1C, 1 to 2 cm; and extension to skin or chest wall is applied to T4 cancers only.

In the fifth edition (1997), *clinical measurement of size applied to both physical examination and mammography, and pathologic tumor size for T applied "only to the invasive component."* Cellular and molecular markers were tabulated acknowledging that 80 putative variables were reported in the literature. Although three prognostic groupings were noted, no specific incorporation of biomarkers was made by the American College of Pathol-

ogists. In the sixth edition (2003), microinvasion is defined at the primary site and regional nodes. The use of scintigraphy for determining the sentinel node(s) has been allowed. More subcategories exist for the primary and regional nodes, but the general parameters of size have remained stable (Fig. 21.2). There have been considerable new data presented for the interested investigator in the latest AJCC sixth edition for evidence-based changes. These are covered in the rules for classification section. The revisions are noted in red in T2 and are more in nature of clarification, most often based on histopathologic evaluation of surgical specimens.

Summary of Changes

- *Micrometastases are distinguished from isolated tumor cells on the basis of size and histologic evidence of malignant activity.*
- *Identifiers have been added to indicate the use of sentinel lymph node dissection and immunohistochemical or molecular techniques.*
- *Major classifications of lymph node status are designated according to the number of involved axillary lymph nodes as determined by routine hematoxylin and eosin staining (preferred method) or by immunohistochemical staining.*
- *The classification of metastasis to the infraclavicular lymph nodes has been added as N3.*

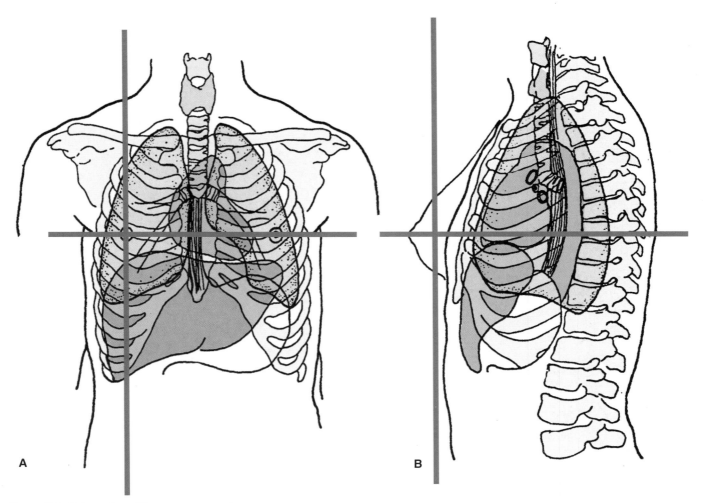

A

B

Figure 21.3 Orientation of T-oncoanatomy. The anatomic isocenter for three-planar oncoanatomy in the coronal view is placed lateral to midline over the breast and in the sagittal view anterior to the chest wall with the transverse view at the T8/T9 level.

- *Metastasis to the internal mammary nodes, based on the method of detection and the presence or absence of axillary nodal involvement, has been reclassified. Microscopic involvement of the internal mammary (parasternal) nodes detected by sentinel lymph node dissection using lymphoscintography but not by imaging studies or clinical examination is classified as N1. Macroscopic involvement of the internal mammary (parasternal) nodes as detected by imaging studies (excluding lymphoscintigraphy) or by clinical examination is classified as N2 if it occurs in the absence of metastases to the axillary lymph nodes or as N3 if it occurs in the presence of metastases to the axillary lymph nodes.*

- *Metastasis to the supraclavicular lymph nodes has been reclassified as N3 rather than M1.*

Orientation of Three-planar Oncoanatomy

The isocenter for the breast three-planar anatomy is customarily at the thoracic T8/T9 level. The planes for re-

gional lymph nodes are midaxillary, midclavicular, and parasternal (Fig. 21.3).

T-oncoanatomy

The mammary gland consists of 15 to 20 lobes of glandular tissue with varying amounts of fat, in a dense fibroareolar stroma, and is attached to the anterior chest wall by pectoral fascia. In cross-sections starting from the nipple, there are openings of the lactiferous ducts and their lactiferous sinuses, which are the conduits for the secretions of the hormonally stimulated breast glands. These ducts are distinct and individual for each lobule; they first run dorsally from the nipple and then spread radially into the glandular tissue.

The three planar views illustrate the breast three dimensionally in terms of its anatomic relationships to other structures. As a superficial structure, the mammary gland is covered by skin. Posteriorly, the underlying pectoral muscles bind the breast to the chest wall. Deep to the glandular tissue, there is usually a small amount of fat, which, along with the breast proper, is bounded by

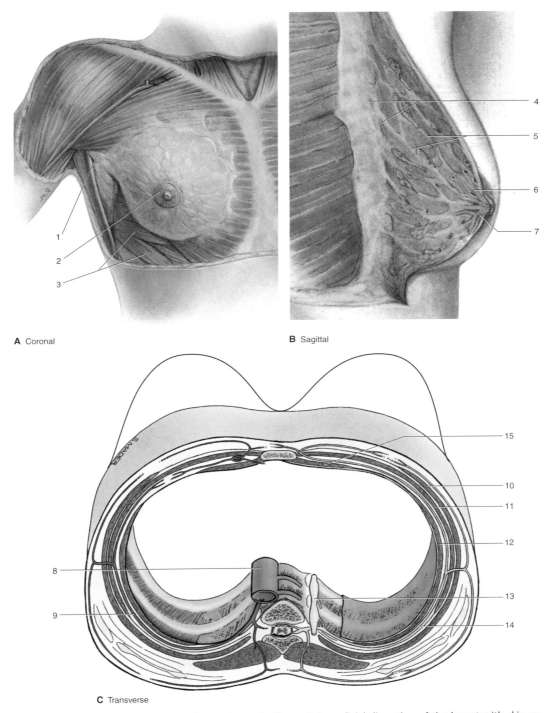

A Coronal

B Sagittal

C Transverse

Figure 21.4 **T-oncoanatomy three-planar views. A.** Coronal. Superficial dissection of the breast with skin removed resting on the pectoralis major fascia and muscle, extending from the second to sixth rib. The skin is attached to with Cooper's ligaments, which is then attached to the pectoralis fascia. **B.** Sagittal. Suspensory ligaments shown with compartmentalization of lobules. Lactiferous ducts, usually 15 to 20, lead to breast lobules. **C.** Transverse. The chest wall is emphasized. The diagram is simplified by showing nerves on the right and arteries on the left. The three musculomembranous layers are the external intercostals muscle and membrane, internal intercostals muscle and membrane, and the innermost intercostal, transverse thoracic muscle, and the membrane connecting them. The intercostals nerves are the anterior rami of spinal nerves T1 to T11; the anterior ramus of T12 is the subcostal nerve. (1) Axillary tail of breast. (2) Areola. (3) Serratus anterior. **B.** (4) Retromammary space. (5) Suspensory ligaments. (6) Lactiferous duct. (7) Lactiferous sinus. **C.** (8) Aorta. (9) Posterior intercostal artery. (10) External intercostals. (11) Internal intercostals. (12) Innermost intercostals. (13) Sympathetic trunk. (14) Anterior ramus–intercostal nerve. (15) Transverse thoracics.

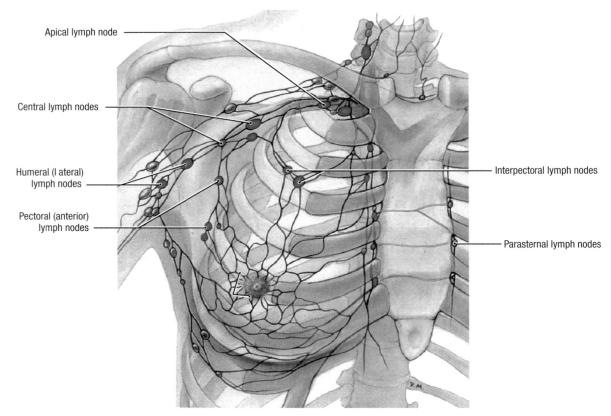

Apical lymph node

Central lymph nodes

Humeral (lateral) lymph nodes

Pectoral (anterior) lymph nodes

Interpectoral lymph nodes

Parasternal lymph nodes

Figure 21.5 N-oncoanatomy. Lymph drained from the upper limb and breast passes through nodes arranged irregularly in groups. **A.** Pectoral, along the inferior border of the pectoralis muscle. **B.** Subscapular, along the subscapular artery and veins. **C.** Brachial, along the distal part of the axillary vein. **D.** Central, at the base of the axilla embedded in axillary fat. **E.** Apical, along the axillary vein between the clavicle and the pectoralis minor muscle.

a deeper layer of superficial fascia. This layer can usually be dissected free from the deep fascia invaginating the pectoralis major muscle. Connective tissue septa called the suspensory ligaments (of Cooper) form subdivisions of the breast, dividing the breast into lobes.

The pectoralis major, the muscle underlying the breast, consists of two heads that arise from the clavicle, sternum, cartilages of the first six ribs, and inserts as a bilaminar structure on the anterolateral aspect of the humeral shaft.

TABLE 21.2	**Lymph Nodes of Breast**
Sentinel nodes	Juxtaregional nodes
Axillary Ipsilateral	Supraclavicular Lateral axilla Parasternal contralateral
Regional nodes	
Axillary low Axillary lateral Axillary mid Axillary apex Internal mammary (parasternal) Interpectoral Infraclavicular	

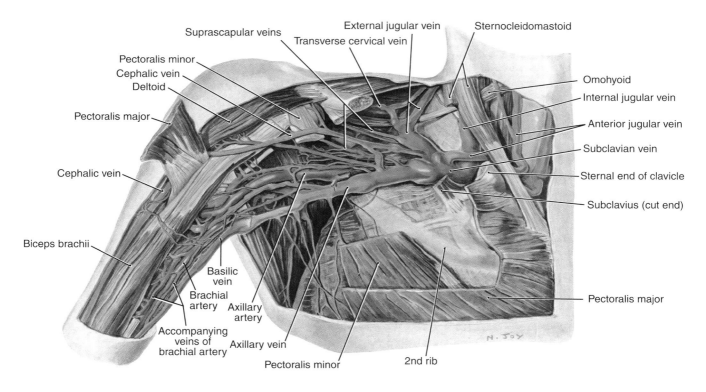

Suprascapular veins
External jugular vein
Sternocleidomastoid
Transverse cervical vein
Pectoralis minor
Cephalic vein
Deltoid
Omohyoid
Internal jugular vein
Pectoralis major
Anterior jugular vein
Subclavian vein
Cephalic vein
Sternal end of clavicle
Subclavius (cut end)
Biceps brachii
Basilic vein
Brachial artery
Axillary artery
Pectoralis major
Accompanying veins of brachial artery
Axillary vein
Pectoralis minor
2nd rib

N. JOY

Anterior view

Figure 21.6 **M-oncoanatomy.** The basilic vein joins the accompanying veins of the brachial artery to become the axillary vein at the inferior border of teres major, the axillary vein becomes the subclavian vein at the lateral border of the first rib, and the subclavian joins the internal jugular to become the brachiocephalic vein posterior to the sternal end of the clavicle. Observe the three suprascapular veins: One entering the axillary vein and two entering the external jugular vein.

The entire chest and breast must be considered as an anatomic unit. This requires knowledge of the underlying bony architecture, the muscles, as well as the nerves and vessels of the region (Fig. 21.4).

- *Coronal:* As a superficial appendage of the chest wall, the mammary gland is covered by skin and its glandular structures are compartmentalized between connective tissue septa—15 to 20 lobes that have their own lacunae and duct opening on the alveolar area of the nipple. Note the axillary tail (of Spence) of the breast.

- *Sagittal:* Most of the breast consists of fat; a region of loose connective tissue between the pectoral fascia muscle and breast—the retromammary bursa—permits mobility because the suspensory ligaments of Cooper allow alteration of shape with movement.

- *Axial:* The T8/T9 level demonstrates the relationship of the breast to chest wall. The diagram is simplified by showing nerves on the right and arteries on the left. The three musculomembranous layers are the external intercostals muscle and membrane, internal intercostals muscle and membrane, and the inner-

most intercostals, transverse thoracic muscle, and the membrane connecting them. The intercostals nerves are the anterior rami of spinal nerves T1 to T11; the anterior ramus of T12 is the subcostal nerve.

N-oncoanatomy

The breast lymphatics drain via four major routes—axillary, transpectoral, internal thoracic parasternal (mammary) trunks, and intercostal into numerous surrounding regional nodes, such as axillary (low, middle), axillary apex, supraclavicular, internal thoracic parasternal, interpectoral, and subclavicular nodes. Other pathways include crossover lymphatic channels to the opposite breast and inferior drainage into diaphragmatic and subdiaphragmatic channels. (Note: Subclavicular nodes are considered juxtaregional on the ipsilateral side.) Disease involvement in all other nodes—cervical, contralateral, supraclavicular, and contralateral internal thoracic, and mammary nodes—are equivalent to distant metastases (Fig. 21.5; Table 21.2).

The axilla is a crucial area to multidisciplinary oncologic decision making. Thorough knowledge of the axillary nodal status requires surgical sampling and/or

TABLE 21.3	Diagnostic Capabilities of Current Imaging Modalities in Breast Cancer	
Method	Diagnosis and Staging Capability	Recommended for Use
Primary Tumor and regional nodes		
Mammography	Visualizes approximately 90% of breast cancers	Film/screen and xeromammography have similar diagnostic accuracies.
Ultrasound (dedicated)	Limited to identification of cystic lesions and evaluation of dense breast	Dedicated unites are expensive and not suitable for stand-alone screening.
CT	Limited to evaluation of chest wall and internal mammary node involvement	Use of dedicated CT breast imaging systems had been abandoned.
MRI	Good for discrete lesions; calcifications are difficult to distinguish	Dedicated units are expensive. Useful for follow-up and for women with implants.
Metastatic breast cancer (as required)		
Chest x-ray film	Adequate for diagnosis; CT usually not needed	Essential for all tumor types.
Radionuclide bone scans	Essential for baseline verification and evaluation of symptomatic patients	Abnormal bone scans require film.
Liver and adrenal imaging	Indicated with abnormal chemistries or symptoms	Initial imaging study: radionuclide scan (requires validation of abnormal scan by ultrasound or CT).

CT, computed tomography; MRI, magnetic resonance imaging.
Modified from Bragg DG, Youker JE (eds): *Oncologic Imaging.* Elmsford, NY: Pergamon Press; 1985.

dissection by the surgical oncologist. The presence of positive axillary nodes often determines the use of adjuvant chemotherapy. And, if the axilla is to be treated by radiation therapy, it needs to be encompassed in its entirely.

The axillary contents consist of a variety of important structures. Damage to vessels can occur if they are injured during dissection. The major vessels include axillary veins, the cephalic vein and its branches, and the axillary artery and its branches. There is a close association between the brachial plexus and these vessels. Although perineural invasion by tumor is uncommon, it can occur.

Although anatomic knowledge of the region of the mammary nodes is quite important in oncologic decision making, internal mammary (parasternal) nodes are most commonly identified in the first three intercostals spaces and/or the xiphisternal angle. These nodes lie laterally to the sternum in an approximately 1- to 2-cm-wide strip and are 3 cm deep to the chest wall. The deeper lymphatics within the thoracic cavity and mediastinum are important pathways for dissemination. They include pleural, vertebral, and mediastinal nodes, and the thoracic duct. Of equal importance clinically are the major lymphatic routes. The lymphatic circulation empties into the general circulation at the junction of the internal jugular and subclavian veins. Therefore, lymphatic metastases often become blood-borne metastases as if direct vascular invasion occurred.

M-oncoanatomy

The rich plexus of veins parallel the lymphatics with the outer quadrants draining into the axillary veins and the inner quadrants draining into the internal mammary (thoracic) veins. The axillary veins enter the subclavian and the internal thoracic veins enter the brachiocephalic veins, which form the superior vena cava (Fig. 21.6).

Rules for Classification and Staging

Clinical Staging

With early and subclinical detection of breast cancer by screening mammography and further evaluation by magnetic resonance imaging (MRI), the clinical staging that relied on physical examination consisting of careful palpation and inspection of the mammary glands and draining lymph nodes has been supplemented by image-guided biopsy of the breast and suspicious nodes. The key feature in staging is in determining the size of the invasive component within 4 months of diagnosis and in the absence of disease progression (Table 21.3).

Pathologic Staging

The importance of pathologic staging (pT) is in its ability to truly assess the invasive component of a nodule

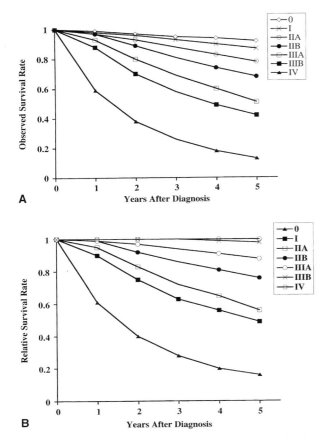

Figure 21.7 Breast cancer survival rates. AJCC figures of (**A**) observed survival rate and (**B**) relative survival rate, up to 5 years after diagnosis.

and evaluate lymph node involvement, often as sentinel nodes determined by scintigraphy. The nodule needs to be completely excised for pT, only microscopic positive margins are allowed, not macroscopic. The intraductal component is not added to the invasive component. Microinvasion is defined as extension beyond the basement membrane, with no focus more than 0.1 cm in diameter. When multiple foci exist, the size of the largest is used to classify microinvasion. Similarly, for multiple primaries only the largest is given a T stage, no stage is assigned to smaller cancers.

- T1a is >1 mm and ≤5 mm in greatest dimension;
- T1b is >5 mm and ≤10 mm in greatest dimension; and
- T1c is >10 mm and ≤20 mm in greatest dimension.

Curiously, microinvasion first defined in cervical uterine cancers is noted differently: T1a$_1$ is stromal invasion 3 mm in depth <7 mm horizontally and T1a$_2$ is >3 mm × ≤7 mm, respectively.

The pN categories are the most detailed in the AJCC manual, noting both the size of micrometastases in nodes as pN1Mi is >0.2 to ≤2 mm and the number of

nodes involved as well as their geographic location. Each pN stage is modified into three subcategories, creating 9 to 12 possibilities. At issue awaiting more data and analysis are:

- Isolated tumor cells (ITCs) detected by immunohistochemical techniques may be as small as 1 mm or 500,000 cells; however, confirmatory hematoxylin and eosin stains are advised.
- ITC is defined as ≤0.2 mm and micrometastases as >0.2 mm but ≤2 mm.
- Reverse transcriptase polymerase chain reaction can identify isolated cancer cells, but pN0 is advised with an appended designation of (mol+) or (mol−) as appropriate.
- The number of positive nodes is well supported by large series: 1 to 3 positive, 4 to 10 positive, and 10 positive show a progressive decline in survival as a function of the number of positive nodes.
- Supraclavicular lymph nodes (SCLN) are considered N3 and not M1 because survival is better with isolated SCLN without disseminated metastatic foci.
- Maturation of 80 potential prognostic variables remains under study, namely, p53, HER2/neu, and Ki-67.

Oncoimaging Annotations

- There are no pathognomonic mammographic signs that a lesion is either benign or malignant. The more irregular a mass is, the greater the likelihood of malignancy. Spiculated masses, however, can be caused by radial scars, postoperative scars, fat necrosis, desmoid tumors, hemorrhage, or abscesses.
- Approximately 10% of breast cancers are not mammographically visible. Only about two thirds of recurrent cancers in the treated breast are visible mammographically.
- On ultrasound, malignancies are typically ill defined, irregular, hypoechoic, taller than wide, and have posterior acoustic shadowing.
- MRI is the most reliable imaging study for assessing the presence of cancer. Contrast enhancement is not needed for this study. Dynamic contrast enhancement is, however, critical in the MRI evaluation of breast masses.

Cancer Statistics and Survival

The 5-year survival rates for women are dramatically different for breast cancer and lung cancer representing the best and worst outcomes. Breast cancer, after continually increasing for more than two decades reaching 200,000 new cases annually, leveled off at the begining of this millennium and has begun decreasing due to cessation of hormones in post-menopausal women. In addition to invasive cancer there are more than 60,000 new cases of *in situ* cancers, 85% of which are ductal cancer *in situ* (DCIS).

By contrast, lung cancer incidence is still above 200,000 new cases annually, decreasing in men and leveling off in women after smoking cessation. However, there are more than 150,000 deaths each year. The incidence of women dying of lung cancer exceeds that of women dying of breast cancer since 1987.

22

Thoracic Esophagus

Although the esophagus is thought of as a thoracic organ, cancers of the esophagus can arise in the neck and abdomen as well as the chest.

Perspective and Patterns of Spread

Esophageal cancers vary in their presentation depending on the anatomic site of origin: Cervical, thoracic, or abdominal. This long, tubular structure is subject to a variety of stresses beginning with smoking and alcohol abuse and terminating with acid reflux and hiatal hernia. The histopathologic types reflect their histiogenic origin (Table 22.1). The thoracic esophagus is largely a stratified squamous epithelium, gives rise to squamous cell carcinomas, and is similar to the mucous membrane of the upper digestive passage, which has a rich network of submucosal lymphatics and capillary loops. The lower esophagus is prone to develop adenocarcinoma owing to Barrett epithelial islands of gastric mucosa. This variety of cancer is presented separately, with digestive system cancers of the abdomen.

The incidence of esophageal cancers is approximately 14,000 new cases with an appalling 90% mortality rate unless the cancer is detected in its early stages. In some regions of the world, there is a very high prevalence, namely, northern provinces of China (20% of all deaths), the Transkei province in South America (50% of all cancers), and the Gonbad region of Northern Iran (200 times that of the United States). Numerous risk factors exist. Of interest is the early esophageal staging system. The Japanese have evolved an early staging system because of their increased and intensive screening, and because this cancer is endemic in the Far East.

The dread in esophageal cancer is ulceration and perforation, which can lead to numerous disastrous complications depending on the surrounding anatomy. In the upper third, tracheoesophageal fistulas, in the middle third, aortoesophageal perforation lead to a fatal and rapid exsanguination, and in the lower third, pericardial tamponade can result in pulsus paradoxus and heart failure.

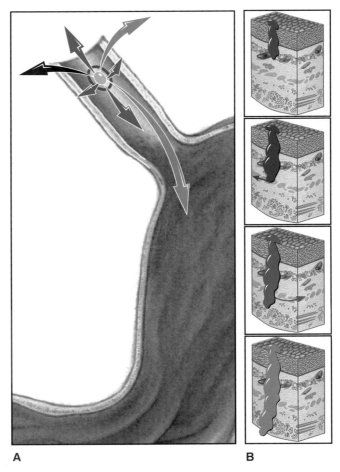

A   B

Figure 22.1 **A. Patterns of spread. B.** T categories. The patterns of spread and the primary tumor classification are similarly color-coded: Tis, yellow, cancer in situ of mucosa; T1, green (infiltrates the submucosa); T2, blue (penetrates to the muscularis propria); T3, purple (reaches the subserosa); and T4, red (invades through the serosa into a neighboring viscera).

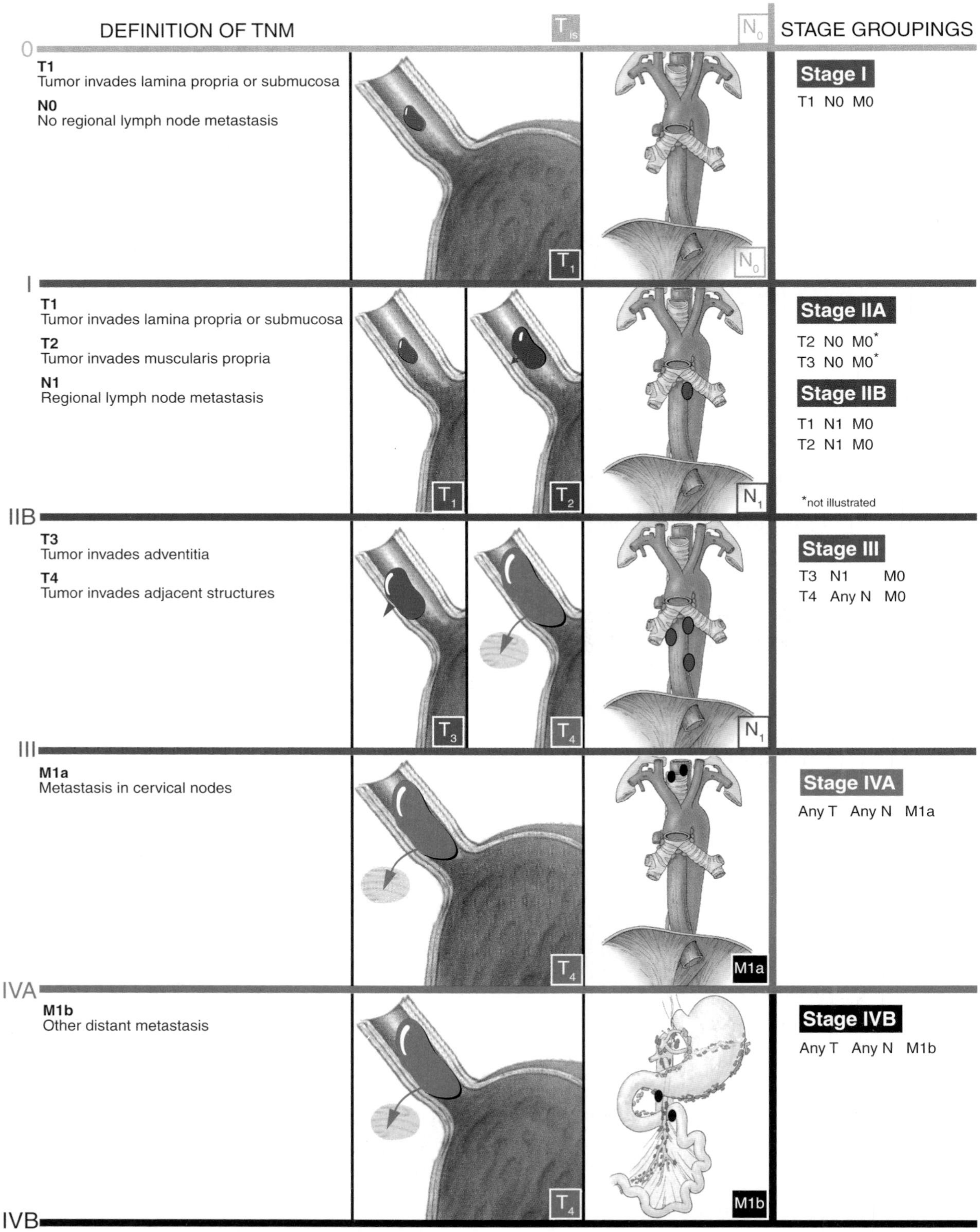

DEFINITION OF TNM

T_{is}

N_0

STAGE GROUPINGS

T1
Tumor invades lamina propria or submucosa

N0
No regional lymph node metastasis

T_1

N_0

Stage I
T1 N0 M0

T1
Tumor invades lamina propria or submucosa

T2
Tumor invades muscularis propria

N1
Regional lymph node metastasis

T_1

T_2

N_1

Stage IIA
T2 N0 M0*
T3 N0 M0*

Stage IIB
T1 N1 M0
T2 N1 M0

*not illustrated

T3
Tumor invades adventitia

T4
Tumor invades adjacent structures

T_3

T_4

N_1

Stage III
T3 N1 M0
T4 Any N M0

M1a
Metastasis in cervical nodes

T_4

M1a

Stage IVA
Any T Any N M1a

M1b
Other distant metastasis

T_4

M1b

Stage IVB
Any T Any N M1b

Figure 22.2 TNM staging diagram. Esophageal cancers are the introduction to hollow organs with multilayered muscle walls lined by an epithelial mucosa on the inside and adentitia or serosa outside. Vertical presentation of stage groupings, which follow same color code for cancer advancement are organized in horizontal lanes: Stage 0, yellow; I, green; II, blue; III, purple; IVA, red; and metastatic stage IVB, black. Definitions of TN on left and stage grouping on right. The histologic section of the esophageal wall illustrates the cancer invasion into and through the wall layers (Fig. 22.1). Note the nodal distribution is from the neck to the abdomen although the esophagus is a thoracic organ.

TABLE 22.1	**Histopathologic Type: Common Cancers of the Esophagus**

Type

The classification applies to all carcinomas. Sarcomas are not included. Worldwide, squamous cell carcinomas are the most common, but the incidence of adenocarcinoma is increasing. In North America and Europe, adenocarcinomas are more common than squamous cell carcinomas. Adenocarcinomas arising from Barrett esophagus are included in the classification.

From Greene FL, Page DL, Fleming ID, et al. (eds): *AJCC Cancer Staging Manual.* 6th ed. New York: Springer; 2002. Used with the permission of the American Joint Committee on Cancer (AJCC) Chicago, Illinois.

The malignant gradient is high throughout, with more survivors in the cervical segment decreasing intrathoracically, and least at the gastroesophageal junction because of the ease of cancer spread to infradiaphragmatic sites (Fig. 22.1).

TNM Staging Criteria

Esophageal staging has remained consistent with no changes in T or N categories. The only histologic difference from other hollow digestive system sites is the presence of an adventitia instead of a serosa. This allows for distensibility of the esophagus to accommodate a food bolus because, in its normal collapsed state, it appears on computed tomography (CT) to have a straw-like lumen of a few millimeters. T1 is mucosal, T2 muscular, T3 adventitial, and T4 is into the surrounding structures (Fig. 22.2).

Summary of Changes

There have been no changes from the fifth edition of the AJCC CSM.

Orientation of Three-planar Oncoanatomy

The isocenter chosen for the esophagus is at the thoracic T10 level to signal the termination of primary sites in the thorax and simultaneously introduce the beginning of the digestive system. T10 is the level of the esophageal opening in the diaphragm; T8 is for the level of the opening for the vena cava; and T12 is the stomal opening for the aorta (Fig. 22.3).

T-oncoanatomy
- *Coronal:* The esophagus consists of three principal regions: Cervical, thoracic, and cardiac portions. The cervical esophagus extends from the pharyngeal–esophageal junction (the cricopharyngeal sphincter) inferiorly to the level of the thoracic inlet, about 18 cm from the upper incisor teeth. The upper and midthoracic esophagus extends from the thoracic inlet to a point 10 cm above the esophagogastric junction, which is usually at the level of the lower border

of the esophagus to the cardiac orifice of the stomach, which is about 40 cm from the upper incisor teeth.
- *Sagittal:* The esophagus is a muscular tube consisting of two layers of smooth muscle, one longitudinal and the other horizontal, and this is carried through into the rest of the gastrointestinal system. Peristalsis is initiated with swallowing and the major function is to propel food into the stomach. There are two sphincters in the esophagus and these are at the cricopharyngeal muscle and the cardiac sphincter at the cardia of the stomach. These sphincters have been extensively studied from the physiologic point of view and are common sites of both benign and neoplastic disease.
- *Transverse:* The esophageal opening of the diaphragm is anterior and to the left (T10) of the aorta (T12) and note the esophagus in between the right and left layer of the mediastinum. The course of the esophagus is from slightly to the right of the midline to the left as it pierces the diaphragm through its own opening. It is in continual contact with the right lung; on the left side, the aorta is in continual contact with the left lung. The azygos vein provides a partial shield on the right side and posteriorly. Pulmonary veins are expected to be in more intimate contact because they drain to the left atrium, which is posterior to the ventricle. The thoracic duct is posterior to the esophagus along its course, which is the reverse of the esophagus coursing from the right side of midline to the left as it ascends. When the esophagus comes in front of the descending aorta, it is suspended by the mesoesophagus, which allows it to curve forward before its escape through the diaphragm (Fig. 22.4).

N-oncoanatomy

The American Joint Committee on Cancer (AJCC)/ International Union Against Cancer numbering of mediastinal and abdominal nodes is unique, but are different from the International Anatomic Terminology.

The regional lymph nodes for the cervical esophagus are the cervical and supraclavicular nodes. For the thoracic esophagus, the regional nodes are the adjacent

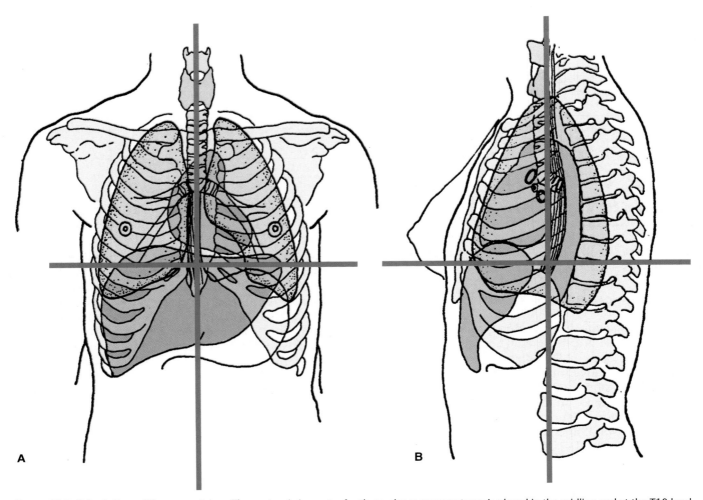

Figure 22.3 Orientation of T-oncoanatomy. The anatomic isocenter for three-planar oncoanatomy is placed in the midline and at the T10 level at the dome of the diaphragm. **A.** Coronal. **B** Sagittal.

mediastinal lymph nodes. Involvement of more distant nodes is considered distant metastasis. Retrograde and prograde lymphatic spread usually places all of the lymph node stations in the neck, mediastinum, and abdomen at risk. One of the major problems with control of this cancer is the frequency with which lymph node invasion occurs and the rapidity of its dissemination to the other distant anatomic areas. Esophageal cancer is therefore not only a disease of the chest, but also of the neck and abdomen. Because of its lymphatic drainage, esophageal cancer is a formidable tumor to encompass by locoregional modalities of therapy (Fig. 22.5).

M-oncoanatomy

A rich plexus of venous anastomoses exists with stomach, liver, pancreas, and adrenals (see Fig. 19.7). Therefore, the liver, lung, and adrenals are the most common sites of distant metastases. Remote metastasis from the carcinoma of the esophagus, although ultimately fa-

tal, often carries a better prognosis than when the primary lesion has extended locally outside the esophagus into mediastinal structures, a condition that is rapidly fatal.

Rules for Classification and Staging

Clinical Staging and Imaging

The esophagus is inaccessible to physical examination and endoscopy is limited as to depth of invasion. Imaging is critical to evaluation of staging (Table 22.2). Endoscopic ultrasound is of greatest value for superficial invasion of the muscular wall. CT provides the assessment of invasion into surrounding structures and regional lymph nodes in the mediastinum. Metastatic disease in lung and liver can be done with spiral CT at the same time. MRI can be useful when invasion of mediastinal lymph nodes and structures are in doubt and need to be resolved. PET can provide an overview if disseminated metastasis is suspected.

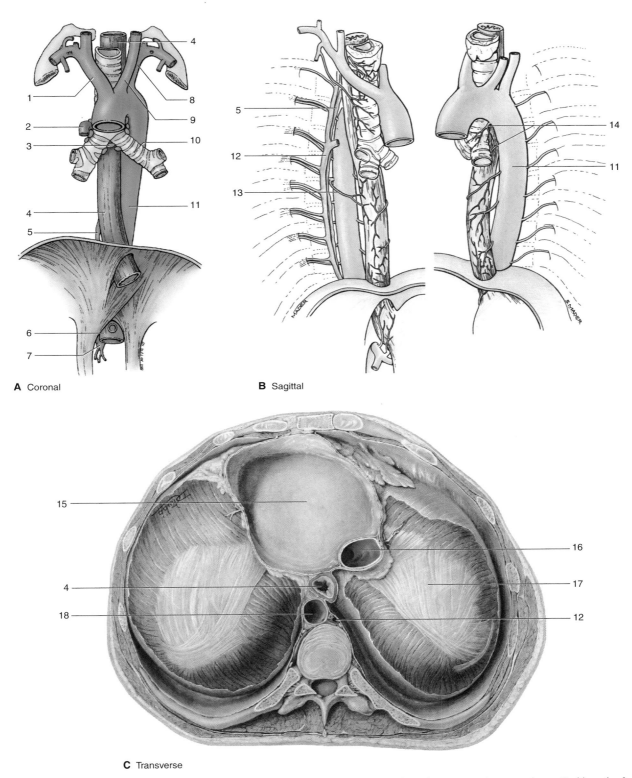

A Coronal

B Sagittal

C Transverse

Figure 22.4 **T-oncoanatomy three-planar views. A.** Coronal. The esophagus is the only structure that runs the vertical length of mediastinum. It originates at the level of the cricoid cartilage in the neck and then courses from right to left entering the abdomen at T10 level at the midline through its own opening. (1) Brachiocephalic artery. (2) Arch of azygos vein. (3) Tracheobronchial lymph node. (4) Esophagus. (5) Thoracic duct. (6) Abdominal aorta. (7) Cisterna chili. (8) Left subclavian artery. (9) Left Common carotid artery. (10) Left Main bronchus. (11) Thoracic aorta. **B.** Sagittal. In the left anterolateral view, note that the aorta is the mediastinal structure maintaining the longest contact and supplies the esophagus directly. (12) Azygos vein. (13) Esophageal artery. (14) Left bronchial artery. **C.** Transverse. Between the inferior part of the esophagus and aorta, the right and left layers of mediastinal pleura from a dorsal mesoesophagus. (15) Pericardial sac. (16) Inferior vena cava. (17) Central tendon of diaphragm. (18) Aorta.

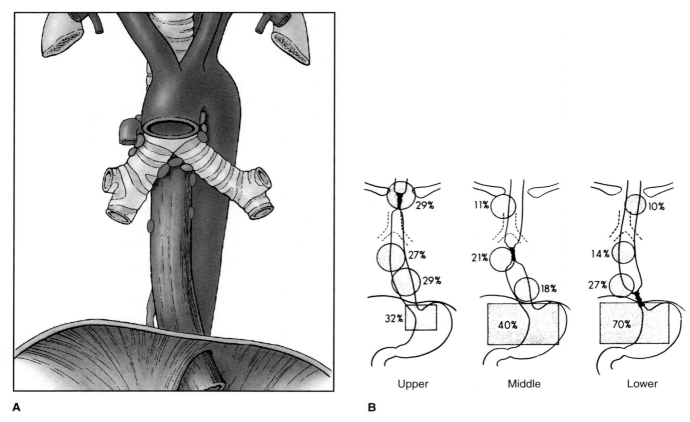

A   **B**

Figure 22.5 **Orientation of N-oncoanatomy. A.** Mediastinal sentinel nodes vary depending on location of cancer. Paracarinal and subcarinal nodes are frequently involved. **B.** The percentage of positive lymph nodes found at surgery for esophageal carcinoma in the upper, middle, and lower esophagus.

TABLE 22.2	Imaging Modalities for Staging for Esophagogastric Junction Cancer	
Method	**Diagnosis and Staging Capability**	**Recommended for Use**
Primary Tumor and regional nodes		
Single-contrast upper GI studies	Useful in detecting and defining primary lesions in stomach	Yes
Double-contrast upper GI studies	Very useful in detecting early gastric cancers	Yes—should be performed along with single contrast
Gastroscopy	Very accurate modality to detect and define primary lesions: ~90% confirmation rate	Yes—use to confirm lesion detected in UGI series and to screen high-risk patients
CT, abdomen ± chest	Most valuable of all modalities for determining degree of extragastric extension and distant metastases	Yes
Endoscopic ultrasound	Most accurate method of determining extension within and beyond gastric wall	Yes, if plan preoperative chemoirradiation
Metastatic tumors		
Chest films	Good for detecting metastases	Yes
Laparoscopy	May allow visualization of small serosal implants or liver metastases	Yes, if plan preoperative chemotherapy or chemoradiation
Bone film	Useful only for confirming metastases	No, unless patient has bone pain
Radionuclide scans—liver, brain, bone	Useful in evaluation of clinically suspected metastases; CT is better than nuclide scan for liver and brain	No, unless suspected bone metastases

GI, gastrointestinal; UGI, upper gastrointestinal; CT, computed tomography.

Pathologic Staging

All pathologic specimens from clinical invasive procedures—bronchoscopy, mediastinoscopy, mediastinotomy, thoracentesis, and thorascopy—are applicable. The thoracotomy and resection of primary and lymph nodes are the mainstay of pathologic staging. Preferably, six nodes should be examined.

Oncoimaging Notations

- Ninety percent of adenocarcinomas occur near the esophagogastric junction.
- Double-contrast studies can recognize mucosal and submucosal lesions.
- CT, endoscopic ultrasound (EUS) and MRI provide a complete picture of invasion. EUS is more accurate in staging penetration of five esophageal layers in its walls and CT is better for detection of invasion to adjacent structures.
- PET is better for finding metastases.
- EUS demonstrates hyperechoic alternately with hypoechoic layers of esophageal wall.
- MRI and Gd-DTPA shows extensions into mediastinal and diaphragmatic tissues.

Cancer Statistics and Survival

The esophagus accounted for 14,250 new cancer cases, 13,300 cancer deaths (93%) with a 5-year survival rate improvement from 1950 to 2000 of 11%. Currently, relative 5-year survival for all stages is 14%, but when localized improves to 29.1%.

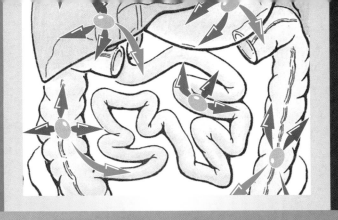

SECTION 3

ABDOMEN PRIMARY SITES

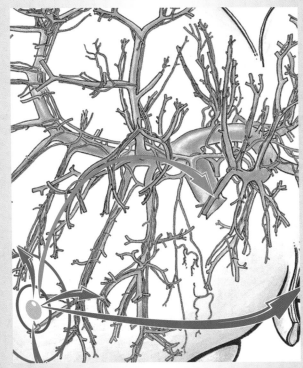

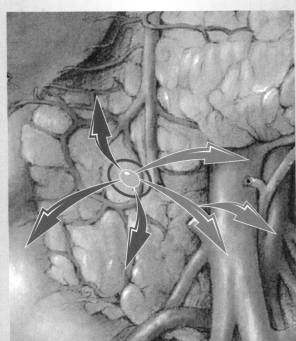

23

Introduction and Orientation

The digestive system anatomy with its multiple layered walls determines the TNM staging and is the model for staging other hollow viscera and structures.

Perspective and Patterns of Spread

Gastrointestinal tract (GIT) neoplasms are among the most common cancers. Colorectal cancers are the third most common cancer in both men and women. Cancer of the colon and rectum affects as many as 150,000 Americans annually; almost a third of this group dies from it. Research stimulating screening and early detection of polyps appears to be reducing mortality rates. Gastric cancers are quite prevalent in some parts of the world, such as Japan, but, curiously, they are decreasing in incidence for unexplained reasons in the United States. Because of the accommodating nature of the GIT, most cancers are insidious in onset and can manifest as subtle changes in digestive and bowel habits or appetite. Unfortunately, the usual presentations of bowel obstruction, ulceration, and bleeding or perforation are signs of considerable advancement.

The digestive system is the longest anatomic structure characterized by the infradiagramatic GIT as a hollow tubular organ, which is largely glandular in nature and gives rise to adenocarcinomas (Table 23.1). The lumen of the small intestines is lined by a single layer of columnar epithelial cells that form an apical membrane of enterocytes that contains numerous microvilli. The villi become less numerous as one transits from the jejunum to the ileum and become more mucous producing and rich in goblet cells in the colon. Polyposis secondary to inflammatory disease or an inherited familial disorder is often the forerunner to frank malignancy. As the benign polyp transforms into an adenocarcinoma it invades the wall of the bowel and spreads in the direction of the muscular layers (Fig. 23.1). First, it encircles the lumen following circular muscles and then is propelled longitudinally with peristalsis by the longitudinal muscle layer. It is important to note that with depth of wall invasion there is propulsion of the cancer by peristalsis in other directions and dimensions. The

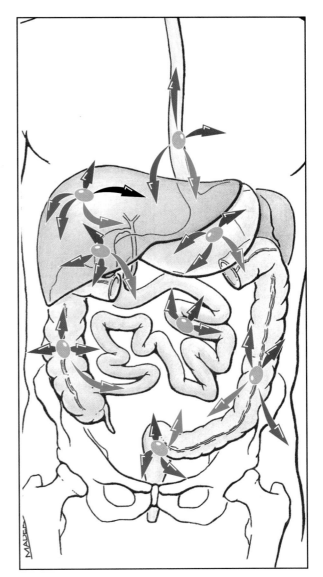

Figure 23.1 **Collage of patterns of spread.** Gastrointestinal cancers and major digestive organ tumors: Color-coded for T stage: Tis, yellow; T1, green; T2, blue; T3, purple; and T4, red.

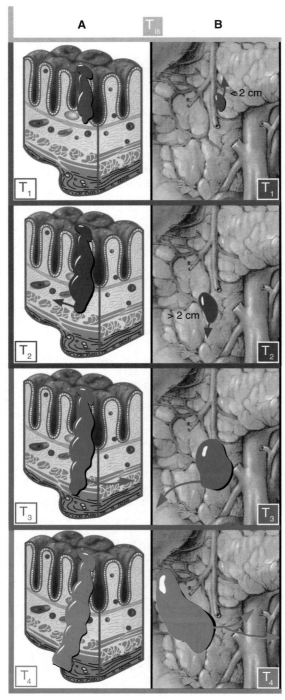

Figure 23.2 TNM staging criteria. A. Hollow organ prototype. Tis (mucosa), yellow; T1 (submucosa), green; T2 (muscularis externa), blue; T3 (serosa), purple; and T4 (perforates into another organ), red. **B.** Solid organ (pancreas) T1, green; T2, blue; T3, purple; and T4, red.

adopted as the molecular biologic basis for carcinogenesis.

The majority of digestive systems neoplasms are successfully treated with multimodal treatment; 65% or 120,000 patients survive long term. In contrast, major digestive gland cancers, whether pancreatic or hepatic, are insidious in onset and rarely cured. Of the estimated 32,000 pancreatic cancers, virtually all (31,000) die annually. Hepatic cancers follow in the wake of hepatitis infection with subsequent scaring, cirrhosis, and neoplastic transformation. Few of the 18,920 patients diagnosed annually survive and most require total hepatectomy and liver transplantation. Recognizing the widespread incidence of hepatitis in China, hepatocarcinomas are among the most common cancers both in Asia and in a global sense, because of China's large population.

TNM Staging Criteria

Gastrointestinal Tract

The pattern of hollow viscus invasion varies with the anatomic location or site of origin of the cancer in the GIT. The size of the lumen and the proximity of the tumor to sphincters determine whether obstruction is an early expression of malignant activity or a sign of an extensive tumor. Adjacent structures are invaded first, particularly those in direct proximity. The bowel loops on mesenteries are more mobile than those that are fixed and can spread their cancer cells intraperitoneally more readily. Tumor behavior is a function of the anatomy and physiology at each of the major sites in the alimentary tract. The GIT is a hollow tubular organ, the penetration of the wall of bowel, the cancers depth of invasion is the commonality for staging at all sites, T1, T2, T3, and T4—mucosal, muscularis, serosa, and adjacent viscera, respectively (Fig. 23.2A). This is also the rule for most other hollow organs in other systems, for example, gallbladder and bile ducts (Table 23.2). Solid organs (pancreas and liver) are based on tumor size T1, T2 and capsular invasion T3 and T4 major vessels.

The lymphoid drainage of the digestive system and major digestive glands (MDG) overlap and reflect both the arterial blood supply and venous drainage, which are not always parallel. The small intestine is a major extranodal site with its Peyer patches and the appendix is an analog for the bursa of Fabricius, the origin for B cells in lower vertebrates. The mesenteric nodes are not acknowledged in the lymphoma staging as a node-bearing region. The para-aortic and paracaval location for lymph nodes relate to the roots of origin of visceral arteries as the celiac, superior, and inferior mesenteric arteries. Smooth metastatic nodules in the pericolic and perirectal fat are considered lymph node metastases and counted in N staging. Irregular nodules are considered as vascular invasion and are either V1 (microscopic) or V2 (macroscopic) when viewed histopathologically.

apocryphal model of genetic instability and gene modifications for the progression of in situ cellular changes from a benign polyp to a locally invasive cancer and then to metastatic behavior was first described by Vogelstein in bowel. This multistep paradigm has been more widely

TABLE 23.1	Histopathologic Type: Digestive System Cancers	
Adenocarcinoma in situ		Squamous cell (epidermoid) carcinoma
Adenocarcinoma		Adenosquamous carcinoma
Medullary carcinoma		Small cell carcinoma
Mucinous carcinoma (colloid type; >50% mucinous carcinoma)		Undifferentiated carcinoma
Signet ring cell carcinoma (>50% signet ring cell)		Carcinoma, NOS

From Greene FL, Page DL, Fleming ID, et al. eds. *AJCC Cancer Staging Manual.* 6th ed. New York: Springer; 2002. Used with the permission of the American Joint Committee on Cancer (AJCC), Chicago, Illinois.

The sentinel lymph nodes for each primary site are also noted.

When the visceral vessels drain into the inferior vena cava, the retroperitoneal lymph nodes cluster along the abdominal aorta and inferior vena cava vessels. When these nodes are involved, they are juxtaregional and can be considered metastatic nodes. The staging of nodes in the gastrointestinal region is extremely varied and one can only speculate as to the lack of more uniform criteria. At most major primary sites, there is only an N1 designation independent of size and number of nodes involved. Thus, N1 is simply a positive node and applies to esophagus, small intestine, liver, pancreas, gallbladder, extrahepatic ducts, and ampulla of Vater. The colon and rectum are similar to the breast in that N1 is one to three nodes and N2 is more than four nodes. The stomach is the most unique site, with an elaborate nodal classification: N1, 1 to 6 nodes; N2, 7 to 15 nodes; and N3, ≥15 nodes.

Major Digestive Glands and Ducts

The major feature in staging cancer of the liver and pancreas is size of the cancer(s) and venous invasion or entrapment of major arteries and veins that render such malignancies unresectable in conventional radical surgery. However, the increasing use of liver transplantation and/or liver–pancreas transplants with their connecting extrahepatic ducts may require the criteria of unresectability to be revamped. For the liver, 5 cm size and for the pancreas, 2 cm size, divides lesions as to early (T1) to advanced (T2, T3; Fig. 23.2B). The gallbladder, the extrahepatic duct cholangiocarcinomas, and the rare cancer of the hepatopancreatic ampulla (of Vater) masquerade as gallstones, presenting with obstructive jaundice. If detected when those duct cancers are contained within their walls it is T1, T2, and the possibility of resection and cure is real. However, once their walls are penetrated by cancer (T3) and enter and invade adjacent and surrounding organs (T4), their resectability decreases and their patient's survival is compromised.

Summary of Changes

Generally, there is no overarching principle or context design for the digestive system (GIT) or MDG as to stage groupings. For gastrointestinal system and major digestive glands there are no overarching rules as to stage groups and definitions of nodal categories. The T categories are consistent for hollow tubular multilayered digestive system sites, i.e., T1 mucosa, T2 submucosa, T3 muscularis, T4 serosa. N1 is the only nodal category in 7 of 10 sites but is variously assigned from stage I to stage III. Stage subgroups A/B are variously assigned in stage I, II, III, IV with an occasional C. The major basis for stage subgroups are supportive survival data, justifying the amalgams of T and N. The color code for progression of stage groups generally defines resectable (purple) versus unresectable (red) cancers and black is reserved for metastatic. Stages are frequently expanded to six by subdividing a stage into A and B. The T and N categories are assigned to a stage grouping, specifically for division of a stage into a (A) more favorable versus a (B) less favorable grouping. This occurs at different stages for different sites. N1, is the only nodal category in 7 of 10 sites but is variously assigned from I, II, III, and IV.

Overview of Oncoanatomy

The digestive system (alimentary tract) is a long hollow tubular organ with multilayered walls and numerous sphincters. Once the upper digestive system passes the esophagus, the mucosa that gives rise to adenocarcinomas is similar for stomach, small intestine, colon, and rectum. The mucosa, the innermost layer, is covered with simple columnar epithelium and has specific variation in villus size, which decreases in size and cell kinetic turnover time as one descends from stomach to rectum. A diagram (Fig. 23.3) of the general organization shows the wall structure for each segment and Table 23.3 lists the derivative cell and respective cancer it gives rise to in the various sections of the digestive system:

- *Esophagus* (Fig. 23.3B): Stratified squamous with islands of gastric mucosa.

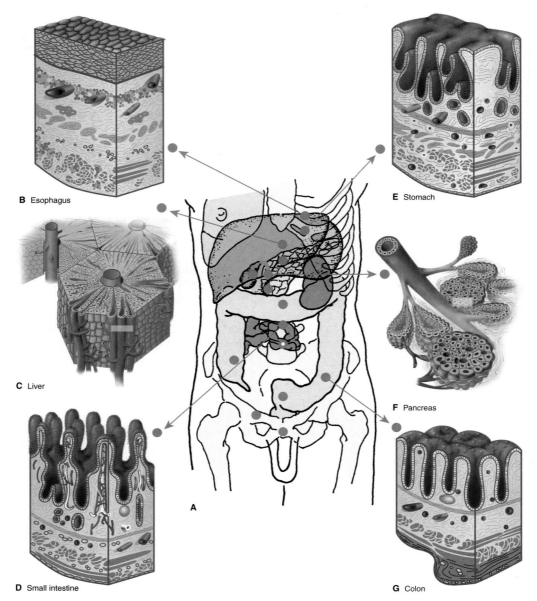

B Esophagus

C Liver

D Small intestine

E Stomach

F Pancreas

G Colon

A

Figure 23.3 **Overview of oncoanatomy.** Histologic structural differences throughout gastrointestinal and major digestive organ systems. **A.** Primary site isocenters. **B.** Esophagus. **C.** Liver. **D.** Small intestine. **E.** Stomach. **F.** Pancreas. **G.** Colon.

- *Stomach* (Fig. 23.3E): Gastric gland: Active divisions are in the neck with its short isthmus compared to the deep pits with mucous (*blue*), parietal (*red*), and chief (violaceous) cells.

- *Small Intestine* (Fig. 23.3D): The small intestinal mucosa is marked with feathery villi and shallow pits with active division being in the neck of the gland with its columnar absorptive cells on the villus and into the pit. The primary function of enterocytes is absorption; goblet cells produce mucin; and paneth cells maintain mucosal immunity with their antimicrobial secretions. Each villus has a central lacteal, a capillary, and venule.

- *Colon* (Fig. 23.3G): The colon has a smooth mucosa without villi or pits. It has shallow glands lined with a simple columnar epithelium that contains goblet cells, absorptive cells, and enteroendocrine cells with active division in its crypts.

- *Liver* (Fig. 23.3C): The liver is a compound tubular gland, each portal triad with its own bile duct, portal vein, and hepatic artery segment.

- *Pancreas* (Fig. 23.3F): The pancreas consists of centroacinar and pancreatic acinar cells with pancreatic islets of α, β and δ cells.

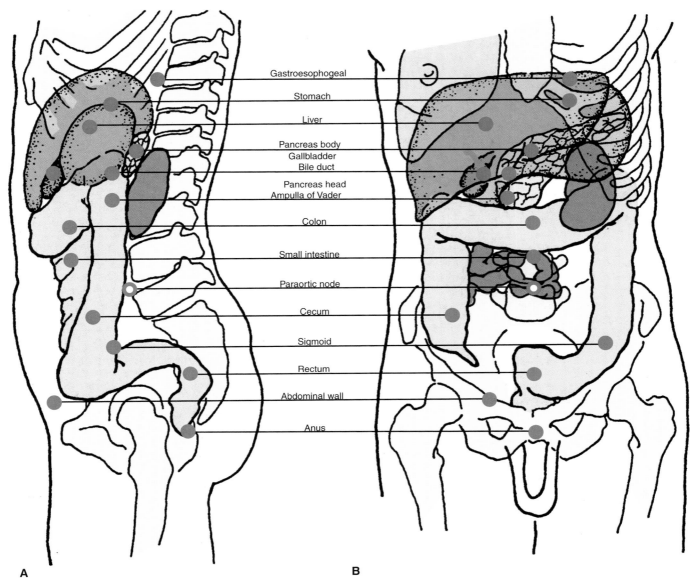

Gastroesophogeal
Stomach
Liver
Pancreas body
Gallbladder
Bile duct
Pancreas head
Ampulla of Vader
Colon
Small intestine
Paraortic node
Cecum
Sigmoid
Rectum
Abdominal wall
Anus

A   B

Figure 23.4 **Orientation of three-3planar T-oncoanatomy.** Anatomic isocenter of 10 GIT primary sites. **A.** Coronal anterior and **B.** sagittal lateral. (*continued*)

The gastrointestinal canal includes that portion of the digestive tract that extends from the stomach to the anus. It is housed within the abdominopelvic cavity, which extends from the thoracic diaphragm to the pelvic diaphragm caudally. The abdominal cavity is lined by peritoneum, an areolar membrane covered with a single layer of mesothelial cells. The peritoneal cavity is a physiologically complex structure containing fluid secretions, which bathe and lubricate the bowel surfaces, and anatomically consists of numerous sacs and folds. Normally, the fluid is absorbed, but when it accumulates as ascites, malignancy with peritoneal seeding is a concern clinically. A double layer of peritoneum connects the stomach with the lesser omentum (from the

lesser curvature) and with the greater omentum (from the greater curvature). The numerous peritoneal folds consist of mesenteries for gut, arteries, and veins, although some do not contain tubes. Peritoneal fossae, recesses, and gutters determine initial pathways of tumor spread both for bowel cancer and ovarian cancer. In addition to the omental bursae, there is a duodenal fossa, a cecal fossa, an intersigmoid fossa, a pelvic fossa, and a paracolic fossa.

Orientation of Three-planar T-oncoanatomy

There are 11 primary cancer sites, including the six GIT hollow structures: Esophagus, stomach, small intestine,

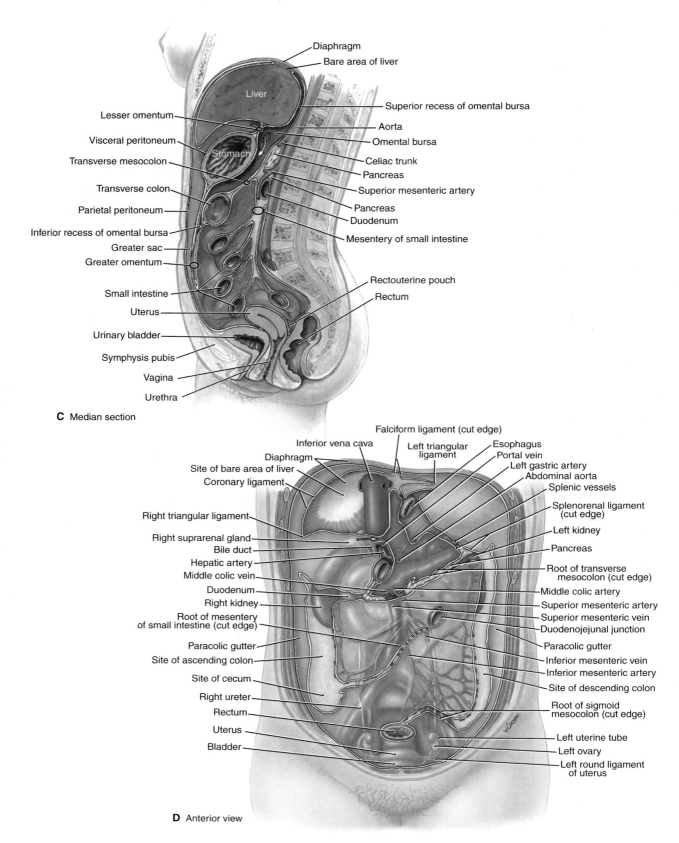

C Median section

D Anterior view

Figure 23.4 *(Continued)* **C.** sectors of abdominal cavity and **D.** roots of peritoneal reflections.

colon, rectum, and anus. In addition, there are five primary sites arising in the MDG: Liver, gallbladder, extrahepatic bile ducts, the ampulla of Vater and pancreas. There are two major anatomic sectors and 11 major primary cancer sites. The abdomen is divided into two sectors based on the peritoneum, that is, the structures are intraperitoneal or extraperitoneal (Fig. 23.4C, D). With the exception of the pancreas, lower rectum, and anus, all major primary sites are intraperitoneal except for that portion of the bowel that is directly attached to the posterior wall of the abdomen and has no mesentery (Fig. 23.4B).

The abdomen superiorly extends under the diaphragm into the lower third of the thorax and inferiorly extends into the pelvis. The GIT and the MDG are the frequent sites of adenocarcinomas. To interweave these 11 primary sites, which are largely intraperitoneal, a multiplanar orientation follows (Fig. 23.4A, B). The presentation of primary site isocenters starts at T11 and T12 near the diaphragmatic insertion and progresses to L1 to L5 and then onto the pelvis S1, S2, and S3.

A cephalad to caudad GIT and MDG tabulation of the cancers, the vertebral levels, and the adjacent anatomic structures to be aware of at the transverse axial level assist in presenting the classification and staging process of the digestive tract cancers. Most GIT and MDG organs occupy many vertebral levels, the three planar views and the axial vertebral assignment is designed to be at the anatomic isocenter of the structure. The anatomic isocenters (Fig. 23.4) for the gastrointestinal tract are displayed in sections transversely at a specific vertebral levels recognizing there is a variablity. The section is more representative than actual. Nevertheless, the oncoanatomy is accurate and allows for aligning surface, musculoskeletal and visceral anatomy. But because most of these cancers are inaccessible to direct clinical examination, they require endoscopy and imaging for diagnosis and evaluation of anatomic extent. Surgical pathologic staging is essential and more accurate, and therefore is most often done for both treatment planning and definitive treatment itself. The GIT primary sites are presented first and then those of the MDG will follow as in the American Joint Committee on Cancer/International Union Against Cancer manuals.

- *Esophagus*: The gastroesophageal junction is at the diaphragmatic level and islands of Barrett mucosa can occur. The ectopic location of gastric mucosa in the distal esophagus is vulnerable for forming adenocarcinomas. The cardioesophageal junction has become increasingly notorious for adenocarcinomas that spread into the thorax as well as the epigastrium.

- *Stomach*: The stomach is divided into three regions: Upper, middle, and lower third. To delineate these regions, the lesser and greater curves of the stomach are divided; the upper third is the cardiac area and fundus, the middle third the body, and the lower third the antrum. Gastric cancers can become large before they produce obstructive symptoms. Avid and aggressive screening in at-risk populations (Japan) has lead to detection of early gastric cancers.

- *Small Intestine*: The small intestine extends from the pylorus of the stomach to the ileocecal valve. It is approximately 25 feet long and divided into three sections: The duodenum, jejunum, and ileum. The duodenum is essentially a midline structure, approximately 1 foot long. It provides some of the most complex anatomy in the upper abdomen as it conforms to and surrounds the head of the pancreas. The small intestine despite its length gives rise to few cancers. Instead, a large variety of neoplastic syndromes occur and unusual tumors is its hallmark.

- *Colon*: The large intestine is the most prevalent site for cancer, particularly with its numerous (eight) subsites at high risk. The large intestine or colon picture frames the abdominal content and is 60 cm long and is divided into an ascending, transverse, descending and sigmoid colon with a hepatic flexure on the right and splenic flexure on the left. Favored subsites for malignancy include the cecum, sigmoid, and rectum. The colon is vulnerable to polyposis and chronic inflammatory disease that can lead to carcinomas.

- *Rectum*: The rectum is the most common site in GIT for malignancies. It is about 12 cm long, extends from a point opposite the third sacral vertebra down to the apex of the prostate in the male and to the apex of the perineal body in the female, that is, to a point 4 cm anterior to the tip of the coccyx. It may be arbitrarily defined as the distal 10 cm of the large intestine, as measured by preoperative sigmoidoscopy from the anal verge. The rectum has no epiploic appendages, no haustrations, and no taeniae. It is covered by peritoneum in front and on both sides in its upper third and on the anterior wall only in its middle third; there is no peritoneal covering in the lower third.

- *Anus*: About 4 cm long, the anal canal courses downward and backward from the apex of the prostate or the perineal body. The anocutaneous line, or white line of Hilton, at the base of the rectal columns marks the site of the original anal membrane that separated the endodermal gut from the ectodermal proctoderm. With the high incidence of anal viral infection, both human papilloma virus and human immunodeficiency virus, the risk of anal cancers is increasing in the homosexual population.

To appreciate the anatomic relationship between the digestive tubular system and the MDG, consider the embryogenesis of the endoderm; there is a foregut, midgut, and hindgut, each with its own arterial blood supply,

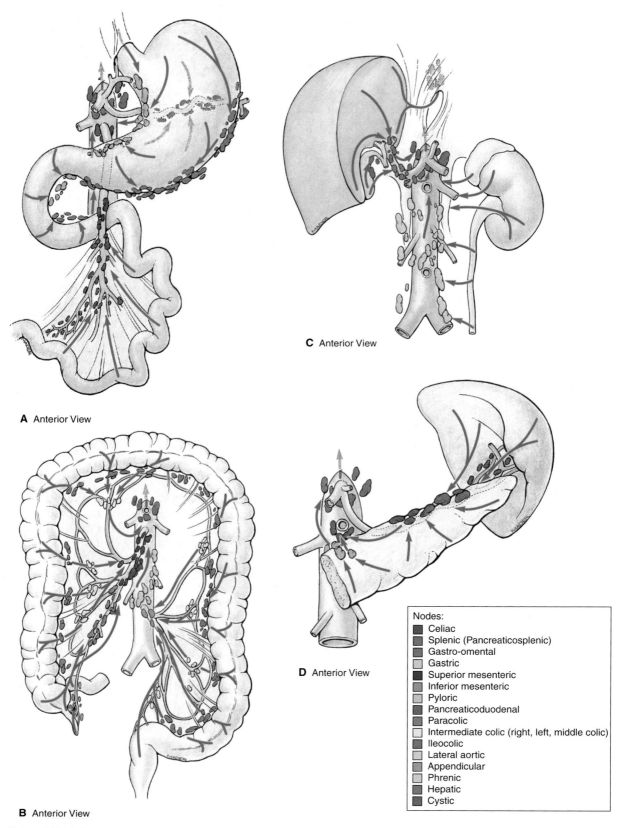

C Anterior View

A Anterior View

Nodes:
- ■ Celiac
- ■ Splenic (Pancreaticosplenic)
- ■ Gastro-omental
- ■ Gastric
- ■ Superior mesenteric
- ■ Inferior mesenteric
- ■ Pyloric
- ■ Pancreaticoduodenal
- ■ Paracolic
- ■ Intermediate colic (right, left, middle colic)
- ■ Ileocolic
- ■ Lateral aortic
- ■ Appendicular
- ■ Phrenic
- ■ Hepatic
- ■ Cystic

D Anterior View

B Anterior View

Figure 23.5 Orientation of N-oncoanatomy. Lymphatic drainage of the abdomen. **A.** Stomach, duodenum, and small intestines to ileum. **B.** Colon and rectum. **C.** Liver. **D.** Pancreas.

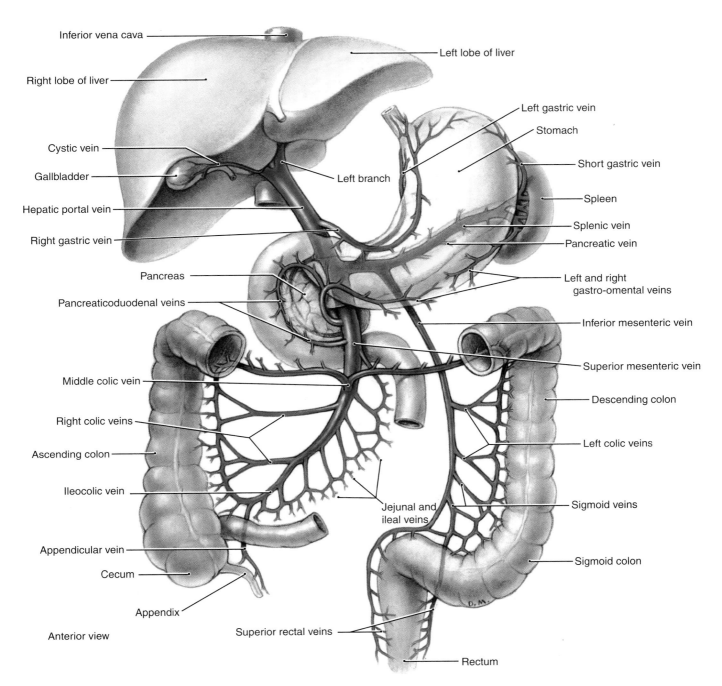

Figure 23.6 **Orientation of M-oncoanatomy.** Portal venous system.

namely, celiac artery, superior mesenteric artery, and inferior mesenteric artery, respectively. As the liver enlarges to the right, the gut rotates clockwise along its midsagittal and midcoronal axes from 12 to 3 o'clock as do the ventral pancreas, gallbladder, and bile ducts around the second part of the duodenum. This clockwise rotation creates the lesser omental bursa with the portal triad of portal vein, hepatic artery, and bile duct in its mouth, the foramen of Winslow. The fusion of mesenteries leads to ligaments, named for their shape or organ they attach and connect. Each of the three arteries with its branches defines the geographic locus of the derivative organs of the foregut, midgut, and hindgut, namely, celiac artery (T12/L1), superior mesenteric artery (L1/L2), and inferior mesenteric artery (L3/L4).

TABLE 23.2	Overview of Histogenesis of Gastrointestinal Tract/Major Digestive Glands Epithelia and Cancers		
Primary Site	**Derivative Cell**	**Cancer Histopathology**	**Axial Level**
Esophagus (see thorax)	Stratified squamous epithelium	Squamous cell	T9/T10
Esophagogastric junction	Ectopic Barrett epithelium, cardiac glands	Adenocarcinoma, papillary, tubular	T9/T10
Stomach	Deep gastric glands, simple columnar, chief and parietal cells	Adenocarcinoma, mucinous	T10/T11/T12
Liver	Hepatocyte	Hepatocellular cancer cholangiocarcinoma	T10/T11/T12, L1
Gallbladder	Hepatic stellate cell, intrahepatic ductal cell	Adenocarcinoma, papillary, mucinous	T12, L1
Extrahepatic ducts	Apical microvilli, simple columnar epithelium	Cholangiocarcinoma	L1/L2
Pancreas	Simple columnar/cuboidal epithelium	Signet ring adenocarcinoma, undifferentiated adenocarcinoma	L1/L2
Ampulla	Acinar, intercalated, interlobular columnar and cuboidal epithelium	Ductal adenocarcinoma; (sclerosing, nodular, papillary) adenosquamous cell	L2
Colon	Simple columnar epithelium	Mucinous adenocarcinoma, Signet ring adenocarcinoma	L2/L3/L4/L5
Small intestine	Simple columnar Goblet cells Plica circularis, microvilli, columnar absorptive cells	Adenocarcinoma, NOS	L3/L4/L5
Rectum	Simple columnar epithelium, mucinous, Goblet cells	Adenocarcinoma, rectal type, mucinous, Signet Ring	S1–S5
Anus	Stratified columnar and stratified squamous epithelium	Squamous cell cancer, basaloid carcinoma	Pubic bone, femoral head

NOS, not otherwise specified.

The MDG constitute five more primary sites, a number of which are quite uncommon cancers.

- *Liver*: By virtue of its weight, the liver is the largest organ in the body. When filled with cancerous nodules, it is often the greatest repository of neoplastic disease, exceeding the primary tumors in the quantity of malignant cells. To understand the anatomy of the liver, it is important to be aware of its internal structure as a gland of compound tubular design. Each lobule is shaped like a cylinder or tubule, with a central vein that drains a rich anatomic sinusoidal network derived from the fine hepatic arterioles and portal vessels. The hepatocyte elaborates both an external/exocrine secretion and an internal/endocrine secretion of enzymes into the blood. The former is referred to as bile and is collected by biliary canaliculi.

- *Gallbladder*: The gallbladder is a small saccular organ located inferior to the liver in its own fossa. It is a harbinger for gallstones and it can undergo dysplastic and then neoplastic changes. As a hollow, pear-shaped organ it simulates bowel, with an epithelial mucosa, smooth muscle layer, and serosa. In contrast to the intestine, there is no submucosa and there is only one muscle layer, muscularis externa.

- *Extrahepatic bile ducts*: The extrahepatic bile ducts are a continuation of the intrahepatic ducts. The confluence of right and left hepatic ducts is the site of most cholangiocarcinomas. Symptoms of obstructive jaundice are invariably present.

- *Ampulla of Vater*: The ampulla of Vater is another confluence junction of both the pancreatic duct and extrahepatic bile ducts as it enters the second part

TABLE 23.3	Overview of T-Oncoanatomy of Gastrointestinal Tract/Major Digestive Glands			
Primary Site	Three Planar Coronal	Sagittal	Transverse	Axial Level
Esophagus (see thorax)	Posterior mediastinum, descending aorta	Sympathetics, parasympathetics	Diaphragmatic stoma	T9/T10
Esophagogastric junction	Zigzag line	Lesser omental bursa, liver	Lesser omental bursa, spleen	T9/T10
Stomach	Fundus, body, pylorus	Lesser and greater omentum	Liver, spleen, kidneys	T10/T11/T12
Liver	Right and left lobes of liver	Eight sectors of liver divided by scissures	H-shaped fissures and fossae, caudate and quadratic lobes	T10/T11/T12, L1
Gallbladder	Gallbladder, cystic duct, bile ducts	Junction of cystic and hepatic ducts	Inferior to liver	T12, L1
Extrahepatic ducts	Extrahepatic bile ducts and pancreatic ducts	Portal triad of bile duct, hepatic artery and portal vein	Relationship to first and second part of duodenum	L1/L2
Pancreas	Head, body, and tail of pancreas	Retroperitoneal	Head and uncinate process wrap around superior mesenteric artery	L1/L2
Ampulla	Relationship of pancreatic duct and bile duct in development	Variation in fusion of bile and pancreatic ducts	Relationship of ventral and dorsal pancreatic bud	L2
Colon	Picture frames abdomen and its intestinal contents	Greater omentum relationship to colon, stomach, and pancreas	Anterior and lateral locations, mesentery	L2/L3/L4/L5
Small intestine	Circular folds variation, duodenum, jejunum, and ileum	Intraperitoneal and mesenteric roots	Fill most of abdomen at this level	L3/L4/L5
Sigmoid colon and rectum	Transition to pelvis exit into sacral hollow	Dorsal vein of male and female pelvis organ	Prostate and bladder anterior Denonvilliers fascia	S1–S5
Anus	Anorectal line, column of Morgagni, pectinate line	Perineal, postanal, presacral, deep, and superficial spaces	Bladder neck, urethra	Pubic bone, femoral head

of the duodenum. This is perhaps the least common malignancy of the MDG.

- *Pancreas*: The pancreas is a long, lobulated structure that lies transversely in the posterior abdomen located retroperitoneally in the concavity of the duodenum on its right end and touching the spleen on its left end. The shape of the pancreas may be compared with the letter J placed sideways. It is divisible into a head with an uncinate process, neck, body, and tail. Each of these sites, when afflicted with cancer, produces a specific set of characteristic signs and symptoms.

Orientation of N-oncoanatomy

The coronal planar oncoanatomy of lymph nodes will present the arrays of regional lymph nodes (Fig. 23.5). The lymphatics and major lymph node stations of the digestive tract are rich and directly related to the vascular arcades that characterize the extensive arterial and venous network. In the upper abdomen, the celiac axis of arteries supplies the stomach along its lesser and greater curvatures and the hepatic and pancreaticosplenic arteries, liver, and pancreas along with its ductal systems. The major lymphatic collecting trunks are parallel with the left gastric artery, splenic artery, and hepatic artery.

TABLE 23.4	**Primary Cancer Sites and Sentinel Nodes**		
Cancer Type	**Axial Level**	**Adjacent Anatomic Structure/Site**	**Sentinel Nodes**
Esophagogastric junction	T9/T10	Diaphragm, pericardium, thoracic duct	Lesser curvature and celiac nodes
Stomach	T10/T11/T12	Crura, liver, spleen, pancreas, greater omentum	Lesser and greater curvative nodes
Liver	T10/T11/T12, L1	Diaphragm, spleen, stomach, lesser omentum sac	Paracaval nodes, porta hepatis nodes
Gallbladder	T12, L1	Liver and intra- and extrahepatic bile ducts, portal vein	Porta hepatis nodes
Extrahepatic bile ducts	L1/L2	Porta hepatic, extrahepatic bile ducts, pancreas, and ampulla of Vater	Porta hepatis nodes
Pancreas	L1/L2	Duodenum, bile ducts, ampulla of Vater, and spleen	Pancreaticoduodenal, pancreaticosplenic nodes
Ampulla of Vater	L2	Duodenum, bile ducts, ampulla of Vater, and spleen	Pancreaticoduodenal nodes
Colon, transverse	L2/L3	Greater omentum, hepatic and splenic flexures, and mesentery	Pericolic, superior and inferior mesenteric nodes
Small intestine	L3/L4/L5	Mesentery, superior mesentery arteric	Superior mesenteric nodes
Cecum	L5	Appendix, sigmoid, small intestine, and ileocecal valve	Iliocecal and pericolic nodes
Sigmoid	S1	Mesentery, small intestine, and gynecologid organs	Pericolic and inferior mesenteric nodes
Rectum	S1–S5	Bladder, male genitourinary, prostate, and vas deferens vs female uterus	Perirectal and sacral nodes
Anus	Pubic bone and femoral head	Perineum/vagina or vulva urethra	Inguinal nodes

The major first station nodes are along the lesser gastropyloric, suprapyloric, pancreatoduodenal, celiac, splenic, and hepatic lymph nodes. The second station nodes include the para-aortic nodes. However, it is the superior and inferior mesenteric arterial and venous arcades that one associates the GIT's rich lymphatics and lymph nodes. The intestinal wall is impregnated with Peyer patches and rich network of lacteals in villi that provide robust drainage of chyme into the cisterna chili then onto the thoracic duct. Each of these regional lymph nodes is discussed separately with the GIT/MDG organ of interest. The sentinel nodes for each site are listed in Table 23.4. The spleen can function as a major systemic lymph node and plays an important immunological role.

Orientation of M-oncoanatomy

The entire portal circulation should be considered as a unit in regard to the venous anatomy of the GIT below the diaphragm. The two major trunks are the inferior mesenteric and superior mesenteric veins. The inferior mesenteric vein drains the left colon and sigmoid colon tributaries, which covers the vascular drainage to the left of the midline originating from the superior rectal veins. On the right side, the superior mesenteric vein originates from the tributaries draining the ileum, jejunum, and ileocolic and right colic veins. The inferior mesenteric vein usually joins the splenic vein, which coalesces with the superior mesenteric vein and forms the portal vein. The splenic vein, which is a major tributary of the portal system in addition, drains much of the stomach

TABLE 23.5	Incidence of Liver Metastases from Various Primary Tumors at Autopsy
Primary Site	**Percentage with Liver Metastases (%)**
Oesophagus	30–100
Stomach	38–100
Colorectal	40–100
Pancreas	50–73
Bile ducts and gall bladder	15–80
Small cell lung cancer	38–67
Breast	19–73
Melanoma	69
Ovary	48–68
Uterus	21–75
Renal cell cancer	40
Urothelial cancer	37–38
Thyroid	20
Prostate	9–71

along its greater curvature and includes the short gastric veins and left gastroepiploic and right gastric epiploic veins. The right gastroepiploic also flows into the superior mesenteric vein. The entire drainage of the lesser curvature of the stomach including the left and right gastric veins drains directly into the portal vein. Because the portal vein then drains directly into the liver, it is the target metastatic organ and the most commonly involved organ in hematogenous spread pattern from the venous system of the GIT as compared with other parts of the body where the drainage is directly into the lung by way of the caval system (Fig. 23.6; Table 23.5).

Rules for Classification and Staging

Clinical Staging and Imaging

Most of the digestive system and MDG are inaccessible to physical examination to detect and diagnose cancer formation and invasion. Endoscopic viewing provides the diagnosis, but to probe and biopsy the wall carries the hazard of perforation. The role and importance of sophisticated imaging are essential to staging. Endoscopic ultrasound can visualize the multilayered wall as rings of hyperechoic and hypoechoic bands and their signal distortion by tumor invasion. Virtual endoscopy as colonoscopy is an improving modality with more

accurate computer displays and reconstructions. Computed tomography (CT) and magnetic resonance imaging (MRI) are valuable to assess solid organs as liver and pancreas as well as adenopathy. Three-planar viewing is widely adopted and available for staging the primary tumor and regional nodes. Hepatic metastases are the greatest concern for all GIT and MDG sites and CT and MRI are excellent modes for searching and identifying lesions. Positron emission tomographic scanning is a sensitive means to total body scan for occult dissemination (Fig. 23.7; Table 23.6).

Pathologic Staging

The surgically resected portion of the GIT and associated lymph nodes removed are noted, numbered, and assessed for tumor. Tumor extension and location of both primary and nodes should be documented. Residual cancer can be R1, microscopic, or R2, macroscopic.

Cancer Statistics and Survival

The multidisciplinary approach has been extremely successful in the digestive system tubular primary sites but without any significant impact on the more solid MDG.

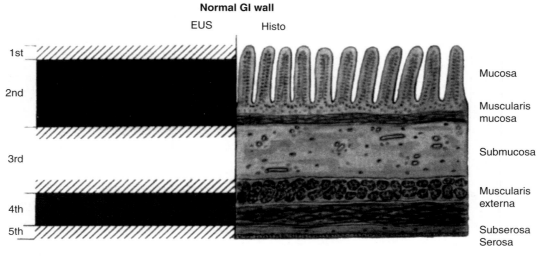

Figure 23.7 Schematic representation of endoscopic ultrasound appearance of the typical five-layered wall pattern and the histologic correlation.

TABLE 23.6	Imaging Modalities for Staging for Abdominal Organs	
Method	**Diagnosis and Staging Capability**	**Recommended for Use**
Primary Tumor ± Regional Nodes		
Barium enema (BE)	Very useful in detecting and defining primary lesions in the colon.	Yes
Endoscopy	Single-contrast study may be less sensitive than double-contrast in detecting polyps.	Yes, if used to confirm lesion detected on BE or to screen high-risk patients
Endorectal ultrasound or coil	Very accurate modality for detecting and defining primary lesions in rectum, sigmoid (flex sigmoidoscopy), or remaining colon (colonoscopy).	
MRI	Useful in defining depth of penetration of the primary lesion.	Yes, if preoperative chemRT is considered
CT	Most valuable of all modalities for determining extrarectal or extracolonic local invasion and nodal metastases.	Yes
PET	Not useful for staging primary cancer.	No
Metastases		
Chest film ± CT	Chest film—best for metastasis screening; CT chest—rules out multiple metastases.	Yes
CT abdomen	Most useful study to define para-aortic node enlargement or liver metastases.	Yes
Liver ultrasound	Can differentiate between cystic and solid lesions.	Yes

chemoRT, chemoradiation; CT, computed tomography; MRI, magnetic resonance imaging.

TABLE 23.7	Cancer Statistics for Abdomen			5-Year Survival Rates (%)	
Site	**New Diagnoses**	**Deaths**	**1950**	**2000**	**Gain**
Digestive	255,640	134,840			
Esophagus	14,250	13,300	4	15.4	11
Stomach	22,710	11,780	12	21.4	9
Liver	18,920	14,270	1	6.8	5.8
Pancreas	31,000	31,270	1	4.4	3.4
Colon	106,370	56,730	41	63	22
Rectum	40,570		40	63	23

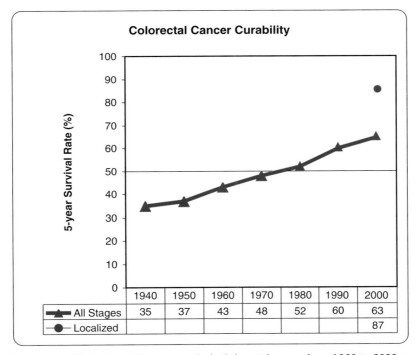

Figure 23.8 Trajectory of 5-year survival. Colorectal cancer from 1950 to 2000, a gain of 25%.

The largest gain in 5-year survival is the most common site for GIT cancers, the colon and rectum, rising from 40% in the 1950s to 63% by 2000, a gain of 23% (Fig. 23.8; Table 23.7). For localized stage I cancers detected by routine screening, survival is 90%, but drops to 65% with nodal involvement. Perhaps the most dramatic gain has been with anal cancers where radiation combined with cisplatin and 5-fluorouracil have not only resulted in complete regressions and high cure rates but anal sphincter preservation (90%). For esophageal cancers, a similar approach has resulted in a more moderate gain from 4% to 15%, but for local stage I/II a doubling to 30% survival with esophageal preservation. Pancreatic cancers and liver cancers are most disconcerting with 1% survival in the 1950s, changing very slightly to 4% and 7%, respectively, in 2000 (Fig. 23.8). Total hepatectomy and liver and pancreas transplantation hold promise.

24

Esophagogastric Junction

Ectopic islands of gastriclike epithelium mucosa referred to as Barrett mucosa have the potential and predisposition to undergo neoplastic change to adenocarcinomas

Perspective and Patterns of Spread

The esophagus in its lower most third is a transitional organ as it passes through the diaphragm exiting the thorax and entering the abdomen. *The stratified squamous epithelium at the cardia becomes glandular as it transforms into the stomach. Ectopic islands of gastriclike epithelium mucosa referred to as Barrett mucosa have the potential and predisposition to undergo neoplastic change to adenocarcinomas (Table 24.1).* These esophagogastric junctional (EGJ) adenocarcinomas often arise in association with a clinical triad: Hiatal hernia, gastric reflux, and persistent ulceration of the cardia junction. There is dispute as to the true origin of EGJ adenocarcinomas particularly without ectopic mucosa. In the sixth edition of the American Joint Committee on Cancer (AJCC) manual, EGJ cancers are referred to as types I, II, and III by Siewert, depending on the amount of esophagus and stomach involvement. In clinical practice, *if >2 cm of the esophagus is involved, it is considered to be esophageal; if the lesion occupies <2 cm of the esophagus, a gastric origin is assigned.*

At one time, adenocarcinomas of the EGJ were uncommon with only 1% to 5% incidence, but have been on the increase and currently account for 34% of all esophageal cancers. Although this has occurred mainly in white males, adenocarcinomas also are on the rise in African Americans. This is attributed to metaplasia of Barrett epithelium becoming dysplastic and then truly neoplastic. The overall risk with Barrett epithelium for giving rise to an adenocarcinoma is 125 times normal.

Alcohol and tobacco abuse are predisposing factors leading to a field carcinogenesis effect and multifocal mucosal lesions. The pattern of spread, once the cancer invades into the wall, follows the muscle layers, encircling the lumen and then migrating longitudinally with the milking action of peristalsis (Fig. 24.1). *Often masquerading as a sliding hiatal hernia with gastric reflux, the diagnosis is made once endoscopic examination reveals islands of pink mucosa in the distal esophagus and biopsy establishes abnormal columnar mucosa with goblet cells similar to gastric mucosa.*

TNM Staging Criteria

The normal EGJ is a zigzag line, which divides the whitish stratified esophageal squamous mucous membranes from the pinkish glandular gastric mucosa. The longitudinal esophageal folds fade into the gastric rugal folds. Spasm, obstruction, and regurgitation occur with cardia dysfunction. Eventually, persistent inflammation results with the mucosal transformation to malignancy. Perforation is rare because thickening of the dual muscular layers of the distal esophagus are reinforced as muscle layers of the stomach. The staging of esophageal cancers has not changed and relates to the standard hollow organ model wherein depth of penetration of the wall rather than size determines stage, that is, T1, mucosa; T2, muscular; T3, serosa; and T4, extraesophageal (Fig. 24.2). Dysplastic Barrett mucosa is substaged in length: Short versus long segment based on whether the lesion is <3 cm or >3 cm long, respectively, from the zigzag line of the EGJ.

Generally, there is no overarching principle or context design for the digestive system (gastrointestinal tract) or major digestive glands. Stages are frequently expanded to six by subdividing a stage into A and B. The T and N categories are assigned to a stage grouping, specifically for division of a stage into a more (a) versus less (b) favorable groupings. This occurs at different stages for different sites.

Specifically, esophagus has six stages; stages II and IV have A and B categories. The initial stage progression (I/II/III) is due to advancement of the primary and late stage progression (III/IV) by nodal involvement: IIB is N1. Regional nodes are either stage II or III and non-regional nodes are stage IVA. There is only one nodal category, N1.

Summary of Changes

There are no changes in the sixth edition of the AJCC CSM.

Orientation of Three-three-planar Oncoanatomy

The anatomic isocenter for the EGJ cancers is at T9/T10. These EGJs are posterior in location, both for the mediastinum and the abdominal cavity (Fig. 24.3).

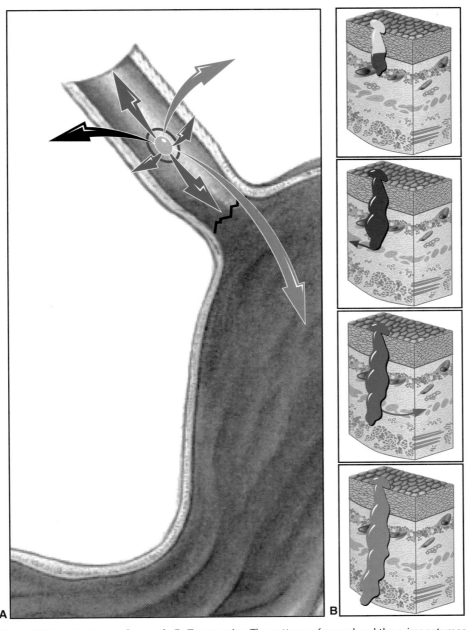

Figure 24.1 **A. Patterns of spread.** **B.** T categories. The patterns of spread and the primary tumor classification are similarly color coded: Tis (cancer in situ of mucosa), yellow; T1 (infiltrates the submucosa), green; T2 (penetrates the muscularis externa), blue; T3 (reaches the adventitia), purple; and T4 (invades through the adventitia into a neighboring viscera), red.

DEFINITION OF TNM

STAGE GROUPINGS

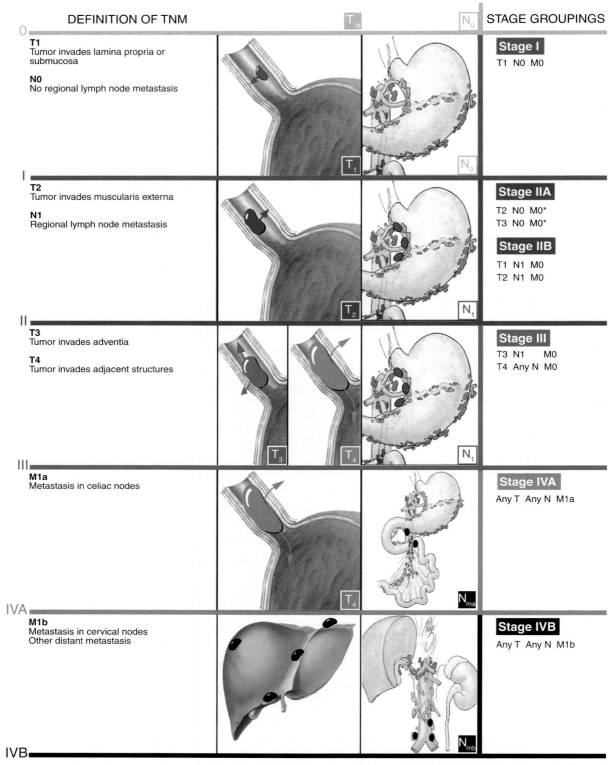

T1
Tumor invades lamina propria or submucosa

N0
No regional lymph node metastasis

Stage I
T1 N0 M0

T2
Tumor invades muscularis externa

N1
Regional lymph node metastasis

Stage IIA
T2 N0 M0*
T3 N0 M0*

Stage IIB
T1 N1 M0
T2 N1 M0

T3
Tumor invades adventia

T4
Tumor invades adjacent structures

Stage III
T3 N1   M0
T4 Any N M0

M1a
Metastasis in celiac nodes

Stage IVA
Any T Any N M1a

M1b
Metastasis in cervical nodes
Other distant metastasis

Stage IVB
Any T Any N M1b

* not illustrated

Figure 24.2 TNM staging diagram presents a vertical arrangement with color bars encompassing TN combinations showing progression. Esophagogastric junction cancers are adenocarcinomas. Note juxtaregional nodes as M1a, celiac nodes although considered metastatic when resected offer a better chance for 5 year survival (10%) than visceral metastases (black). Stage 0, yellow; stage I, green; stage II, blue; stage III, purple; stage IV, red; and stage IV (metastatic), black. Definitions of TN on left and stage grouping on right.

TABLE 24.1	Histopathologic Type: Common Cancers of the Esophagogastric and Junction and Stomach

Type

Adenocarcinoma
  Papillary adenocarcinoma
  Tubular adenocarcinoma
  Mucinous adenocarcinoma
  Signet ring cell carcinoma

Adenosquamous carcinoma
Squamous cell carcinoma
Small cell carcinoma
Undifferentiated carcinomas

From Greene FL, Page DL, Fleming ID, et al. eds.: *AJCC Cancer Staging Manual.* 6th ed. New York: Springer; 2002. Used with the permission of the American Joint Committee on Cancer (AJCC), Chicago, Illinois.

T-oncoanatomy

The esophagus consists of three principal regions: The cervical, thoracic, and cardiac portions.

- Cervical esophagus extends from the pharyngeal-esophageal sphincter to the level of the thoracic inlet, about 18 cm from upper incisor teeth (UIT).
- Upper thoracic esophagus extends from the thoracic inlet to the level of the tracheal bifurcation, about 24 cm from UIT.
- Mid thoracic esophagus extends from the tracheal bifurcation toward the esophagogastric junction, about 32 cm from UIT.
- Lower thoracic esophagus is ductal, 3–8 cm in length, and includes the esophageal gastric junction and is about 40 cm from UIT.

The esophagus is a muscular tube that consists of two layers of smooth muscle—one longitudinal and the other horizontal—and this is carried through into the rest of the gastrointestinal system. Peristalsis is initiated with swallowing and the major function is to propel food into the stomach. There are two sphincters in the esophagus and these are at the cricopharyngeous muscle at its inlet and the cardiac sphincter at the cardia of the stomach. These sphincters have been extensively studied from the physiologic point of view and are common sites of both benign and neoplastic disease.

The course of the esophagus is from slightly to the right of the midline to the left as it pierces the diaphragm through its own opening. It is in continual contact with the right lung; on the left side, the descending aorta is in continual contact. The azygos vein provides a partial shield on the right and posteriorly. Pulmonary veins would be expected to be in more intimate contact because they drain to the left auricle, which is posterior to the ventricle. *The thoracic duct is posterior to the esophagus along its course, which is the reverse of the esophagus coursing from the right side of midline to the left as it ascends. When the esophagus comes anterior to the descending aorta, it is suspended by the mesoesophagus,* which allows it to curve forward before its escape through the diaphragm (Fig. 24.4).

- *Coronal:* The EGJ is usually located to the left of the midline, at the 11th thoracic vertebra, and the py-

lorus is usually located at the L1 vertebral level to the right of the midline at the transpyloric plane; the angular incisura separates the body from the pyloric region of the stomach.

- *Sagittal:* The peritoneal cavity consists of the greater sac and omental bursa. The superior recess of the omental bursa is between the liver and the posterior attachment of the diaphragm. The inferior recess of the omental bursa is between the two double layers of the greater omentum. In the adult, the inferior recess usually only extends inferiorly as far as the transverse colon because of fusion of the two double peritoneal layers at birth.
- *Transverse:* The gastrosplenic and splenorenal ligaments tether the spleen in place between the stomach and the kidney; the ligaments from a pedicle (stalk) through which blood vessels run to and from the hilum of the spleen. These ligaments are double layers of peritoneum that form the left boundary of the omental bursa (lesser sac); the inner layer consists of peritoneum lining the omental bursa, and the outer layer consists of peritoneum lining the peritoneal cavity (greater sac).

N-oncoanatomy

Esophagogastric cancers frequently lead to lymphatic involvement not only of mediastinal nodes, but celiac and para-aortic nodes (Table 24.2). The AJCC/International Union Against Cancer numbering of mediastinal and abdominal nodes is unique, and is different from the International Anatomy Terminology (Fig. 24.5). The percentage of positive lymph nodes in the coeliac area increases as the cancer location migrates from the upper esophagus to the EGJ (Fig. 24.5B), namely, 32% to 70%.

The regional lymph nodes for the cervical esophagus are the cervical and supraclavicular nodes. For the thoracic esophagus, the regional nodes are the adjacent mediastinal lymph nodes. Involvement of more distant nodes is considered distant metastasis. *Retrograde and prograde lymphatic spread usually places all of the lymph node stations in the neck, mediastinum, and abdomen at risk.*

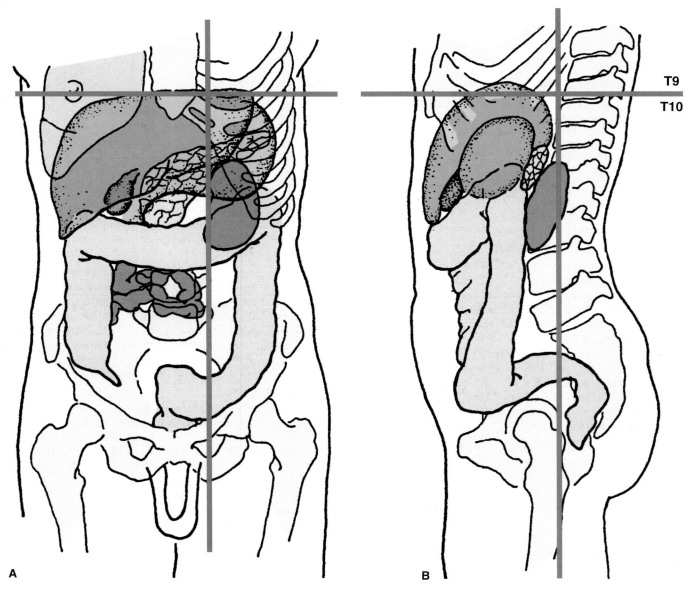

T9
T10

A   **B**

Figure 24.3 Orientation and overview of oncoanatomy. The anatomic isocenter for the esophagogastric junction (EGJ) cancers is at T9/T10. **A.** Coronal. **B.** Sagittal.

One of the major problems with control of this cancer is the frequency with which lymph node invasion occurs and the rapidity of its dissemination to other, distant anatomic areas. Esophageal cancer is therefore not only a disease of the chest, but also of the neck and abdomen. Because of its lymphatic drainage, esophageal cancer is a formidable tumor to encompass by locoregional modalities of therapy. The percentage of positive nodes found at surgery staging—both mediastinal and abdominal—indicates at all levels of the primary, infradiaphragmatic nodes are frequently involved (Fig. 24.5B).

M-oncoanatomy

A rich plexus of venous anastomoses exists with stomach, liver, pancreas, and adrenals (Fig. 24.6). Therefore, the liver, lung, and adrenals are the most common sites of distant metastases. Remote metastasis from the carcinoma of the esophagus, although ultimately fatal, often carries a better prognosis than when the primary lesion has extended locally outside the esophagus into mediastinal structures, a condition that is rapidly fatal. The incidence of liver metastases exceeds other sites. According to a variety of reports in the literature, the range is

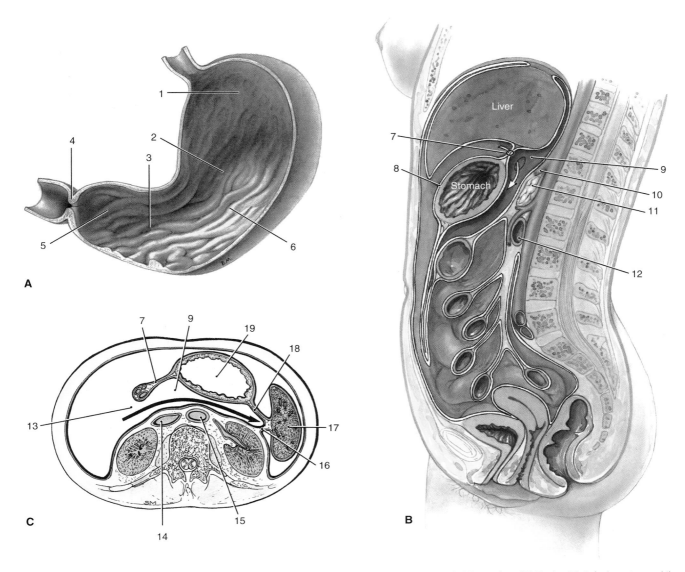

Figure 24.4 **T-oncoanatomy: Esophagogastric junction three-planar views. A.** Coronal. (1) Fundus. (2) Body. (3) Pyloric antrum. (4) Pyloric sphincter. (5) Pyloric canal. (6) Rugae (gastric folds). **B.** Sagittal. (7) Lesser omentum (hepatogastric ligament). (8) Visceral peritoneum. (9) Omental bursa (lesser sac). (10) Celiac trunk. (11) Pancreas. (12) Duodenum. **C.** Transverse. (13) Omental (epiploic) foramen. (14) Inferior vena cava. (15) Aorta. (16) Splenorenal ligament. (17) Spleen. (18) Gastrosplenic ligament. (19) Stomach.

30% to 100% at autopsy. Other sites are mainly bone metastases (20%–35%) and lung metastases (40%–60%), with only occasional metastases to brain.

Rules for Classification and Staging

Clinical Staging and Imaging

Because the esophagus is not accessible to direct physical examination, endoscopy and imaging play a vital role in determining the stage of esophageal cancer. Barium esophagram with air contrast is able to detect the cancer, but to determine the depth of penetration, endoluminal ultrasound (EUS) can define the layers of the esophageal wall. Computed tomography (CT) of the chest and abdomen can determine invasion of surrounding structures as well as metastatic lesions in lung and liver (Table 24.3).

Pathologic Staging

The surgically resected esophagus and associated lymph nodes removed are assessed. Tumor extension and

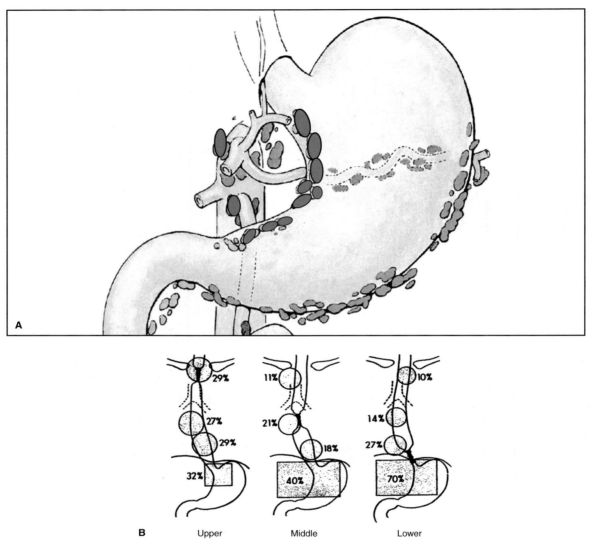

Figure 24.5 N-oncoanatomy. A. Sentinel nodes of esophagogastric junction include thoracic and abdominal nodes. **B.** The percentage of positive lymph nodes found at surgery for esophageal carcinoma in the upper, middle, and lower esophagus.

TABLE 24.2	Lymph Nodes of Esophagogastric Junction

Sentinel nodes include lesser curvature and celiac nodes

Regional nodes	Juxtaregional nodes
Lower esophageal	Internal jugular
Left gastric	Cervical
Posterior mediastinal	Para-aortic
Pericardial	
Diaphragmatic	

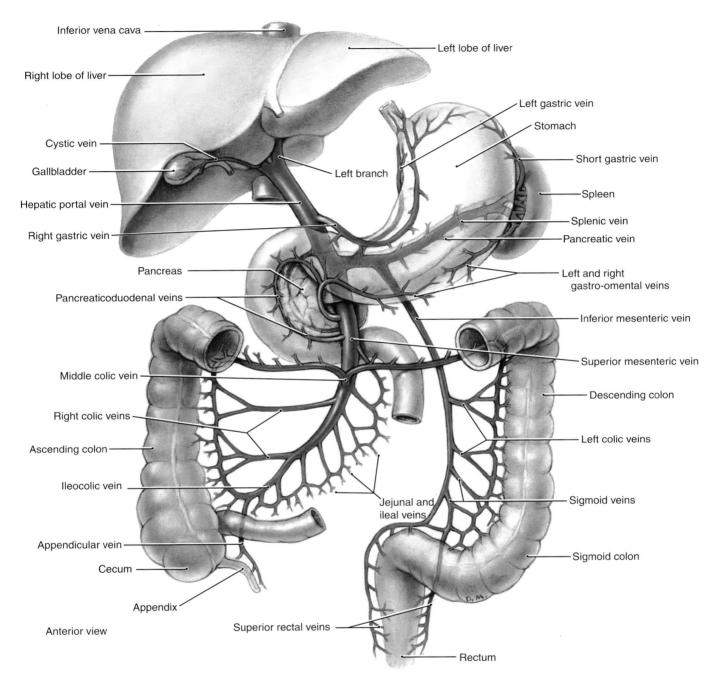

Figure 24.6 **M-oncoanatomy.** Portal venous system.

location of both primary and nodes should be documented. Accurate radial margins should be marked and recorded and are defined "as the surgically dissected surface adjacent to the deepest point of tumor invasion beyond the wall of the gut." The completeness of resection depends on the clearing of the deepest point of invasion R0 (complete), R1 (microscopic), and R2 (macroscopic).

Oncoimaging Annotations

- Ninety percent of adenocarcinomas occur near the EGJ.
- Recognizing early mucosal and submucosal lesions can be found with double-contrast studies.
- CT, EUS, and magnetic resonance imaging (MRI) provide a complete picture of invasion. EUS is more

TABLE 24.3 — Imaging Modalities for Staging for Esophagogastric Junction Cancer

Method	Diagnosis and Staging Capability	Recommended for Use
Primary tumor and regional nodes		
Single-contrast upper GI studies	Useful in detecting and defining primary lesions in stomach	Yes
Double-contrast upper GI studies	Very useful in detecting early gastric cancers	Yes—should be performed along with single contrast
Gastroscopy	Very accurate modality to detect and define primary lesions: ~90% confirmation rate	Yes—use to confirm lesion detected in UGI series and to screen high-risk patients
CT-abdomen ± chest	Most valuable of all modalities for determining degree of extragastric extension and distant metastases	Yes
Endoscopic ultrasound	Most accurate method of determining extension within and beyond gastric wall	Yes—if plan preoperative chemoirradiation
Metastatic tumors		
Chest films	Good for detecting metastases	Yes
Laparoscopy	May allow visualization of small serosal implants or liver metastases	Yes—if plan preoperative chemotherapy or chemoradiation
Bone film	Useful only for confirming metastases	No—unless patient has bone pain
PET scans—liver, brain, bone	Useful in evaluation of clinically suspected metastases	Yes—if metastases are suspected

CT, computed tomography; GI, gastrointestinal; UGI, upper gastrointestinal.

accurate in staging penetration of five esophageal layers in its walls and CT is better for detection of invasion to adjacent structures.

- PET is better for finding metastases.
- EUS demonstrates hyperechoic alternately with hypoechoic layers of esophageal wall.
- MRI and Gd-DTPA shows extensions into mediastinal and diaphragmatic tissues.

Cancer Statistics and Survival

Cancer of the digestive system or gastrointestinal tract, which includes major digestive glands, accounts for 255,640 new patients annually, with colon and rectum responsible for >50% with 146 new diagnoses annually. Approximately half eventually die of these cancers. Major digestive gland cancers as a group are more lethal; only a handful of patients becoming long-term

TABLE 24.4 — Cancer Curability by Stages at Diagnosis (1992–1998)

Site	5-Year Survival Rate (%)			
	All Stages	Local	Regional	Advanced
Esophagus	15.6	33.6	16.8	2.6
Stomach	23.9	61.9	22.2	3.4
Liver	10.5	21.9	7.2	3.3
Pancreas	5.0	19.6	8.2	1.9
Colorectum	64.1	90.4	68.1	9.8

survivors. Fortunately, colon and rectal cancers are the most common, with the majority of patients becoming 5-year survivors (63%), responding to chemoradiation programs often with the sparing of the rectal sphincter with conservative surgery. Anal cancers are the most responsive to chemoradiation (5-fluorouracil and cisplatin), eliminating the need for. surgery. The 5-year survival is >90% with anal sphincter preservation. This regimen has been proven effective in clinical trials and results in more long-term survivors, which is currently reflected in the literature. Liver, bile duct, and pancreatic cancers are among the poorest in the terms of sur-

vival, often measured in months rather than years (see Table 23.7).

Specifically, the esophagus accounted for 14,250 new cancer cases, 13,300 cancer deaths (93%) with a survival (5-year) rate improvement over the past 5 decades of (1950–2000) of 11%. Currently, relative 5-year survival for all stages is 14%, but when localized improves to 29.1% (Table 24.4). Chemoradiation in RTOG trials has resulted in 27% 5 yr. survival with local control at 68% and with esophageal preservation. For adenocarcinoma of the EJG, the best 5-year survival after chemoradiation and surgery is 40%, in an intergroup study.

25

Stomach

The predisposing carcinogenic factors remain atrophic gastric mucosa and intestinal metaplasia that transit into neoplasia from Menetriere disease or hypertrophic gastritis.

Perspective and Patterns of Spread

Gastric cancers have undergone a decline in deaths and incidence since the 1950s; however, its stature as an aggressive and highly malignant neoplasm has not changed. In the United States and the Western world, although it has steadily declined in incidence, there are 23,000 new cases annually with an overall 5-year survival rate of 23%. There is a tremendous variation worldwide; Japan has the highest incidence, accounting for 20% to 30% of all stomach cancers. The predisposing factors remain atrophic gastric mucosa and intestinal metaplasia that transit into neoplasia from Menetriere disease or hypertrophic gastritis. Fundic and adenomatous polyps as in Gardner and Peutz–Jeghers syndrome tend to undergo carcinogenic change. Because of the large, saclike nature of the stomach, this part of the digestive system can accommodate large neoplasms before onset of symptoms. *Presentations range from fungating and ulcerative process to a widely infiltrative process resulting in a linitis plastica, stomach almost devoid of peristalsis.* The patterns of invasion into and through the stomach wall are shown in Figure 25.1.

Early diagnosis is essential to cure and when camera imaging and frequent endoscopic screens are employed, as in Japan, precancerous and small lesions are being found. An Early Gastric Cancer (ECG) classification of minimal microscopic lesions has been introduced. ECG in Japan constitute 25% to 50% of all gastric adenocarcinomas as compared to 5% to 15% in Western countries. ECG is noted to have three types of presentation: Type I (elevated) protrudes in lumen >5 cm; type II are superficial lesions with elevations or depressions; and type III resembles ulcers or craters and amputate gastric folds. The staging recommendations apply to carcinomas not lymphomas or sarcomas. A tabulation of cell types reflects the varied surface epithelia and secretory glandular cells. Once the mucosa is breeched, invasion of the muscle cell wall occurs with dissemination along these muscle layers (see Table 24.1).

TNM Staging Criteria

Gastric cancers are confined and accommodated in the stomach and can reach large size as compared with other, narrower parts of the intestine. Bormans originally described the various appearance of advanced cancer including the criteria to distinguish a malignant versus a benign gastric ulcer: I, polypoid; II, ulcerative; III, infiltrative ulcerated; and IV, linitis plastica.

The major American Joint Committee on Cancer staging criteria are based on depth of invasion of a hollow viscus. T1 (mucosal) invades lamina propria; T2 has been modified as T2a (invades muscularis propria) and T2b (subserosa). Subserosa stage applies to tumors extending into gastrocolic or gastrohepatic ligament or lesser or greater omentum. The omentum consists of two layers of peritoneum. *An infiltrating cancer sandwiched between the two layers of omental peritoneum is considered subserosal despite being extragastric because the serosa is not penetrated.* T3 means penetration of serosa or visceral peritoneum, and T4 implies invasion of surrounding viscera as spleen, transverse colon, liver, diaphragm, pancreas, or other structure. (Fig. 25.2).

Intramural extension to esophagus or duodenum follows the depth of invasion rules for staging rather than advancing in stage.

Generally, there is no overarching principle or context design for stage groupings in the digestive system (gastrointestinal tract) or major digestive glands. Stages are frequently expanded to six by subdividing stages into A and B. The T and N categories are assigned to a stage grouping, specifically for division of a stage into more (a) versus less (b) favorable groupings. This occurs at different stages for different sites.

Specifically, this site has the most unorthodox staging with its six stages; I and III are divided into A and B. It is the only anatomic site in which positive nodes (T1 N1) is still stage I, assigned to B. The T and N progression together advances stages II, III, and IV. Curiously, adding subscript numbers of T and N categories together correlates with stage; that is, stage IA = 1, stage IB = 2, stage II = 3, stage IIIA = 4, stage IIIB = 5, and stage IV = >5. The nodal categories are unique: N1, 1 to 6 nodes; N2, 7 to 15 nodes; and N3 >15 nodes. By contrast to many digestive system sites where N1 encompasses all nodal categories, the stomach is the most

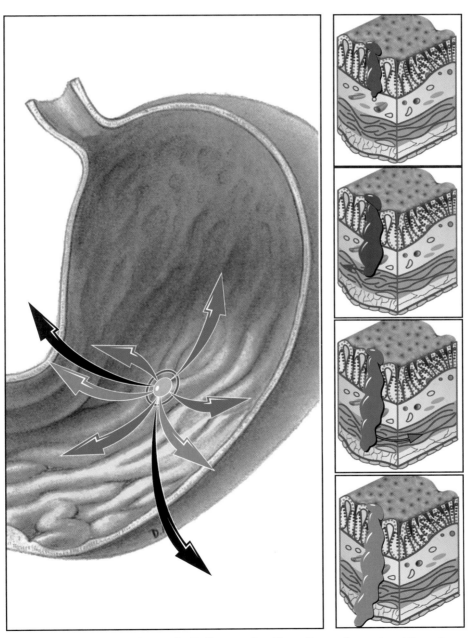

Figure 25.1 **A. Patterns of spread.** **B.** T categories. The patterns of spread and the primary tumor classification are similarly color coded: Tis (cancer in situ of mucosa), yellow; T1 (infiltrates the submucosa), green; T2 (penetrates the muscularis externa), blue; T3 (reaches the subserosa), purple; and T4 (invades through the serosa into a neighboring viscera), is red.

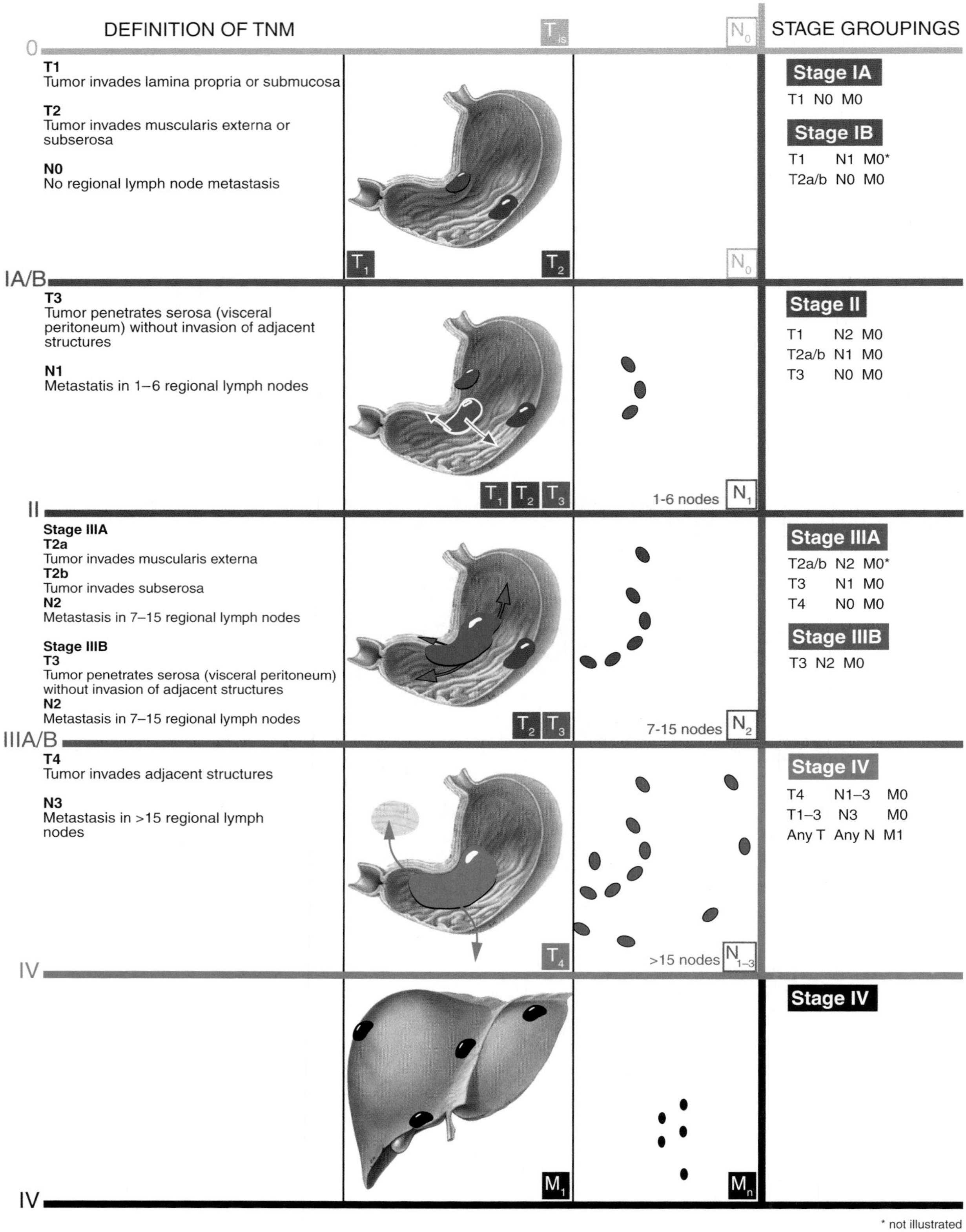

Figure 25.2 **TNM staging diagram presents a vertical arrangement with color bars encompassing TN combinations showing progression.** The stomach has the most elaborate nodal staging categories and despite < or > 15 regional nodes (N2/N3) resections allow for 20% vs 8% 5-year survival, i.e., IIIA ≠ B vs IV or purple vs red lane respectively, Stage 0, yellow; I, green; II, blue; III, purple; IV, red; and stage IV (metastatic), black. Definitions of TN on left and stage grouping on right.

TABLE 25.1	Lymph Nodes of Stomach

Sentinel nodes include lesser and greater curvature nodes

Regional nodes	Juxtaregional nodes
Celiac	Para-aortic
Left gastropancreatic	Mediastinal
Lesser curvature	Retrocaval
Juxta cardiac	
Splenic	
Hepatic	
Gastroduodenal	
Right gastropyloric	
Suprapyloric	
Pancreatic–duodenal	

elaborate. Nevertheless, there are survival curve data supporting subdividing I and III into A and B (see last section).

Summary of Changes

Changes in the sixth edition are minor.

* *T2 lesions have been divided into T2a and T2b.*
* *T2a is defined as a tumor that invades the muscularis externa.*
* *T2b is defined as a tumor that invades into subserosa.*

Orientation of Three-planar Oncoanatomy

The isocenter for the three-planar anatomy is to the left of the midline anteriorly and at the T10/T11 level posteriorly (Fig. 25.3).

T-oncoanatomy

The stomach is divided into three regions: Upper, middle, and lower third. To delineate these regions, the lesser and greater curves of the stomach are divided; *the upper third is the cardia and the fundus, the middle third the body, and the lower third the antrum.*

The stomach is an organ with numerous metamorphic shapes: Hypertonic contracted stomach is often high in the upper quadrant; hypotonic to atonic viscus drops into the pelvis; and normal orthotonic viscus reaching to the umbilicus. *The stomach mucosa begins at the zigzag line of the cardia defined by the pinkish glandular mucosa with its chief and parietal cells (Fig. 25.4).*

* *Coronal*: The body of the stomach has a lesser and greater curvature, a fundus superior to the body and a pyloric region divided into an antrum and a pyloric canal. Extensions into adjacent or contiguous structures as esophagus or duodenum are staged according to the depth of invasion in their wall. *Gastric rugae or magenstrasse are the villous mucosal folds with their*

secretory epithelia with parietal (HCl), chief (pepsin), and mucous (mucin) cells, which constitute their make up and their varied secretions. In addition to an inner circular layer and an outer longitudinal layer, there is a middle zone of both circular and oblique muscle layers. The cardia and pylorus have sphincteric activity and control the entry and departure of swallowed food.

* *Sagittal*: The arrow passes from the greater sac into the omental foramen into the lesser sac or omental bursa.

* *Transverse*: The gastrosplenic and splenorenal ligaments tether the spleen in place between the stomach and the kidney; the ligaments form a pedicle (stalk), through which blood vessels run to and from the hilum of the spleen. These ligaments are double layers of peritoneum that form the left boundary of the omental bursa (lesser sac); the inner layer consists of peritoneum lining the omental bursa and the outer layer consists of peritoneum lining the peritoneal cavity (greater sac).

N-oncoanatomy

The major lymphatic collecting trunks are parallel with the left gastric artery, the splenic artery, and the hepatic artery. The major first station nodes are along the lesser and greater curvatures, consisting of the left gastropancreatic, juxtacardiac, gastroduodenal, gastropyloric, suprapyloric, pancreatoduodenal, celiac, splenic, and hepatic lymph nodes. The second station nodes include the para-aortic nodes (Fig. 25.5; Table 25.1).

M-oncoanatomy

The entire portal circulation should be considered as a unit in regard to the venous anatomy of the gastrointestinal tract below the diaphragm. The two major trunks are the inferior mesenteric and superior

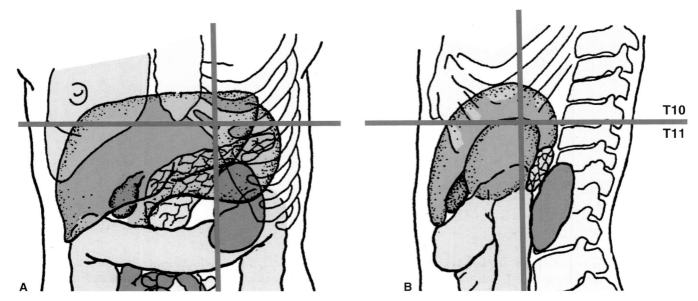

Figure 25.3 Orientation and overview of oncoanatomy. The anatomic isocenter for stomach cancers is at T10/T11. **A.** Coronal. **B.** Sagittal.

mesenteric veins. The inferior mesenteric vein drains the left colon and sigmoid colon tributaries, which covers the vascular drainage to the left of the midline originating from the superior rectal veins. On the right side, the superior mesenteric vein originates from the tributaries draining the ileum, jejunum, and the ileocolic and right middle colic veins. *The inferior mesenteric vein usually joins the splenic vein, which coalesces with the superior mesenteric vein and forms the portal vein.* The splenic vein, which is a major tributary of the portal system, also drains much of the stomach along its greater curvature and includes the short gastric veins and left and right gastric epiploic veins. The right gastric epiploic also flows into the superior mesenteric vein. The entire drainage of the lesser curvature of the stomach including the left and right gastric veins drains directly into the portal vein. Because the portal vein then drains directly into the liver, it is the target metastatic organ and the most commonly involved organ in hematogenous spread pattern from the venous system of the gastrointestinal tract as compared with other parts of the body where the drainage is directly into the lung by way of the caval system.

The incidence of liver metastases exceeds other sites. According to a variety of reports in the literature, the range is 38% to 100% at autopsy. Other sites are mainly bone metastases 20% to 35% and lung metastases 40% to 60%, with only occasional metastases to brain.

Rules for Classification and Staging

Clinical Staging and Imaging

The stomach, as are all digestive tract viscera, when involved with cancer can be detected by endoscopy and double-contrast studies. The challenge is accurate delineation of gastric cancer, which is penetrating the many layers composing the stomach wall. Endoscopic ultrasound (EUS) is the most favored method of determining the cancer's extent in and through the stomach wall. Computed tomography (CT) is excellent for diagnosing both extragastric extension and distant metastases. Magnetic resonance imaging (MRI) is not helpful because of organ motion. Single photon emission CT scans of liver and bone are useful, but CT is better for assessing liver and lung metastases and MRI is superior for brain foci (Table 25.2).

Pathologic Staging

The surgically resected stomach and associated lymph nodes removed are assessed. Tumor extension and location of both primary and nodes should be documented. Accurate radial margins should be marked and recorded, and are defined "as the surgically dissected surface adjacent to the deepest point of tumor invasion beyond the wall of the stomach." The completeness of resection depends on the clearing of the deepest point of invasion R0 (complete), R1 (microscopic), and R2 (macroscopic). This aspect of number of regional nodes involved exceeds most cancer sites in which a more limited number of nodes determines substages.

Oncoimaging Annotations
* Screening for early gastric cancers is best done using double-contrast (barium–air) coupled with endoscopy.

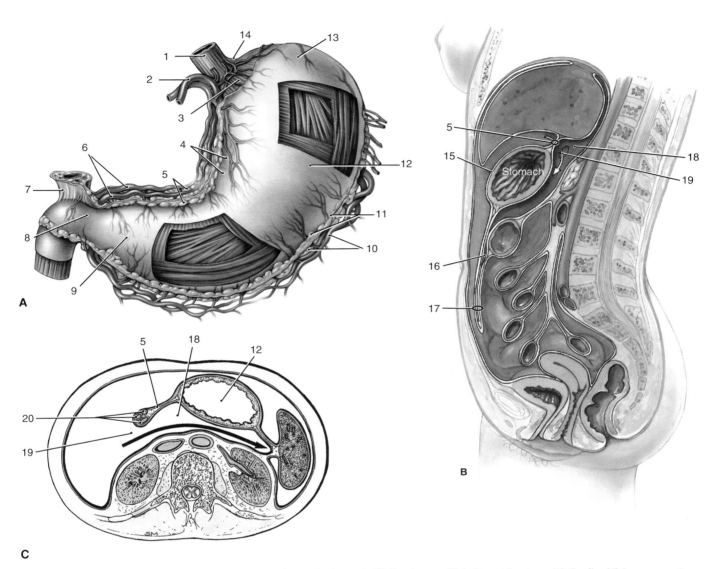

Figure 25.4 **T-oncoanatomy: Stomach three-planar views. A.** Coronal. (1) Esophagus. (2) Left gastric artery. (3) Cardia. (4) Lesser curvature. (5) Lesser omentum. (6) Right gastric vessels. (7) Hepatoduodenal ligament. (8) Pylorus. (9) Pyloric canal. (10) Left gastro-omental vessels. (11) Greater curvature. (12) Body of stomach. (13) Fundus. (14) Cardia notch. **B.** Sagittal. (15) Visceral peritoneum. (16) Inferior recess of omental bursa. (17) Greater omentum. (18) Omental bursa. (19) Omental (epiploic) foramen. **C.** Transverse. (20) Portal triad (hepatic artery proper, common bile duct, and portal vein) in hepatoduodenal ligament.

- Staging is performed by EUS and CT for extensions beyond the wall.
- Lymph node invasion is reliably determined in surgical pathologic assessment of excised nodes rather than imaging.
- Distinguishing malignant from benign ulcers depends on features as the meniscus sign, nodular and irregular folds around the ulcer.
- Dissemination into lesser and greater omentum, peritoneal implants, and ascites are detectable by CT.
- EUS of value in analyzing cancer invasion of five-layered stomach wall. In linitis plastica, the layers

are preserved but the wall is thickened, especially the fourth layer, corresponding to the muscularis externa.

Cancer Statistics and Survival

The digestive system or gastrointestinal tract, which includes major digestive glands, accounts for 255,640 new patients annually with colon and rectum responsible for >50% with 146 new diagnoses annually. Approximately half eventually die of these cancers. Major digestive gland cancers as a group are more lethal; only a handful of patients becoming long-term survivors.

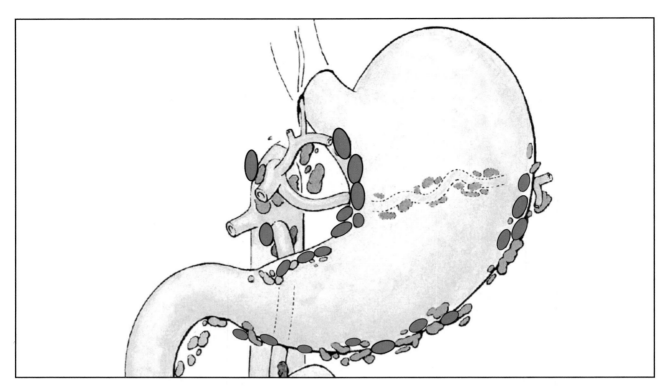

Figure 25.5 **N-oncoanatomy.** Sentinel nodes of stomach are along the lesser and greater curvature.

TABLE 25.2	Imaging Modalities for Staging for Gastric Cancer	
Method	**Diagnosis and Staging Capability**	**Recommended for Use**
Primary Tumor and Regional Nodes		
Single-contrast upper GI studies	Useful in detecting and defining primary lesions in stomach	Yes
Double-contrast upper GI studies	Very useful in detecting early gastric cancers	Yes—should be performed along with single contrast
Gastroscopy	Very accurate modality to detect and define primary lesions: ~90% confirmation rate	Yes—use to confirm lesion detected in UGI series and to screen high-risk patients
CT-abdomen ± chest	Most valuable of all modalities for determining degree of extragastric extension and distant metastases	Yes
Endoscopic ultrasound	Most accurate method of determining extension within and beyond gastric wall	Yes—if plan preoperative chemoirradiation
Metastatic tumors		
Chest films	Good for detecting metastases	Yes
Laparoscopy	May allow visualization of small serosal implants or liver metastases	Yes—if plan preoperative chemotherapy or chemoradiation
Bone film	Useful only for confirming metastases	No—unless patient has bone pain
PET—liver, brain, bone	Useful in evaluation of clinically suspected metastases	Yes—if suspected metastases

CT, computed tomography; GI, gastrointestinal; UGI, upper gastrointestinal.

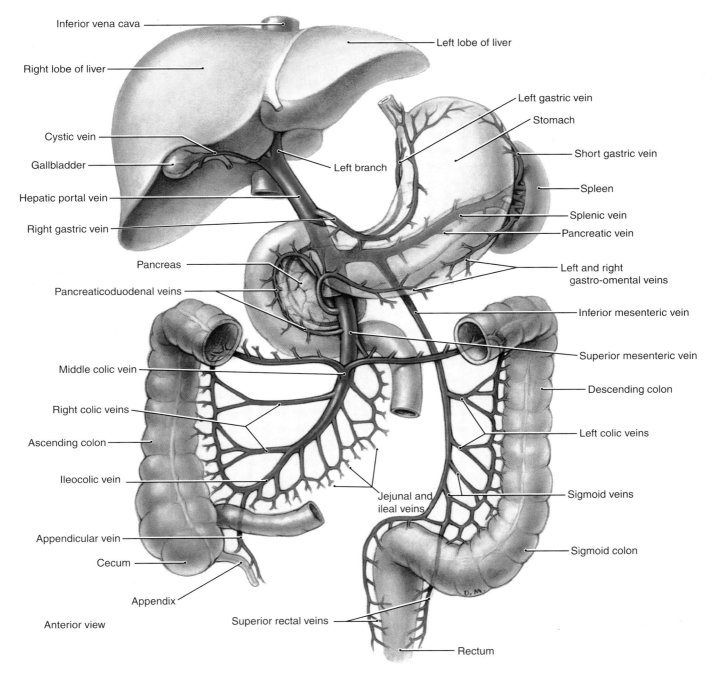

Figure 25.6 **M-oncoanatomy.** Portal venous system.

Fortunately, colon and rectal cancers are the most common, with the majority of patients becoming 5-year survivors (63%) responding to chemoradiation programs often with the sparing of the rectal sphincter with conservative surgery. Anal cancers are the most responsive to chemoradiation (5-fluorouracil and cisplatin) eliminating the need for surgery. The 5-year survival rate is >90% with anal sphincter preservation. This regimen has been proven effective in clinical trials and results in more long-term survivors, which is currently reflected in the literature. Liver, bile duct, and pancreatic cancers are amongst the poorest in the terms of survival often measured in months rather than years (see Table 23.7 and Table 24.5).

Specifically, the stomach accounted for 22,710 new cancer cases and 11,780 cancer deaths (52%) with a survival (5-year) rate improvement over the last 5 decades of (1950–2000) of 9%. Currently, relative 5-year survival for all stages is 22.5%, but when localized improves to 59% (Table 23.7). The basis for subdividing stages I and III is supported by American Joint Committee on Cancer survival data. An intergroup trial by the gastrointestinal group has established chemoradiation post-operatively doubling survival from 20 to 40% at 5 years (Fig. 29.2–7).

Because of the higher incidence of hepatitis B viral infections, wider ingestion of aflatoxins from moldy peanuts, and intestinal parasites as schistosomiasis, hepatocellular cancers are extremely common among Asians and the Bantu.

Perspective and Patterns of Spread

Cancers of the major digestive glands (MDG) remain a challenge to diagnose and treat. The 5-year survival rates have remained at 1% to 2% for decades, reflecting the advanced stages in which this disease is detected. Masquerading as nonspecific complaints such as epigastric fullness or mild distress, vague abdominal or back pain, or unexplained weight loss, it is no surprise that these neoplasms are recognized when they have become extensive replacing much of their organ of origin. Both cancer of the pancreas and liver are increasing in incidence. Incidence of pancreatic cancers has tripled over the past 40 years and they are the second most common tumors in the alimentary tract. By contrast, liver neoplasms are relatively uncommon in the North American hemisphere; however, in Southeast Asia and Africa, because of the higher incidence of hepatitis B viral infections, wider ingestion of aflatoxins from moldy peanuts, and intestinal parasites as schistosomiasis, hepatocellular cancers are extremely common among Asians and the Bantu. In fact, the high incidence of hepatomas in China and Asia makes this tumor, by sheer size of the population involved, a common cancer globally.

With an annual rate of almost 20,000 new patients, liver cancers are becoming a problem in the United States. Most patients succumb to either their hepatoma or the cirrhotic liver that hepatitis virus B and C induce. Liver failure is inevitable. The only viable alternative most often is liver transplantation. *The histopathology of hepatic malignancy originates from either hepatocyte or intrahepatic duct lining cell, that is, hepatocellular carcinoma (HCC) or cholangiocarcinoma, respectively (Fig. 26.1; Table 26.1).* Propagation and proliferation of cancers spread within the liver pursuing paths of infiltrating low-pressure zones as central veins or into bile ducts.

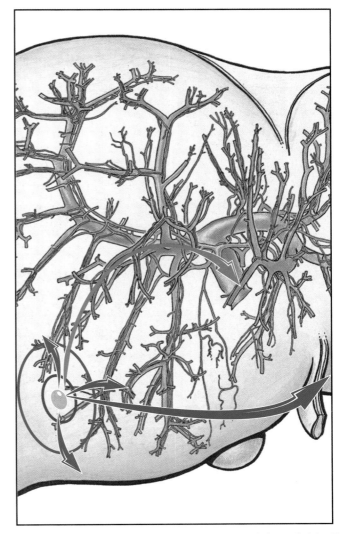

Figure 26.1 **Patterns of spread for liver cancer.** Color-coded for T stage: Tis, yellow; T1, green; T2, blue; T3, purple; and T4, red.

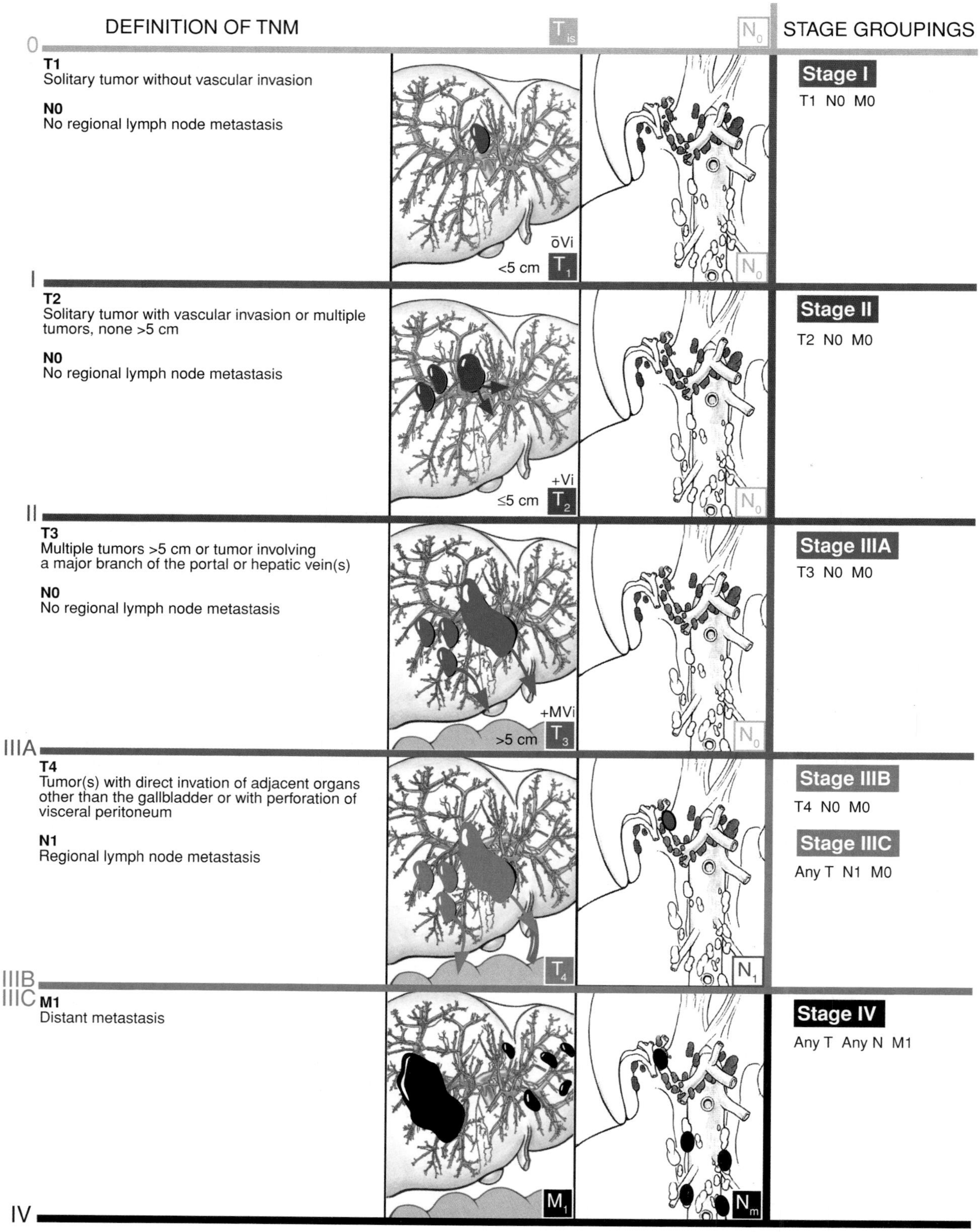

DEFINITION OF TNM

STAGE GROUPINGS

T1
Solitary tumor without vascular invasion

N0
No regional lymph node metastasis

Stage I
T1 N0 M0

ōVi
<5 cm T₁

T2
Solitary tumor with vascular invasion or multiple tumors, none >5 cm

N0
No regional lymph node metastasis

Stage II
T2 N0 M0

+Vi
≤5 cm T₂

T3
Multiple tumors >5 cm or tumor involving a major branch of the portal or hepatic vein(s)

N0
No regional lymph node metastasis

Stage IIIA
T3 N0 M0

+MVi
>5 cm T₃

T4
Tumor(s) with direct invation of adjacent organs other than the gallbladder or with perforation of visceral peritoneum

N1
Regional lymph node metastasis

Stage IIIB
T4 N0 M0

Stage IIIC
Any T N1 M0

T₄

N₁

M1
Distant metastasis

Stage IV
Any T Any N M1

M₁

Nₘ

Figure 26.2 TNM staging diagram presents a vertical arrangement with color bars encompassing TN combinations showing progression. Liver cancers are generally advanced stages. Stage IIIA is borderline resectable (purple), stage IIIB (red) is unresectable as is stage IV metastatic (black). Stage 0, yellow; I, green; II, blue; III, purple; IV, red; and IV (metastatic), black. Definitions of TN on left and stage grouping on right.

TABLE 26.1	Histopathologic Type: Common Cancers of the Liver	
Type		**% Incidence**
Hepatocellular carcinoma (liver cell carcinoma)		85–95
Cholangiocarcinoma (intrahepatic bile duct carcinoma)		5–15
Mixed hepatocellular cholangiocarcinoma		<1
Undifferentiated		<1

From Rubin P ed. *Clinical Oncology.* 8th ed. Philadelphia: WB Saunders; 2001.

TNM Staging Criteria

Hepatomas or hepatocellular cancers of the liver tend to remain localized in the liver for long periods of time. They often tend to invade various lobes of the liver, deep into its substance, entering sinusoidal channels and producing satellite lesions. Although some encapsulation occurs, it tends to be diffuse and does not respect lobar boundaries.

As the liver substance is replaced, the cancer penetrates through Glisson's capsule. It can invade other vital viscera, such as the stomach and intestine, although this is very uncommon. The size of the liver nodules and their volume have influenced the establishment of a staging system. The size of T1 cancer is solitary, <5 cm, and lacks vascular invasion. T2 are multiple nodules in aggregate <5 cm in size but with vascular invasion. T3 are multiple tumors >5 cm, or evidence of invasion of a major branch of the portal or hepatic system must be present. T4 is penetration of the visceral peritoneum or direct invasion of surrounding abdominal viscera excluding the gallbladder (Fig. 26.2).

Generally, there is no overarching principle or context design for the digestive system (gastrointestinal tract) or MDG. Stages are frequently expanded to six by subdividing stages into A and B. The T and N categories are assigned to a stage grouping, specifically for division of a stage into more (A) versus less (B) favorable grouping. This occurs at different stages for different sites.

Specifically, there is a direct relationship of T category advancement and stage. Stage III is divided into A/B/C: IIIA = T3, IIIB = T4, and IIIC = N1.

Summary of Changes

The changes in the sixth edition are major.

- *The T categories in this edition have been redefined and simplified.*
- *All solitary tumors without vascular invasion, regardless of size, are classified as T1 because of similar prognosis.*

- *All solitary tumors with vascular invasion (again regardless of size) are combined with multiple tumors ≤5 cm and classified as T2 because of similar prognosis.*
- *Multiple tumors >5 cm and tumors with evidence of major vascular invasion are combined and classified as T3 because of similarly poor prognosis.*
- *Tumor(s) with direct invasion of adjacent organs other than the gallbladder or with perforation of visceral peritoneum are classified separately as T4.*
- *The separate subcategory for multiple bilobar tumors has been eliminated because of a lack of distinct prognostic value.*
- *T3 N0 tumors and tumors with lymph node involvement are combined into stage III because of similar prognosis.*
- *Stage IV defines metastatic disease only. The subcategories IVA and IVB have been eliminated.*

Orientation of Three-planar Oncoanatomy

The anatomic isocenter for the liver is to right of midline at the T10 to T12 level (Fig. 26.3).

T-oncoanatomy

By virtue of its weight, the liver is the largest visceral organ in the body. When filled with cancerous nodules, it is often the greatest repository of neoplastic disease, exceeding primary tumors in the quantity of malignant cells. To understand the anatomy of the liver, *it is important to be aware of its internal structure as a gland of compound tubular design. Each lobule is shaped like a cylinder or tubule, with a central vein that drains a rich anatomic sinusoidal network derived from the fine hepatic anterioles and portal vessels (Fig. 26.4). The hepatocyte* elaborates both an external/exocrine secretion and an internal/endocrine secretion of enzymes into the blood. The former is referred to as *bile* and is collected by biliary canaliculi.

At the porta hepatis, the bile ducts coalesce into a right and left main duct, via the common hepatic duct

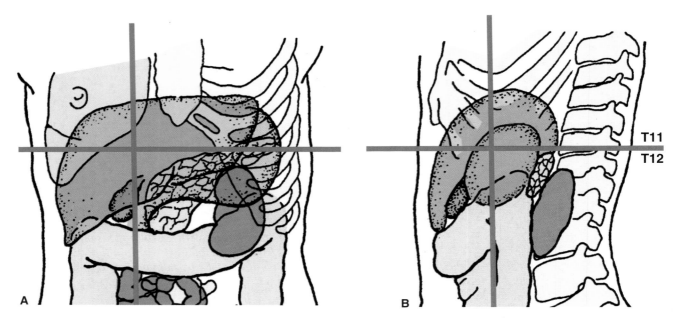

Figure 26.3 **Orientation and overview of oncoanatomy.** The anatomic isocenter of the 3planar anatomy is placed to right in the epigastrium and between T11 and T12 posteriorly. **A.** Coronal. **B.** Sagittal.

to the gallbladder and the cystic ducts below, as common bile duct courses toward the second portion of the duodenum where it fuses with the pancreatic duct at the ampulla of Vater. The gallbladder and its cystic duct is to the right and below the porta hepatis.

The liver sits under and is virtually surrounded by the diaphragm, superiorly, most of which is covered by peritoneum. Inferiorly, it is partially attached to the retroperitoneum. Abdominal viscera are in contact with its undersurface.

There are two major vascular systems in the liver. The major blood supply to the organ consists of the hepatic artery and vein. The portal system results from a fusion of the splenic vein with the superior mesenteric vein to form a portal vein that also enters the liver parenchyma via the porta hepatis. This brings the products of the intestine for detoxification and metabolic activation. The lymphatics follow the hepatic and portal veins and drain into the high para-aortic nodes, particularly around the celiac axis.

The new anatomic terminology refined by Couinaud is based on dividing the liver into four sectors by virtual/oblique planes referred to as *scissura*. The sectors are divided by a horizontal scissura thereby increasing the number of liver segments to eight. The eight segments are numbered clockwise in the frontal plane (Fig. 26.5).

• *Coronal*: The liver is divided into a right and a left half, if one judges by its blood supply for both the hepatic artery and portal veins that bifurcate at the porta hepatis. The left side usually includes the quadrate and caudate lobes of the liver.

• *Sagittal*: The new anatomic terminology refined by Couinaud is based on dividing the liver into four sectors by virtual/oblique planes referred to as *scissura*. The sectors are divided by a horizontal scissura thereby increasing the number of liver segments to eight. The eight segments are numbered in a clockwise in the frontal plane (Fig. 26.5) and are based on hepatic vein branching and determine portal liver resections.

• *Transverse*: There is an H-shaped group of fissures and fossae that describe these aforementioned lobes on either side of the H with other lobes positioned on the right and left sides. The porta hepatis represents the letter's crossbar, where the hepatic artery, portal vein, and major bile ducts enter, as well as nerves and lymphatics. The falciform ligament holds the liver in its position anteriorly and is attached to the superior and anterior surfaces as well as the dome of the diaphragm. The stomach and bowel are in contact on its inferior surface.

N-oncoanatomy

The lymphatics follow the hepatic and portal veins and drain into the paraortic or paracaval nodes, particularly around the celiac axis (Fig. 26.5; Table 26.2).

M-oncoanatomy

The entire portal circulation should be considered as a unit with regard to the venous anatomy of the gastrointestinal tract below the diaphragm (see Fig. 25.6). The two major trunks are the inferior mesenteric and superior mesenteric veins. The inferior mesenteric vein

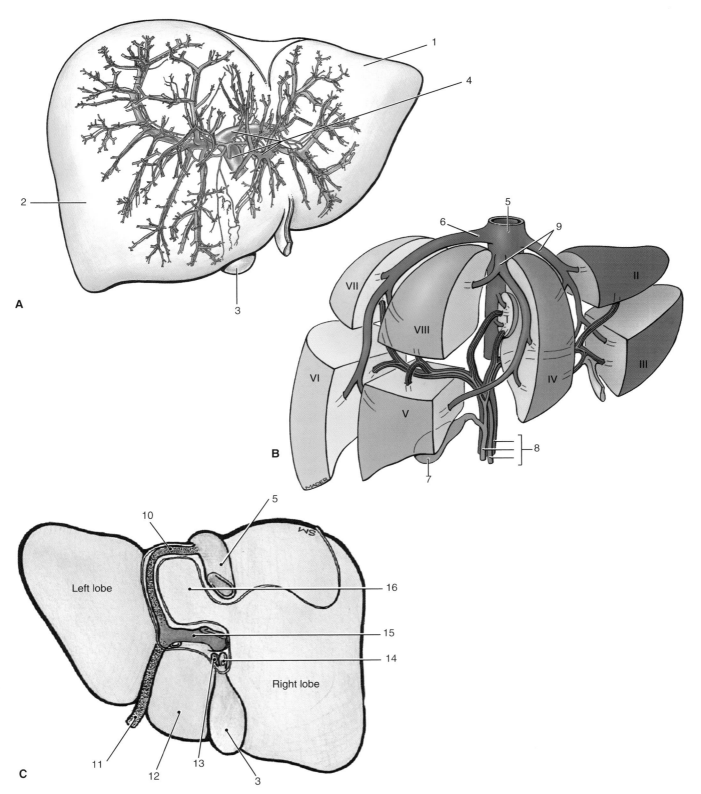

Figure 26.4 T-oncoanatomy. Liver three-planar views. **A.** Coronal. (1) Left lobe. (2) Right lobe. (3) Gallbladder. (4) Intrahepatic branches of portal vein. **B.** Sagittal. (5) Inferior vena cava. (6) Right hepatic vein. (7) Gallbladder. (8) Portal triad (portal vein, common bile duct, hepatic artery proper). (9) Left and middle hepatic veins. **C.** Transverse (inferior surface). (10) Ligamentum venosum (ductus venosus). (11) Round ligament of liver (ligamentum teres hepatis). (12) Quadrate lobe. (13) Hepatic artery. (14) Bile passage. (15) Portal vein. (16) Caudate lobe.

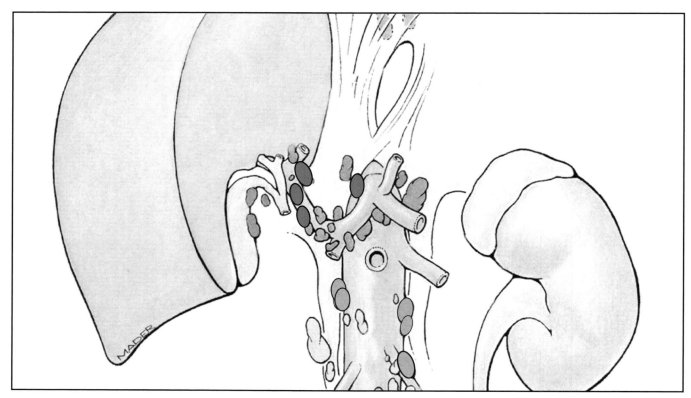

Figure 26.5 N-oncoanatomy. Sentinel nodes of the liver include the paracaval and paraortic nodes.

drains the left colon and sigmoid colon tributaries, which covers the vascular drainage to the left of the midline originating from the superior rectal veins. On the right side, the superior mesenteric vein originates from the tributaries draining the ileum, jejunum, and the ileocolic and right and middle colic veins. *The inferior mesenteric vein usually joins the splenic vein, which coalesces with the superior mesenteric vein and forms the portal vein.* The splenic vein, which is a major tributary of the portal system, also drains much of the stomach along its greater curvature and includes the short gastric veins and left and right gastric epiploic veins. The right gastroepiploic also flows into the superior mesenteric vein. The entire drainage of the lesser curvature of the stomach, including the left and right gastric veins, drains directly into the portal vein. Because the portal vein then drains directly into the liver, it is the target metastatic organ and

the most commonly involved organ in a hematogenous spread pattern from the venous system of the gastrointestinal tract as compared with other parts of the body, where the drainage is directly into the lung by way of the caval system.

Rules of Classification and Staging

Clinical Staging and Imaging

Imaging is essential for clinical staging of HCC. Because the liver is diseased due to hepatitis B and C infection and its associated cirrhosis, it is a challenge to uncover dysplastic nodules believed to be precursors to HCC. Computed tomography is favored to determine tumor size and if vascular invasion is present. Only 10% to 20% of HCC patients are surgically resected, preferably with

TABLE 26.2	Lymph Nodes of Liver	
Sentinel nodes include paracaval and porta hepatis nodes	
Regional nodes	Juxtaregional nodes
Hepatic vein Paracaval Celiac	Mediastinal Iliac Superior mesentery Pericardial and diaphragmatic

TABLE 26.3	Imaging Modalities for Evaluating Carcinoma of the Liver	
Method	Capability	Recommended for Use
CT	CT with IV contrast using dynamic changes in tumor enhancement multiphase.	Yes—Helical CT preferred
MRI	Dynamic study increases specificity to 85%–95% using gadolinium (T1 and T2 weighted).	Yes
CT	CT Arterial portography for determining major vessel invasion	No
Ultrasonography	Ultrasonography is useful for guiding needle biopsies, also Doppler and ultrasound angiography	Yes

T1 nodules, preferably <2 cm and not >5 cm. Numerous additional adverse factors can be found to contraindicate surgery, namely, presence of nodules in other lobes, lymphadenopathy, or major vessel invasion (Table 26.3).

Pathologic Staging

The surgically resected liver segments and associated lymph nodes removed are assessed. Tumor extension and location of both primary and nodes should be documented. Complete surgical staging consists of evaluation of primary tumor and underlying associated liver disease as severity of fibrosis/cirrhosis (F_0 = Ishak score 0–4 or F_1 = Ishak score 5–6) for better versus worse prognosis. Histologic grade and lymph node if any are recorded. If surgical margins are not released, total hepatectomy and liver transplantation are required for survival.

Oncoimaging Annotations

* HCC nodules receive blood via hepatic artery versus dysplastic nodules are supplied by portal veins.
* HCC classified on imaging as nodular, massive, and diffuse.

Cancer Statistics and Survival

The digestive system or gastrointestinal tract, which includes MDG, accounts for 255,640 new patients annually with colon and rectum responsible for >50%, with 146 new diagnoses annually. Approximately half eventually die of these cancers. MDG cancers as a group are more lethal; only a handful of patients becoming long-term survivors. Fortunately, colon and rectal cancers are the most common, with the majority of patients becoming 5-year survivors (63%) responding to chemoradiation programs often with the sparing of the rectal sphincter with conservative surgery. Anal cancers are the most responsive to chemoradiation (5-flourouracil and cisplatin) eliminating the need for surgery and 5-year survival is >90% with anal sphincter preservation. This regimen has been proven to be very effective in clinical trials and to result in more long-term survivors, which is currently reflected in the literature. Liver, bile duct, and pancreatic cancers are amongst the poorest in the terms of survival often measured in months rather than years (see Table 23.7).

Specifically, the liver accounted for 18,920 new cancer cases, 14,270 cancer deaths (88%), with a 5-year survival rate improvement over the past 5 decades of 5.8%. Currently, relative 5-year survival for all stages is 6.9%, but when localized improves to 16.3% (see Table 24.5). Remarkably overall survival at 5 years has steadily improved with total hepatectomy and liver transplantation. From 30% survival in 1988 to 57%. For all liver transplantations in USA, a 74% 5-year survival is reported.

Cancer of gallbladder is insidious in onset and associated with gallstones in 75% of presentations.

Perspective and Patterns of Spread

An elaborate bile ductal system originates in the liver, which becomes extrahepatic at the porta hepatis. The gallbladder can be viewed as a bile reservoir that responds to fat in meals and is connected by a cystic duct to the common bile duct (CBD). The CBD joins the pancreatic duct and forms an ampulla within the head of the pancreas referred as the ampulla of Vater, which terminates in a papilla that empties into the second part of the duodenum. This complex of branching bile ducts and fusion with the pancreatic duct is best appreciated diagrammatically (Fig. 27.1). Altogether these sites give rise to a variety of cancers, but the most common are adenocarcinomas.

The gallbladder and the extrahepatic biliary ducts account for 1,000 new cancer cases annually, approximately 50% of whom survive. Cancer of gallbladder is insidious in onset and associated with gallstones in 75% of presentations. Many gallbladder cancers are unsuspected and found incidentally by the surgeon who may be operating because of cholelithiasis. Although extrahepatic bile duct cancers can arise anywhere in its network, it is worth noting that 70% to 80% are found at the confluence of the right and the left hepatic ducts and the other 20% to 30% arise more distally. Obstructive jaundice is a frequent consequence and can occur even with small tumors. The main reason for identifying the ampulla of Vater separately is that obstruction at the site induces severe pain and causes jaundice and a most disconcerting reflux pancreatitis.

TNM Staging Criteria

The gallbladder and the extrahepatic bile ducts terminating at the ampulla of Vater share a hollow structure with thin walls. With the exception of the gallbladder, most bile duct cancers can obstruct and still be small. Whereas

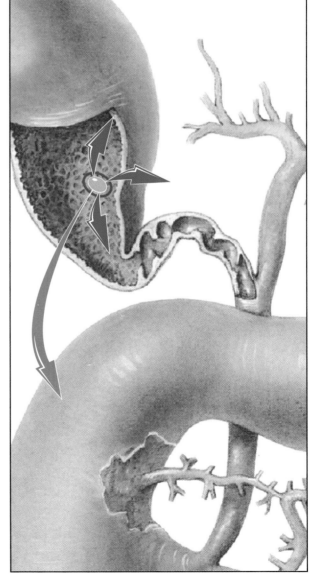

Figure 27.1 **Patterns of spread for gallbladder.** Color-coded for T stage: Tis, yellow; T1, green; T2, blue; T3, purple; T4, red.

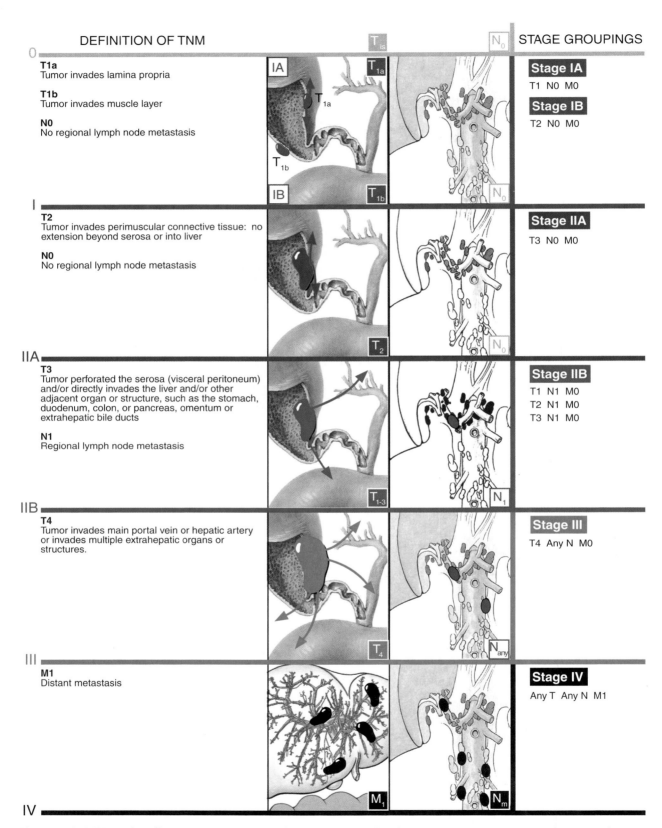

DEFINITION OF TNM

T1a
Tumor invades lamina propria

T1b
Tumor invades muscle layer

N0
No regional lymph node metastasis

IA

IB

T2
Tumor invades perimuscular connective tissue: no extension beyond serosa or into liver

N0
No regional lymph node metastasis

T3
Tumor perforated the serosa (visceral peritoneum) and/or directly invades the liver and/or other adjacent organ or structure, such as the stomach, duodenum, colon, or pancreas, omentum or extrahepatic bile ducts

N1
Regional lymph node metastasis

T4
Tumor invades main portal vein or hepatic artery or invades multiple extrahepatic organs or structures.

M1
Distant metastasis

STAGE GROUPINGS

Stage IA
T1 N0 M0

Stage IB
T2 N0 M0

Stage IIA
T3 N0 M0

Stage IIB
T1 N1 M0
T2 N1 M0
T3 N1 M0

Stage III
T4 Any N M0

Stage IV
Any T Any N M1

Figure 27.2 TNM staging diagram presents a vertical arrangement with color bars encompassing TN combinations showing progression. Gallbladder cancers are discovered incidentally to gallstones with Stage IIA (blue) being most resectable, Stage IIB (purple) borderline N1 nodes, and Stage III (red) is unresectable. Stage 0, yellow; I, green; II, blue; III, purple; IV, red; and IV (metastatic), black. Definitions of TN on left and stage grouping on right.

TABLE 27.1	Histopathologic Type: Common Cancers of the Gallbladder and the Bile Duct	
Type		**% Incidence**
Carcinoma		96
Adenocarcinoma		86
Adenocarcinoma, NOS		71
Papillary adenocarcinoma		6
Mucinous and mucin producing		5
Other adenocarcinoma		4
Squamous cell carcinoma		0.2
Carcinoma, NOS		7
Other specific carcinomas		0.5
Sarcoma		0.2
Other unspecified		0.8

NOS, not otherwise specified.
Modified from Carriaga MT, Henson DE: Liver, gallbladder, extrahepatic bile ducts, and pancreas. *Cancer* 1995;75(Suppl):171.

cancer of the ampulla of Vater can be confused with primary duodenal and/or pancreatic cancer of the head of the gland, their relative infrequency suggests this diagnosis is made by exclusion.

Each of these staging systems has been revised and simplified. Each of these primary sites are hollow structures with their muscular walls sharing common staging criteria (Fig. 27.2). T1 is a tumor that invades the lamina propria muscle layer and is contained within the wall. In stage T2, the tumor penetrates to the serosa. T3 tumor invades and penetrates the wall, through the serosa to a surrounding structure as liver or pancreas. T4 is an advanced cancer with invasion of multiple adjacent sites and into blood vessels. The staging criteria attempt to stage cancers of extrahepatic ducts as T3 to indicate resectability versus T4, which are nonresectable. Two of these three cancer sites are presented together to enable comparisons.

The malignant gradient of the gallbladder is highest at the surface in contact with the liver and decreases on the free side and the cystic duct. For the extrahepatic ducts, the malignant gradient is close to liver at the confluence of the right and left hepatic ducts and decreases peripherally.

Generally, there is no overarching principle or context design for the digestive system (gastrointestinal tract) or major digestive glands (MDG). Stages are frequently expanded to six by subdividing stages into A and B. The T and N categories are assigned to a stage grouping, specifically for division of a stage into more

(a) versus less (b) favorable groupings. This occurs at different stages for different sites.

Specifically, there is a direct relationship between T categories and stage progression that is, T1 = IA, T2 = IIA, T3 = IIB, and T4 = IV.

Summary of Changes

The changes in the sixth edition are moderate.

- *The T and N classifications have been simplified in an effort to separate locally invasive tumors into potentially resectable (T3) and unresectable (T4).*
- *There is no longer a distinction between T3 and T4 based on depth of liver invasion.*
- *Lymph node metastasis is now classified as stage IIB; stage IIA is reserved for large invasive tumors (resectable) without lymph node metastasis.*
- *Stage grouping has been changed to allow stage III to signify locally unresectable disease and stage IV to indicate metastatic disease.*

Orientation of Three-planar Oncoanatomy

The anatomic isocenter for the three-planar oncoanatomy for the gallbladder is to the right of the midline (pararectus plane) at the subcostal region anteriorly and T12/L1 posteriorly (Fig. 27.3). The bile ducts are in a similar locale but inferior at L1/L2.

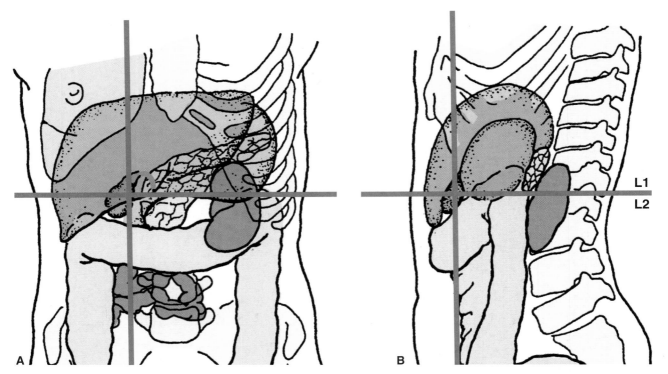

Figure 27.3 Orientation and overview of oncoanatomy. The anatomic isocenter for the three-planar oncoanatomy for the gallbladder is the right of the midline (pararectus plane) at the subcostal region anteriorly and L1/L2 posteriorly. **A.** Coronal. **B.** Sagittal.

T-oncoanatomy

Figure 27.4 provides orientation of three-planar views of these interrelated sites, anatomically as well as functionally.

- *Coronal*: The gallbladder is a pearlike organ with four layers: A lining epithelium, which is simple columnar consisting of common clear cells and occasional brush cells, the lamina propria, a layer of smooth muscle with connective tissue, and cone of a serosa on the free caudad tail side; and the adventitia on the cephalad head side juxtaposed to the liver. When empty the gallbladder is folded into tall parallel ridges; filled, the folds are reduced.

- *Sagittal*: The extrahepatic ducts unite with the cystic duct to become the CBD. Again, there are four layers or sphincter muscles of Oddi that control the flow of bile and move pancreatic secretions in the correct directions without reflux of bile into the pancreas. The ampulla of Vater opens at a duodenal papilla to always maintain a prograde flow into the small bowel.

- *Transverse*: The gallbladder at the inferior margin of the right lobe of the liver to which it is juxtaposed on its superior surface and to bowel on its inferior surface. The cystic duct drains to the left, toward the midline where it coalesces with the extra hepatic bile ducts to form the CBD at the porta hepatis.

N-oncoanatomy

The distance between the porta hepatis and the head of the pancreas ranges between 5 and 10 cm. The region is abundant in lymphatics with the cisterna chyli located posterior to the head of the pancreas. The gallbladder drains toward the porta hepatis (Fig. 27.5; Table 27.2) and the extrahepatic bile ducts drain into the pancreatic duodenal nodes (Fig. 27.5B).

M-oncoanatomy

The entire portal circulation should be considered as a unit in regard to the venous anatomy of the gastrointestinal tract below the diaphragm (see Fig. 25.6). The two major trunks are the inferior mesenteric and superior mesenteric veins. The inferior mesenteric vein drains the left colon and sigmoid colon tributaries, which covers the vascular drainage to the left of the midline originating from the superior rectal veins. On the right side, the superior mesenteric vein originates from the tributaries draining the ileum, jejunum, the ileocolic, and right middle colic veins. *The inferior mesenteric vein usually joins the splenic vein, which coalesces with the superior mesenteric vein and forms the portal vein. The*

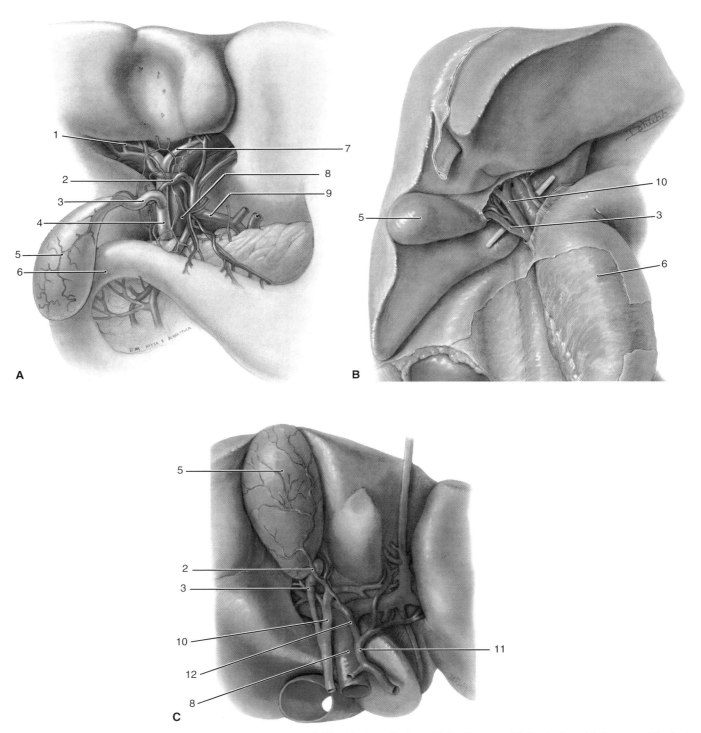

Figure 27.4 **T-oncoanatomy: Three-planar views. A.** Coronal. (1) Right hepatic duct. (2) Cystic artery. (3) Cystic duct. (4) Common bile duct. (5) Gallbladder. (6) Duodenum. (7) Left hepatic duct. (8) Portal vein. (9) Common hepatic artery. **B.** Sagittal. (10) Common hepatic duct. **C.** Transverse (Inferior view). (11) Hepatic artery proper. (12) Right hepatic artery.

splenic vein, which is a major tributary of the portal system, also drains much of the stomach along its greater curvature and includes the short gastric veins and left and right gastroepiploic veins. The right gastric epiploic vein also flows into the superior mesenteric vein. The

entire drainage of the lesser curvature of the stomach, including the left and right gastric veins, drains directly into the portal vein. Because the portal vein then drains directly into the liver, the liver is the target metastatic organ and most commonly involved in hematogenous

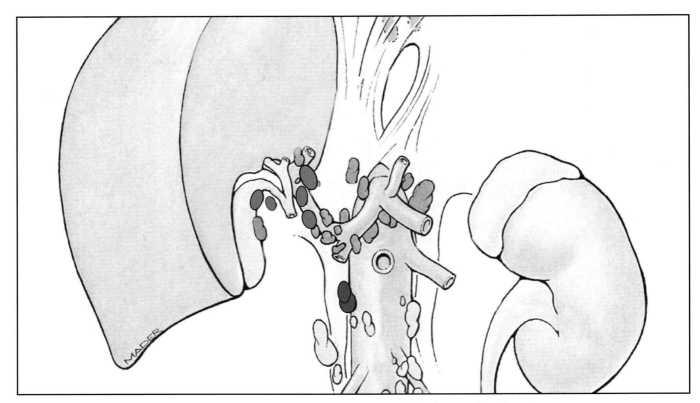

Figure 27.5 **N-oncoanatomy.** Sentinel nodes of the gallbladder and bile ducts include the porta hepatis nodes.

spread pattern from the venous system of the gastrointestinal tract as compared with other parts of the body, where the drainage is directly into the lung by way of the caval system.

Rules of Classification and Staging

Clinical Staging and Imaging

The inability to evaluate the gallbladder, its ducts, and the ampulla of Vater has led the American Joint Committee on Cancer to simplify the staging so that both clinical and surgical criteria are the same. Imaging procedures include abdominal ultrasound, which is surpassed

by computed tomography (CT) in defining biliary obstruction. Endoscopic retrograde cholangiopancreatography (ERCP) and percutaneous transhepatic cholangiography define biliary tree anatomy. Magnetic resonance imaging (MRI) with gadolinium is also useful (Table 27.3).

Pathologic Staging

The surgically resected gallbladder and/or bile ducts with associated lymph nodes removed are assessed. Tumor extension and location of both primary and nodes should be documented. Accurate radial margins should be marked and recorded and are defined "as the surgically

TABLE 27.2	Lymph nodes of Gallbladder and the Bile Duct
Sentinel nodes include porta hepatis nodes	
Regional nodes	Juxtaregional nodes
Hepatic vein	Mediastinal
Paracaval	Iliac
Celiac	Superior mesentery
	Pericardial and diaphragmatic

TABLE 27.3	Imaging Modalities for Staging Biliary Tree Tumors	
Method	**Capability**	**Recommended for Use**
CT	Minimally invasive with IV contrast. Most useful for determining local invasion, extent of tumor, defining site of biliary ductal obstruction and evaluating for distant metastases.	Yes
Ultrasound	Excellent for evaluating metastatic disease and the biliary tract. Even when the primary tumor is not seen, the bile ducts may be visualized.	Yes
ERCP/PTC	Defines biliary anatomy. PTC is preferred for proximal lesions, ERCP for distal.	Yes
Angiography	To determine surgical resection for pancreatic cancers.	No

CT, computed tomography; ERCP/PTC, endoscopic retrograde cholangiopancreatography/percutaneous transhepatic cholangiography; IV, intravenous.

dissected surface adjacent to the deepest point of tumor invasion beyond the wall of the gallbladder." The completeness of resection depends on the clearing of the deepest point of invasion: R0, complete; R1, microscopic; and R2, macroscopic.

Oncoimaging Annotations

- Imaging is used for tumor detection and evaluation of tumor resectability: Ultrasonography (including Doppler, and ultrasound angiography), contrast-enhanced CT (intravenous bolus injection), multiple (early arterial, portal, and delayed scanning), and MRI (including T1 weighted, T2 weighted, and dynamic contrast enhanced) are all used.

- MRI is considered to have higher sensitivity for detection of smaller lesions.

- Ten percent to 20% of carcinomas of the gallbladder are found incidentally in resected gallbladder specimens.

- *Imaging approaches*: Ultrasonography with color Doppler, CT with bolus intravenous, contrast material injection and multiphase scanning. T1- or T2-weighted MRI and dynamic scanning with gadolinium and ERCP are all helpful.

- CT-guided biopsy is essential.

- Staging is excellent with either CT or MRI.

Cancer Statistics and Survival

The digestive system or gastrointestinal tract, which includes MDG, accounts for 255,640 new patients annually with colon and rectum responsible for >50% with 146 new diagnoses annually. Approximately half eventually die of these cancers. MDG cancers as a group are more lethal; only a handful of patients becoming long-term survivors. Fortunately, colon and rectal cancers are the most common, with the majority of patients becoming 5-year survivors (63%) responding to chemoradiation programs often with the sparing of the rectal sphincter with conservation surgery. Anal cancers are the most responsive to chemoradiation (5-fluorouracil and cisplatin), eliminating the need for surgery. The 5-year survival rate is >90% with anal sphincter preservation. This regimen has been proven to be very effective in clinical trials and to result in more long-term survivors, which is currently reflected in the literature. Liver, bile duct, and pancreatic cancers are among the poorest in the terms of survival often measured in months rather than years.

Specifically, the gallbladder and bile ducts accounted for 6,950 new cancer cases and 3,540 cancer deaths (51%). Survival rates (5-year) as a function of stage following and extended cholecystectomy ± extended lobectomy of liver are by stage: T1 90–100%, T2 30–80%, and T3T4 10–25%.

28

Extrahepatic Bile Ducts

The commonest site for cancers of the extrahepatic bile ducts is at the confluence of the right and left ducts; the Klatskin tumor or hilar cholangiosarcoma.

Perspective and Patterns of Spread

The onset of jaundice is the common provocative symptom that requires attention and may lead to an early diagnosis of an extrahepatic cholangiocarcinoma. An unusually high serum bilirubin (>10–20 mg) should suggest malignancy because bilirubin levels of 2 to 4 mg are normal for obstructive cholelithiasis. This uncommon malignant entity is a disease of elderly populations, peaking late in 80 year olds. As with hepatocellular carcinoma where hepatitis B and C virus infection is predisposing factors, the presence of infection in the form of primary sclerosing cholangitis is most often associated with cholangiocarcinoma. Primary sclerosing cholangitis is an autoimmune process and produces multifocal strictures in both extrinsic and intrinsic hepatic bile ducts. Although the incidence of cancer is only detected in 10% of infected patients, it can be as high as 30% to 40% at autopsy. Another source of chronic infection, especially in the far East, that leads to hepatolithiasis and eventuates from hepatic pigment stone formation to strictures, then to recurrent cholangitis and carcinogenesis, biliary parasites can increase the risk of cholangiocarcinomas. Another well-recognized risk factor is Canoli disease or congenital choledochal cysts. Canoli disease patients have a predisposition for harboring infection, which has been shown in adults and even when excised to have incidental rates of 15% to 20% bile duct cancers.

Patterns of spread depend on the site of origin in the biliary tree (Fig. 28.1). The extrahepatic cholangiocarcinoma can arise anywhere along its length. *By far the commonest site is at the confluence of the right and left hepatic ducts*, which has an incidence of 40% to 60% and includes *the Klatskin tumor or the hilar cholangiocarcinomas*. Multifocality is rare with ≤10% occurring throughout the biliary tree. The overwhelming majority are well-differentiated, mucin-producing adenocarcinomas (see Table 27.1).

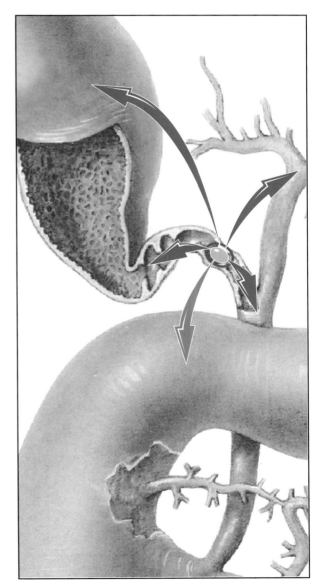

Figure 28.1 **Patterns of spread for extrahepatic bile ducts.** Color coded for T stage: Tis, yellow; T1, green; T2, blue; T3, purple; and T4, red.

DEFINITION OF TNM

STAGE GROUPINGS

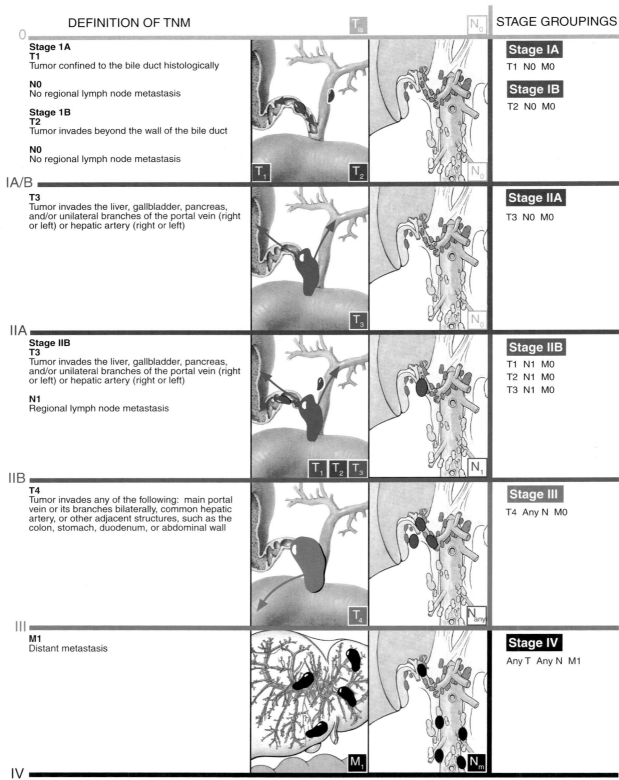

0

Stage 1A
T1
Tumor confined to the bile duct histologically

N0
No regional lymph node metastasis

Stage 1B
T2
Tumor invades beyond the wall of the bile duct

N0
No regional lymph node metastasis

Stage IA
T1 N0 M0

Stage IB
T2 N0 M0

IA/B

T3
Tumor invades the liver, gallbladder, pancreas, and/or unilateral branches of the portal vein (right or left) or hepatic artery (right or left)

Stage IIA
T3 N0 M0

IIA

Stage IIB
T3
Tumor invades the liver, gallbladder, pancreas, and/or unilateral branches of the portal vein (right or left) or hepatic artery (right or left)

N1
Regional lymph node metastasis

Stage IIB
T1 N1 M0
T2 N1 M0
T3 N1 M0

IIB

T4
Tumor invades any of the following: main portal vein or its branches bilaterally, common hepatic artery, or other adjacent structures, such as the colon, stomach, duodenum, or abdominal wall

Stage III
T4 Any N M0

III

M1
Distant metastasis

Stage IV
Any T Any N M1

IV

*not illustrated

Figure 28.2 **TNM staging diagram presents a vertical arrangement with color bars encompassing TN combinations showing progression.** Note Stage I and II are divided into substages A/B. Resectability is possible with Stage IA/B and Stage IIA, decreases with Stage IIB (purple) when nodes are involved and invasion of gallbladder occurs. Stage III is unresectable and Stage IV is metastatic and not treatable. Stage 0, yellow; I, green; II, blue; III, purple; IV, red; and stage IV (metastatic), black. Definitions of TN on left and stage grouping on right.

Hilar or confluens cholangiocarcinomas can readily penetrate through the thin muscular walls of extrahepatic bile ducts and have immediate access to the major vessels of the porta hepatis, portal vein, and hepatic artery. Distal biliary duct cancers represent the other 20% to 30% of cholangiocarcinomas; mid-duct occurrence is rare. These cancers are discussed with periampullary cancers or cancers of ampulla of Vater.

TNM Staging Criteria

A single classification is offered for both the clinical and pathologic staging. This site was added in the fourth edition (1992) of the American Joint Committee on Cancer (AJCC). Recognize that the extrahepatic bile duct on cross-section is lined by a single layer of columnar cells. In its collapsed state, the mucosa is pleated with longitudinal folds, and a thin subepithelial layer of fibrous and muscle cells is surrounded by serosal cells. For these reasons, T1 is confined to the bile duct, T2 is tumor beyond its confines, and both require histologic verification. T3 relates to the immediate surrounding anatomy in the porta hepatis being invaded as liver, gallbladder, and unilateral branches of the hepatic artery and portal vein, whereas T4 is further spread into the common portal vein or hepatic artery or into colon, stomach, duodenum—essentially the other viscera (Fig. 28.2).

Nodal involvement is simply N1 and refers to the hilar nodes near the gallbladder and around the portal vein, hepatic artery, cystic ducts, and so on.

Summary of Changes

With the sixth edition, the T and N classification has been simplified and includes:

- *Invasion of the subepithelial fibro (muscular) connective tissue is classified as T1 irrespective of muscular invasion, which cannot always be noted because of the scarcity of muscle fibers in some bile duct segments.*
- *T2 is defined as invasion beyond the wall of the bile duct.*
- *The T classification allows one to separate locally invasive tumors into resectable (T3) and unresectable (T4).*
- *Invasion of branches of the portal vein (right or left), hepatic artery, or liver is classified as T3.*
- *Invasion of the main portal vein, common hepatic artery, and/or regional organs is classified as T4.*
- *The stage grouping has been changed to allow stage III to signify locally unresectable disease and stage IV to indicate metastatic disease.*

Orientation of Three-planar Oncoanatomy

The anatomic isocenter for the extrahepatic biliary tree is at the hilar level and (a) the bullet is to the right of the midsagittal plane and (b) and in the midcoronal plan, the bullet is anterior to the 12th rib (Fig. 28.3).

T-oncoanatomy

The complexity in understanding the oncoanatomy of the extrahepatic biliary tree is the precise details in each individual as to the potential variations in the arrangements of the gallbladder, cystic duct, and the confluens, which can be a low or high union, or swerving in its course (Fig. 28.4). In addition, the resectability relates to the arrangements of hepatic artery and portal vein as well as its branching. Optimally, a confluens carcinoma with a low lying union and separation of the right and left hepatic artery would be more resectable than a high union with the main hepatic artery lying anterior to confluens.

- *Coronal*: The extrahepatic bile ducts and pancreatic bile ducts and pancreatic ducts are dissected free. The left and right hepatic ducts collect bile from the liver and unite with the cystic duct superior to the pancreas and the duodenum.
- *Sagittal*: The extrahepatic bile duct lies posterior to the gallbladder and passes posterior to the first part of the duodenum at the porta hepatis. The portal triad of the common bile duct, hepatic artery, and portal vein lies in the hepatoduodenal ligament, at the entrance to the lesser omental sac.
- *Transverse*: The inferior surface of the liver exposes the intimate relationship at the porta hepatis of the cystic duct to the common bile duct and its confluens in addition to medially placed hepatic artery and portal vein.

N-oncoanatomy

The lymphatic drainage of the extrahepatic bile duct are the lymph nodes at the porta hepatis and include hilar, coeliac, periduodenal, and peripancreatic nodes as well as nodes around the gallbladder and the hepatic triad. The sentinel nodes are the porta hepatis nodes. Nodal metastases are common and occur in 30% of cases (Fig. 28.5; see Table 27.2).

M-oncoanatomy

The venous drainage of the extrahepatic bile ducts joins the cystic vein and drains into the right gastric vein and posterior superior pancreaticoduodenal vein, and then into the portal vein, returning to the liver. In addition to hematogenous spread, perineural and neural invasion are common (see Fig. 25.6).

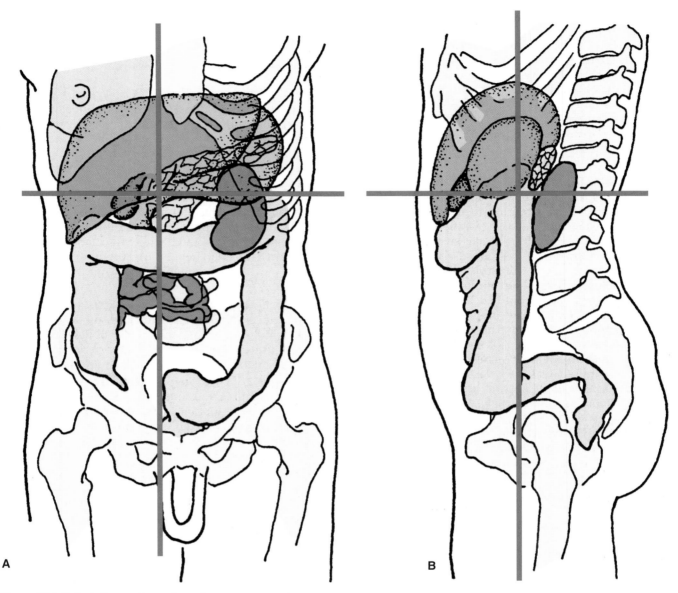

A

B

Figure 28.3 **Orientation and overview of oncoanatomy.** The anatomic isocenter for the three-planar oncoanatomy for the gallbladder is the right of the midline (pararectus plane) at the subcostal region anteriorly and L1/L2 posteriorly. The bile ducts are in a similar locale, but inferior at L1/L2. **A.** Coronal. **B.** Sagittal.

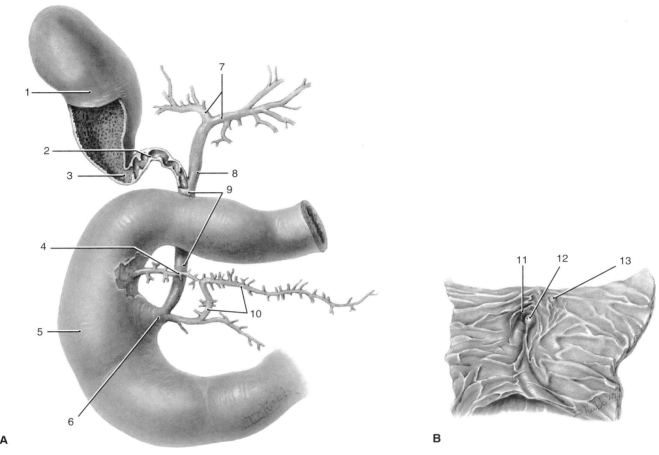

Figure 28.4 **T-Oncoanatomy: Bile ducts three-planar views. A.** Coronal. (1) Gallbladder (body). (2) Spiral fold in cystic duct. (3) Neck of gallbladder. (4) Accessory pancreatic duct. (5) Second part of duodenum. (6) Hepatopancreatic ampulla. (7) Right and left hepatic ducts. (8) Common hepatic duct. (9) Common bile duct. (10) Main pancreatic duct. **B.** Sagittal. (11) Hood. (12) Major duodenal papilla. (13) Minor duodenal papilla.

Rules of Classification and Staging

Clinical Staging and Imaging

The inability to evaluate the gallbladder, its ducts, and the ampulla of Vater has led the AJCC to simplify the staging so that both clinical and surgical criteria are the same. Imaging procedures include abdominal ultrasound, which is surpassed by computed tomography (CT) in defining biliary obstruction. Endoscopic retrograde cholangiopancreatography (ERCP) and percutaneous transhepatic cholangiography define biliary tree anatomy. Magnetic resonance imaging with gadolinium is also useful (see Table 27.3).

Pathologic Staging

The surgically resected gallbladder and/or bile ducts with associated lymph nodes removed are assessed. Tu-

mor extension and location of both primary and nodes should be documented. Accurate radial margins should be marked and recorded and are defined "as the surgically dissected surface adjacent to the deepest point of tumor invasion beyond the wall of the extrahepatic bile duct." The completeness of resection depends on the clearing of the deepest point of invasion: R0, complete; R1, microscopic; and R2, macroscopic.

Oncoimaging Annotations

- Ultrasound initially reveals a dilated extrahepatic duct and intrahepatic duct system.
- Helical multiplanar CT with five 1- to 2-mm cuts best shows the mass. ERCP is an optional procedure that may show the common bile duct cancer without involvement of the pancreatic duct, but

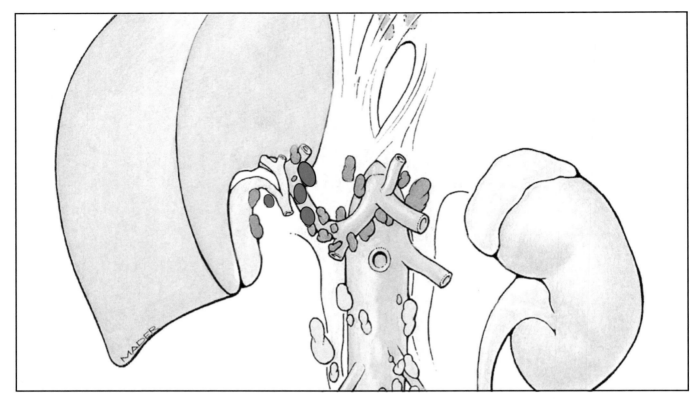

Figure 28.5 **N-Oncoanatomy.** Sentinel nodes of the bile ducts include the porta hepatis nodes.

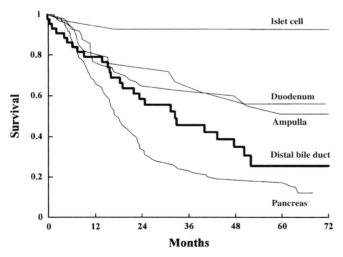

Figure 28.6 Survival for patients with various peripancreatic tumors.

surgical evaluation followed by resection and microscopy is critical to both diagnosis and staging.

• When direct cholangiograms are needed, a percutaneous transhepatic cholangiogram identifies the common bile duct cancer site and is preferred over ERCP.

Cancer Statistics and Survival

Complete resection is critical for survival. Node-negative patients do better, as anticipated; low recurrence is seven times more common without positive nodes. Survival for periampullary cancers is highly dependent on true anatomic site of origin. Liver resections with negative margins are the key to survival for hilar and confluens bile duct cancer (Fig. 28.6).

Painless jaundice suggests the head of the pancreas; pain in the back, worse at night, suggests the body of the pancreas. Invasion of the pancreas tail is usually silent.

Perspective and Patterns of Spread

Cancer of the pancreas has been increasing over the past decades, currently there are >30,000 new patients annually, most of whom die within 1 to 2 years, having a dismal 3% 5-year survival rate. The causative factors remain obscure; no dietary relationship is evident and no high-risk group has been identified to offer more intensive screening of the pancreas. Painless jaundice suggests the head of the pancreas; pain in the back, worse at night, relieved by sitting up or rolling to the side suggests the body of the pancreas is involved. Invasion of the pancreas tail is usually silent and invariably found at post mortem in patients dying with severe cachexia. Cancer of the pancreas ranks as the fifth leading cause of cancer deaths.

The histogenesis of pancreatic cancers applies to its exocrine cell activities, not endocrine, which relate to Islands of Langerhans cells. The World Health Organization Tabulation of carcinomas is long and varied (Fig. 29.1; Table 29.1).

TNM Staging Criteria

The pancreas is both intraperitoneal and retroperitoneal in location. Situated in the epigastrium, the cancer can and does invade adjacent structures. Size is the major factor in staging: T1, <2 cm and T2, >2 cm, limited to pancreas. Involvement of the celiac axis and superior mesenteric artery (SMA) renders the cancer T4 and nonresectable (Fig. 29.2).

Each section of the pancreas has a critical adjacent structure that determines the clinical course as mentioned, but does not affect staging. Despite the intimate contact anteriorly with stomach, duodenum, colon, spleen, and kidneys, pancreatic cancers rarely invade these viscera; however, peritoneal seeding is common and can lead to massive ascites.

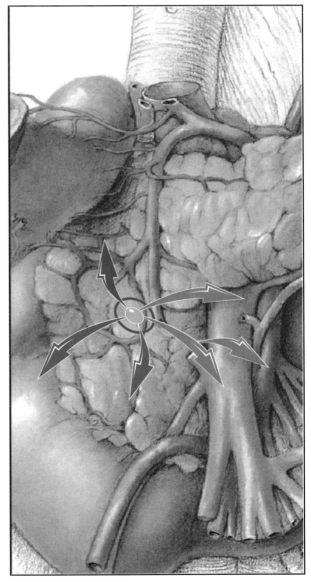

Figure 29.1 **Patterns of spread for pancreas.** Color coded for T stage: Tis, yellow; T1, green; T2, blue; T3, purple; T4, red.

DEFINITION OF TNM

STAGE GROUPINGS

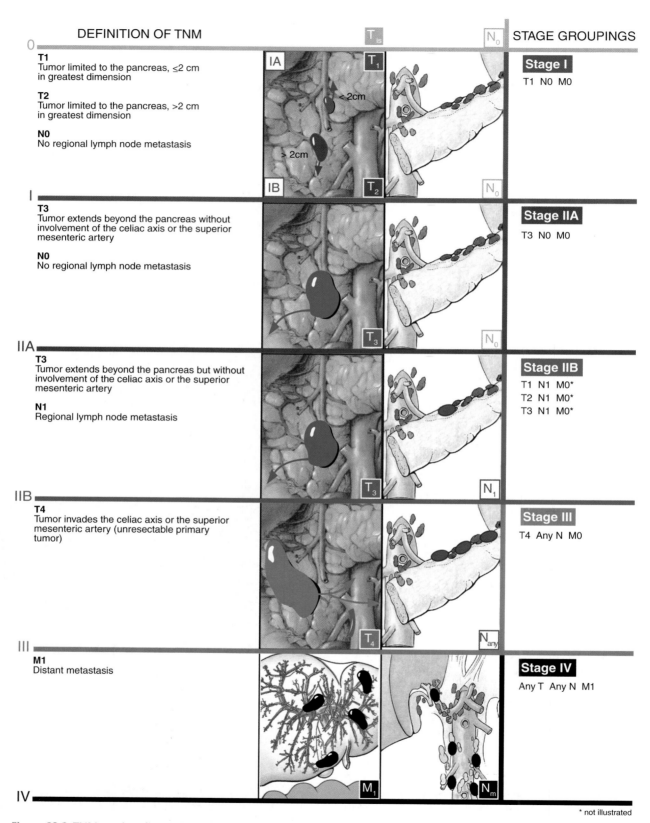

T1
Tumor limited to the pancreas, ≤2 cm in greatest dimension

T2
Tumor limited to the pancreas, >2 cm in greatest dimension

N0
No regional lymph node metastasis

T3
Tumor extends beyond the pancreas without involvement of the celiac axis or the superior mesenteric artery

N0
No regional lymph node metastasis

T3
Tumor extends beyond the pancreas but without involvement of the celiac axis or the superior mesenteric artery

N1
Regional lymph node metastasis

T4
Tumor invades the celiac axis or the superior mesenteric artery (unresectable primary tumor)

M1
Distant metastasis

Stage I
T1 N0 M0

Stage IIA
T3 N0 M0

Stage IIB
T1 N1 M0*
T2 N1 M0*
T3 N1 M0*

Stage III
T4 Any N M0

Stage IV
Any T Any N M1

* not illustrated

Figure 29.2 **TNM staging diagram presents a vertical arrangement with color bars encompassing TN combinations showing progression.** Pancreas cancers are generally advanced Stage IIB (purple) and N1 borderline resectable, Stage III (red) are unresectable and Stage IV (black) metastatic. Stage 0, yellow; I, green; IIA, blue; IIB, purple; III, red; and stage IV (metastatic), black. Definitions of TN on left and stage grouping on right.

TABLE 29.1	Histopathologic Type: Common Cancers of the Pancreas

Type	
Severe ductal dysplasia/carcinoma in situ (PanIn; pancreatic intraepithelial neoplasia)	Intraductal papillary mucinous carcinoma with or without invasion
Ductal adenocarcinoma	Acinar cell carcinoma
Mucinous noncystic carcinoma	Acinar cell cystadenocarcinoma
Signet ring cell carcinoma	Mixed acinar-endocrine carcinoma
Adenosquamous carcinoma	Pancreaticoblastoma

Undifferentiated carcinoma
    Spindle and giant cell types
    Small cell types
	Solid pseudopapillary carcinoma

Mixed ductal-endocrine carcinoma	Borderline (uncertain malignant potential) tumors
	    Mucinous cystic tumor with moderate dysplasia
	    Intraductal papillary-mucinous tumor with moderate dysplasia
	    Solid pseudopapillary tumor

Osteoclast-like giant cell tumor	Other
Serous cystadenocarcinoma	
Mucinous cystadenocarcinoma	

Generally, there is no overarching principle or context design for the digestive system (gastrointestinal tract) or major digestive glands (MDG). Stages are frequently expanded to six by subdividing stages into A and B. The T and N categories are assigned to a stage grouping, specifically for division of a stage into more (a) versus less (b) favorable groupings. This occurs at different stages for different sites.

Specifically, there is a direct relationship between N category and stage II progression with stage: IIA = N0 and IIB N1.

Summary of Changes

The changes in the sixth edition are moderate.

- *The T classification reflects the distinction between potentially resectable (T3) and locally advanced unresectable (T4) primary pancreatic tumors.*
- *Stage grouping has been changed to allow stage III to signify unresectable, locally advanced pancreatic cancer, whereas stage IV is reserved for patients with metastatic disease.*

Orientation of Three-planar Oncoanatomy

The anatomic isocenter for the three-planar oncoanatomy for the pancreas is at the L1/L2 level deep in the epigastrium (Fig. 29.3).

T-oncoanatomy

- *Coronal*: The pancreas is a long, lobulated structure that lies transversely in the posterior abdomen, located retroperitoneally in the concavity of the duodenum on its right end and touching the spleen on its left end. The shape of the pancreas may be compared to the letter J placed sideways. It is divisible into a head with an uncinate process, a neck, a body, and a tail (Fig. 29.4). The acinous glands of the pancreas secrete into a branching ductal network, which forms the main horizontal pancreatic duct that runs the length of the pancreas and terminates in the second portion of the duodenum after it creates a common junction with the hepatic duct at the ampulla of Vater. There is often a small accessory pancreatic duct, which has a separate opening into the duodenum. The uncinate process of the head wraps around the SMA and is hugged by the duodenum.
- *Sagittal*: The midsagittal plane shows the intimate relationship of the head of the pancreas to the SMA inferiorly. Note the retroperitoneal location of the pancreas posterior to the lesser omental bursa. However, the transverse mesocolon arising from its anterior surface allows pancreatic cancers to spread intraperitoneally and seed the peritoneal surface, once invaded.
- *Transverse*: The pancreas lies in the midcoronal plane and is at the divide of the retroperitoneum from

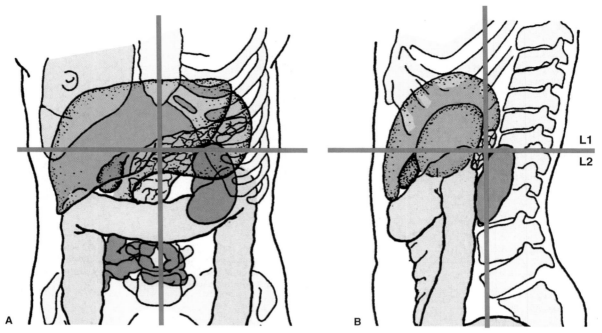

Figure 29.3 **Orientation and overview of oncoanatomy.** The anatomic isocenter for the three-planar oncoanatomy for the pancreas is at the L1/L2 level, deep in the epigastrium. **A.** Coronal. **B.** Sagittal.

peritoneal cavity. The pancreas stretches from right kidney hilum to left renal hilum.

N-oncoanatomy

A rich lymphatic network surrounds the pancreas with a left splenic and superior and inferior right side truncal drainage. The first station nodes include the celiac, splenic, suprapancreatic, left gastropancreatic, and hepatic arteries, and inferior pancreatic, juxta-aortic, anterior pancreatic duodenal, and posterior pancreatic duodenal lymph nodes. Juxtaregional nodes include the inferior portion of the para-aortic nodal drainage and mediastinal and mesenteric nodes. Distant spread occurs mainly to liver and lungs, with a lesser degree of involvement of bones and brain as well as to other anatomic sites (Fig. 29.5; Table 29.2).

M-oncoanatomy

The rich venous anastomoses of pancreas and its juxtaposition to the liver makes portal vein invasion and liver metastases as the favored target organs. The entire portal circulation should be considered as a unit with regard to the venous anatomy of the gastrointestinal tract below the diaphragm (see Fig. 25.6). The two major trunks are the inferior and superior mesenteric veins. The inferior mesenteric vein drains the left colon and sigmoid colon tributaries, which covers the vascular drainage to the left of the midline originating from the superior rectal veins. On the right side, the superior mesenteric vein originates from the tributaries draining the ileum, jejunum, and ileocolic and right middle colic veins. *The inferior mesenteric vein usually joins the splenic vein, which coalesces with the superior mesenteric vein and forms the portal vein.* The splenic vein, which is a major tributary of the portal system, also drains much of the stomach along its greater curvature and includes the short gastric veins and left and right gastroepiploic veins. The right gastroepiploic also flows into the superior mesenteric vein. The entire drainage of the lesser curvature of the stomach, including the left and right gastric veins, drains directly into the portal vein. Because the portal vein then drains directly into the liver, it is the target metastatic organ and the most commonly involved organ in hematogenous spread pattern from the venous system of the gastrointestinal tract as compared with other parts of the body, where the drainage is directly into the lung by way of the caval system.

The incidence of liver metastases exceeds other sites. According to a variety of reports in the literature, the range is 45% to 80% at autopsy. Other sites are mainly bone metastases (20%–35%) and lung metastases (40%–60%), with only occasional metastases to the brain.

Rules for Classification and Staging

Clinical Staging and Imaging

Clinical and pathologic classifications have been combined into a single staging system. It is important to

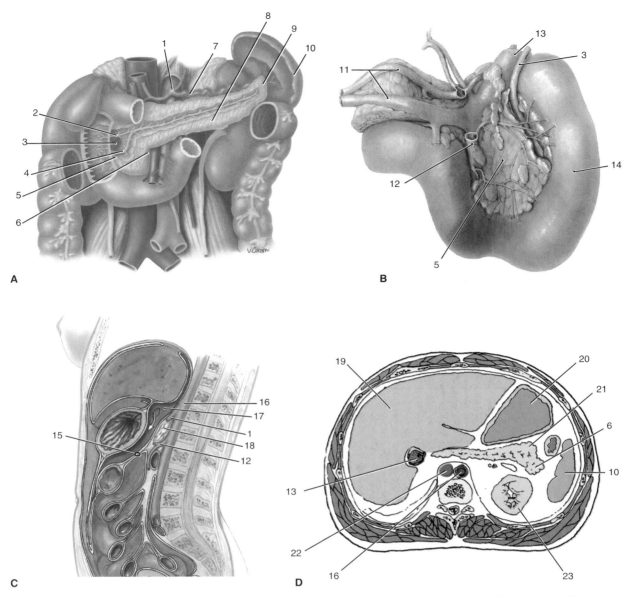

Figure 29.4 T-oncoanatomy. Pancreas three-planar views. **A.** Anterior Coronal. **B.** Posterior Coronal. **C.** Sagittal. The greater omentum divides over the surface of the transverse colon and its mesocolon is suspended from the pancreas. To appreciate the head of the pancreas and its uncinate process wrapping around the SMA, a posterior view is added. **D.** Once the cancer traps the SMA the cancer is no longer resectable. Note the peritoneum separates the pancreas from the renal artery and vein, and the kidneys. **D.** Transverse. (1) Celiac trunk. (2) Accessory pancreatic duct. (3) Common bile duct. (4) Main pancreatic duct. (5) Head. (6) Uncinate process. (7) Splenic artery. (8) Body. (9) Tail. (10) Spleen. (11) Splenic vessels. (12) Superior mesenteric artery. (13) Portal vein. (14) Second part of duodenum. (15) Transverse mesocolon. (16) Aorta. (17) Omental bursa. (18) Pancreas. (19) Liver. (20) Stomach. (21) Pancreas. (22) Inferior vena cava. (23) Left kidney.

distinguish resectable (T1, T2, and T3) from unresectable (T4). The critical feature is reliance on contrast enhanced computed tomography (CT) to assess whether the adjacent arterial structures—namely, the SMA or celiac axes—are involved. Portal vein involvement can also occur. Endoscopic ultrasound (EUS) can be used for guiding needle biopsies. Laparoscopy is useful for detecting peritoneal seeding. Endoscopic retrograde cholangiopancreatography (ERCP) is useful to place shunts when obstructions of bile ducts are present. Surgical pathologic staging requires definition of margins (Table 29.3).

Pathologic Staging

The surgically resected esophagus and associated lymph nodes removed are assessed. Tumor extension and location of both primary and nodes should be documented.

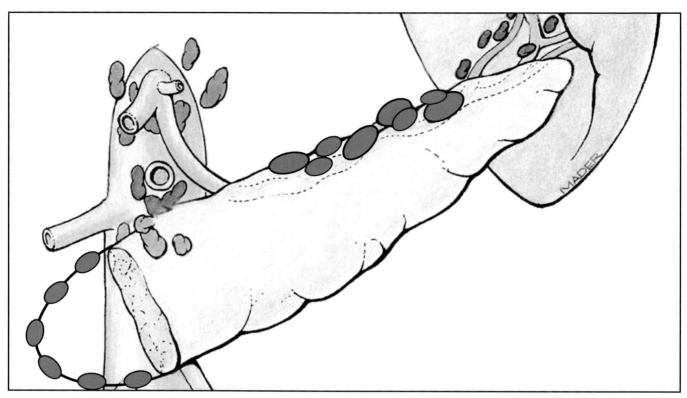

Figure 29.5 N-oncoanatomy. Sentinel nodes of the head of the pancreas and ampulla of Vater include the pancreatic duodenal nodes as shown in a circle on the right and those of the body and tail of the pancreas as shown on the left.

Both partial and complete resection of pancreas and regional nodes, as well as bile ducts and pancreatic ducts, need to be examined for margins and include the common bile duct, pancreatic neck, retroperitoneal margin, other soft tissue margins (such as posterior pancreatic), duodenum, and stomach. Special attention is required to the retroperitoneal margin adjacent to SMA. The uncinate process of head should be marked. Record the microscopic clearance of tumor in millimeters.

The surgically resected pancreas, ampulla of Vater, and associated lymph nodes removed are assessed. Tumor extension and location of both primary and nodes should be documented. Accurate radial margins should be marked and recorded and are defined "as the surgically dissected surface adjacent to the deepest point of tumor invasion." The completeness of resection depends on the clearing of the deepest point of invasion: R0, complete; R1, microscopic; and R2, macroscopic.

Oncoimaging Annotations
- *EUS*: When combined with needle biopsy, EUS is highly sensitive and specific.

TABLE 29.2	**Lymph Nodes of Pancreas**
Sentinel nodes include pancreatic duodenal and pancreatosplenic nodes	
Regional nodes	**Juxtaregional nodes**
Splenic hilum	Mediastinal
Suprapancreatic	Mesenteric
Left gastropancreatic fold	Iliac
Hepatic artery	
Inferior pancreatic	
Juxta-aortic	
Anterior pancreatic-duodenal	
Posterior pancreatic-duodenal	
Celiac	

TABLE 29.3	Imaging Modalities for Evaluating Carcinoma of the Pancreas and Ampulla of Vater	
Method	Diagnosis and Staging Capability	Recommended for Use
Abdominal ultrasound	Helpful in defining primary tumor and evaluating dilated bile ducts and ascites. Useful for evaluating suspected abdominal metastases, especially hepatic.	Yes
CT	Most useful of all imaging modalities in determining local invasion and distant metastases.	Yes
ERCP/PTC	Very accurate in defining deformity of bile and pancreatic duct and localizing site of obstruction.	No
MRI	Useful in jaundiced patient. Morphologic imaging of pancreas and peripancreatic duct for local and distant metastases.	No

CT, computed tomography; ERCP/PTC, endoscopic retrograde cholangiopancreatography/percutaneous transhepatic cholangiography; MRI, magnetic resonance imaging.

- *Multiplanar*: CT is highly effective in determining arterial and venous involvement and for staging.
- Magnetic resonance imaging (MRI) with gadolinium is excellent for defining extrapancreatic spread.
- ERCP in combination with other imaging approaches are very valuable.
- CT-guided biopsy is essential.
- Staging is excellent with either CT or MRI.

Cancer Statistics and Survival

The digestive system (gastrointestinal tract), which includes the MDG, accounts for 255,640 new patients annually with colon and rectum responsible for >50%, with 146 new diagnoses annually. Approximately half eventually die of these cancers. MDG cancers as a group are more lethal; only a handful of patients become long-term survivors. Fortunately, colon and rectal cancers are the most common, with the majority of patients be-

coming 5-year survivors (63%) responding to chemoradiation programs, often with the sparing of the rectal sphincter with conservative surgery. Anal cancers are the most responsive to chemoradiation (5-flourouracil and cisplatin), eliminating the need for surgery. The 5-year survival rate is >90% with anal sphincter preservation. This regimen has been proven to be very effective in clinical trials and to result in more long-term survivors, which is currently reflected in the literature. Liver, bile duct, and pancreatic cancers are among the poorest in the terms of survival, which is often measured in months rather than years (see Table 23.7).

Specifically, the pancreas accounted for 31,860 new cancer cases and 31,270 cancer deaths (98%), with a survival (5-year) rate improvement over the past 5 decades of 3.4%. Currently, relative 5-year survival for all stages is 4.4%, but when localized improves to 16.6% (see Table 23.8 and Fig. 28.6). The best positive results are limited to surgical resected T1 and T2 cancers of which 50% are alive at 1 year decreasing to 15–20% at 5 years.

30

Ampulla of Vater

Carcinomas of the *arrondissement* of the ampulla of Vater reflect its complex anatomy.

Perspective and Patterns of Spread

Cancers in the distal portion of the bile duct at its confluens with the pancreatic duct is uncommon. The reason for being aware of these periampullary cancers is they may offer a chance for survival, which is better than the more common cancer of its neighborhood, cancer of the pancreas. The onset is insidious and unexplained persistent itching; slight alterations in the color of stool and urine are the precursors to frank jaundice. Mirizzi syndrome, idiopathic focal stenosis, or sclerosing cholangitis, referred as the "malignant masquerade," is a hopeful entity in the differential diagnosis. Classically, Mirizzi syndrome is caused by a large gallstone impacted in the neck of the gallbladder causing biliary obstruction because of periductal inflammation.

Three distinct macroscopic subtypes occur: Sclerosing, nodular, and papillary. With the sclerosing variety, diffuse or annular thickening or stricturing of the bile duct occurs, often associated with inflammatory disease. Nodular cancers project into the lumen, and papillary cancers are soft and friable but with a better prognosis because transmural invasion is less often seen. These tumors are more often encountered in the ductal part of the bile duct. Adenocarcinomas are most frequent at the site and have been referred to as periampullary or peripapillary reflecting the normal anatomy (Fig. 30.1, Table 30.1).

TNM Staging Criteria

The accuracy in staging is most often apparent after resection and dissection of the specimen. T1 is limited to the ampulla of Vater or the sphincter of Oddi, T2 invades the duodenal wall, T3 the pancreas, and T4 invades more extensively in peripancreatic tissues and adjacent organs

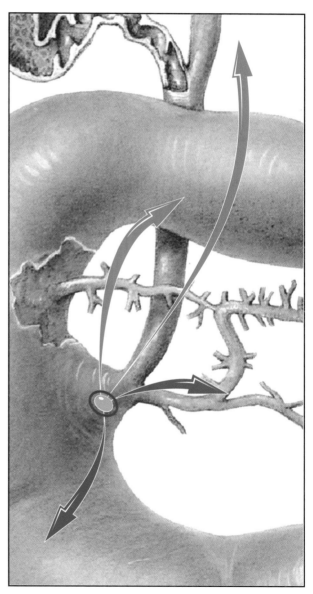

Figure 30.1 **Patterns of spread for the ampulla of Vater,** color coded for T stage: Tis, yellow; T1, green; T2, blue; ,T3 purple; T4, red.

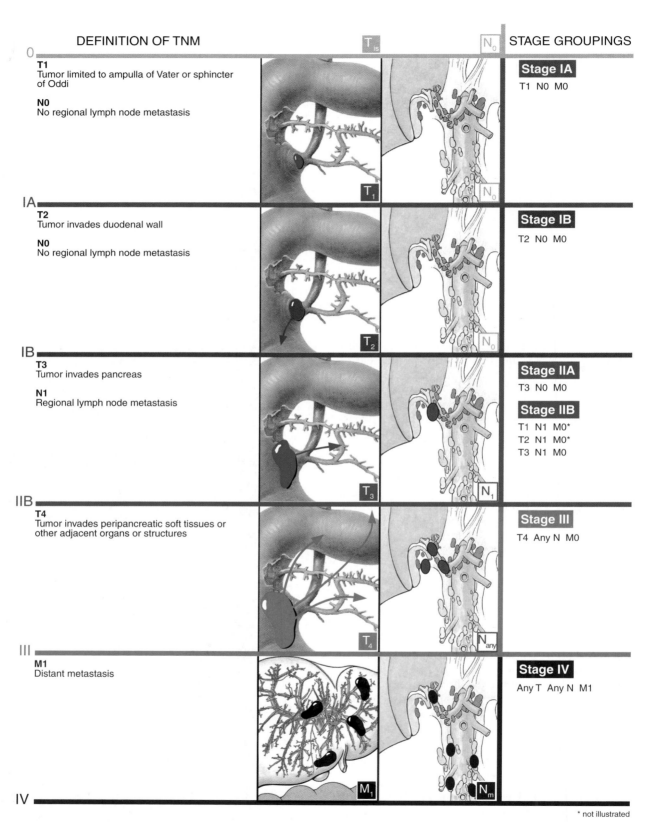

DEFINITION OF TNM

0

T1
Tumor limited to ampulla of Vater or sphincter of Oddi

N0
No regional lymph node metastasis

IA

T2
Tumor invades duodenal wall

N0
No regional lymph node metastasis

IB

T3
Tumor invades pancreas

N1
Regional lymph node metastasis

IIB

T4
Tumor invades peripancreatic soft tissues or other adjacent organs or structures

III

M1
Distant metastasis

IV

STAGE GROUPINGS

Stage IA
T1 N0 M0

Stage IB
T2 N0 M0

Stage IIA
T3 N0 M0

Stage IIB
T1 N1 M0*
T2 N1 M0*
T3 N1 M0

Stage III
T4 Any N M0

Stage IV
Any T Any N M1

* not illustrated

Figure 30.2 TNM staging diagram presents a vertical arrangement with color bars encompassing TN combinations showing progression. Ampulla of vater cancers masquerade as pancreatic head cancers and are resectable as Stage I and IIA with Stage IIB (purple) borderline resectable, Stage III (red) is often unresectable, Stage IV is metastatic (black). Stage 0, yellow; IA, green; IB, blue; IIB, purple; III, red; and IV (metastatic), black. Definitions of TN on left and stage grouping on right.

TABLE 30.1	Histopathologic Type: Common Cancers of the Ampulla of Vater	
Type		
Carcinoma in situ	Papillomatosis
Adenocarcinoma, NOS	Papillary carcinoma, non-invasive
Adenocarcinoma, intestinal type	Papillary carcinoma, invasive
Clear cell carcinoma	Carcinoma, NOS
Mucinous carcinoma	Other (specify)
Signet ring cell carcinoma	
Squamous cell carcinoma	
Adenosquamous carcinoma	
Small cell carcinoma	

Undifferentiated carcinoma
  Spindle and giant cell types
  Small cell types	

NOS, not otherwise specified.

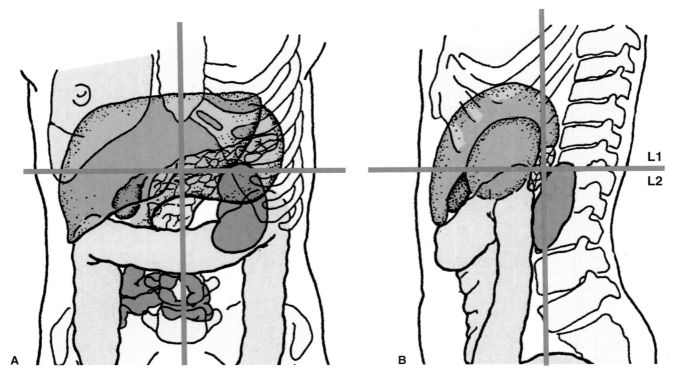

Figure 30.3 Orientation and overview of oncoanatomy. The anatomic isocenter for the three-planar oncoanatomy for the pancreas is at the L1/L2 level deep in the epigastrium. **A.** Coronal. **B.** Sagittal.

and structures as stomach, colon, and small intestines (Fig. 30.2).

The nodal designation is simply N1 and the sentinel nodes are the pancreaticoduodenal lymph nodes. The regional nodes are in the porta hepatis region surrounding the hepatic artery and portal vein and juxtaregional paracaval and para-aortic nodes.

Summary of Changes

The site was added in the fourth edition (1992) and has been reorganized in the sixth edition as follows.

*   *There is no longer a distinction between T3 and T4 on the basis of depth of pancreatic invasion.*
*   *The stage grouping has been revised.*
*   *Stage I has been replaced with stages IA and IB.*
*   *Stage II has been replaced with stages IIA and IIB.*
*   *Node-positive disease has been moved to stage IIB to retain consistency with the staging of tumors of the bile duct and of the pancreas.*

Orientation of Three-planar Oncoanatomy

The anatomic isocenter is at the L2 level surrounded by pancreas and duodenum. (A) The anterior bullet enters to right of the midline at the subcostal plane and

(B) the lateral bullet enters at the midcoronal plane anterior to the bodies of the upper lumbar vertebrae (Fig. 30.3).

T-oncoanatomy

The variation in the pancreatic duct and bile duct fusion are understandable if one reviews the developmental stages of this region (Fig. 30.4).

*   *Coronal:* The gallbladder, bile duct, and ventral pancreas bud rotate when the duodenum rotates clockwise on its long axis during embryonic development. The fusion of the ventral and dorsal pancreatic buds results in numerous possible unions of the bile duct and pancreatic duct as it forms the ampulla of Vater.
*   *Transverse:* The clockwise rotation is best appreciated in this view as the ventral pancreatic bud, which becomes the uncinate process and the dorsal pancreatic bud forms the head, body, and tail of the pancreas.
*   *Sagittal:* A variety of ampulla of Vater formations are shown emphasizing the different fusions of the common bile duct and the main and accessory pancreatic ducts.

N-oncoanatomy

The lymphatics are particularly rich with numerous nodes surrounding the head of the pancreas. These

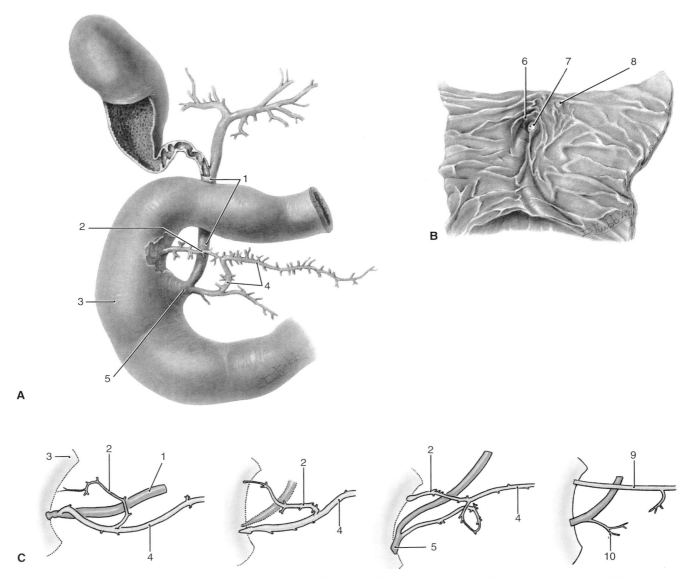

Figure 30.4 **T-oncoanatomy.** Three-planar views. **A.** Coronal. **B.** Sagittal. The greater omentum divides over the surface of the transverse colon and its mesocolon is suspended from the pancreas. **C.** Variations in duct anatomy. To appreciate the head of the pancreas and its uncinate process wrapping around the superior mesenteric artery (SMA), a posterior view is substituted for the axial view. Once the cancer traps the SMA, the cancer is no longer resectable. Note the peritoneum separates the pancreas from the renal artery, vein, and kidneys. (1) Common bile duct. (2) Accessory pancreatic duct. (3) Second part of duodenum. (4) Main pancreatic duct. (5) Hepatopancreatic ampulla of Vater. (6) Hood. (7) Major duodenal papilla. (8) Minor duodenal papilla. (9) Primitive dorsal duct. (10) Primitive ventral duct.

include the pancreaticoduodenal nodal arcade and superior mesenteric nodes and porta hepatis nodes (Fig. 30.5; see Table 29.2).

M-oncoanatomy

The pancreaticoduodenal veins drain into the superior mesenteric vein, then the portal vein so that the liver is the target metastatic organ (see Fig. 25.6).

Rules of Classification and Staging

Clinical Staging and Imaging

The inability to evaluate the gallbladder, its ducts, and the ampulla of Vater has led the American Joint Committee on Cancer to simplify the staging so that both clinical and surgical criteria are the same. Imaging procedures include abdominal ultrasound, which is surpassed by computed tomography (CT) in defining biliary

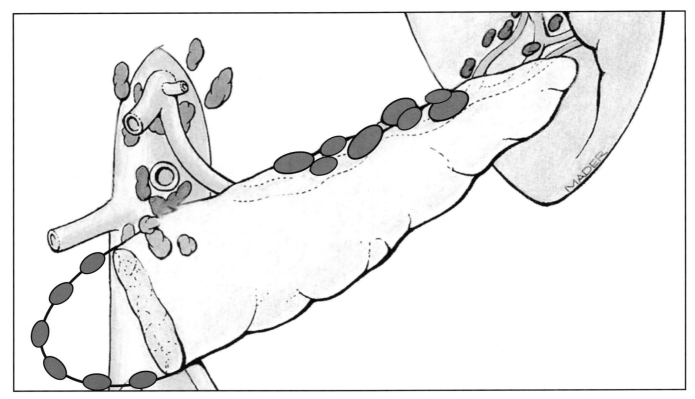

Figure 30.5 **N-oncoanatomy.** Sentinel nodes of the ampulla of Vater include the pancreatic duodenal nodes as shown in a circle on the right.

obstruction. Endoscopic retrograde cholangiopancreatography (ERCP) and percutaneous transhepatic cholangiography define biliary tree anatomy. Magnetic resonance imaging with gadolinium is also useful (see Table 29.3).

Pathologic Staging

The surgically resected gallbladder and/or bile ducts with associated lymph nodes removed are assessed. Tumor extension and location of both primary and nodes should be documented. Accurate radial margins should be marked and recorded and are defined "as the surgically dissected surface adjacent to the deepest point of tumor invasion beyond the wall of the large bowel." The completeness of resection depends on the clearing of the deepest point of invasion: R0, complete; R1, microscopic; and R2, macroscopic.

Oncoimaging Annotations

- Ultrasound initially reveals a dilated extrahepatic duct and intrahepatic duct system.
- Helical CT with five multiplanar 1- to 2-mm cuts most shows the mass.
- ERCP is an optional procedure that may show the common bile duct cancer without involvement of

the pancreatic duct, but surgical evaluation followed by resection and microscopy are critical to both diagnosis and staging.

- When direct cholangiograms are needed, a percutaneous transhepatic cholangiogram identifies the common bile duct cancer site and is preferred over ERCP.

Cancer Statistics and Survival

The digestive system, or gastrointestinal tract, which includes major digestive glands (MDG), accounts for 255,640 new patients annually with colon and rectum responsible for >50% with 146 new diagnoses annually. Approximately half eventually die of these cancers. MDG cancers as a group are more lethal, with only a handful of patients becoming long-term survivors. Fortunately, colon and rectal cancers are the most common, with the majority of patients becoming 5-year survivors (63%) responding to chemoradiation programs often with the sparing of the rectal sphincter with conservative surgery. Anal cancers are the most responsive to chemoradiation (5-flourouracil and cisplatin), eliminating the need for surgery. The 5-year survival is >90% with anal sphincter preservation. This regimen has been proven to be very effective in clinical trials and to result in more long-term survivors, which is currently reflected in the literature. Liver, bile duct, and pancreatic cancers are among the poorest in the terms of survival, which is often measured in months rather than years.

Specifically, the cancer survival curves depend on the site of origin of cancers in the neighborhood of peri-ampullary malignancies. Islet cell cancers are the most benign and assure long-term survival. Duodenal adeno-carcinomas yield 50% long-term survival, whereas am-pullary cancers tend to range between 30% and 45%.

Distal bile duct cancers tend to be in the 20% to 30% range, whereas cancers of bile duct confluens tend to be poorer at 10% to 20%. Pancreatic cancers are the poorest in overall survival, most often with few survivors at 5 years, most often <5% (see Fig. 28.6). Note that the survival for Ampulla of vater cancers are indeterminate in prognosis with approximately 50% 5-year survival but superior to extrahepatic bile ducts (25% 5-year survival) and pancreas cancers poorest (< 10% 5-year survival).

31

Colon

There have been intensive studies of adenomas as to genetic defects that lead to their transformation from benign polyps to dysplasia and neoplasia.

Perspective and Pattern of Spread

The colon, including the rectum, accounts for the majority of digestive system cancers. There have been intensive studies of adenomas as to genetic defects that lead to their transformation from benign polyps to dysplasia and neoplasia. Portions of chromosomes 5, 17, and 18 are mutated or deleted. The gene deletion associated with the multistep process leading to malignancy and metastases has been documented by Fearon and Vogelstein. *Large intestine has no villi and the feathered mucosa is characterized by haustral markings. Except for the absence of paneth cells the cellular makeup of the crypts of Lieberkuhn are similar. The number of goblet cells increases from cecum to sigmoid colon.* The major colon function is to absorb water and electrolytes; it also compacts feces. The array of histopathology is largely similar to intestinal tumors, but the staging system applies only to carcinomas, not lymphomas, sarcomas, or carcinoids (Table 31.1).

TNM Staging Criteria

The patterns of cancer spread are predetermined by the mucosal and muscle layers until it penetrates the serosa and invades adjacent structures. Because the posterior wall is often without serosa, direct infiltration of abdominal wall is possible (Fig. 31.1). Polyps are mucosal tumors that are either pedunculated on stalks or sessile with a broad base. Adenomatous polyps are more likely to progress than hyperplastic polyps. Risk factors are size >2 cm, sessile, and villous features with evidence of dysplasia. Colon cancers invade their wall and the staging system (Fig. 31.2) reflects the cancer penetration in depth: T1, mucosal; T2, muscular; and T3, serosal. T4 is transmural into adjacent structures and surrounding organs. *As cancers encircle the bowel wall, it is important to recognize the absence of peritoneal lining and mesentery in the ascending and descending colons on their posterior surfaces.* Such anatomic features reduce the size of margins of resection as compared to mobile mesenteric portions, that is, the transverse and sigmoid segments.

Generally, there is no overarching principle or context design for the digestive system (gastrointestinal tract) or major digestive glands (MDG). Stages are frequently expanded to six by subdividing stages into A and B. The T and N categories are assigned to a stage grouping, specifically for division of a stage into more (A) versus less (B) favorable groupings. This occurs at different stages for different sites.

Specifically, this site has a clear separation of T progression I/II from N progression III/IV. Stages IIIA and B node progression and stage IIIC for venous invasion (V1) and IV for metastatic. Because this site is the dominant cancer, this staging system impacts other gastrointestinal sites and MDG sites.

Summary of Changes

Changes in the sixth edition are moderate:

- *A revised description of the anatomy of the colon and rectum better delineates the data concerning the boundaries between colon, rectum, and anal canal. Adenocarcinomas of the vermiform appendix are classified according to the TNM staging system, but should be recorded separately, whereas cancers that occur in the anal canal are staged according to the classification used for the anus.*

- *Smooth metastatic nodules in the pericolic or perirectal fat are considered lymph node metastases and are counted in N staging. In contrast, irregularly contoured metastatic nodules in the peritumoral fat are considered vascular invasion and are coded as an extension of the T category as either a V1 (microscopic vascular invasion) if only microscopically visible or a V2 (macroscopic vascular invasion) if grossly visible.*

- *Stage group II is subdivided into IIA and IIB on the basis of whether the primary tumor is T3 or T4, respectively.*

- *Stage group III is subdivided into IIIA (T1–T2 N1 M0), IIIB (T3–T4 N1 M0), or IIIC (any T N2 M0).*

Orientation of Three-planar Oncoanatomy

The three-planar anatomic isocenter for the colon occupies the L2/L3 level in the abdomen (Fig. 31.3).

T-oncoanatomy

- *Coronal*: The colon is a large structure that picture frames the entire abdominal visceral contents. It

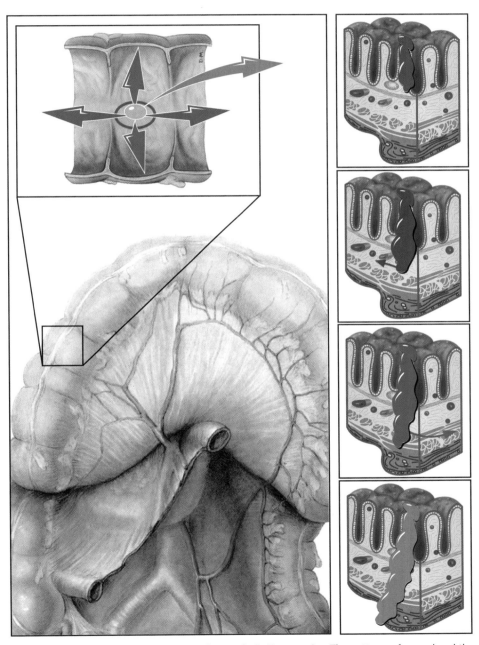

Figure 31.1 **A. Colon cancer patterns of spread. B.** T categories. The patterns of spread and the primary tumor classification are similarly color coded: Tis (cancer in situ of mucosa), yellow; (infiltrates the submucosa), green; T2 (penetrates the muscularis externa), blue; T3 (reaches the subserosa), purple; and T4 (invades through the serosa into a neighboring viscera), red.

DEFINITION OF TNM

STAGE GROUPINGS

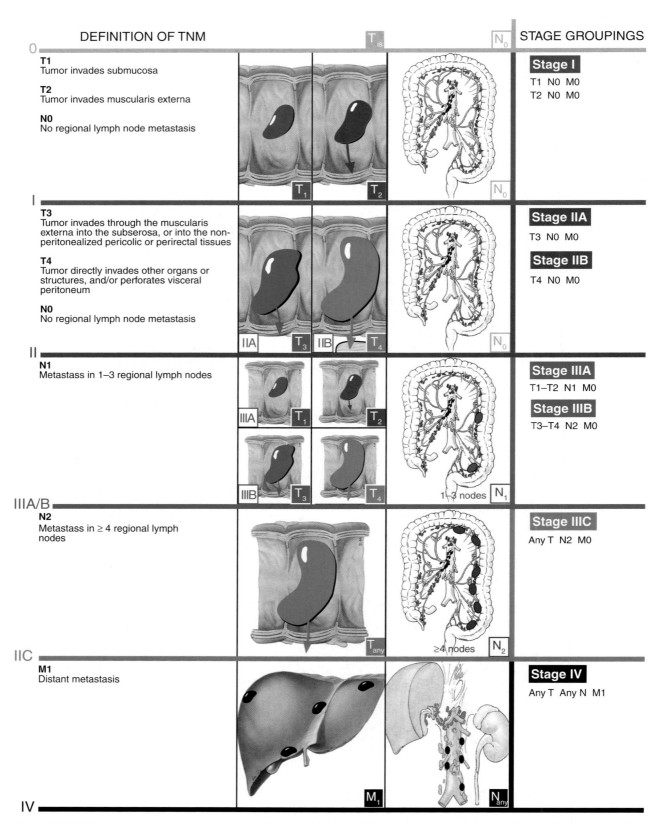

T1
Tumor invades submucosa

T2
Tumor invades muscularis externa

N0
No regional lymph node metastasis

Stage I
T1 N0 M0
T2 N0 M0

T3
Tumor invades through the muscularis externa into the subserosa, or into the non-peritonealized pericolic or perirectal tissues

T4
Tumor directly invades other organs or structures, and/or perforates visceral peritoneum

N0
No regional lymph node metastasis

Stage IIA
T3 N0 M0

Stage IIB
T4 N0 M0

N1
Metastass in 1–3 regional lymph nodes

Stage IIIA
T1–T2 N1 M0

Stage IIIB
T3–T4 N2 M0

N2
Metastass in ≥ 4 regional lymph nodes

Stage IIIC
Any T N2 M0

M1
Distant metastasis

Stage IV
Any T Any N M1

Figure 31.2 TNM staging diagram presents a vertical arrangement with color bars encompassing TN combinations showing progression. Colon cancers are resectable. Stage IIIA/B (purple) N1 and become more advanced with nodal progression N2 and Stage III (red) less resectable and Stage IV (black) metastatic. Stage 0, yellow; I, green; II, blue; III, purple; IV, red; and IV (metastatic), black. Definitions of TN on left and stage grouping on right.

TABLE 31.1	Histopathologic Type: Common Cancers of the Colon
Type	
Adenocarcinoma in situ	Squamous cell (epidermoid) carcinoma
Adenocarcinoma	Adenosquamous carcinoma
Medullary carcinoma	Small cell carcinoma
Mucinous carcinoma (colloid type; >50% mucinous carcinoma)	Undifferentiated carcinoma
Signet ring cell carcinoma (>50% signet ring cell)	Carcinoma, NOS

NOS, not otherwise specified.
From Greene FL, Page DL, Fleming ID, et al. eds. *AJCC Cancer Staging Manual.* 6th ed. New York: Springer; 2002. Used with the permission of the American Joint Committee on Cancer (AJCC), Chicago, Illinois.

begins at the cecum and continues as the right ascending, transverse, left descending, and sigmoid segments of the colon. The colon is partially covered by a peritoneal surface. Tumors follow the pattern of arising on their mucosal surface penetrating into the muscularis and into the serosa; therefore, their manifestations relate to their location. *Depending on where the cancer arises, it can invade into the surrounding structures such as the liver at the hepatic flexure, which is at the junction of the ascending and transverse colon.* The stomach and spleen are at risk when the cancer arises at the splenic flexure or the junction of the transverse and descending colon. The large intestine, or colon, extends from the terminal ileum to the anal canal. *It may be subdivided into five sections, exclusive of the rectum: Right, middle, and left or ascending, transverse, descending and sigmoid portions, respectively. The large intestine may also be divided into the intraperitoneal colon and the rectum (Fig. 31.4).*

- *Sagittal*: The peritoneal cavity consists of the greater sac and omental bursa. The superior recess of the omental bursa is between the liver and the posterior attachment of the diaphragm. The inferior recess of the omental bursa is between the two double layers of the greater omentum. *In the adult, the inferior recess usually only extends inferiorly as far as the transverse colon because of fusion of the two double peritoneal layers at birth.*
- *Transverse*: The transverse colon is located anteriorly, with the ascending colon on right and descending colon on left. Note this is at the lower pole of the kidney.

N-oncoanatomy

Regional nodes follow the vascular arcades for each colon segment along its marginal arteries on the mesocolic border. Specifically, the regional lymph nodes for each segment are shown and listed. The recent major revisions in staging relate to nodules in the pericolic fat: If such nodules are smooth they are considered to be nodes, if irregular they are considered to be vascular or venous invasion (Fig. 31.5, Table 31.2).

M-oncoanatomy

The entire portal circulation should be considered as a unit with regard to the venous anatomy of the gastrointestinal tract below the diaphragm (see Fig. 25.6). The two major trunks are the inferior mesenteric and superior mesenteric veins. The inferior mesenteric vein drains the left colon and sigmoid colon tributaries, which covers the vascular drainage to the left of the midline originating from the superior rectal veins. On the right side, the superior mesenteric vein originates from the tributaries draining the ileum, jejunum, and ileocolic right and middle colic veins. *The inferior mesenteric vein usually joins the splenic vein, which coalesces with the superior mesenteric vein and forms the portal vein.* The splenic vein, which is a major tributary of the portal system, also drains much of the stomach along its greater curvature and includes the short gastric veins and left and right gastric epiploic veins. The right gastroepiploic vein also flows into the superior mesenteric vein. The entire drainage of the lesser curvature of the stomach, including the left and right gastric veins, drains directly into the portal vein. Because the portal vein then drains directly into the liver, it is the target metastatic organ and the most commonly involved organ in hematogenous spread pattern from the venous system of the gastrointestinal tract as compared with other parts of the body where the drainage is directly into the lung by way of the caval system.

The incidence of liver metastases exceeds other sites. According to a variety of reports in the literature the range is 40% to 100% at autopsy. Other sites are mainly bone metastases 20% to 35% and lung metastases 40% to 60%, with only occasional metastases to brain.

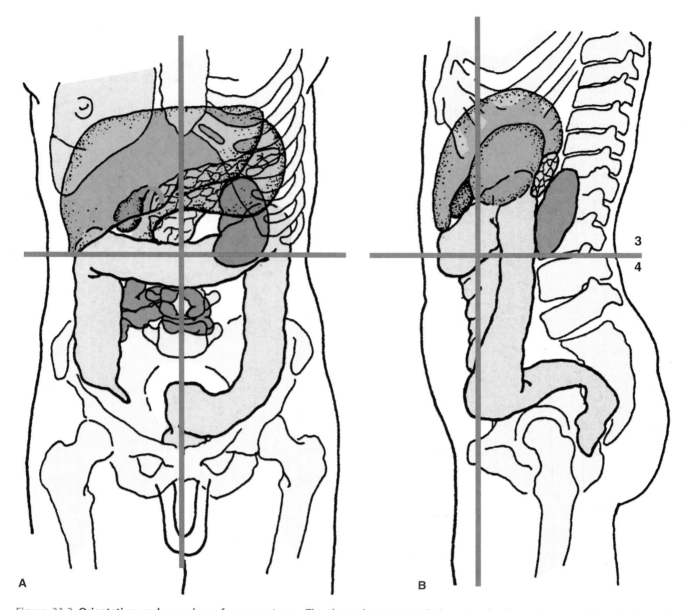

Figure 31.3 Orientation and overview of oncoanatomy. The three-planar anatomic isocenter for the colon is at L3/L4. **A.** Coronal. **B.** Sagittal.

Rules of Classification and Staging

Clinical Staging and Imaging

Extension of diagnostic imaging to staging is gaining in popularity. Virtual colonoscopy and sigmoidoscopy are challenging endoscopic colonoscopy as to accuracy in diagnosing adenocarcinomas. Endoscopic ultrasound shows the layers of the colon and rectal wall and their penetration by cancer. Endorectal magnetic resonance imaging (MRI) is most valuable to demonstrate extracolonic and extrarectal invasion into adjacent struc-

tures. Computed tomography (CT) is preferred to detecting liver and lung metastases (Table 31.3).

Pathologic Staging

The surgically resected colon and associated lymph nodes are assessed. Tumor extension and location of both primary and nodes should be documented. Accurate radial margins should be marked and recorded and are defined "as the surgically dissected surface adjacent to the deepest point of tumor invasion beyond the wall of the large bowel." The completeness of resection

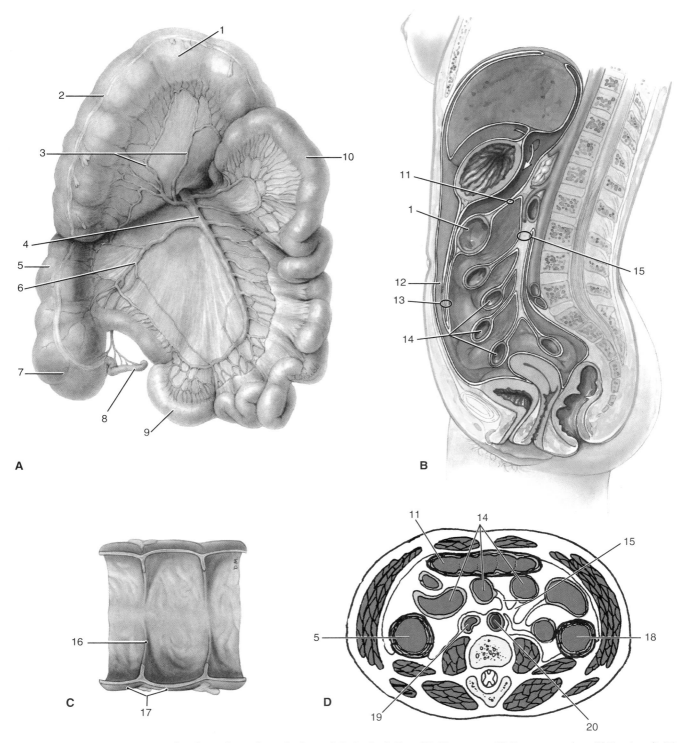

Figure 31.4 T-oncoanatomy. Colon three-planar views. **A.** Coronal. **B.** Sagittal. **C and D.** Transverse. (1) Transverse colon. (2) Taenia coli. (3) Middle colic artery. (4) Superior mesenteric artery. (5) Ascending colon. (6) Ileocolic artery. (7) Cecum. (8) Appendix. (9) Ileum. (10) Jejunum. (11) Transverse mesocolon. (12) Greater sac. (13) Greater omentum. (14) Loops of small intestine. (15) Mesentery of small intestine. (16) Semilunar fold. (17) Haustra. (18) Descending colon. (19) Inferior vena cava. (20) Abdominal aorta.

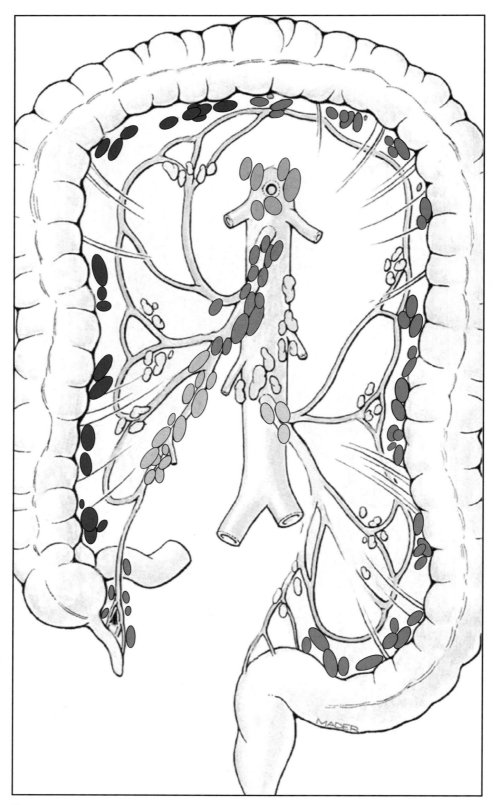

Figure 31.5 N-oncoanatomy. Sentinel nodes of the colon include the pericolic nodes of the superior mesenteric (blue) and inferior mesenteric (red) nodes. Depending upon the T site colon segment of origin, the pericolic nodes adjacent are the sentinel nodes (Table 31.2). Paraortic nodes are gray.

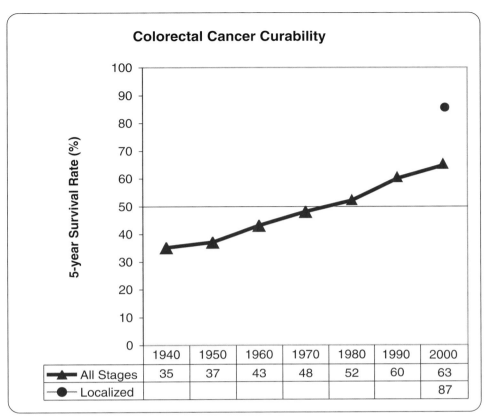

Figure 31.6 Cancer statistics and survival rates.

TABLE 31.2	Lymph Nodes of Colon

Sentinel nodes include pericolic nodes

Segment	Regional Nodes
Cecum	Pericolic anterior cecal, posterior cecal, ileocolic, right colic
Ascending colon	Pericolic, ileocolic, right colic, middle colic
Hepatic flexure	Pericolic, middle colic, right colic
Transverse colon	Pericolic, middle colic
Splenic flexure	Pericolic, middle colic, left colic, inferior mesenteric
Descending colon	Pericolic, left colic, inferior mesenteric sigmoid
Sigmoid colon	Pericolic, inferior mesenteric, superior rectal (hemorrhoidal), sigmoidal, sigmoid mesenteric
Rectosigmoid	Pericolic, perirectal, left colic, sigmoid mesenteric, sigmoidal, inferior mesenteric, superior rectal (hemorrhoidal), middle rectal (hemorrhoidal)

Juxtaregional nodes
 Para-aortic
 Portal
 Rectal

TABLE 31.3	Imaging Modalities for Staging for Colon Cancer	
Method	Diagnosis and Staging Capability	Recommended for Use
Primary tumor ± regional nodes		
BE	Very useful in detecting and defining primary lesions in the colon. Single-contrast study may be less sensitive than double-contrast in detecting polyps.	Yes
Endoscopy	Very accurate modality for detecting and defining primary lesions	Yes, if used to confirm lesion detected on BE or to screen high-risk patients
Endorectal ultrasound or coil	In rectum, sigmoid (flex sigmoidoscopy), or remaining colon (colonoscopy).	Yes, if preoperative chemoRT is considered.
MRI	Useful in defining depth of penetration of the primary lesion.	Yes
CT	Most valuable of all modalities for determining extrarectal or extracolonic local invasion and nodal metastases	Yes
PET	Not useful for staging primary cancer. Useful for suspected metastasis.	No
Metastases		
Chest film ± CT	Chest film—best for metastasis screening; CT chest—rules out multiple metastases.	Yes
CT abdomen	Most useful study to define para-aortic node enlargement or liver metastases.	Yes
Liver ultrasound	Can differentiate between cystic and solid lesions.	Yes

BE, barium enema; CT, computed tomography; chemoRT, chemoradiation; MRI, magnetic resonance imaging.

depends on the clearing of the deepest point of invasion: R0, complete; R1, microscopic; and R2, macroscopic.

Oncoimaging Annotations

- Although colonoscopy is more accurate in assessment for small polyps, overall cost effectiveness is greater when double-contrast barium enema examinations are used.
- CT colonography is a recent addition to the modalities used to screen for colorectal cancer and polyps. This modality requires further refinement and testing before being more widely adopted.
- Transrectal ultrasonography and MRI are able to demonstrate the extent of tumor through the rectal wall and provide some assessment for lymphadenopathy.
- If there is clinical suspicion of metastasis or elevated carcinoembryonic antigen level, CT and MR scanning are useful for determining the presence and site of recurrent disease. Overall accuracy for the detection of recurrent disease with these modalities is 90% to 95%. This evaluation may require fine-needle aspiration biopsy under direct CT guidance.
- Other noninvasive means to determine the presence or absence of recurrent or metastatic tumor are nuclear medicine scanning techniques with radiolabeled monoclonal antibodies and positron emission tomography techniques using fluorodeoxyglucose. Some of these have shown great potential.

Cancer Statistics and Survival

The digestive system, or gastrointestinal tract, which includes the MDG, accounts for 255,640 new patients annually with colon and rectum responsible for >50%, with 146 new diagnoses annually. Approximately half eventually die of these cancers. MDG cancers as a group are more lethal; only a handful of patients become long-term survivors. Fortunately, colon and rectal cancers are the most common, with the majority of patients becoming 5-year survivors (63%) responding to chemoradiation programs often with the sparing of the rectal sphincter with conservative surgery (Fig. 31.6). Anal cancers are the most responsive to chemoradiation (5-fluorouracil and cisplatin) eliminating the need for surgery. The 5-year rate survival is >90% with anal sphincter preservation. This regimen has been proven to be very effective in clinical trials and to result in more long-term survivors, which is currently reflected in the literature. Liver, bile duct, and pancreatic cancers are among the poorest in the terms of survival, which is often measured in months rather than years (see Table 23.7).

Specifically, the colon accounted for 106,370 new cancer cases and 56,730 cancer deaths (53%) with a 5-year survival rate improvement over the last 5 decades of 22%. Currently, relative 5-year survival for all stages is 62.3% but when localized improves to 90.1% (see Table 23.8). Colon cancer (T3T4) when resected plus multi-nodal therapy decreases from 70–80% for N0 to 50% ± 3% for N1, N2 nodal involvement.

32

Small Intestine

Adenocarcinomas are more common in the duodenum, lymphomas in the jejunum, and sarcomas and carcinoids in the ileum, with its most favored site being the vermiform appendix.

Perspective and Pattern of Spread

Consider the contradictory paucity of neoplasms in the small intestine in view of the extreme length of the small bowel, which exceeds in its length all other regions of the digestive system combined. It has a rich variety of metabolically active cells with high and rapid turnover rates of its regenerative cells. *Their stem cells are estimated to have cell turnover times of 24 hours and have cell travel times of 5 to 7 days to rise from the crypt of Lieberkuhn to the tip of villus.* The absence of malignancy is attributed to rapid transport of carcinogens in luminal contents, abundant surface immunoglobulin A expression and active enzymes. The annual rate of new cases is barely at 4,500 new cases, with a high survival rate. *The surface columnar epithelial cells have brush borders for absorption of fluids and chyme with numerous lymphoid cells, neuroendocrine cells, goblet cells, and paneth cells with loose connective tissue filling the microvilli with its lacteal.* What the small intestine lacks in numbers of cancers, it makes up for by their variety. Table 32.1 lists them succinctly and one notes a predilection for specific tumors in different bowel segments: *Adenocarcinomas are more common in the duodenum, lymphomas in the jejunum and sarcomas, and carcinoids in the ileum with its most favored site being the vermiform appendix (T1 histopathology versus distribution).* Predisposing factors include celiac disease, Crohn disease, familial adenomatosis polyposis, Gardner syndrome, and Peutz–Jaeger syndromes, all beginning with hyperplasia, then dysplasia, and finally neoplasia. The patterns of cancer spread follow the mucosal and muscle layers of the bowel wall (Fig. 32.1).

TNM Staging Criteria

There has been no change or revision with depth of wall penetration determining the stage: T1, mucosal; T2, muscularis; T3, serosa; and T4 other viscera (Fig. 32.2).

Generally, there is no overarching principle or context design for the digestive system (gastrointestinal tract) or major digestive glands (MDG). Stages are frequently expanded to six by subdividing stages into A and B. The T and N categories are assigned to a stage grouping, specifically for division of a stage into more (a) versus less (b) favorable groupings. This occurs at different stages for different sites.

Specifically, this site is staged in the same fashion as colorectal cancers. Stages I and II are due to T progression, whereas stages III and IV are related solely to N progression: >T4 = N1.

Summary of Changes

There are no changes in the sixth edition of the AJCC CSM.

Orientation of Three-planar Oncoanatomy

The anatomic isocenter for the small intestine is at L3 to L5 (Fig. 32.3).

T-oncoanatomy

The small intestine extends from the pylorus of the stomach to the ileocecal valve. *It is approximately 25 feet long and divided into three sections: the duodenum, jejunum, and ileum.* The duodenum is essentially a midline structure, approximately 1 foot long. It provides some of the most complex anatomy in the upper abdomen as it bends at two right angles and loops around the pancreas, accepting the insertion of pancreatic main duct into its second portion via the ampulla of Vater. The visceral relationships of the stomach, duodenum, pancreas, and liver are in multiple layers, separated by the omental bursa, lesser omentum, and greater omentum (Fig. 32.4).

- *Coronal*: The jejunum starts in the left side of the abdomen as the duodenal loop terminates posteriorly and to the left side of the superior mesenteric artery and vein. It occupies the left upper quadrant of the abdomen mainly leading into the ileum, which, in turn, terminates in the cecum and occupies most of the right lower quadrant. *The internal mucosal markings are like bowel fingerprints and when seen on film vary from the duodenum, which is relatively smooth to the jejunum with multiple circular folds that are narrow, feathery, and thin; they gradually thicken and separate in the ileum (Fig. 32.4A, B).* The small intestine is mainly concerned with

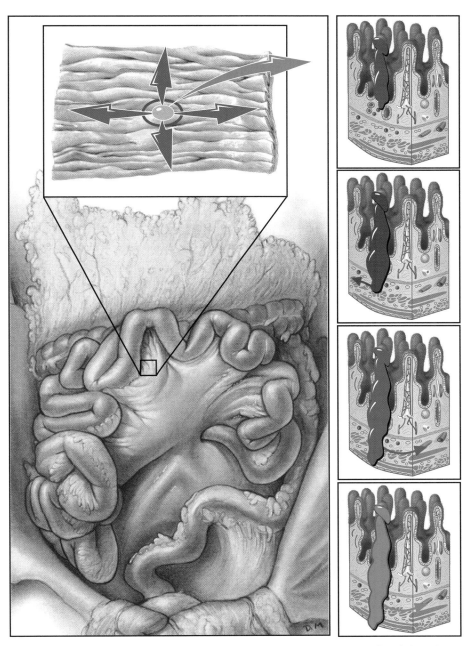

Figure 32.1 **A. Patterns of spread. B.** T categories. The patterns of spread and the primary tumor classification are similarly color coded: Tis (cancer in situ of mucosa), yellow; T1, (infiltrates the submucosa), green; T2, (penetrates the muscularis externa), blue; T3 (reaches the subserosa), green; and T4 (invades through the serosa into a neighboring viscera), red.

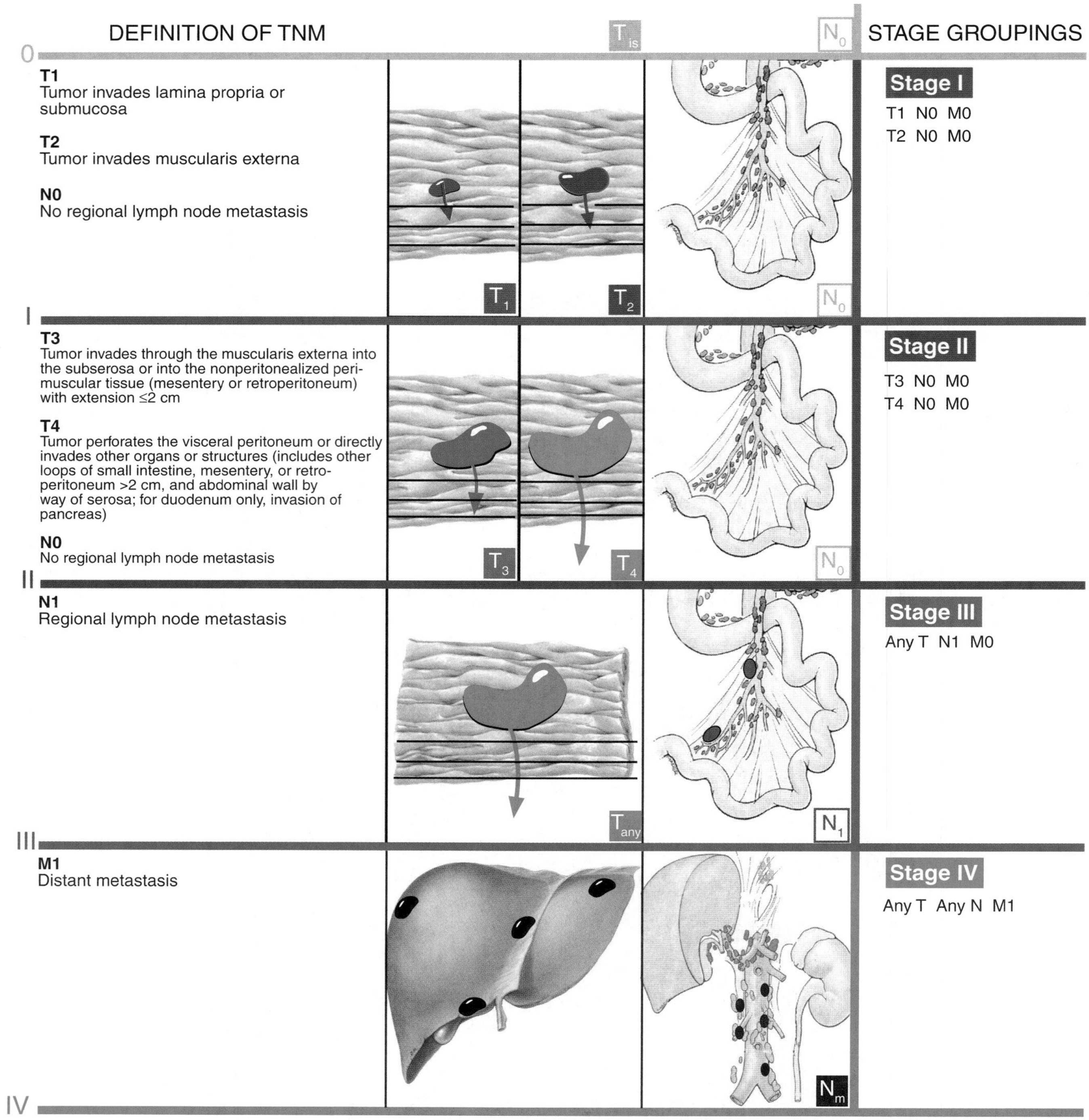

DEFINITION OF TNM

STAGE GROUPINGS

T1
Tumor invades lamina propria or submucosa

T2
Tumor invades muscularis externa

N0
No regional lymph node metastasis

Stage I

T1 N0 M0
T2 N0 M0

T3
Tumor invades through the muscularis externa into the subserosa or into the nonperitonealized perimuscular tissue (mesentery or retroperitoneum) with extension ≤2 cm

T4
Tumor perforates the visceral peritoneum or directly invades other organs or structures (includes other loops of small intestine, mesentery, or retroperitoneum >2 cm, and abdominal wall by way of serosa; for duodenum only, invasion of pancreas)

N0
No regional lymph node metastasis

Stage II

T3 N0 M0
T4 N0 M0

N1
Regional lymph node metastasis

Stage III

Any T N1 M0

M1
Distant metastasis

Stage IV

Any T Any N M1

Figure 32.2 **TNM staging diagram presents a vertical arrangement with color bars encompassing TN combinations showing progression.** Small intestine cancers are both uncommon and unique. They are simply staged I to IV without substages, an exception for the digestive system. Stage 0, yellow; I, green; II, blue; III, purple; IV, red; and IV (metastatic), black. Definitions of TN on left and stage grouping on right.

Type of Neoplasm	Duodenum	Jejunum	Ileum	Total
Adenocarcinoma	427 (40%)	408 (38%)	241 (22%)	1076 (46%)
Sarcoma	46 (10%)	162 (36%)	239 (54%)	447 (19%)
Lymphoma	4 (16%)	9 (36%)	12 (48%)	25 (1%)
Carcinoid	48 (6%)	78 (10%)	682 (84%)	808 (34%)
Total	525 (22%)	660 (28%)	1171 (50%)	2356 (100%)

TABLE 32.1 Distribution of Malignant Neoplasms in the Small Intestine

Number and Percentage by Region

From Sindelar WF: Cancer of the small intestine. In: De Vita VT Jr, Hellman S. Rosenberg SA eds. *Cancer, Principles and Practice of Oncology*, 3rd ed, 875–894. Philadelphia: JB Lippincott Co.; 1989, with permission.

fine absorption of the variety of products of digestion, the large intestine with fluid reabsorption.

- A. *Proximal jejunum.* The circular folds (plicae circulares) are tall, closely packed, and commonly branched. B. *Proximal ileum.* The circular folds are low and becoming sparse. The caliber of the gut is reduced, and the wall is thinner. C. *Distal ileum.* Circular folds are absent, and solitary lymph nodules stud the wall. D. *Intestines in situ,* greater omentum reflected. The ileum is reflected to expose the appendix in the lower right quadrant. The appendix usually lies posterior to the cecum (retrocecal) or, as in the case, projects over the pelvic brim. Note the extensive coiling of the jejunum and ileum of the small intestine (together approximately 6 meters long). Also observe the distinguishing features of the large intestine: Its position around the small intestine; the teniae coli or longitudinal muscle bands; the sacculations or haustra; and fatty omental appendices.

- *Sagittal*: The peritoneal cavity consists of the greater sac and omental bursa. The superior recess of the omental bursa is between the liver and the posterior attachment of the diaphragm. The inferior recess of the omental bursa is between the two double layers of the greater omentum. In adults, the inferior recess usually only extends inferiorly as far as the transverse colon because of fusion of the two double peritoneal layers at birth.

- *Transverse*: The small intestine loops fills most of the abdomen. The inferior vena caval and aorta are located anterior to the vertebral column.

N-oncoanatomy

Despite a large variety and number of regional lymph nodes following the superior mesenteric artery and vein,

the lymph node classification is simply N1, positive regional node, without qualification as to number or size of lymph nodes (Fig. 32.5; Table 32.2).

M-oncoanatomy

The entire portal circulation should be considered as a unit in regard to the venous anatomy of the gastrointestinal tract below the diaphragm (see Fig. 25.6). The two major trunks are the inferior and superior mesenteric veins. The inferior mesenteric vein drains the left colon and sigmoid colon tributaries, which covers the vascular drainage to the left of the midline originating from the superior rectal veins. On the right side, the superior mesenteric vein originates from the tributaries draining the ileum, jejunum, and the ileocolic and right and middle colic veins. *The inferior mesenteric vein usually joins the splenic vein, which coalesces with the superior mesenteric vein and forms the portal vein.* The splenic vein, which is a major tributary of the portal system, also drains much of the stomach along its greater curvature and includes the short gastric veins and left and right gastroepiploic veins. The right gastroepiploic also flows into the superior mesenteric vein. The entire drainage of the lesser curvature of the stomach including the left and right gastric veins drains directly into the portal vein. Because the portal vein then drains directly into the liver, it is the target metastatic organ and the most commonly involved organ in hematogenous spread pattern from the venous system of the gastrointestinal tract as compared with other parts of the body, where the drainage is directly into the lung by way of the caval system.

Venous drainage is by way of the tributaries of the superior mesenteric vein and fusion with the splenic vein to give rise to the portal vein. Liver metastases are the most common site.

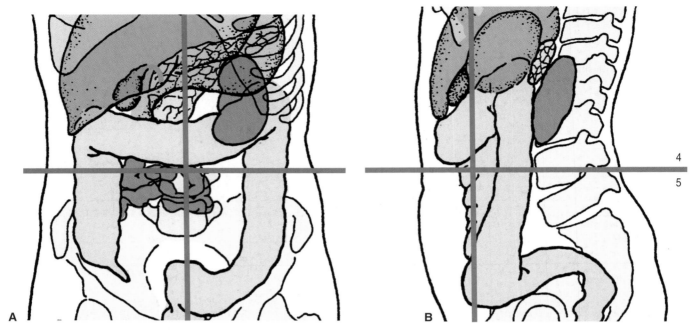

Figure 32.3 Orientation and overview of oncoanatomy. The anatomic isocenter for the small intestine is at L3 to L5. **A.** Coronal. **B.** Sagittal.

Rules of Classification and Staging

Clinical Staging and Imaging

Cancers of the small intestines are uncommon and although imaging may be useful for staging, the diagnosis realistically is often uncovered at laparotomy. At the time of surgery and resection an accurate view of penetration of bowel wall is possible. Computed tomography (CT) and magnetic resonance imaging (MRI) may be useful; however, most small bowel neoplasia are carcinoids, lymphomas, or leiomyosarcomas and not applicable to the TNM staging system (Table 32.3).

Pathologic Staging

The surgically resected small intestine and associated lymph nodes removed are assessed. Tumor extension and location of both primary and nodes should be documented. Accurate radial margins should be marked and recorded and are defined as the surgically dissected surface adjacent to the deepest point of tumor invasion beyond the wall of the small bowel. The completeness of resection depends on the clearing of the deepest point of invasion: R0, complete; R1, microscopic; and R2, macroscopic.

Oncoimaging Annotations
* Adenocarcinomas occur in the duodenum; decreasing in frequency are jejunum and ileum.

* Enteroclysis has a 90% success rate in imaging small bowel tumors although it is 30% to 40% of small bowel follow-through studies.

* CT is best for determining penetration of bowel into surrounding viscera; MRI is useful for detecting liver metastases.

* CT is reported to have accuracy of detection rate between 70% and 80%. CT misses tumors <2 cm. Mucosal detail is absent. CT is best for staging and follow-up.

* At present, the role of MRI is limited to the search for liver metastases, but enthusiasm for MRI enteroclysis is increasing.

Cancer Statistics and Survival

The digestive system, or gastrointestinal tract, which includes MDG, accounts for 255,640 new patients annually with colon and rectum responsible for >50% with 146 new diagnoses annually. Approximately half eventually die of these cancers. MDG cancers as a group are more lethal; only a handful of patients become long-term survivors. Fortunately, colon and rectal cancers are the most common, with the majority of patients becoming 5-year survivors (63%) responding to chemoradiation programs often with the sparing of the rectal sphincter with conservative surgery. Anal cancers are the most responsive to chemoradiation (5-flourouracil and cisplatin), eliminating the need for surgery. The 5-year survival rate is >90% with anal

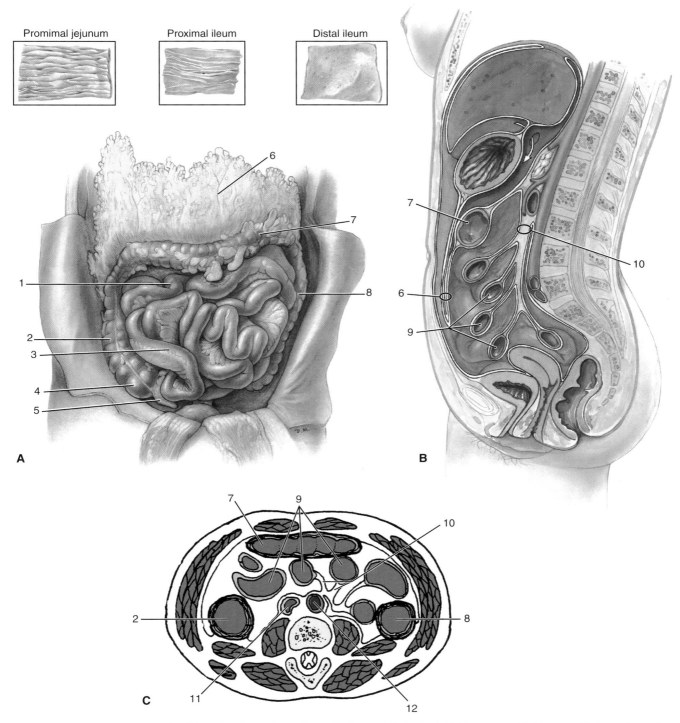

Figure 32.4 **T-oncoanatomy:** Small intestine three-planar views. **A.** Coronal. **B.** Sagittal, **C.** Transverse. (1) Jejunum. (2) Ascending colon. (3) Ileum. (4) Cecum. (5) Appendix. (6) Greater omentum. (7) Transverse colon. (8) Descending colon. (9) Loops of small intestine. (10) Mesentery of small intestine. (11) Inferior vena cava. (12) Aorta.

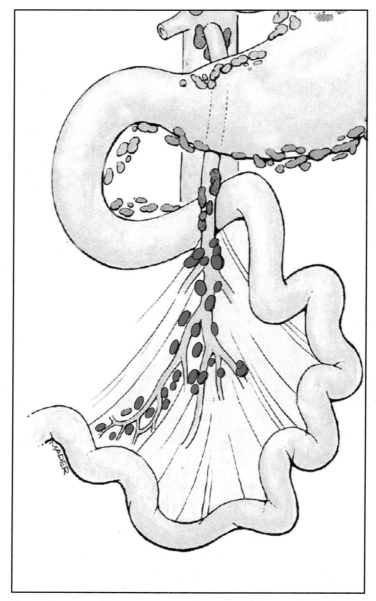

Figure 32.5 N-oncoanatomy. Sentinel nodes of small intestine include the mesenteric nodes.

TABLE 32.2	Lymph Nodes of Small Intestine
Sentinel nodes include superior mesenteric nodes	
Segment	**Regional Nodes**
Duodenum	Duodenal, hepatic, pancreaticoduodenal, infrapyloric, gastroduodenal, pyloric, superior mesenteric, pericholedochal
Ileum and jejunum	Posterior cecal (terminal ileum only), ileocolic (terminal ileum only), superior mesenteric, mesenteric
Juxtaregional nodes Para-aortic Portal Rectal	

TABLE 32.3	Imaging Modalities for Staging for Small Intestine	
Method	**Diagnosis and Staging Capability**	**Recommended for Use**
Primary tumor and regional nodes		
Single-contrast GI studies*	Useful in detecting and defining primary lesions in small intestine: 90%	Yes
Double-contrast GI studies*	Very useful in detecting early gastric cancers	Yes—should be performed along with single contrast
Endoscopy	Very accurate modality to detect and define primary lesions: ~90% confirmation rate	Yes—use to confirm lesion detected in UGI series and to screen high-risk patients
CT-abdomen ± chest	Most valuable of all modalities for determining degree of extrabowel extension and distant metastases	Yes
Endoscopic ultrasound	Most accurate method of determining extension within and beyond gastric wall	Yes—if plan preoperative chemoirradiation
Metastatic tumors		
Chest films	Good for detecting metastases	Yes
Laparoscopy	May allow visualization of small serosal implants or liver metastases	Yes—if plan preoperative chemotherapy or chemoradiation
Bone film	Useful only for confirming metastases	No—unless patient has bone pain
PET—liver, brain, bone	Useful in evaluation of clinically suspected metastases; CT is better than nuclide scan for liver and brain	No—unless suspected metastases

CT, computed tomography; GI, gastrointestinal; UGI, upper gastrointestinal.
*Enteroclysis.

sphincter preservation. This regimen has been proven to be very effective in clinical trials and to result in more long-term survivors, which is currently reflected in the literature. Liver, bile duct, and pancreatic cancers are among the poorest in the terms of survival, which is often measured in months rather than years (see Table 23.7).

Specifically, the small intestine accounted for 5,260 new cancer cases and 1,130 cancer deaths (21%).

33

Rectum

Nevertheless, the rectum considering its length, is perhaps the most common site for intestinal cancer with 40,000 cases annually, equally divided by gender.

Perspective and Pattern of Spread

Rectal cancers present according to the "early warning" signs of cancer, that is, change in bowel habits, bleeding into stools, and narrowing or pencil stools. However, such signs are not in keeping with "early detection." Rectal cancers should be uncovered in their asymptomatic stage during annually performed rectal examinations and testing for hemoccult blood in the stool. Nevertheless, the rectum considering its length, is perhaps the most common site for intestinal cancer with 40,000 cases annually, equally divided by gender. Fortunately, the vast majority of patients are controlled and become cancer survivors, often with rectal sphincter preservation. More than 90% of patients become 5-year survivors and mortality rates have been trending downward, more dramatically in females then males. The histopathology of rectal cancers are mainly adenocarcinomas and the staging system is not applicable to lymphomas or sarcomas (Table 33.1). Cancer spread patterns are both intraperitoneal and extraperitoneal because of its pelvic location (Fig. 33.1).

TNM Staging Criteria

The staging of rectal cancer is relatively unchanged and based on the depth of penetration of its wall and whether lymph nodes are involved. Because the rectum lies in the sacral hollow, it has no peritoneum on its lateral or posterior surfaces, with direct access to the sacral plexus of nerves. The rectum has been variously defined anatomically because only for half of its length is it an extraperitoneal organ. Its relationship to genitourinary organs differs in the male and female pelvis (Fig. 33.2). The cancer invades the mucosa (T1), muscularis (T2), and serosa (T3) anteriorly; however, posteriorly it has no barrier to invasion of the sacral hollows. Perineural invasion of the sacral plexus is T4.

Generally, there is no overarching principle or context design for the digestive system (gastrointestinal tract) or major digestive glands (MDG). Stages are frequently expanded to six by subdividing stages into A

and B. The T and N categories are assigned to a stage grouping, specifically for division of a stage into more (a) versus less (b) favorable groupings. This occurs at different stages for different sites.

Specifically, this site has a clear separation of T progression I/II from N progression III/IV. Stages IIIA and IIIB show node progression and stage IIIC, venous invasion (V1); IV is metastatic. Because this site is the dominant cancer, this staging system impacts on other gastrointestinal sites and major digestive gland sites.

Summary of Changes

Changes with the sixth edition are moderate:

- *A revised description of the anatomy of the colon and rectum better delineates the data concerning the boundaries between colon, rectum, and anal canal. Adenocarcinomas of the vermiform appendix are classified according to the TNM staging system, but should be recorded separately. Cancers that occur in the anal canal are staged according to the classification used for the anus.*

- *Smooth metastatic nodules in the pericolic or perirectal fat are considered lymph node metastases and are counted in the N staging. In contrast, irregularly contoured metastatic nodules in the peritumoral fat are considered vascular invasion and are coded as an extension of the T category as either a V1 (microscopic vascular invasion) if only microscopically visible or a V2 (macroscopic vascular invasion) if grossly visible.*

- *Stage II is subdivided into IIA and IIB on the basis of whether the primary tumor is T3 or T4, respectively.*

- *Stage III is subdivided into IIIA (T1–T2 N1 M0), IIIB (T3–T4 N1 M0), or IIIC (any T N2 M0).*

Orientation of Three-planar Oncoanatomy

The three-planar anatomic isocenter for the rectum occupies the sacral hollow (S1–S5) inside the true pelvis, retropubically located from an anterior view (Fig. 33.3).

T-oncoanatomy

The rectum, about 12 cm long, extends from a point opposite the third sacral vertebra down to the apex of the prostate in the male and to the apex of the perineal

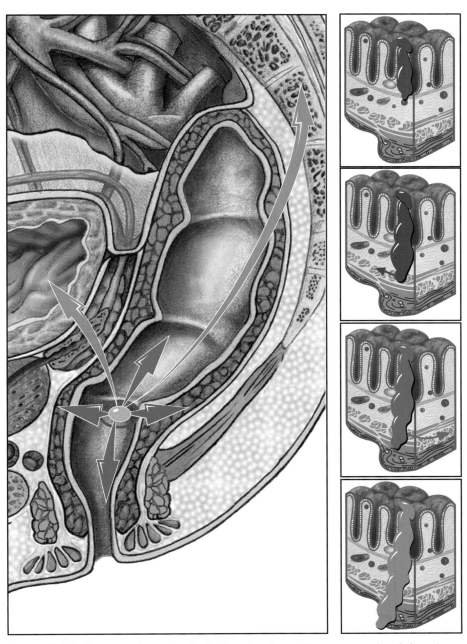

Figure 33.1 **A. Patterns of spread. B.** T categories. The patterns of spread and the primary tumor classification are similarly color coded: Tis (cancer in situ of mucosa), yellow; T1 (infiltrates the submucosa), green; T2 (penetrates the muscularis externa), blue; T3 (reaches the subserosa), purple; and T4 (invades through the serosa into a neighboring viscera), red.

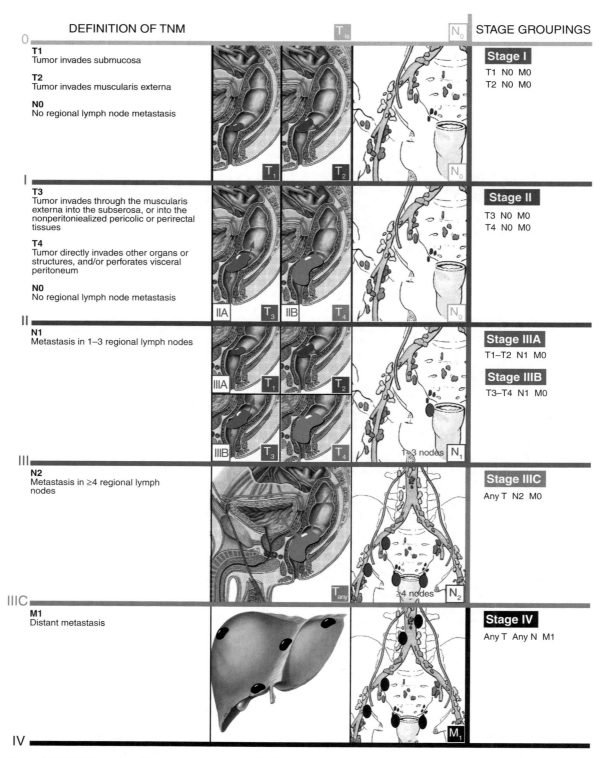

DEFINITION OF TNM

T1
Tumor invades submucosa

T2
Tumor invades muscularis externa

N0
No regional lymph node metastasis

T3
Tumor invades through the muscularis externa into the subserosa, or into the nonperitoniealized pericolic or perirectal tissues

T4
Tumor directly invades other organs or structures, and/or perforates visceral peritoneum

N0
No regional lymph node metastasis

N1
Metastasis in 1–3 regional lymph nodes

N2
Metastasis in ≥4 regional lymph nodes

M1
Distant metastasis

STAGE GROUPINGS

Stage I
T1 N0 M0
T2 N0 M0

Stage II
T3 N0 M0
T4 N0 M0

Stage IIIA
T1–T2 N1 M0

Stage IIIB
T3–T4 N1 M0

Stage IIIC
Any T N2 M0

Stage IV
Any T Any N M1

Figure 33.2 TNM staging diagram presents a vertical arrangement with color bars encompassing TN combinations showing progression. Rectal cancers can be resected as Stage II A/B (purple) with N1 nodes but are less favorable and borderline resectable stage IIIC (red) as N2 nodes (>4) are found, stage IV are (black) metastatic. Stage 0, yellow; I, green; II, blue; III, purple; IV, red; and IV (metastatic), black. Definitions of TN on left and stage grouping on right.

TABLE 33.1	Histopathologic Type: Common Cancers of the Rectum
Type	
Adenocarcinoma in situ	Squamous cell (epidermoid) carcinoma
Adenocarcinoma	Adenosquamous carcinoma
Medullary carcinoma	Small cell carcinoma
Mucinous carcinoma (colloid type; >50% mucinous carcinoma)	Undifferentiated carcinoma
Signet ring cell carcinoma (>50% signet ring cell)	Carcinoma, NOS

NOS, not otherwise specified.
From Greene FL, Page DL, Fleming ID, et al. eds. *AJCC Cancer Staging Manual*. 6th ed. New York: Springer; 2002. Used with the permission of the American Joint Committee on Cancer (AJCC) Chicago, Illinois.

body in the female; that is, to a point 4 cm anterior to the tip of the coccyx. It may be arbitrarily defined as the distal 10 cm of the large intestine, as measured by preoperative sigmoidoscopy from the anal verge (Fig. 33.4).

- *Coronal*: The rectum extends approximately 10 to 12 cm; the rectosigmoid area is 10 to 15 cm from this junction. *The rectum has no epiploic appendages, no haustrations, and no taeniae. It is covered by peritoneum in front and on both sides in its upper third and on the anterior wall only in its middle third; there is no peritoneal covering in the lower third.*

- *Sagittal*: In the lower rectum, the mucosa is thrown into longitudinal folds, known as the rectal columns or the columns of Morgagni. Between them, just above the white line of Hilton, are the anal pits or sinuses. About 4 cm long, the anal canal courses downward and backward from the apex of the prostate or the perineal body. The anocutaneaous line (pectinate line), or white line of Hilton, at the base of the rectal columns marks the site of the original anal membrane that separated the endodermal gut from the ectodermal proctoderm. The transition from colon to rectum has been explicitly defined by the American Joint Committee on Cancer as marked by the fusion of the tenia of the sigmoid colon to the circumferential longitudinal muscle of the rectum. This occurs 12 to 15 cm from the dentate line. The upper third is covered anteriorly and at its sides by peritoneum, which is completely absent in its lower third.

- *Transverse*: The rectouterine cul-de-sac (pouch of Douglas) in females is the rectovesical pouch in males and inferiorly becomes the Denonvier fascia, separating and shielding the rectum from direct prostate cancer invasion. The rectal mucosa is smooth and is characterized by transverse folds, the valves of Houston that divide the rectum into thirds. In the three-dimensional, three-planar views of the female and male pelvises, the axial views are most informative (Fig. 33.4C, D). Compare the location of the female cervix with the male prostate and their critical relationship to the rectum and bladder presents a specific challenge to radiation oncologists to avoid injuring this important viscera.

N-oncoanatomy

The nodal drainage and distribution follows its blood supply, which is complicated because of its anatomy as both a pelvic and an abdominal organ. The superior third follows the superior rectal lymph nodes, which follow inferior mesenteric node to the portal and caval nodes. The middle portion drains directly into the pelvic internal iliac nodes. The lower third drains into inguinal lymph nodes (Fig. 33.5; Table 33.2).

M-oncoanatomy

The venous drainage is different for each third of the rectum owing to its anatomic position as an abdominal and pelvic organ. Superiorly, the superior rectal vein drains into the inferior mesenteric vein then portal vein resulting in a high probability of liver metastases. The middle and inferior third drain into the internal and external iliac veins, the inferior vena cava, and then to the right side of the heart and into lung. The middle rectal vein may predispose to osseous pelvic metastases because of anastomoses of perirectal veins with intervertebral veins (see Fig. 25.6).

The incidence of liver metastases exceeds other sites. According to a variety of reports in the literature the range is 40% to 100% at autopsy. Other sites are mainly bone metastases 25% to 40% and lung metastases with occasional and a lesser percentage of bone metastasis.

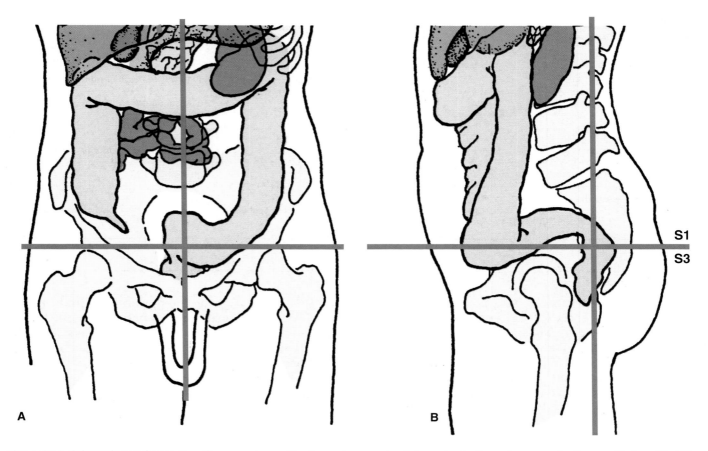

A

B

S1
S3

Figure 33.3 Orientation and overview of oncoanatomy. The three-planar anatomic isocenter for the rectum occupies the sacral hollow (S1–S5) inside the true pelvis, retropubically located from an anterior view. **A.** Coronal. **B.** Sagittal.

Rules of Classification and Staging

Clinical Staging and Imaging

Extension of diagnostic imaging to staging is gaining in popularity. Virtual colonoscopy and sigmoidoscopy are challenging endoscopic colonoscopy as to accuracy in diagnosing adenocarcinomas. Endoscopic ultrasound shows the layers of the colon and rectal wall and their penetration by cancer. Endorectal magnetic resonance imaging (MRI) is most valuable to demonstrate extracolonic and extrarectal invasion into adjacent structures. Computed tomography (CT) is preferred for detecting liver and lung metastases (Table 33.3).

Pathologic Staging

The surgically resected rectum and associated lymph nodes removed are assessed. Tumor extension and location of both primary and nodes should be documented. Accurate radial margins should be marked and recorded and are defined "as the surgically dissected surface adjacent to the deepest point of tumor invasion beyond the wall of the rectum." The completeness of resection depends on the clearing of the deepest point of invasion: R0, complete; R1, microscopic; and R2, macroscopic.

Oncoimaging Annotations

- Although colonoscopy is more accurate in assessment for small polyps, overall cost effectiveness is greater when double-contrast barium enema examinations are used.

- CT colonography is a recent addition to the modalities used to screen for colorectal cancer and polyps. This modality requires further refinement and testing before being more widely adopted.

- Transrectal ultrasonography and MRI are able to demonstrate the extent of tumor through the rectal wall and provide some assessment for lymphadenopathy.

- If there is clinical suspicion of metastasis or elevated carcinoembryonic antigen level, CT and MRI are useful for determining the presence and site of recurrent disease. Overall accuracy for the detection of recurrent disease with these modalities is 90% to 95%.

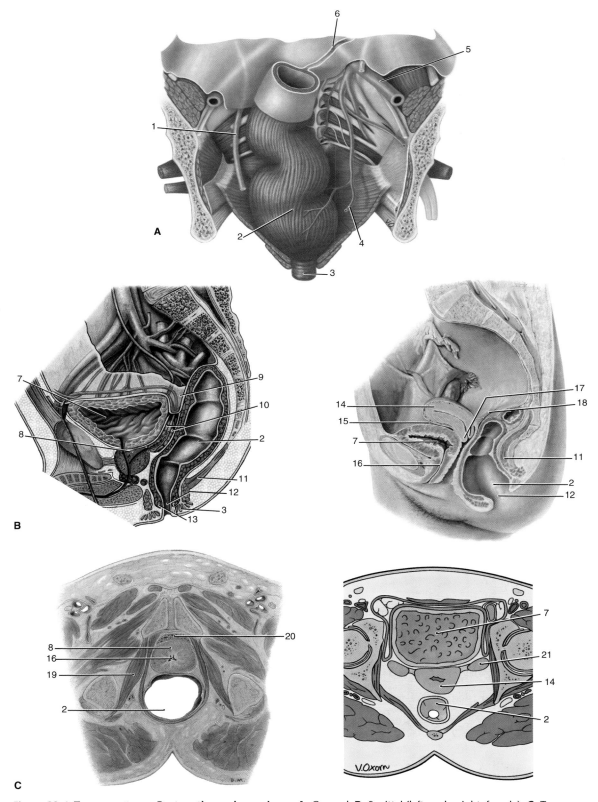

Figure 33.4 **T-oncoanatomy: Rectum three-planar views. A.** Coronal. **B.** Sagittal (left, male; right, female). **C.** Transverse (left, male; right, female). (1) Right ureter. (2) Rectum. (3) External anal sphincter. (4) Middle rectal artery. (5) Left external iliac artery. (6) Roof of sigmoid mesocolon. (7) Urinary bladder. (8) Prostate. (9) Rectovesical pouch. (10) Seminal vesicle. (11) Levator ani. (12) Anal canal. (13) Internal anal sphincter. (14) Uterus. (15) Vesicouterine pouch. (16) Urethra. (17) Cervix of uterus. (18) Rectouterine pouch (of Douglas). (19) Obturator internus. (20) Prostatic venous plexus. (21) Ovary.

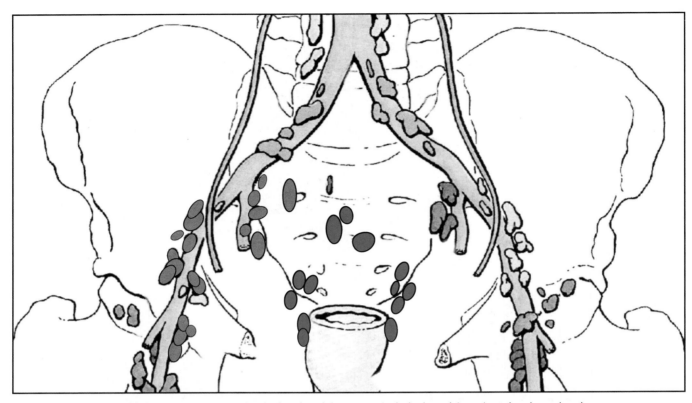

Figure 33.5 N-oncoanatomy. Sentinel nodes of the rectum include the pelvic perirectal and sacral nodes.

This evaluation may require fine-needle aspiration biopsy under direct CT guidance.

- Other noninvasive means to determine the presence of absence of recurrent or metastatic tumor are nuclear medicine scanning techniques with radiolabeled monoclonal antibodies and positron emission tomography techniques using fluorodeoxyglucose. Some of these have shown great potential.

Cancer Statistics and Survival

The digestive system, or gastrointestinal tract, which includes MDG, accounts for 255,640 new patients annu-

ally with colon and rectum responsible for >50% with 146 new diagnoses annually. Approximately half eventually die of these cancers. MDG cancers as a group are more lethal; only a handful of patients become long-term survivors. Fortunately, colon and rectal cancers are the most common, with the majority of patients becoming 5-year survivors (63%) responding to chemoradiation programs often with the sparing of the rectal sphincter with conservative surgery (see Fig. 31.6). Anal cancers are the most responsive to chemoradiation (5-fluorouracil and cisplatin) eliminating the need for surgery. The 5-year survival rate is >90% with anal sphincter preservation. This regimen has been proven to be very effective in clinical trials and to result in more

TABLE 33.2	Lymph Nodes of Rectum	
Sentinel nodes include perirectal and sacral nodes.		
Regional nodes		**Juxtaregional nodes**
Perirectal		External iliac
Sigmoid mesenteric		Common iliac
Inferior mesenteric		Para-aortic
Lateral sacral presacral		
Internal iliac		
Superior rectal (hemorrhoidal)		
Middle rectal (hemorrhoidal)		
Inferior rectal (hemorrhoidal)		

TABLE 33.3	Imaging Modalities for Staging for Rectum and Anus	
Method	**Diagnosis and Staging Capability**	**Recommended for Use**
Primary tumor ± regional nodes		
BE	Very useful in detecting and defining primary lesions in the colon.	Yes
Endoscopy	Single-contrast study may be less sensitive than double-contrast in detecting polyps.	Yes, if used to confirm lesion detected on BE or to screen high-risk patients.
Endorectal ultrasound or coil	Very accurate modality for detecting and defining primary lesions. In rectum, sigmoid (flex sig), or remaining colon (colonoscopy).	Yes, if preoperative chemoRT is considered
MRI	Useful in defining depth of penetration of the primary lesion.	Yes
CT	Most valuable of all modalities for determining extrarectal or extracolonic local invasion and nodal metastases.	Yes
PET	Not useful for staging primary cancer.	No
Metastases		
Chest film ± CT	Chest film—best for metastasis screening; CT chest—rules out	Yes
CT abdomen	Multiple metastases. Most useful study to define para-aortic node enlargement or liver metastases.	Yes
Liver ultrasound	Can differentiate between cystic and solid lesions.	Yes

BE, barium enema; CT, computed tomography; chemoRT, chemoradiation; MRI, magnetic resonance imaging; PET, positron emission tomography.

long-term survivors, which is currently reflected in the literature. Liver, bile duct, and pancreatic cancers are among the poorest in the terms of survival, which is often measured in months rather than years (see Table 23.7).

Specifically, the rectum accounted for approximately 40,570 new cancer cases with a 5-year survival rate improvement over the last 5 decades of 23%. Cur-

rently, relative 5-year survival for all stages is 62.3%, but when localized improves to 90.1% (see Table 23.8). Local recurrence is highly dependent on site in the rectum, i.e., 18% overall for tumors <7 cm from the anal verge. Stage is a strong prognosticator for local recurrence, i.e., T1 T2 38% and T3 T4 30% but with positive node failure doubles to 65%.

Anal cancers provide new evidence for the role of immunosuppression and viral infections in carcinogenesis.

Perspective and Pattern of Spread

Anal cancers provide new evidence for the role of immunosuppression and viral infections in carcinogenesis. Of the 4,000 new patients expected annually, there is a bioassociation with condylomata (human papilloma virus and human immunodeficiency virus; with a higher incidence of anal cancer in homosexuals with acquired immunodeficiency syndrome). *The anal canal is a transitional zone marked by the pectinate line, or mucocutaneous junction. The two predominant histologic types of anal carcinoma are variants of squamous cell cancers.* Basaloid (cloacogenic) cancers arise at this junction, whereas more typical epidermoid cancers occur on the skin. The epicenter of the cancer determines its origin. According to the American Joint Committee on Cancer, cancers are anal tumors if their epicenter is ≤2 cm from the pectinate line; otherwise, they are rectal cancers with epicenters >2 cm proximal to the dentate line (Fig. 34.1; Table 34.1).

Anal sphincter preservation with radiochemotherapy is the standard of treatment for most patients with anal cancers. In fact, the application of similar treatment regimens to rectal and esophageal cancers has improved their survival outcomes with normal tissue and organ conservation. Size of tumor determines the staging categories rather than depth of invasion similar to the skin cancer classification.

TNM Staging Criteria

The anatomy reflects the spread pattern. *There is an important distinction between those cancers of the anal canal (extending from rectum to the pectinate line) versus cancers on the perineal aspect of the anus to the pectinate line.* Anal margin lesions are distal to the anal verge, where hair-bearing skin occurs. Cancers of the anal canal are of greater concern because they are more likely to invade

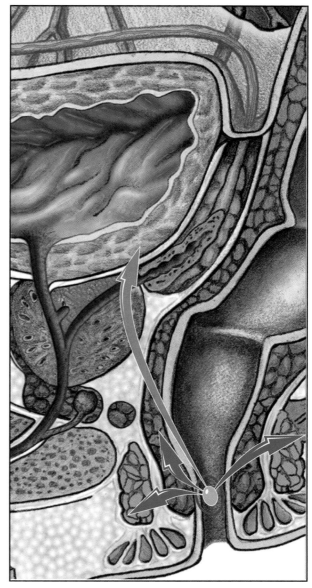

Figure 34.1 **Patterns of spread for anal cancer are color coded for T stage:** Tis, yellow; T1, green; T2, blue; T3, purple; and T4, red.

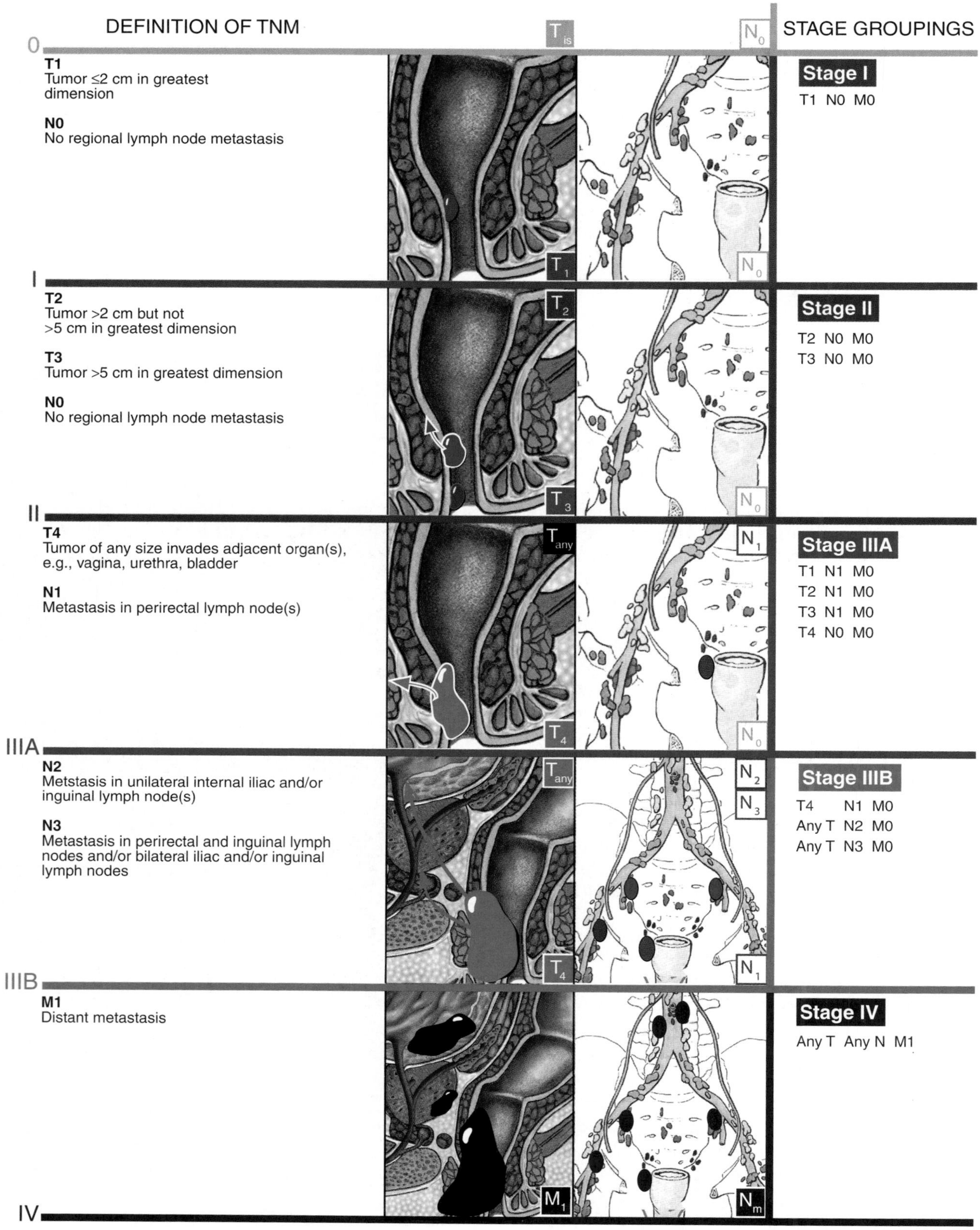

DEFINITION OF TNM

STAGE GROUPINGS

0

T1
Tumor ≤2 cm in greatest
dimension

N0
No regional lymph node metastasis

T_{is} N_0

Stage I

T1 N0 M0

I

T2
Tumor >2 cm but not
>5 cm in greatest dimension

T3
Tumor >5 cm in greatest dimension

N0
No regional lymph node metastasis

T_2 T_3

Stage II

T2 N0 M0
T3 N0 M0

II

T4
Tumor of any size invades adjacent organ(s),
e.g., vagina, urethra, bladder

N1
Metastasis in perirectal lymph node(s)

T_{any} T_4 N_1 N_0

Stage IIIA

T1 N1 M0
T2 N1 M0
T3 N1 M0
T4 N0 M0

IIIA

N2
Metstasis in unilateral internal iliac and/or
inguinal lymph node(s)

N3
Metastasis in perirectal and inguinal lymph
nodes and/or bilateral iliac and/or inguinal
lymph nodes

T_{any} T_4 N_2 N_3 N_1

Stage IIIB

T4   N1 M0
Any T N2 M0
Any T N3 M0

IIIB

M1
Distant metastasis

M_1 N_m

Stage IV

Any T Any N M1

IV

Figure 34.2 TNM staging diagram presents a vertical arrangement with color bars encompassing TN combinations showing progression: Anal cancers are very chemoradiation sensitive and response and survival rates are high with anal preservation. Stage 0, yellow; I, green; II, blue; III, purple; IV, red; and IV (metastatic), black. Definitions of TN on left and stage grouping on right.

TABLE 34.1	World Health Organization Classification of Carcinoma of the Anal Canal
Type	
Squamous cell carcinoma	

Adenocarcinoma
    Rectal type
    Of anal glands
    Within anorectal fistula	

Mucinous adenocarcinoma	
Small cell carcinoma	
Undifferentiated carcinoma	

From Greene FL, Page DL, Fleming ID, et al. eds. *AJCC Cancer Staging Manual.* 6th ed. New York: Springer; 2002. Used with the permission of the American Joint Committee on Cancer (AJCC) Chicago, Illinois.

the rectal sphincters and open more pathways of spread deep into the pelvis via lymphatics and hemorrhoidal veins.

The TNM staging of anal cancer has not changed. Primary anal cancers are staged based on size of the cancer rather than depth. However, it should be noted that direct invasion of the rectal wall, or anal and rectal sphincter invasion are T3 and T4 cancers. Evidence of an adjacent organ, such as vagina, urethra, or bladder, is required (Fig. 34.2).

Generally, there is no overarching principle or context design for the digestive system (gastrointestinal tract) or major digestive glands. Stages are frequently expanded to six by subdividing stages into A and B. The T and N categories are assigned to a stage grouping, specifically for division of a stage into more (a) versus less (b) favorable groupings. This occurs at different stages for different sites. Specifically, this site has similar pattern of T stage progression than N stage progression, with T3/T4 = N1; stage III is divided into A/B/C (i.e., IIIA = T3, IIIB = T4); and IIIC is N1.

Summary of Changes

There are no changes in the sixth edition of the AJCC CSM.

Orientation of Three-planar Oncoanatomy

The anatomic isocenter for the anus is below the coccyx in line with pubic bone and femoral heads and readily identified on physical examination (Fig. 34.3).

T-oncoanatomy

Orientation views are presented in Figure 34.3 and three-planar views in Figure 34.4A–C. The terminal portion of

the digestive system has a complex anatomy and is best viewed in:

- *Coronal*: Defines the anorectal line, the columns of Morgagni, and the pectinate line at the mucocutaneous junction. The anal canal extends from the dentate or pectinate line to the hair bearing skin.
- *Sagittal*: Differentiates the anatomy of the female and male pelvises. It offers views of the various spaces of the perineopelvic region: Perianal, postanal, superficial and deep, and submucosal and presacral. *The axial views relate the female and male genitalia to the anus.*

N-oncoanatomy

The nodal drainage again depends on which side of the pectinate line the anal cancer has its epicenter. For cancers of the anal verge, the lymphatic drainage is into inguinal nodes and then external iliac nodes. For cancers of the anal canal, particularly involving the rectum, the drainage is into internal iliac nodes. Both external and internal iliac nodes eventually drain into the common iliacs and para-aortic nodes (Fig. 34.5; Table 34.2).

Rules of Classification and Staging

Clinical Staging and Imaging

Clinical staging is commonly used because effective chemoradiation regimens have allowed for cure with anal sphincter preservation. The imaging tools, such as endorectal magnetic resonance imaging (EMRI) and endoluminal ultrasound (EUS), are most useful for assessing deeper invasion especially to pelvic structures as bladder and rectum, vagina and uterus when the cancer is extensive (see Table 33.3).

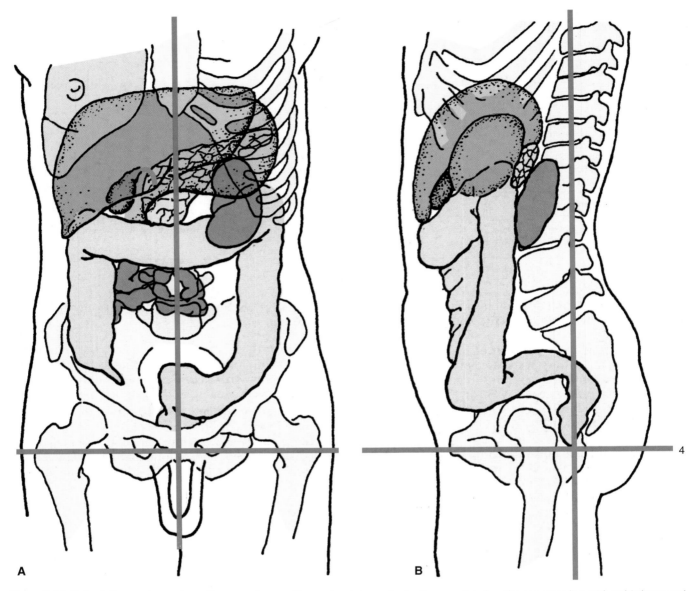

Figure 34.3 Orientation and overview of oncoanatomy. The anatomic isocenter for the anus is below the coccyx in line with pubic bone and femoral heads and readily identified on physical examination. **A**. Coronal. **B**. Sagittal.

Pathologic Staging

The surgically resected anus and associated lymph nodes removed are assessed. Tumor extension and location of both primary and nodes should be documented. Accurate radial margins should be marked and recorded and are defined as the surgically dissected surface adjacent to the deepest point of tumor invasion beyond the wall of the anus. The completeness of resection depends on the clearing of the deepest point of invasion: R0, complete; R1, microscopic; and R2, macroscopic.

Oncoimaging Annotations

• Computed tomography is useful for advanced stages and deeper invasion of surrounding structures.

• EUS and EMRI are valuable to assess depth of wall penetration.

Cancer Statistics and Survival

The digestive system, or gastrointestinal tract, which includes MDG, accounts for 255,640 new patients annually with colon and rectum responsible for >50% with 146 new diagnoses annually. Approximately half eventually die of these cancers. MDG cancers as a group are more lethal; only a handful of patients become long-term survivors. Fortunately, colon and rectal cancers are the most common, with the majority of patients becoming 5-year survivors (63%) responding to

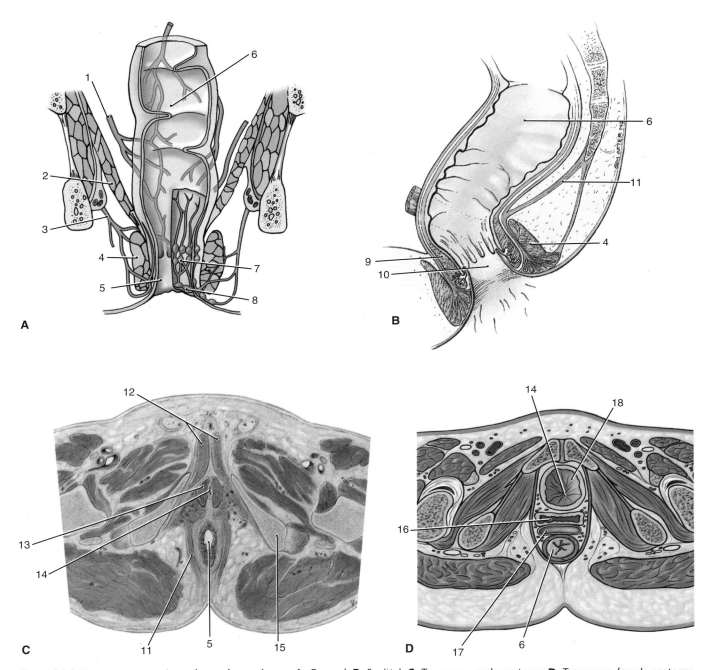

Figure 34.4 **T-oncoanatomy: Anus three-planar views.** **A.** Coronal. **B.** Sagittal. **C.** Transverse, male anatomy. **D.** Transverse, female anatomy. (1) Middle rectal artery. (2) Obturator internus. (3) Inferior rectal artery. (4) External anal sphincter. (5) Anal canal. (6) Rectum. (7) Internal rectal venous plexus. (8) External rectal venous plexus. (9) Internal anal sphincter. (10) Pectin of anal canal. (11) Levator ani. (12) Corpus cavernosum penis. (13) Bulb of penis. (14) Urethra. (15) Ischial tuberosity. (16) Vagina. (17) Rectouterine pouch (of Douglas). (18) Urinary bladder.

TABLE 34.2	**Lymph Nodes of Anus**	

Sentinel nodes include perirectal and inguinal nodes

Regional nodes	Juxtaregional nodes
Perirectal	External iliac
Anorectal	Common iliac
Perirectal	Para-aortic
Lateral sacral	
Internal iliac (hypogastric)	
Inguinal	
Superficial	
Deep femoral	

chemoradiation programs often with the sparing of the rectal sphincter with conservative surgery. Anal cancers are the most responsive to chemoradiation (5-fluorouracil and cisplatin), eliminating the need for surgery. The 5-year survival rate is >90% with anal sphincter preservation. This regimen has been proven to be very effective in clinical trials and to result in more long-term survivors, which is currently reflected in the literature. Liver, bile duct, and pancreatic cancers are amongst the poorest in the terms of survival, which is often measured in months rather than years (see Table 23.7).

Specifically, the anus accounted for approximately 4,000 new cancer cases and 580 cancer deaths (15%). Survival rates vary as a function of stage i.e., T1 T2 at 75–80% and T3 T4 at 40–60%.

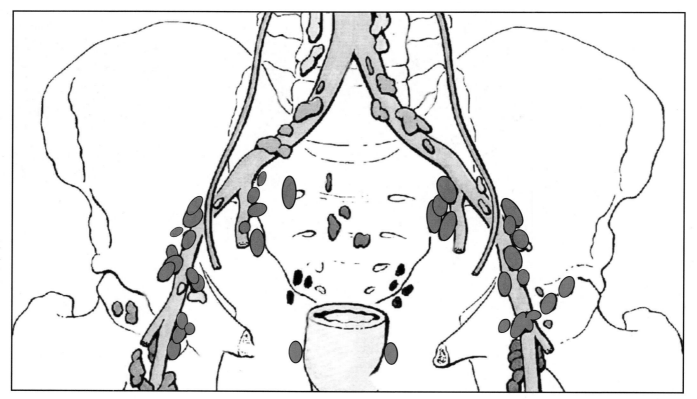

Figure 34.5 **N-oncoanatomy.** Sentinel nodes of the anus are inguinal nodes.

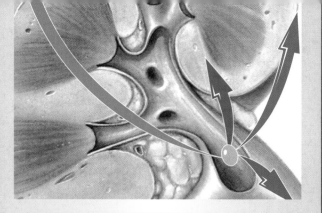

SECTION 4

MALE GENITAL TRACT AND URINARY SYSTEM PRIMARY SITES

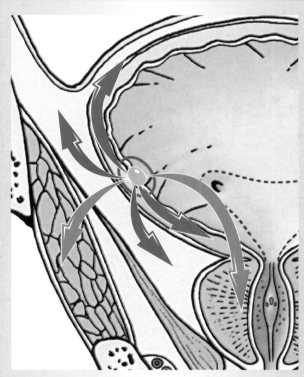

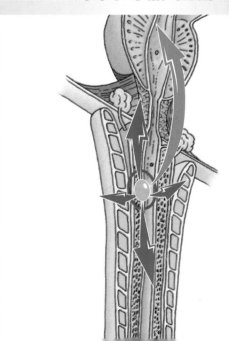

35

Introduction and Orientation

The TNM staging system of male genitourinary tract (MGU) depends on whether the organ oncoanatomy is solid and encapsulated or hollow and tubular.

Perspective and Patterns of Spread

The urinary tract of kidney, renal pelvis and ureter, urinary bladder, and urethra can frequently be involved with carcinogenesis owing to the excretion of toxic antigenic products or proteins, which can be harmful and transform their epithelial lining. Carcinogenic field effects, cancer in situ, and seeding of the excretory urinary system are major concerns; instead of a single tumor, there can be multiple cancers. Curiously, patterns of spread are limited often to the urinary system; however, juxtaposed structures are at risk (Fig. 35.1). Prostate cancer, which is the dominant malignancy in males particularly among those >50 years of age, is included with cancers of the MGU. With each decade of age it increases in incidence, affecting every other male in his 80s. In contrast, testicular cancer is the most common tumor in younger males (30–50 years). Both prostate cancer and testicular cancers are among the most highly curable tumors owing to both early diagnosis and advances in multimodal treatment.

Male genital cancers are among the first to incorporate the leading edge advances in molecular biomarker prognosticators. The development of serum prostatic antigen (PSA) into a universal serum screening test has completely changed prostate cancer from a clinically palpable tumefaction to a nonpalpable early stage disease where in fact histologic confirmation by needle biopsy is necessary to establish the existence of this malignant disease (i.e., T1c). Serum PSA is a powerful prognosticator and most useful clinical biomarker for prostate cancer, which includes its rate of increase or doubling time. Both bound and free PSA levels are useful. Although the PSA has not been incorporated officially into the staging system, pathology by Gleason grading has. In testicular tumors, several serum markers exist, namely, alpha fetoprotein, human chorionic gonadotropin, and lactate dehydrogenase. Staging of

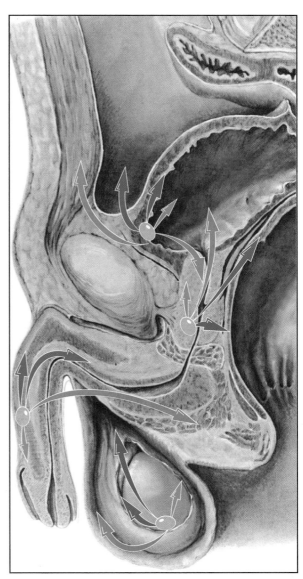

Figure 35.1 **Patterns of spread.** The cancer crab at each primary site is presented at the different anatomical locations of the MGU, color-coded as to stage: T0, Tis, Ta yellow; T1, green; T2, blue; T3, purple; T4, red. The primary sites shown are from superior to inferior: The urinary bladder, the prostate, the penis, and the testes.

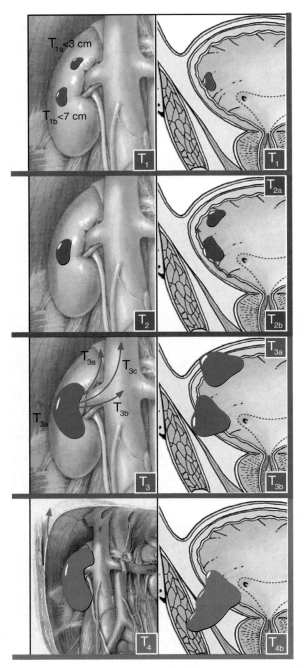

Figure 35.2 TNM staging systems. A. Kidney represents a solid organ. **B.** Urinary bladder represents a hollow organ. The T category determines the stage. Color-coded with bars: Stage T0, yellow; I, green; II, blue; III, purple; and IV, red (see text for legend).

TNM Staging Criteria

The staging system is based on the patterns of spread, which depends on whether the organ oncoanatomy is solid and encapsulated or hollow and tubular. With solid organs, tumor growth within the capsule has a good prognosis; however, once the capsule is breeched or penetrated, the likelihood of a successful outcome decreases (Fig. 35.2A). The solid organs are kidney, prostate, and testes. Urinary tract cancers of the renal pelvis, ureters, and bladder follow the classification and staging of thin-walled, hollow organs lined with transitional epithelium over their musculature. That is, the depth of penetration of the layers in their wall determines the T stage (Fig. 35.2B). The adoption of the alphabetical American Urological Association classification into the TNM language allowed for unifying the literature. The poorly differentiated variety of cancers, especially in solid organs, can result in widespread lymphatic and hematogenous metastases. Virtually every remote and distant site can be involved. Kidney has a predilection for lung, as do most testicular cancers, but bone and brain are often sites for dissemination.

The most unique metastatic pattern is the predilection of prostate cancer to form axial vertebral metastases. The extensive osteoblastic sclerosis of bone is virtually pathognomonic when pelvis, lumbar, and thoracic vertebral bodies appear uniformly positive first on bone scans and then as white, dense bones in radiographs. This has been attributed to retrograde venous spread of prostate cancer cells from the periprostatic plexus of veins to the Batson's vertebral venous plexus.

Summary of Changes

The classification of solid organs, the kidney, prostate, and testes depends on whether the tumor is confined (T1T2) or invasion through their adventitial fibrous capsule (T3) and into surrounding adjacent structures or fixation to bone (T4) has occurred (Fig. 35.2A). The renal pelvis and ureter are staged similar to the bladder and their cancers follow the same pattern for staging hollow viscera as in the digestive system: T1, mucosal; T2, submucosal muscle layer; T3, fibrous outer wall or peritoneum; and T4, invasion into adjacent tissues (Fig. 35.2B).

Overview of the Histogenesis in the Male Genitourinary System

The urinary system consists of two kidneys, each with a renal pelvis that drains into two separate ureters, which enter the urinary bladder with its single urethral exit. The male genital system consists of the prostate, seminal vesicles, the testes, and the penis (Fig. 35.3A). The cancer histopathology relates to the epithelium of the different sections (Fig. 35.3, Table 35.1).

testicular cancers is unique because they are the first durable instance of biomarkers inclusion in the TNM staging system. Furthermore, these molecular markers are useful in determining "cure" or control of the cancer and are often the first evidence of relapse if their elevation occurs in follow-up visits.

TABLE 35.1	Orientation of Histogenesis of Primary Cancer Sites of the MGU	
Primary Site Normal Anatomic Structures	Derivative Normal Cell	Cancer Histopathologic Type Primary Site
Renal parenchyma	Simple cuboidal epithelium	Clear cell renal adenocarcinoma
Renal pelvis and urether	Transitional cell epithelium	Uroepithelial transitional cell cancer
Urinary bladder	Transitional cell epithelium	Transitional cell cancer Squamous cell cancer
Prostate	Pseudostratified columnar epithelium	Adenocarcinoma, Gleason grading
Testes	Germ cells	Seminomas, embryonal cell cancer, teratocarcinoma
Penis	Stratified squamous	Squamous cell cancer
Urethra, spongy	Pseudostratified columnar epithelium	Squamous cell cancer Transitional cell cancer

- The majority of renal cancers arise in epithelium of the proximal or distal convoluted tubule. The functional unit of each kidney is the convoluted tubule, which consists of a nephron and a collecting duct (Fig. 35.3B).
- Cancers of the renal pelvis arise in the excretory portion of the urinary system, which is lined with a transitional epithelium covering a multilayered wall consisting of a submucosa, a circular and longitudinal muscle layer, and most often a fibrous adventitia or a serosalike external covering (Fig. 35.3C).
- In the bladder, the epithelium is transitional when empty but flattened, almost squamouslike, when full and distended. Most cancers are transitional cell (Fig. 35.3C), although squamous cell cancers and adenocarcinomas can and do occur in the bladder.
- Cancers of the penis and urethra tend to be squamous cell cancers arising from stratified squamous cell mucosal lining and skin (Fig. 35.3D)
- Cancers of the prostate arise from tubuloalveolar glandular epithelium and transit into adenocarcinoma of varying grade (Fig. 35.3E).
- Cancers of the testes are highly varied owing to their unique genetic and gonadal function (Fig. 35.3F).

The separation of two juxtaposed abdominal and pelvic cavity systems is by a single layer of mesothelial cells. The peritoneum is sufficient to protect the genitourinary system from invasion by gastrointestinal cancers and vice versa. MGU cancers tend to spread within their system involving or complicating their function. Seeding of ureters and bladder with renal pelvis cancer is a common concern. MGU tumors never seed out into the peritoneal cavity in contrast with gastrointestinal tract (GIT) cancers, which may. Except for the kidney

and ureters the rest of the genitourinary system is confined to the true pelvis. The two anatomic sectors are intraperitoneal and retroperitoneal.

Orientation of T-oncoanatomy: Odyssey of Primary Sites

In the orientation of pelvic organs it is important to view the osseous anatomy (Fig. 35.4A), the cavities in the musculoskeletal anatomy (Fig. 35.4B), and the different anatomic sectors that house the viscera and neurovasculature (Fig. 35.4C). The bony pelvis above the pelvic brim is referred to as the greater or false pelvis because it houses and contains the contents of the peritoneal cavity. The true pelvis on coronal section is below the pelvic brim, shaped like a wine glass, and houses the male and female genital organs and the urinary bladder. The floor of the true pelvis is the levator ani muscle covered with superior and inferior parietal fascia and its roof is the peritoneal covering over the pelvic viscera. The obturator lymph nodes (green) are in the true pelvis with the obturator nerve, artery, and vein as it penetrates the levator ani. The perineum roof (levator ani muscle) is perforated by the urethra and houses the corpus cavernosum of the penis in the male and the vagina in the female.

The anatomic isocenters of the seven primary sites in the male genitourinary system are presented in multiplanar orientation diagrams (Fig. 35.4D, E). Each of the primary sites is presented in three planes—coronal, sagittal, and axial—as well as their sentinel and regional lymph nodes and adjacent organs.

The odyssey of the seven MGU primary sites is presented from cephalad to caudad (Table 35.2). The tabulation aligns each primary site with associated surrounding structures and osseous landmarks when feasible. The sentinel node for each primary site is also noted. The

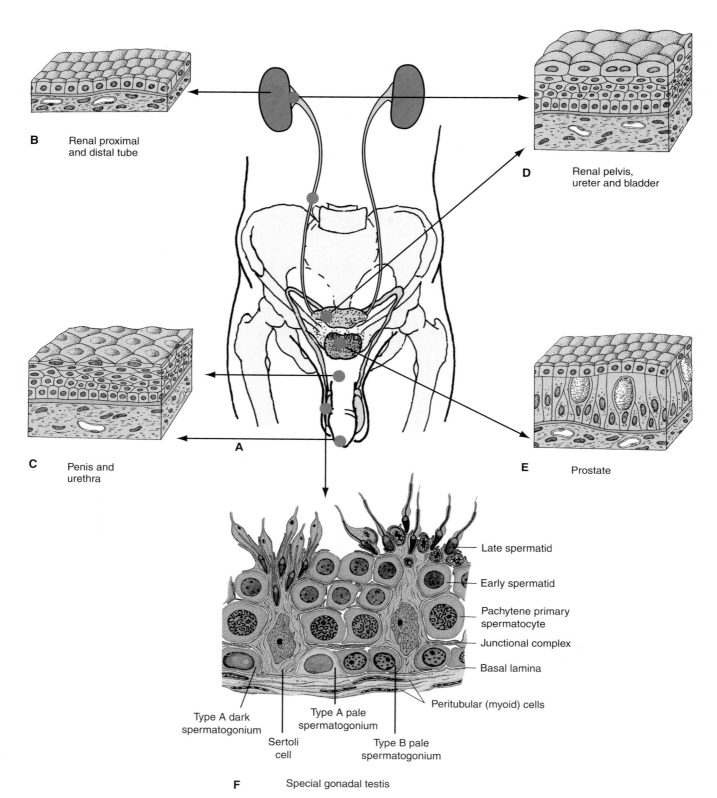

B Renal proximal and distal tube

D Renal pelvis, ureter and bladder

C Penis and urethra

A

E Prostate

Late spermatid

Early spermatid

Pachytene primary spermatocyte

Junctional complex

Basal lamina

Peritubular (myoid) cells

Type A dark spermatogonium

Sertoli cell

Type A pale spermatogonium

Type B pale spermatogonium

F Special gonadal testis

Figure 35.3 **Overview of the histogenesis. A.** The cancer originates in the various histogenic phenotypes of epithelial cells of MGU organs. **B.** Renal **C.** Renal pelvis, ureter, and bladder **D.** Penis and urethra **E.** Prostate **F.** Special gonadal testis.

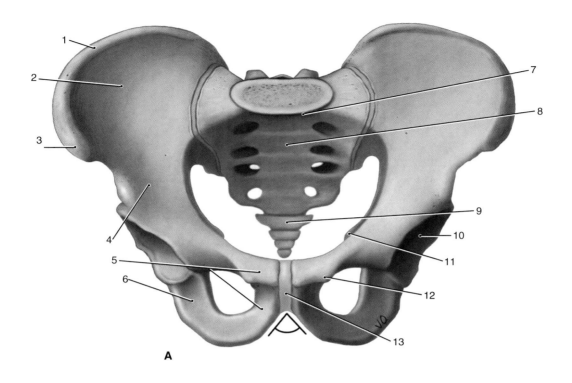

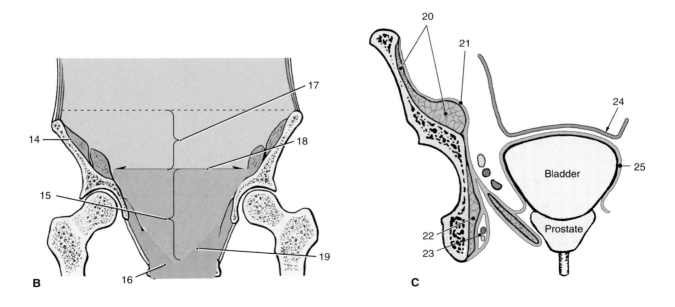

Figure 35.4 **Orientation of three-planar T-oncoanatomy.** **A.** Three pelvic bones: Ilium holds false pelvis or peritoneal cavity, pelvic inlet is framed by ilium, and the perineum by pubic arch. **B.** Greater and lesser pelvis and perineum are color coded. **C.** Peritoneal cavity and extraperitoneal pelvic cavity and perineum with their contents are shown. The anatomic isocenters for the seven different primary sites are shown in (**D**) coronal and (**E**) sagittal views with primary sites presented from cephalad to caudad at specific transverse levels related to vertebrae. (1) Iliac crest. (2) Iliac fossa. (3) Anterior superior iliac spine. (4) Ilium. (5) Pubis. (6) Ischium. (7) Sacral promontory. (8) Sacrum. (9) Coccyx. (10) Acetabulum. (11) Ischial spine. (12) Pubic tubercle. (13) Pubic symphysis. (14) Ala of ilium. (15) Lesser pelvis (pelvic cavity). (16) Perineum. (17) Greater brim. (18) Pelvic brim. (19) Pelvic diaphragm (levator ani muscle). (20) Iliopsoas muscle. (21) Parietal abdominal fascia. (22) Obturator internus muscle. (23) Pudendal canal. (24) Peritoneum. (25) Visceral pelvic fascia. (*continued*)

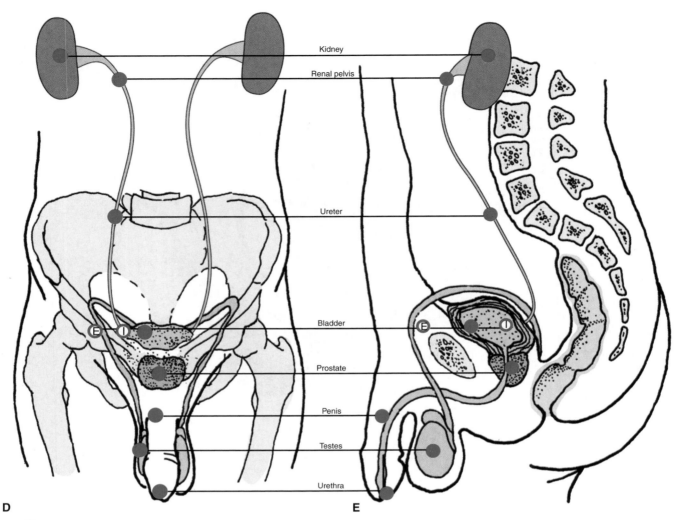

E External iliac inguinal node

I Internal iliac obturator node

Figure 35.4 *(Continued)*

TABLE 35.2	**Orientation of Three-planar T-oncoanatomy Nexi**			
Primary Site	**Coronal**	**Sagittal**	**Transverse**	**Axial Level**
Renal parenchyma and renal pelvis	Renal pelvis, artery and vein	12th rib	Lesser omental sac	T12–L3
Ureter	Adrenal, liver, spleen	Major/minor calyces	Quadratus lumborum	L1–S4
Urinary bladder	Pancreas	Psoas muscle	Pubis	S3–S5
Prostate	Primary Large and small intestine	Prostate, seminal vesicles, rectum	Prostatic plexus	Cx Coccyx
Testes	Prostate trigone	Bladder	Denonviere fascia	Femoral head
Penile	Bladder seminal vesicles, levator ani muscle Peritoneal layers within scrotum Corpus Spongiosum and cavernosum	Rectum Vas deferens Inguinal canal Prostate	Hilum, epididymis Corpus Spongiosum and cavernosum	Pubis Femoral Neck — —

MGU tract includes highly vascular organs, placing them at high risk for hematogenous dissemination.

The MGU are in the true pelvis in juxtaposition to the alimentary system. The orientation three-dimensional/three-planar diagram is presented in from cephalad to caudad, with the kidney ranging from T12 to L3, the ureters from L3 to S4, and the urinary bladder from S3 to S5. The prostate is at the coccyx and the penis and testes are outside the bony pelvis and are perineal structures.

- The *kidney* is encased by a fibrous capsule and is surrounded by perinephric fat. The kidney is composed of the cortex, which includes glomeruli, convoluted tubules; and the medulla, which consists of the pyramids of converging tubules and the loops of Henle. The exterior two thirds of the kidney substance is the cortex in contrast to the inner third, which is the medulla. The medulla contains 8 to 18 striated pyramids that send fingerlike rays into the cortex and end in the minor calices. The minor calices unite and form the major calices, which drain into the renal pelvis. The hilus of the kidney has the pelvis, ureter, renal artery and veins, nerves, and lymphatics.

   There are many structures that overlie the kidney; however, they are of little concern oncologically because the peritoneal lining essentially excludes the visceral structures it contains from direct invasion. Nevertheless, it is important to recognize the intimate relationships of the stomach on the left and the duodenum on the right, and the location of the hepatic and splenic flexures of the colon in relationship to the midportions of the kidneys. The lung overlies the upper poles of both kidneys due to the low insertion of the diaphragm, particularly during deep inspiration. One should be aware of the position of the pancreas, particularly of its head and tail and in regard to the right and left hila of the kidneys, respectively.

- The *renal bed* consists of renal fascia, which overlies the psoas major muscle and the quadratus lumborum musculature. The superior poles of both kidneys also lie in contact with the diaphragm. Usually, the 12th rib overlies the superior portion of the kidneys and is the only bone that is intimate anatomically. The kidney also lies opposite the transverse processes of T12 to L3.

- The course of the *ureter* is such that it is first crossed anteriorly by the renal artery and vein and then the testicular artery and vein in the male or the ovarian artery and vein in the female. In its continued descent retroperitoneally, the ureter passes anterior to the major iliac vessels. Before its insertion in the bladder, the vesical arteries and veins as well as the uterine artery and vein pass anteriorly to the ureter ("water under the bridge"). There are considerable variations in the anatomic relationships of the renal ureters with renal arteries and veins owing to normal anatomic variations of embryologic development that lead to different locations of the kidneys. In addition, anomalies in their development are common and include multiple renal arteries, fetal lobulations of the kidney, deflected and bifid ureters and pelves, and horseshoe and pelvic kidneys.

   The urinary bladder is the major collecting organ of urine. It is central to the anatomy and function of the urologic tract. The location of the bladder is inside the true pelvis when empty; however, it is an abdominal organ when full. It relates to the pubic bone and musculature of the anterior abdominal wall and to the levator ani muscle laterally and inferiorly, and to the content of the peritoneal cavity superiorly. The bladder's location requires knowledge of adjacent genital structures and disease. Symptomology depends, in some part, on gender. The relationship of the ureters to surrounding blood vessels is important. The bladder is not a fixed structure, but has considerable capacity and mobility altering its contour contact with the colointestinal viscera as it fills with urine.

- The *urinary bladder* is a hollow viscus consisting of three layers: the mucosa and submucosa, the muscularis, and the serosa. The thickness of the wall depends on whether the bladder is expanded or contracted. In the male, the bladder is intimately related to the seminal vesicles posteriorly, the prostate inferiorly, and the pubis and peritoneum anteriorly. The seminal vesicles are situated between the bladder and the rectum. In the female, the vagina and cervix are located posteriorly to the bladder and the body of the uterus superiorly. The bladder is extraperitoneal, although the sigmoid colon and terminal portions of the ileum can be in contact with its superior surface intraperitoneally.

- The *prostate gland* is in the central location of the male pelvis and anatomically is positioned similar to the cervix in the female pelvis. The prostate gland, the largest accessory sex gland, is divided into several morphologic and functional zones. It consists of 30 to 50 tubuloalveolar glands arranged in three concentric layers: inner mucosal, an intermediate submucosal, and the peripheral layer containing the main prostatic glands.

- The peripheral zone corresponds to the main prostatic gland, constitutes 70% of glandular tissue, and gives rise to the majority of cancers. This is the most palpable part of the gland, which has a sulcus and feels bilobed after the major internal branching of the glands.

- The central zone contains less glandular tissue and is more resistant to both inflammation and cancer.

- The transitional zone contains the mucosal glands and this zone has a tendency to undergo extensive division or hyperplasia, forming benign nodular

TABLE 35.3	Primary Cancer Sites and Sentinel Nodes		
Cancer Type	**Axial Level**	**Adjacent Anatomic Structure/Site**	**Sentinel Nodes (Assigned Number)**
Renal adenocarinoma	T12–L3	Kidney, renal artery and vein, adrenal, pancreas, liver, spleen	Renal hilar (1), paracaval (2), and para-aortic (3) nodes
Renal pelvis transitional cell cancer	L1–S5	Abdominal contents	Renal hilar (1), paracaval (2), and para-aortic (3) nodes
Ureteral transitional cell cancer	L1–L5	Small and large intestine	Paracaval (2), para-aortic (3), and common iliac (4) nodes
Urinary bladder transitional cell cancers	S5	Prostate, distal, ureters	Common iliac (4) and internal iliac (6a) nodes
Prostate adenocarcinomas	Coccyx	Rectum, bladder, ureters	Internal (6) iliac, obturator (6'), and sacral (4) nodes
Penile squamous cell cancer		Scrotum, testes, dorsal vein, periprostatic venous plexus	Inguinal nodes, superficial (8) and deep (7), femoral (9) nodes
Testicular cancer		Vas deferens and inguinal canal	Left renal hilar (1) and right paracaval (2) nodes

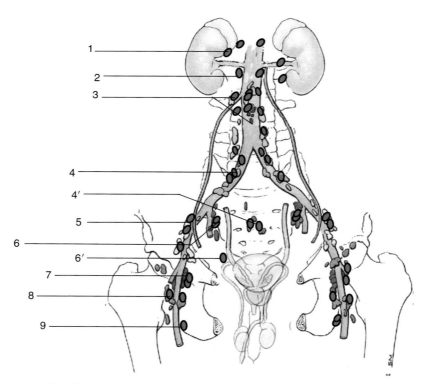

Figure 35.5 **Orientation of N-oncoanatomy.** The lymphoid drainage of the major MGU organs in the male pelvis overlap. Lymphatic drainage of the ureters, urinary bladder, prostate, and urethra and lymphatic drainage of the testis, deferent duct, prostate, and seminal vesicles. (1) Renal hilar. (2) Renal pelvis and ureter. (3) Para-aortic and paracaval. (4) Common iliac. (4') Presacral. (5) External iliac. (6) Internal iliac. (6') Obturator. (7) Deep inguinal. (8) Superficial inguinal. (9) Femoral.

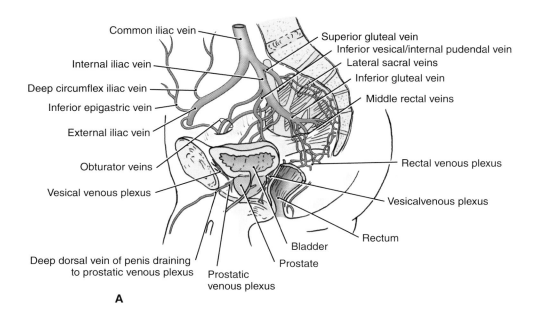

Common iliac vein
Internal iliac vein
Deep circumflex iliac vein
Inferior epigastric vein
External iliac vein
Obturator veins
Vesical venous plexus
Deep dorsal vein of penis draining
to prostatic venous plexus
Prostatic
venous plexus
Prostate
Bladder
Rectum
Vesicalvenous plexus
Rectal venous plexus
Middle rectal veins
Inferior gluteal vein
Lateral sacral veins
Inferior vesical/internal pudendal vein
Superior gluteal vein

A

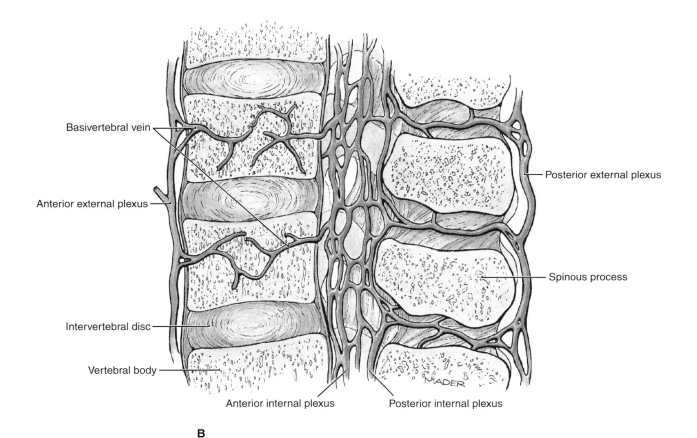

Basivertebral vein
Anterior external plexus
Intervertebral disc
Vertebral body
Anterior internal plexus
Posterior internal plexus
Spinous process
Posterior external plexus

MADER

B

Figure 35.6 **Orientation of M-oncoanatomy.** **A.** The pelvic veins and venous plexuses. **B.** Vertebral venous plexus (Batson's).

masses of epithelial cells. This benign prostate hyperplasia (BPH) produces difficulty voiding, but is not the site of most malignant transformations.

* The periurethral zone contains mucosal and submucosal glands and may participate in BPH.

The prostate is firmly fixed in position by a dense capsule and ligamentous attachments. The urethra courses from the base of the bladder to the bulb of the penis. The cortical structure of the prostate's apex is directed below the perineum. Its flat base touches the base of the bladder, which has no fascia separating these two sites. Thus, the bladder is prone to direct invasion by prostate cancers as they advance. Posteriorly, Denonvillier fascia separates the prostate gland from the rectum and acts as a major resistance to tumor invasion because it is composed of obliterated layers of the peritoneal cavity that extend downward. The ductus vas deferens and the seminal vesicles lie posterior to the bladder. They drain into the ejaculatory duct, which has the diameter of a lead pencil.

The *penis* is not a common cancer site and neoplasms tend to locate around the glans or foreskin. It is considered to be associated with sexually transmitted papilloma virus and may frequently be manifested with partners who have cervical cancers. Penile cancers are squamous or basal cell.

Urethral cancers are more rare and tend to arise from the prostate urethral epithelium. Such malignancies can arise in females as well as males, but are quite rare.

The *testis* is a favored site for malignant disease in young adults, predominantly male, but account for only 1% of all male malignancies. Undescended testes (cryptorchidism) is a predisposing situation and is often corrected by puberty to avoid spermatogonia degeneration. A large variety of tumor types exist because of the germ cell origin and their different paths of differentiation and maturation. Two main categories are commonly noted: Seminoma and nonseminoma, which include embryonal cancer and teratocarcinomas. The regional nodes are not regional and their para-aortic location can be traced back to the gubernaculums during embryologic development when the testes are abdominal organs.

The *scrotum* also contains the vas deferens and its surrounding capsule, which includes all the layers of the abdominal wall, which extend and envelope the testis. The muscular and fascial scrotal wall surrounding the testes is an extension of the anterior abdominal wall with similar layers of fascia and muscle.

Orientation of N-oncoanatomy: Regional Lymph Nodes

The renal hilar nodes are the first involved and the renal lymphatics then follow the renal vein and enter paracaval and para-aortic nodes. Nodes in the retroperitoneal area inferior to the kidney are considered distant metastatic. Renal pelvis and ureters are similar except that pelvic nodes are considered regional nodes (Table 35.3 and Fig. 35.5).

The spermatic lymphatic collecting ducts on the right side tend to follow the vascular components of the spermatic cord and drain into the paracaval lymph nodes in the area where the spermatic vein enters the inferior vena cava and the artery arises from the aorta. The spermatic lymphatic collecting ducts on the left side also tend to follow the vascular components of the cord and drain into the para-aortic nodes in the region where the spermatic and the inferior mesenteric arteries arise out of the aorta and into the nodes of the left renal hilum in the region where the left spermatic vein joins the left renal vein. Juxtaregional nodes are those of the pelvis but mediastinal and supraclavicular nodes are metastatic (Fig. 35.5).

The bladder's rich lymphatic network of numerous small anterior vesical lymph nodes drains into three major routes: (i) the trigone, (ii) posterior and lateral walls, and (iii) anterior wall trunks. The regional or pelvic lymph nodes, located below the bifurcation of the common iliac arteries include the internal iliacs, the hypogastric, the common iliac located above the pelvic basin, and the lateral, sacral, and anterior perivesicular nodes. The juxtaregional lymph nodes are the inguinal nodes, the high common iliac nodes, and the para-aortic nodes. The vessels, nerves, and lymphatics lie on the inner wall of the true pelvis, below the pelvic rim on the obturator muscle.

The regional nodes are true pelvis nodes for the prostate gland. The lymphatic drainage of the prostate gland is to the obturator node, which is the sentinel node in the hypogastric or internal iliac chain. The obturator node is in the true pelvis, located alongside the obturator blood vessels and is not in the medial chain of the external iliac chain in the false pelvis. The confusion is due to the projection in an anteroposterior pelvis radiograph, where the location of the obturator node appears to lie in a medial position but is actually posterior in the sagittal plane to the external iliac nodes, which are more anterior.

In addition, there is a rich network of lymphatics that drain into internal and external iliac nodes along the superior rectal veins and a posterior sacral trunk, which drains directly into para-aortic nodes. The nerves of the prostate are derived from the pelvic sympathetic plexuses.

M-oncoanatomy

Regional Veins Each of the MGU organs has a distinct pattern of dissemination dictated in part by its anatomic location and in part by its venous drainage (Fig. 35.6).

* *Kidney*: Renal cancers are highly vascular and may invade directly into the renal vein and into the inferior vena cava. They most often spread to the lung, extending into the heart as a tumor thrombus.

TABLE 35.4	Imaging Modalities for Staging Prostate Cancer	
Method	**Diagnosis and Staging Capability**	**Recommended for Use**
Primary (T) Staging		
TRUS	Accurate for tumor localization but not for assessing T stage	Routine use for guiding biopsies of the prostate gland
CTe	Not useful for stage T1–T3 disease but for evaluation of stage T4 disease (e.g., bladder, rectum invasion)	Recommended only for patients with clinically suspected stage T3–T4 disease
MRI	Probably the most accurate technique available for assessing T stage, anatomy well shown	May be cost effective in evaluating patients at intermediate and high clinical risk of having extraprostatic disease
MRS	An adjunct to MRI for improved tumor localization and staging	Under investigation; early results useful as a helpful adjunct to MRI
Nodal (N) staging		
CTe	Excellent for detecting enlarged nodes >1 cm vs. large blood vessels	Yes, less expensive and time consuming than MRI
MRI	Excellent if node is replaced by cancer; yields positive intense signal	Yes, but more expensive and time consuming than CTe
Metastases (M) staging		
Bs-Tc	Identifies bone metastases	Recommended for patients with PSA >10 ng/mL, Gleason score >8, or clinical stage T3–T4 disease
CT-Ch	Identifies hematogenous or lymphatic metastases to chest, more sensitive than chest radiograph	May be used to confirm abnormal findings on the chest radiograph or to evaluate patients with pulmonary symptoms
CT-Ab	Identifies hematogenous metastases to liver, abdominal viscera or lymphatic metastases to para-aortic lymph nodes	Not cost effective in the evaluation of patients with PSA <20 ng/mL because of low yield of abnormal studies
CT-Pv	Identifies invasion of adjacent organs (i.e., bladder, rectum, pelvic sidewall)	Not cost effective in patients with PSA <20 ng/mL or clinical stage T1–T2 because of low yield of abnormal studies
PET	May increase the sensitivity for detecting lymph node and visceral metastases	Under investigation; early results show promise

BS-Tc, bone scintigraphy; CT, computed tomography; CTe, CT enhanced with IV contrast; CT-Ab, abdominal CT; CT-Ch, chest CT; CT-Pv, pelvic CT; MRI, magnetic resonance imaging; MRS, magnetic resonance spectroscopic imaging; PET, positron emission tomography; TRUS, transrectal ultrasound.
Modified from Bragg DG, Rubin P, Hricak H, eds. *Oncologic Imaging*. 2nd ed. Philadelphia: Elsevier; 2002:579.

- *Bladder*: Cancers tend to be locally invasive and recur locally and metastasize late. Lymphatic spread is more frequent than distant metastases.
- *Prostate*: The veins are branches of the rectal (hemorrhoidal) and inferior vesical veins. The thin-walled veins are set inside and outside the prostatic capsule forming a plexus of prostatic-vesical veins. Prostate cancers preferentially seek bone. The osteoblastic distribution of metastases is largely confined to pelvic and vertebral bones and has been attributed to the Batson's vertebral venous plexus link to the periprostatic plexus.

- *Testes*: The spermatic artery and vein on the right side drains directly into the inferior vena cava. On the left side, it drains into the renal vein. This causes a higher pressure gradient in the left spermatic vein, which leads to a slight dilatation of the pampiniform venous plexus that accounts for the lower lying position of the left testicle as compared with the right. The testes target the para-aortic lymph nodes and then the mediastinal nodes.
- *Penis*: The dorsal vein of the penis drains into the periprostatic and perivesicular plexus and then the internal iliac vein whereas the scrotum drains into

TABLE 35.5	Male Genital and Urinary Systems: Cancer Statistics				
			5-Year Survival Rates (%)		
Site	Incidence	Mortality	1950	2000	Gain
Prostate	232,090	30,350	43	99	**+56**
Testis	8,010	390	57	96	**+39**
Penis and associated structures	1,470	270	—	—	**—**
Urinary bladder	63,210	13,180	53	82	**+29**
Kidney	36,160	12,660	34	64	**+30**
Ureter	2,510	750	—	—	**—**

Modified from American Cancer Society. *Cancer Facts and Figures 2005*. Atlanta: American Cancer Society; 2005:18.

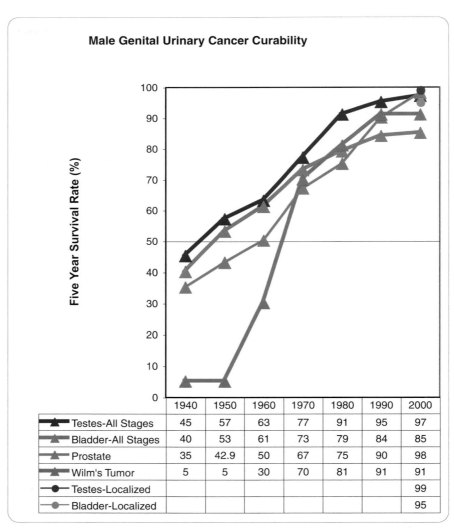

Figure 35.7 **Trajectory of cancer survival for MGU organs:** Prostate, bladder, testes, and Wilms tumor.

TABLE 35.6	Cancer Curability by Stages at Diagnosis (1995–2001)			
	5-Year Survival Rates (%)			
Site	All Stages	Local	Regional	Distant
Prostate	97	**100**	50	34
Testis	95	**99**	95	74
Urinary Bladder	82	**94**	48	6
Kidney	62	**90**	60	9

Modified from Ries LAG, Eisner MP, Kosary CL, et al., eds. *SEER Cancer Statistics Review, 1975–2001.* National Cancer Institute. Bethesda, MD. Available: http://seer.cancer.gov/csr/1975_2001/, 2004; Tables XI, XXIII, XXV, XXVII.

the external iliac via the femoral and inguinal venous branches (Fig. 35.6).

Rules of Classification and Staging

Clinical Staging and Imaging

Clinical examination is limited and reliance on imaging is critical to properly stage cancer of the male genitourinary tract. Fortunately, modern imaging is superb and includes computed tomography (CT), magnetic resonance imaging (MRI), and selective arteriography. If the primary tumor is a renal parenchymal cancer, CT of chest for lung and mediastinal nodal metastases is advised. An intravenous pyelogram and routine laboratory studies are worthwhile. Bone scans are essential for suspected osseous metastases (Table 35.4).

With radiologic imaging, the prostate's four compartments are visualized, the peripheral zone, the central zone, a transitional zone, and the periurethral zone. MRI allows for appreciating their relationship in axial, sagittal, and coronal views. The peripheral zone houses the majority of the branching tubuloalveolar glands and gives rise to 70% of adenocarcinomas, the submucosal glands in the central zone account for 10%, and transitional zone of mucosal glands 20% of cancers. The imaging procedures for the prostate gland adenocarcinoma serves as a model for the MGU because it is by far the commonest cancer.

Pathologic Staging

Careful assessment of resected primary tumor should be done with appropriate lymph nodes. All specimens should be carefully studied for clear margins.

Oncoimaging Annotations

- Cross-sectional imaging is essential in staging and treatment guidance.
- Although the reported staging accuracy for CT and MRI is similar, CT is used as a primary imaging approach; MRI complements CT and is most useful in defining the presence and extent of intravenous tumor extension.
- Doppler ultrasonography is also recommended for the evaluation of vascular invasion.
- Pretreatment use of chest radiography versus chest CT is controversial. The use of chest CT is recommended when there is vascular tumor extension, the patient has chest symptoms, or a suspicious nodule is seen on the chest film.

Cancer Statistics and Survival

The MGU constitutes almost half of all malignancies in males. Malignancies of the male genital system are dominated by prostate cancer accounting for approximately 350,000 new cancers and the urinary system for almost another 100,000 patients. Cancer deaths have been dramatically reduced but prostate cancer still claims 30,000 lives as does bladder cancer at 26,000.

When considered together, the MGU are the major sites of malignancy. Prostate cancer alone accounts for 200,000 new patients annually. There are 100,000 new urinary tract cancers and two and half fold more of male genital cancers: 250,000 cases annually (Table 35.5).

The most dramatic gains in survival are due to multidisciplinary approaches to both diagnosis and detection and a transdisciplinary attack on MGU cancer. Reviewing the last 50 years, prostate cancer 5-year survival rates improved by 50%, testes 39%, urinary bladder, kidney, and renal pelvis 30%. Even more impressive are the MGU survival rates for stage I localized cancers, all 90% to 100% curable according to latest Surveillance Epidemiology and End Results data: kidney, 90%; bladder, 94%; testis, 99%; and prostate, 100%. These 5-year results are plotted in Figure 35.7 and Table 35.6. The pediatric Wilms' tumor of the kidney was the first solid malignancy cured by combining modalities in childhood neoplasms achieving >90% long-term survival along with Hodgkin disease at around 70%. The reversal of a death sentence for these pediatric tumors is strikingly plotted in Figure 35.7. Equally important are improvements of quality of life owing to organ function preservation of the majority of prostate cancer patients.

36

Kidney: Renal Cancer

In the more advanced stages, the staging features relate to the patterns of spread to the surrounding anatomy and, to a degree, criteria of resectability.

Perspective and Patterns of Spread

Renal cancers are of obscure etiology. Painless hematuria is the most common symptom, but by itself is nonspecific and can occur with other genitourinary tumors. An estimated 20,000 new cases are diagnosed annually, 40% of whom are destined to die. *An unusual aspect of this highly angioinvasive malignancy is its ability to metastasize widely and its peculiarity to undergo spontaneous regression.* It has triggered intensive investigation into both specific and nonspecific immunobiologic effects for diagnostic and therapeutic purposes. The challenge to contain and cure this neoplasm remains unmet.

In contrast, Wilms tumor was the first pediatric success story of the multimodal era. A very unique neoplasm of the renal parenchyma, the nephroblastoma is most often seen in children. Abdominal mass is the presenting complaint, and there is a tendency to develop metastases. *There have been interesting hypotheses developed relating Wilms tumor to doubling times and cancer curability using mathematical modeling.* The addition of effective chemotherapy to radiation therapy and extirpative surgery stimulated the combined modality approach to other pediatric and adult tumors. Within three decades, this relatively incurable malignancy has become 90% curable through carefully organized clinical trials. More effective treatment has become less intensive to reduce toxicity and late effects in the process of optimization. Currently, therapy reduction tailored to each stage of the tumor's advancement is under study in clinical protocols.

Renal adenocarcinomas arise in the renal parenchyma mainly from the proximal renal tubule in contrast with to transitional cell cancers from the renal pelvis and its intrarenal collecting system. Their incidence ratio is 90% to 10%, respectively. A number of different histopathologic types of renal cancer have been identified with subtypes clear cell and granular cell or a mixture (Table 36.1).

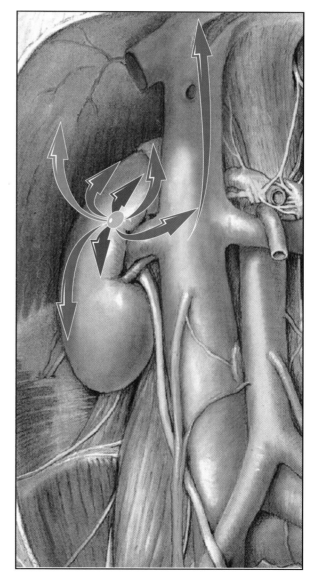

Figure 36.1 **Patterns of spread (cancer crab) of renal cancer are color-coded for stage:** T0, yellow; T1, green; T2, blue; T3, purple; and T4, red.

DEFINITION OF TNM

STAGE GROUPINGS

T1
Tumor ≤7 cm in greatest dimension, limited to the kidney
(T1a) Tumor ≤4 cm in greatest dimension, limited to the kidney
(T1b) Tumor >4 cm but not >7 cm in greatest dimension, limited to the kidney

N0
No regional lymph node metastasis

T2
Tumor >7 cm in greatest dimension, limited to the kidney

N0
No regional lymph node metastasis

T3
Tumor extends into major veins or invades adrenal gland or perinephric tissues but not beyond Gerota's fascia
(T3a) Tumor directly invades adrenal gland or perirenal and/or renal sinus fat but not beyond Gerota's fascia
(T3b) Tumor grossly extends into the renal vein or its segmental (muscle-containing) branches, or vena cava below the diaphragm
(T3c) Tumor grossly extends into vena cava above diaphragm or invades the wall of the vena cava

N1
Metastasis in a single regional lymph node

T4
Tumor invades beyond Gerota's fascia

N2
Metastasis in >1 regional lymph node

Stage I
T1 N0 M0

Stage II
T2 N0 M0

Stage III
T1	N1	M0*
T2	N1	M0*
T3	N0	M0*
T3	N1	M0
T3a	N0	M0*
T3a	N1	M0
T3b	N0	M0
T3b	N1	M0
T3c	N0	M0*
T3c	N1	M0*

Stage IV
T4	N0	M0*
T4	N1	M0*
Any T	N2	M0
Any T	Any N	M1

* not illustrated

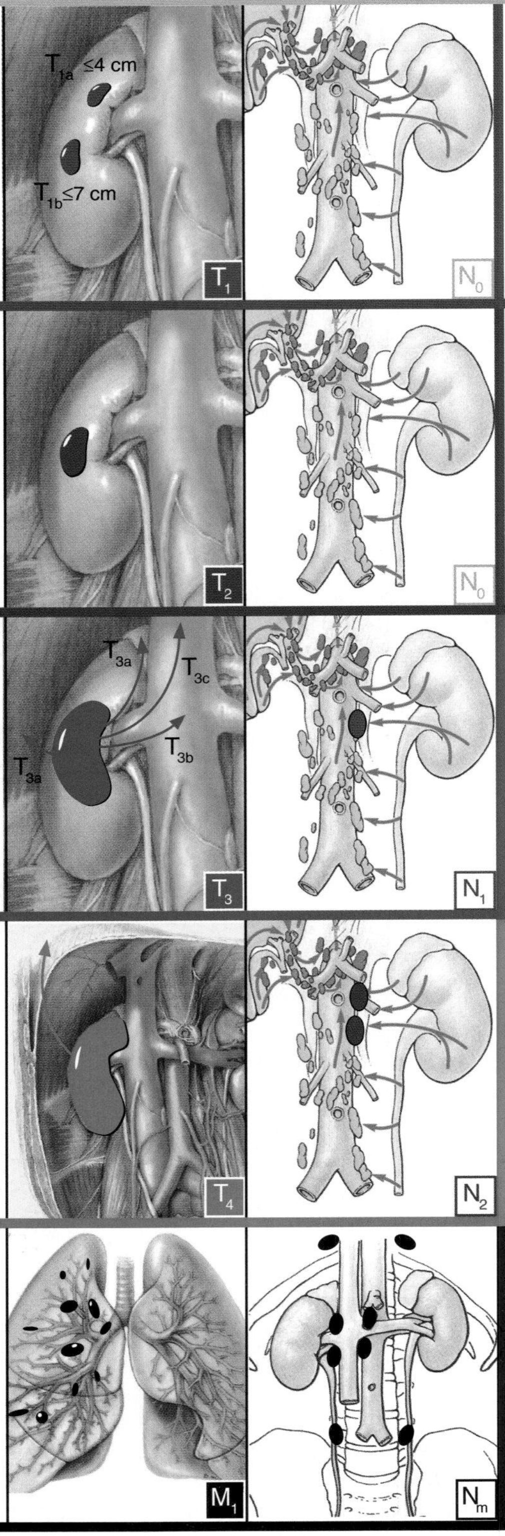

Figure 36.2 TNM renal cancer diagram. Renal cancers are well vascularized, when invasive stage III T3a, 3b, 3c, (purple) are resectable, stage IV (red) T4 are unresectable and stage IV is also metastatic. Vertically arranged with T definitions on left and stage groupings on right. Color bars are coded for stage: Stage I, green; II, blue; III, purple; IV, red; and metastatic, black.

TABLE 36.1	Histopathologic Type: Common Cancers of the Kidney

Type

Conventional (clear cell) renal carcinoma	Collecting duct carcinoma
Papillary renal cell carcinoma	Unclassified
Chromophobe renal carcinoma	

Adapted from Rubin P, Williams J, eds. *Clinical Oncology: A Multidisciplinary Approach for Physicians and Students.* 8th ed. Philadelphia: Elsevier; 2001:524.

In the early stages, tumor size is the dominant criterion for renal cancer (Fig. 36.1) whereas in the more advanced stages, the staging features relate to the patterns of spread to the surrounding anatomy and, to a degree, criteria of resectability.

TNM Staging Criteria

In the early stages, tumor size is the dominant criterion for renal cancer (Fig. 36.1) whereas in the more advanced stages, the staging features relate to the patterns of spread to the surrounding anatomy and, to a degree, criteria of resectability. The TNM staging has been undergoing subtle changes reflecting the advances of imaging hypernephromas because the radiologic appearance is virtually pathognomic. Renal cancers show a supervascularity when computed tomography (CT) with contrast is used, that is characteristic when compared to cysts. Initially in the first to third editions (1978–1980), T1 was distinguished from T2 by absence of deformity in contour of pelvis calyces structures and T3 from T4 by a medial venous spread to the renal vein and/or renal pelvis invasion compared to lateral spread through the renal capsule into perirenal fat versus penetrating to Gerota fascia. With the fourth edition in 1992, the tumor size and more specific patterns of invasion were defined to modify stage III into substages A/B/C (Fig. 36.2).

T2 tumors measure >7 cm and are limited to the kidney or have no renal capsule invasion. T3 cancers are subdivided according to patterns of spread. Once the renal capsule is penetrated, T3a means the cancer has spread into perirenal fat laterally or adrenal gland superiorly. T3b cancers invade medially into renal vein and inferior vena cava and T3c cancers extend into the vena cava above diaphragm. T4 cancer applies to posterior and lateral invasion beyond Gerota fascia. With a few exceptions, stage reflects the primary categories.

Summary of Changes

Stage I has been divided into tumor sizes of (a) ≤4 cm and (b) 4 to 7 cm limited to the kidney. The evidence has been compelling based on the excellent survival and low recurrence rate of partial nephrectomy for T1a. Based on surgical series, T1a patients had similar outcomes with nephron-sparing surgery rather than nephrectomies.

Orientation of Three-planar Oncoanatomy

The isocenter of kidney is the renal bed, which consists of Gerota fascia, which overlies the psoas major muscle and the quadratus lumborum musculature. The superior poles of both kidneys also lie in contact with the diaphragm. Usually, the 12th rib overlies the superior portion of the kidneys and is the only bone that is intimate anatomically. The kidney also lies opposite the transverse processes of T12 to L3 (Fig. 36.3).

T-oncoanatomy

- *Coronal*: There are many structures that overlie the kidney; however, they are of little concern oncologically because the *peritoneal lining essentially excludes the visceral structures it contains from direct invasion.* Nevertheless, it is important to recognize the intimate relationships of the stomach on the left and the duodenum on the right, and the location of the hepatic and splenic flexures of the colon in relationship to the midportions of the kidneys. The lung overlies the upper poles of both kidneys owing to the low insertion of the diaphragm, particularly during deep inspiration. One should be aware of the position of the pancreas, particularly of its head and tail and in regard to the right and left hila of the kidneys, respectively (Fig. 36.4). The course of the ureter is such that it is first crossed anteriorly by the renal artery and vein and then the spermatic artery and vein in the male or the ovarian artery and vein in females. In its continued descent retroperitoneally, the ureter passes anterior to the major iliac vessels.
- *Sagittal*: The kidney is encased by a fibrous capsule and is surrounded by perinephric fat. The kidney is composed of the cortex, which includes glomeruli, convoluted tubules, and the medulla, which consists

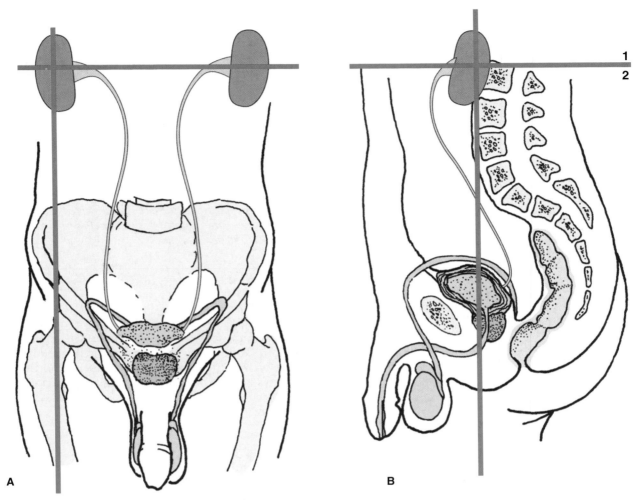

Figure 36.3 Orientation of T-oncoanatomy. The anatomic isocenter for three-planar anatomy of kidney is at the T12 to L3 level. **A.** Coronal. **B.** Sagittal.

of the pyramids of converging tubules and the loops of Henle. *The exterior third of the kidney substance is the cortex in contrast to the inner two thirds, which is the medulla.* The medulla contains 8 to 18 striated pyramids that send finger-like rays into the cortex and end in the minor calices. The minor calices unite and form the major calices that drain into the renal pelvis. *The hilus of the kidney has the pelvis, ureter, and renal artery and veins.*

- *Transverse*: *Before its insertion in the bladder, the vesical arteries and veins as well as the uterine artery and vein pass anteriorly to the ureter ("water under the bridge").* There are considerable variations in the anatomic relationships of the renal ureters with renal arteries and veins owing to normal anatomic variations of embryologic development that lead to different locations of the kidneys. In addition, anomalies in their development are common and include multiple renal arteries, fetal lobulations of the kidney, deflected and

bifid ureters and pelves, and horseshoe and pelvic kidneys.

N-oncoanatomy

The regional nodes are anterior to and surround the renal artery and vein and at the midline, para-aortic and paracaval in location. It is important to note *the left testis drains to the left hilar area of the kidney and the right testis drains to paracaval nodes at the lower pole on the right*. The cisterna chyli is located on the right side near the upper pole.

There are considerable variations in the anatomic relationships of the renal ureters with renal arteries and veins owing to normal anatomic variations of embryologic development that lead to different locations of the kidneys. In addition, anomalies in their development are common and include multiple renal arteries, fetal lobulations of the kidney, deflected and bifid ureters

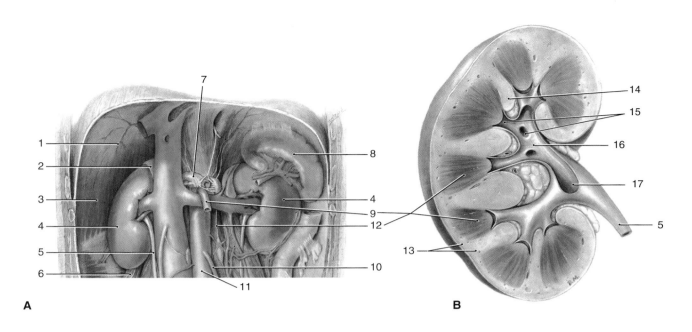

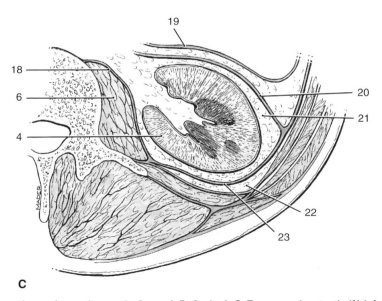

Figure 36.4 **T-oncoanatomy three-planar views.** **A.** Coronal. **B.** Sagittal. **C.** Transverse (see text). (1) Inferior vena cava. (2) Suprarenal (adrenal) gland. (3) Diaphragm. (4) Kidney. (5) Ureter. (6) Psoas muscle. (7) Celiac ganglion. (8) Spleen. (9) Superior mesenteric artery. (10) Inferior mesenteric artery. (11) Aorta. (12) Renal pyramids. (13) Renal cortex. (14) Renal columns. (15) Minor calix. (16) Major calix. (17) Renal pelvis. (18) Psoas fascia. (19) Peritoneum. (20) Renal fascia (anterior layer). (21) Perirenal fat. (22) Pararenal fat. (23) Renal fascia (posterior layer).

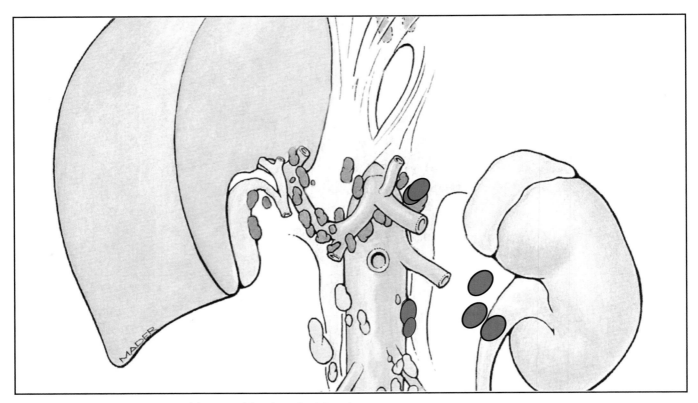

Figure 36.5 N-oncoanatomy: Renal (para-aortic) and renal pelvis and ureter.

and pelves, and horseshoe and pelvic kidneys (Fig. 36.5; Table 36.2).

M-oncoanatomy

Common metastatic sites reflect the vascular drainage of the kidney. As noted in the patterns of spread, invasion in the renal vein and inferior vena cava is common. Pulmonary spread is very common. With continued circulation of tumor cells through the left heart, metastases to bone, brain, and liver become possible. Unfortunately, *remote metastases frequently occur with this tumor owing to the rich neovascularization.*

Renal pelvis transitional cell cancers are characterized similarly to transitional cell cancers of uroepitheleum of bladder in their ability to "seed" throughout the urinary tract. Endoscopic assessment is important to determine when renal pelvis cancer is a primary or part of a disseminated urological cancer (Fig. 36.6).

TABLE 36.2	Lymph Nodes of Kidney	
Sentinel nodes		Juxtaregional nodes
Renal hilar		Common iliac
Paracaval		External iliac
Para-aortic		
Regional nodes		Metastatic nodes
Renal vein (left)		Mediastinal
Para-aortic (high infrarenal a.)		Left supraclavicular
Para-aortic (high suprarenal a.)		
Para-aortic low		
Lateral caval (right)		

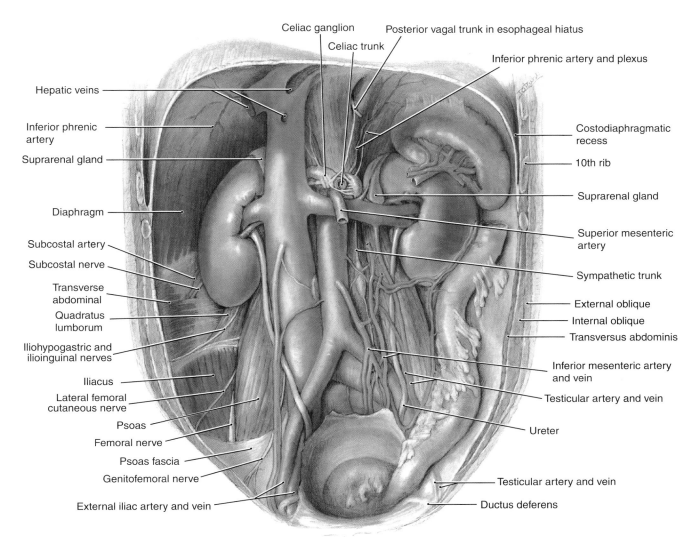

Celiac ganglion

Celiac trunk

Posterior vagal trunk in esophageal hiatus

Inferior phrenic artery and plexus

Hepatic veins

Inferior phrenic artery

Suprarenal gland

Diaphragm

Subcostal artery

Subcostal nerve

Transverse abdominal

Quadratus lumborum

Iliohypogastric and ilioinguinal nerves

Iliacus

Lateral femoral cutaneous nerve

Psoas

Femoral nerve

Psoas fascia

Genitofemoral nerve

External iliac artery and vein

Costodiaphragmatic recess

10th rib

Suprarenal gland

Superior mesenteric artery

Sympathetic trunk

External oblique

Internal oblique

Transversus abdominis

Inferior mesenteric artery and vein

Testicular artery and vein

Ureter

Testicular artery and vein

Ductus deferens

Figure 36.6 **M-oncoanatomy:** Renal venous drainage.

Rules of Classification and Staging

Clinical Staging and Imaging

Clinical examination is limited and reliance on imaging is critical. Fortunately, modern imaging is superb and includes CT, magnetic resonance imaging (MRI), and selective arteriography. If the primary tumor is advanced, CT of chest for lung and mediastinal nodal metastases is advised. An intravenous pyelogram and routine laboratory studies are worthwhile (Table 36.3).

Pathologic Staging

Careful assessment of resected primary which includes primary tumor, kidney, appropriate lymph nodes contained within the renal (Gerota's) fascia, perinephric fat and renal vein/artery. Partial nephrectomy needs careful study for margins.

Oncoimaging Annotations

- Renal carcinomas are more conspicuous in the CT nephrogram phase than in the early arterial or corticomedullary phase of imaging.

- Cross-sectional imaging is essential in staging and treatment guidance.

- Although the reported staging accuracy for CT and MRI is similar, CT is used as a primary imaging approach; MRI complements CT and is most useful in defining the presence and extent of intravenous tumor extension.

- Doppler ultrasonography is also recommended for the evaluation of vascular invasion.

- Pretreatment use of chest radiography versus chest CT is controversial. The use of chest CT is recommended when there is renal-vascular tumor

TABLE 36.3	Imaging Modalities for Staging Renal Cancer	
Method	Diagnosis and Staging Capability	Recommended for Use
Primary (T) staging		
CTe	Most accurate cross-sectional imaging and with IV contrast during vascular phase appears as hypervascular lesion and a decrease in attenuation in nephrogram and excretory phase	Yes, advantage is detecting renal cancer neovascularization
MRI	Plays a complimentary role to CT and with gadolinium hypernephromas appear hyperintense on T1 and T2	Yes
TAUS	Renal cancers appear as large hypoechoic masses and can guide biopsy	No
Nodal (N) staging		
CTe	Identifies nodal metastases at hilum of kidney	Yes, recommended only for patients with clinically suspected stage T3–T4 disease
MRI	Better for detecting gross vascular invasion than nodes	Yes, may be cost effective in evaluating patients at intermediate and high clinical risk of having extrarenal disease
Metastases (M) staging		
CT-Ch	Identifies hematogenous or lymphatic metastases to chest, more sensitive than chest radiograph. Liver metastases can also often be evaluated.	Yes, may be used to confirm abnormal findings on the chest radiograph or to evaluate patients with pulmonary symptoms
PET	May increase the sensitivity for detecting lymph node and visceral metastases	No, under investigation; early results show promise

CT, computed tomography; CTe, CT enhanced with IV contrast; CT-Ch, chest CT; MRI, magnetic resonance imaging; PET, positron emission tomography; TAUS, transabdominal ultrasound.

extension, the patient has chest symptoms, or a suspicious nodule is seen on the chest film.

Cancer Statistics and Survival

When considered together, the genital and urinary system in males are the major sites of malignancy. Prostate cancer alone accounts for 200,000 new patients annually. There are 100,000 new urinary tract cancers and 2.5-fold more of male genital cancers: 250,000 cases annually (see Table 35.5).

The dramatic gains in survival are due to multidisciplinary achievements in screening, early detection, precise diagnoses, and effective multimodal therapies. The

TABLE 36.4	Cancer Curability by Stages at Diagnosis (1995–2001)			
	5-Year Survival Rates (%)			
Site	All Stages	Local	Regional	Distant
Prostate	100	100	—	34
Testis	96	99	96	72
Urinary bladder	82	94	48	6
Kidney	**65**	**91**	**60**	**10**

Modified from Ries LAG, Eisner MP, Kosary CL, et al., eds. *SEER Cancer Statistics Review, 1975–2002.* Bethesda, MD: National Cancer Institute. Available: http://seer.cancer.gov/csr/1975_2002; Tables XI-4, XXIII-4, XXV-4, XXVII-4.

cancer statistics are revealing of perhaps the greatest gains in survival in oncology over the past five decades. In local stage I, male genitourinary tumors are 90% to 100% curable according to the latest Surveillance Epidemiology and End Results data: Kidney, 90%; bladder, 94%; testes, 99%; and prostate, 100% (Table 36.4).

Death and mortality rates are declining. The pediatric Wilms tumor was the first malignancy in childhood to be cured, achieving >90% long-term survival and heralded the success of multimodal treatment that would be achieved in adult tumors in urology (see Fig. 35.7).

37

Renal Pelvis and Ureters

Multifocality is a significant attribute of cancers of the renal pelvis and ureter.

Perspective and Patterns of Spread

Multifocality is a significant attribute of cancers of the renal pelvis and ureter. Once a cancer appears and progresses, the issue of seeding versus field cancerization is a concern. The probability of an associated bladder cancer reaches 75% if both the renal pelvis and ureter have lesions versus half that with single cancers. Smokers and analgesic abusers (phenacetin) are at risk. The majority of cancers are transitional cell (90%); the rest are squamous cell cancers often associated with chronic inflammation or infection of the renal pelvis (Table 37.1). Adenocarcinomas are extremely rare. Gross hematuria is the presenting sign in most patients (75%–90%), with the associated triad of flank mass, pain, and hematuria occurring in fewer than one fifth (20%) of patients. The diagnosis is readily made with either intravenous or retrograde urography and the absence of the usual abundant tumor neovascularization suggest renal pelvic cancer. The issue of multifocal disease is addressed on surgical resection; that is, nephrectomy with total ureterectomy including a cuff of the urinary bladder. Isolated ureteral cancers are rare (1%) and predominate in males (2:1).

The renal pelves is akin to a hollow structure with a thin wall. The pattern of spread is into the muscle wall and then through the wall into the peripelvic fat and periureteral junction. As it advances, the renal parenchyma may be invaded. Seeding into the ureters and bladder are quite common (Fig. 37.1).

TNM Staging Criteria

Cancers of the renal pelvis and ureters were distinguished in the fourth edition and have followed the tradition of staging hollow organs, similar to the digestive system (Fig. 37.2); that is, depth of renal pelvis wall invasion rather than size.

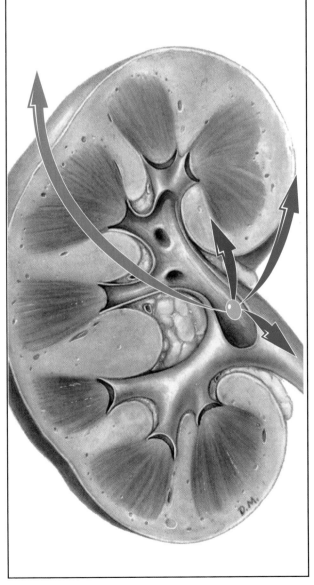

Figure 37.1 **Patterns of spread (cancer crab) of renal pelvis and ureter cancer are color coded for stage:** Tis or Ta, yellow; T1, green; T2, blue; T3, purple; and T4, red.

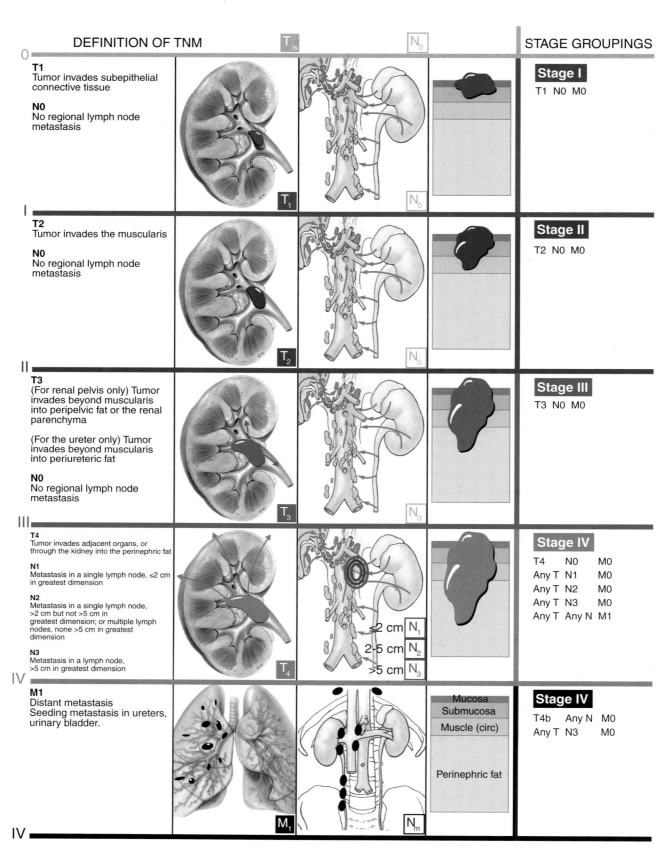

DEFINITION OF TNM

T1
Tumor invades subepithelial connective tissue

N0
No regional lymph node metastasis

T2
Tumor invades the muscularis

N0
No regional lymph node metastasis

T3
(For renal pelvis only) Tumor invades beyond muscularis into peripelvic fat or the renal parenchyma

(For the ureter only) Tumor invades beyond muscularis into periureteric fat

N0
No regional lymph node metastasis

T4
Tumor invades adjacent organs, or through the kidney into the perinephric fat

N1
Metastasis in a single lymph node, ≤2 cm in greatest dimension

N2
Metastasis in a single lymph node, >2 cm but not >5 cm in greatest dimension; or multiple lymph nodes, none >5 cm in greatest dimension

N3
Metastasis in a lymph node, >5 cm in greatest dimension

≤2 cm N1
2-5 cm N2
>5 cm N3

M1
Distant metastasis
Seeding metastasis in ureters, urinary bladder.

Mucosa
Submucosa
Muscle (circ)
Perinephric fat

STAGE GROUPINGS

Stage I
T1 N0 M0

Stage II
T2 N0 M0

Stage III
T3 N0 M0

Stage IV
T4   N0   M0
Any T N1   M0
Any T N2   M0
Any T N3   M0
Any T Any N M1

Stage IV
T4b   Any N M0
Any T N3   M0

Figure 37.2 **TNM renal pelvis and ureter cancer diagram:** Renal pelvis cancers and ureteral cancers are often detected early and resectable when confined Stages I, II or minimal penetrations of their walls into perinephric fat Stage III (purple) with extensive invasion Stage IV (red) they become unresectable as well as become metastic by seeding out. Vertically arranged with T definitions on left and stage groupings on right. Color bars are coded for stage: Stage Tis or Ta, yellow; I, green; II, blue; III, purple; IV, red; and metastatic, black.

TABLE 37.1	Histopathologic Type: Common Cancers of the Renal Pelvis and Ureter
Type	
Urothelial (transitional cell) carcinoma	Epidermoid carcinoma
Squamous cell carcinoma	Adenocarcinoma

Adapted from Greene FL, Page DL, Fleming ID, et al. eds. *AJCC Cancer Staging Manual.* 6th ed. New York: Springer; 2002:330.

Stage T1 cancer invades into subepithelial connective tissue and stage T2 cancer into the muscular layer. Stage T3 cancer invades into perinephric fat through the renal pelvis wall and T4 cancer invades into adjacent organs (Fig. 37.2).

The regional nodes are the same for renal cancers and renal pelvis cancers. However, their definitions are different in the fourth edition. In renal cancers, the major criterion is node number: N1 is single and N2 is multiple nodes. In contrast, in renal pelvis cancers, size of nodes is the critical criterion: N1 ≤2 cm; N2 2 to 5 cm, and N3 >5 cm. Although lymph node stages defined in the fourth edition were the same, they have diverged as noted for renal parenchymal versus renal pelvis cancers.

Summary of Changes

No changes have been made from the fifth edition of the AJCC CSM.

Orientation of Three-planar Oncoanatomy

The isocenter of renal cancer is the renal bed, which consists of renal (Gerota's) fascia, which overlies the psoas major muscle and the quadratus lumborum musculature. The superior poles of both kidneys also lie in contact with the diaphragm. Usually, the 12th rib overlies the superior portion of the kidneys and is the only bone that is intimate anatomically. *The kidney also lies opposite the transverse processes of T12 to L3 (Fig. 37.3).*

T-oncoanatomy

- *Coronal*: There are many structures that overlie the kidney; however, they are of little concern oncologically because the *peritoneal lining essentially excludes the visceral structures it contains from direct invasion.* Nevertheless, it is important to recognize the intimate relationships of the stomach, on the left and the duodenum, on the right, and the location of the hepatic and splenic flexures of the colon in relationship to the midportions of the kidneys. The lung overlies the upper poles of both kidneys owing to the low insertion of the diaphragm, particularly during deep inspiration. One should be aware of the position of the pancreas, particularly of its head and tail and in

regard to the right and left hila of the kidneys, respectively (Fig. 37.4).

- *Sagittal*: The kidney is encased by a fibrous capsule and is surrounded by perinephric fat. The kidney is composed of the cortex, which includes glomeruli; convoluted tubules; and the medulla, which consists of the pyramids of converging tubules and the loops of Henle. *The exterior third of the kidney substance is the cortex in contrast to the inner two thirds, which is the medulla.* The medulla contains 8 to 18 striated pyramids that send fingerlike rays into the cortex and end in the minor calices. The minor calices unite and form the major calices that drain into the renal pelvis. *The hilus of the kidney has the pelvis, ureter, renal artery, and veins.*

- *Transverse*: The ureteropelvic interface serves as the variable junction between pelvis and ureter, which courses inferiorly into the pelvis. The course of the ureter is such that it is first crossed anteriorly by the renal artery and vein and then the spermatic artery and vein in the male or the ovarian artery and vein in the female. In its continued descent retroperitoneally, the ureter passes anterior to the major iliac vessels. Before its insertion in the bladder, the vesical arteries and veins as well as the uterine artery and vein pass anteriorly ("water under the bridge") to the ureter. There are considerable variations in the anatomic relationships of he renal ureters with renal arteries and veins owing to normal anatomic variations of embryologic development that lead to different locations of the kidneys. In addition, anomalies in their development are common and include multiple renal arteries, fetal lobulations of the kidney, deflected and bifid ureters and pelves, and horseshoe and pelvic kidneys.

N-oncoanatomy

The regional nodes are anterior to and surround the renal artery and vein and at the midline, para-aortic and paracaval in location. It is important to note the left testis drains to the left hilar area of the kidney and the right testis drains to paracaval nodes at the lower pole on the right. The cisterna chyli is located on the right side near the upper pole.

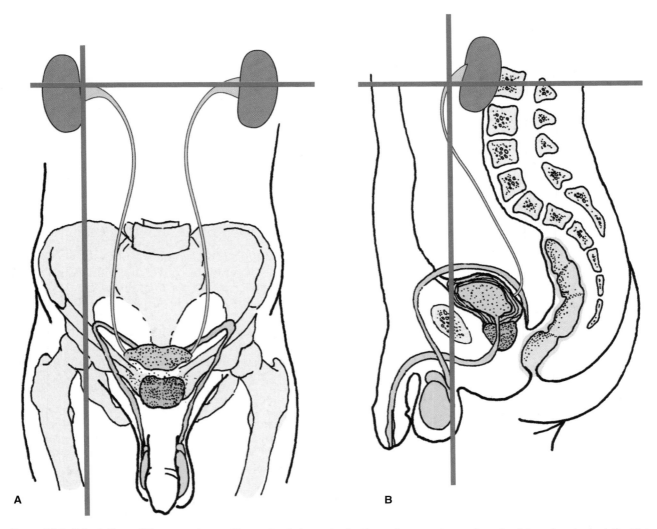

Figure 37.3 Orientation of T-oncoanatomy: The anatomic isocenter for three-planar anatomy of renal pelvis and ureter is at the L1 to S5 level. **A.** Coronal. **B.** Sagittal.

There are considerable variations in the anatomic relationships of the renal ureters with renal arteries and veins because of normal anatomic variations of embryologic development that lead to different locations of the kidneys. In addition, anomalies in their development are common and include multiple renal arteries, fetal lobulations of the kidney, deflected and bifid ureters and pelves, and horseshoe and pelvic kidneys (Fig. 37.5; Table 37.2).

M-oncoanatomy

Common metastatic sites reflect the vascular drainage of the kidney. As noted in the patterns of spread, invasion in the renal vein and inferior vena cava is common. Pulmonary spread is very common. With continued circulation of tumor cells through the left heart, metastases to bone, brain, and liver become possible. Unfortunately,

remote metastases frequently occur with this tumor because of its rich neovascularization.

Renal pelvis transitional cell cancers are characterized similarly to transitional cell cancers of uroepitheleum of bladder in their ability to "seed" throughout the urinary tract. Endoscopic assessment is important to determine when renal pelvis cancer is a primary or part of a disseminated urological cancer (see Fig. 36.6).

Rules of Classification and Staging

Clinical Staging and Imaging

Clinical examination is limited and reliance on imaging is critical. The intravenous or retrograde pyelogram are essential for diagnosis. Fortunately, modern imaging is superb and includes computed tomography

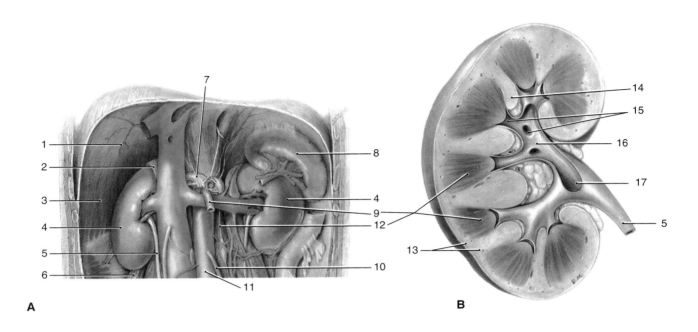

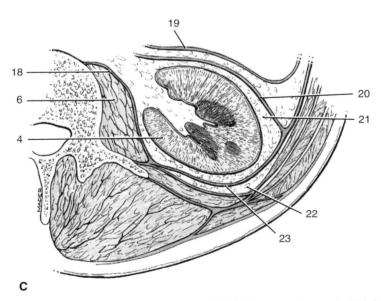

Figure 37.4 **T-oncoanatomy:** Three-planar views. **A.** Coronal. **B.** Sagittal. **C.** Transverse (see text). (1) Inferior vena cava. (2) Suprarenal (adrenal) gland. (3) Diaphragm. (4) Kidney. (5) Ureter. (6) Psoas muscle. (7) Celiac ganglion. (8) Spleen. (9) Superior mesenteric artery. (10) Inferior mesenteric artery. (11) Aorta. (12) Renal pyramids. (13) Renal cortex. (14) Renal columns. (15) Minor calyx. (16) Major calyx. (17) Renal pelvis. (18) Psoas fascia. (19) Peritoneum. (20) Renal fascia (anterior layer). (21) Perirenal fat. (22) Pararenal fat. (23) Renal fascia (posterior layer).

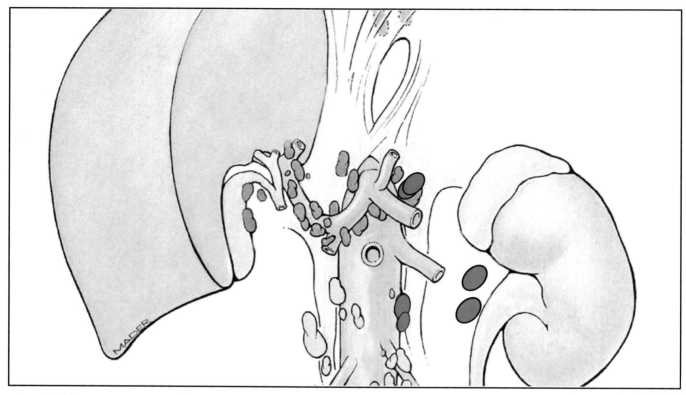

Figure 37.5 N-oncoanatomy: Renal (para-aortic) and renal pelvis and ureter.

(CT), magnetic resonance imaging and selective arteriography. If the primary tumor is advanced, CT of chest for lung and mediastinal nodal metastases is advised (Table 37.3).

Pathologic Staging

Careful assessment of resected primary tumor, including kidney, appropriate lymph nodes contained within renal (Gerota's) fascia, perinephric fat, and renal vein/artery, is necessary. Partial nephrectomy needs careful study for margins.

Oncoimaging Annotations

• Intravenous pyelography and retrograde studies are still considered to be the mainstay of transitional cell carcinoma imaging, but CT is slowly replacing conventional radiographic studies.

• In a patient with transitional cell carcinoma, staging by CT is recommended.

Cancer Statistics and Survival

When considered together, the male genital and urinary system are the major sites of malignancy. Prostate

TABLE 37.2	Lymph Nodes of Renal Pelvis and Ureters	
Pelvis and Ureters		
Sentinel nodes		Juxtaregional nodes
Renal hilar Paracaval Para-aortic nodes		External iliac Mediastinal
Regional nodes		Metastatic nodes
Renal hilar Para-aortic Common iliac Internal iliac		Supraclavicular

TABLE 37.3	Imaging Modalities for Staging Renal Pelvis and Ureter Cancer	
Method	**Diagnosis and Staging Capability**	**Recommended for Use**
Primary (T) staging		
Pyelography	Retrograde superior to IV for cancer confined to renal pelvis and ureters	Yes, cost effective and useful for diagnosis
CTe	Cross-sectional imaging superior for detecting extensions beyond renal pelvis (L3–L4) and into urinary bladder	Yes, most accurate for staging
MRI	Accurate for staging	No, unless CTe is not clear
Nodal (N) staging		
CTe-Abd	Identifies renal nodal metastases >1 cm and para-aortic nodes	Yes, cost effective; can also assess visceral metastases
Metastases (M) staging		
CTe-Abd	Accurate for detecting liver and visceral metastases	Yes, cost effective
PET	May increase the sensitivity for detecting lymph node and visceral metastases	No, under investigation

CT, computed tomography; CTe, CT enhanced with IV contrast; CTe-Abd, abdominal CTe; MRI, magnetic resonance imaging; PET, positron emission tomography.

cancer alone accounts for 200,000 new patients annually. There are 100,000 new urinary tract cancers and 2.5-fold more of male genital cancers: 250,000 cases annually.

The dramatic gains in survival are due to multidisciplinary achievements in screening, early detection, precise diagnoses, and effective multimodal therapies. The cancer statistics are revealing of perhaps the greatest gains in survival in oncology over the past five decades.

In local stage I, male genitourinary tumors, all are 90% to 100% curable according to the latest Surveillance Epidemiology and End Results data: Kidney, 90%; bladder, 94%; testes, 99%; and prostate, 100%. Mortality rates are declining. The pediatric Wilms' tumor was the first malignancy in childhood to be cured, achieving >90% long-term survival and heralded the success of multimodal treatment that would be achieved in adult tumors in urology.

38

Urinary Bladder

The uroepithelium is subject to numerous excretory products and responds with a proliferative process, often as a benign papilloma, which can become multiple covering most of the bladder epithelium representing a field carcinogenesis.

Perspective and Patterns of Spread

Bladder cancer is a neoplasm of the elderly, peaking at 60 to 80 years of age. Despite its highly varied gross appearance in the bladder, intermittent hematuria, either macroscopic or microscopic, is the major manifestation. Occasionally, it presents as a bladder infection with irritability and dysuria, particularly recurrent in character, that suggests some underlying pathology or tumor. This is the most frequent cancer of the urinary tract with an estimated 60,000 new cases reported annually. Bladder cancer accounts for 2.5% of all tumors or 13,000 cancer deaths annually. Although aniline dyes have been implicated as well as other industrial agents or some carcinogenic metabolite secreted in urine, no true cause of bladder cancer is known. Some infectious agents, however, such as *Schistosoma haematobium* have been implicated in Egypt, where the more commonly squamous cell cancer results (Table 38.1).

Worldwide, bladder cancer is among the most common malignancies, in 11th place. North Africa and western Asia are considered high-risk areas. Males predominate in a 3:1 ratio to females.

The uroepithelium is subject to numerous excretory products and responds with a proliferative process, often as a benign papilloma, which can become multiple covering most of the bladder epithelium representing a field carcinogenesis. The transformation to cancer depends on three criteria: Cell type, pattern of growth, and grading. The majority are transitional cell carcinomas that change from mucosal exophytic lesions (grade I) to endophytic invading into muscle (grades II–III). The patterns of spread are determined by muscular contraction of the bladder; as the tumor penetrates the wall, it spreads circumferentially. Squamous cell cancers are mainly associated with schistosomiasis. Primary adenocarcinomas tend to develop in the dome of the bladder often from urachal epithelium rests. The various cancers

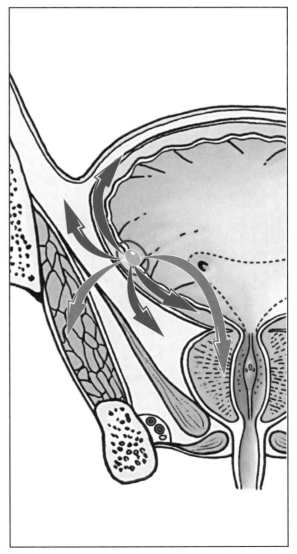

Figure 38.1 **Patterns of spread (cancer crab) of urinary bladder cancer are color coded for stage:** Tis or Ta, yellow; T1, green; T2, blue; T3, purple; T4, red; and metastatic, black.

DEFINITION OF TNM

STAGE GROUPINGS

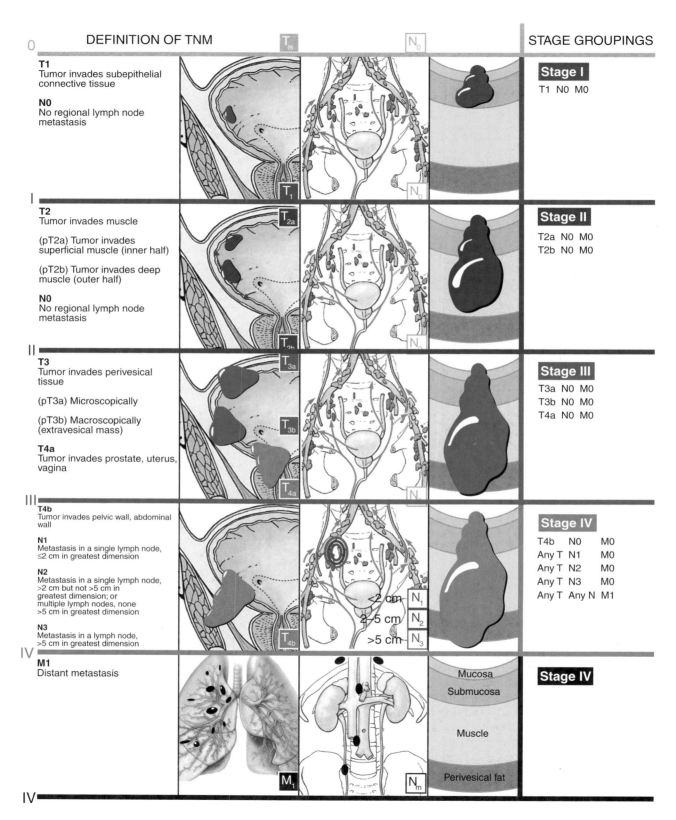

T1
Tumor invades subepithelial connective tissue

N0
No regional lymph node metastasis

Stage I

T1 N0 M0

T2
Tumor invades muscle

(pT2a) Tumor invades superficial muscle (inner half)

(pT2b) Tumor invades deep muscle (outer half)

N0
No regional lymph node metastasis

Stage II

T2a N0 M0
T2b N0 M0

T3
Tumor invades perivesical tissue

(pT3a) Microscopically

(pT3b) Macroscopically (extravesical mass)

T4a
Tumor invades prostate, uterus, vagina

Stage III

T3a N0 M0
T3b N0 M0
T4a N0 M0

T4b
Tumor invades pelvic wall, abdominal wall

N1
Metastasis in a single lymph node, ≤2 cm in greatest dimension

N2
Metastasis in a single lymph node, >2 cm but not >5 cm in greatest dimension; or multiple lymph nodes, none >5 cm in greatest dimension

N3
Metastasis in a lymph node, >5 cm in greatest dimension

Stage IV

T4b   N0   M0
Any T N1   M0
Any T N2   M0
Any T N3   M0
Any T Any N M1

M1
Distant metastasis

Mucosa
Submucosa
Muscle
Perivesical fat

Stage IV

Figure 38.2 **TNM urinary bladder cancer diagram:** Urinary bladder cancers can be solitary but are often multiple in a field of epithelial carcinogenesis. Stage I (green) papillomas are conservatively resected transurethrally, Stage II (blue) with partial cystectomies, Stage III (purple) require total cystectomy and urethral diversion, Stage IV (red) are no longer completely resectable. Vertically arranged with T definitions on left and stage groupings on right. Color bars are coded for stage: Stage 0is and 0a, yellow; I, green; II, blue; III, purple; IV, red; and metastatic, black.

TABLE 38.1	Histopathologic Type: Common Cancers of the Bladder

Type

Urothelial (transitional cell) carcinoma
    In situ
        Papillary
        Flat
        With squamous metaplasia
        With glandular metaplasia
        With squamous and glandular metaplasia
        Squamous cell carcinoma

Adenocarcinoma

Undifferentiated carcinoma

Adapted from Greene FL, Page DL, Fleming ID, et al., eds. *AJCC Cancer Staging Manual.* 6th ed. New York: Springer; 2002:337.

of the urinary bladder are tabulated (Table 38.1) and their grading is noted.

The pattern of spread is into its wall and then its surrounding structures (Fig. 38.1).

TNM Staging Criteria

In their initial phase, bladder cancers tend to be multiple, superficial mucosal, and submucosal lesions (stage T1; Fig. 38.2). With invasion into the muscular wall (T2), the tumor spreads, first in depth and then, circumferentially in the submucosal and muscular lymphatics. *There is a relationship between depth of invasion and circumferential spread; the tumor infiltration in the wall is massaged due to the contractility of this viscus.* The capacity of the bladder to expand and contract is altered somewhat as the tumor invades its walls. *When circumferential spread is extensive (T2B) akin to linitis plastica of the stomach, a permanently contracted bladder results with little capacity.*

Once the tumor reaches the serosal surface, invasion of perivesical fat (T3) and adjacent structures occurs (T4). Anteriorly, it can become fixed to, but rarely destroys, the bony pubis; laterally, the cancer can extend to the pelvic wall and invades lymphatics and enlarged pelvic lymph nodes can compress the iliac vessels. Direct posterior invasion into the rectum rarely occurs in the male; the same is true of direct invasion of posterior gynecological structures in females. This pattern of invasion is more representative of late or recurrent disease.

Tumors of the trigone usually result in ureteral obstruction owing to the entry of the ureters at this juncture. If secondary infection and edema cause the obstruction, it may be reversible. Once unilateral obstruction of the ureter occurs, hydronephrosis results; if unrelieved, the kidney stops functioning and atrophies. Secondary infection may lead to an ascending pyelonephritis and septicemia. Bilateral obstruction can result in renal failure and uremia.

Summary of Changes

No changes have been made from the fifth edition of the AJCC CSM.

Orientation of Three-planar Oncoanatomy

The isocenter for the urinary bladder varies depending on its fullness or when it is empty. Most often it is depicted empty and as a pelvic organ at the S4/S5 level (Fig. 38.3).

T-oncoanatomy

The bladder's location requires knowledge of adjacent genital structures and disease. Symptomology depends, in some part, on gender (Figs. 38.4 and 38.5: Male and Female).

- *Coronal: In the male, the bladder is intimately related to the seminal vesicles posteriorly, the prostate inferiorly, and the pubis and peritoneum anteriorly.*

- *Sagittal:* The relationship of the ureters to surrounding blood vessels is important. *The bladder is not a fixed structure, but has considerable capacity and mobility, altering its contour and contact with the colointestinal viscera as it fills with urine.* The bladder is a retroperitoneal structure, whereas the GIT is intraperitoneal except for the rectum.

- *Transverse*: The seminal vesicles are situated between the bladder and rectum. *In the female, the vagina and cervix are located posterior to the bladder and the body of the uterus, superiorly.* The bladder is extraperitoneal, although the sigmoid colon and terminal portions of the ileum can be in contact with its superior surface.

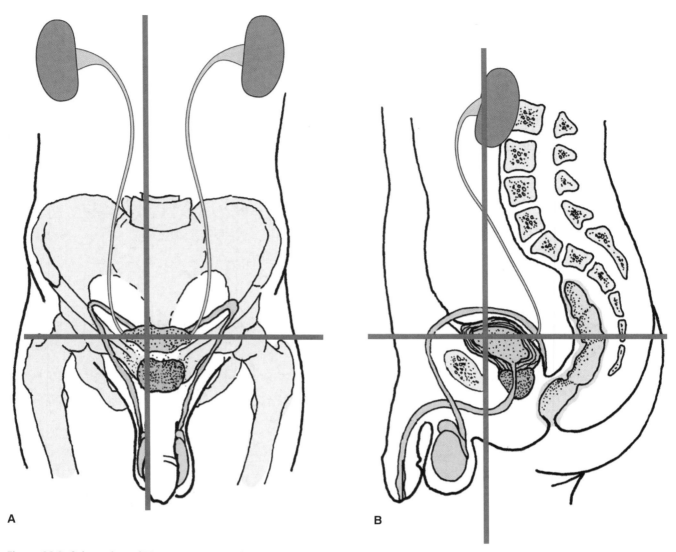

Figure 38.3 **Orientation of T-oncoanatomy:** The anatomic isocenter for three-planar anatomy of renal pelvis and ureter is at the S1 to S5 level. **A.** Coronal. **B.** Sagittal.

In the female, the bladder is intimately related to the uterus and vagina. The trigone of the bladder is in direct contact with on its posterior surface with the anterior lip of the cervix and anterior fornix of the vagina. The urethra is located in the anterior wall of the vagina. *Cancers of the bladder rarely invade the female genital tract, but cancers of the cervix infiltrate and invade the bladder.* The ureters, which have a horizontal course, straddle the cervix and are commonly strapped and obstructed by parametrial invasion.

- *Coronal view*: The opened bladder is situated above the pubis. The trigone and ureteral orifices are noted in the corners with the ureter coursing superiorly alongside the cervix. The uterus is anteflexed and rests on the bladder.

- *Sagittal view*: The bladder is anterior, the rectum posterior to the female genital organs.

- *Axial view*: The superior axial section shows the intimate relationship of cervix to the bladder wall. The inferior axial section shows the relationship of the urethra in the anterior wall of the vagina.

N-oncoanatomy

Lymph node invasion is common once the tumor has penetrated into the deep muscular layer and the serosa. *The lymph nodes most commonly involved are the obturator or hypogastric nodes and the internal iliacs on the pelvic wall.* All of these first station nodes are bilateral; however, the node at risk depends on the location of the primary tumor in the bladder. Eventually, invasion of the common

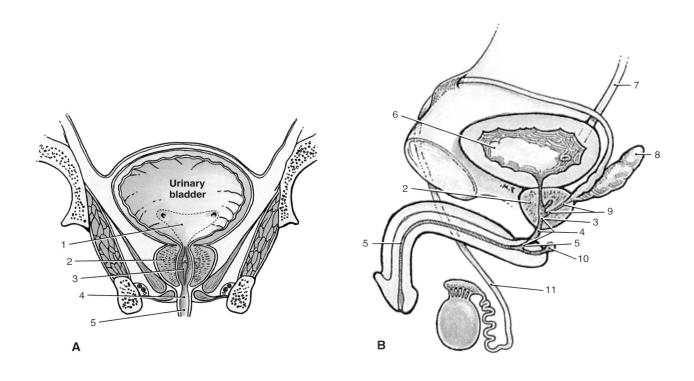

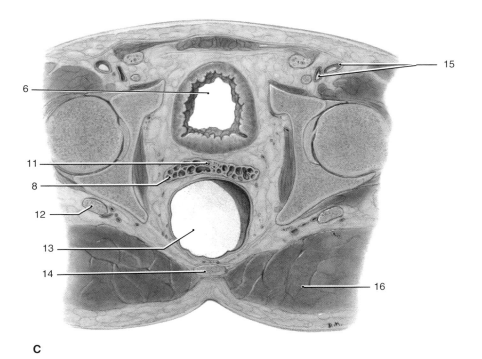

Figure 38.4 T-oncoanatomy. Male: Three-planar views. **A.** Coronal. **B.** Sagittal. **C.** Transverse (see text). (1) Trigone of bladder. (2) Prostate gland. (3) Prostatic urethra. (4) Membranous urethra. (5) Spongy urethra. (6) Urinary bladder. (7) Ureter. (8) Seminal vesicle. (9) Ejaculatory duct. (10) Bulbourethral gland. (11) Ductus deferens. (12) Sciatic nerve. (13) Rectum. (14) Coccyx. (15) Femoral nerve, artery, and vein. (16) Gluteus maximus.

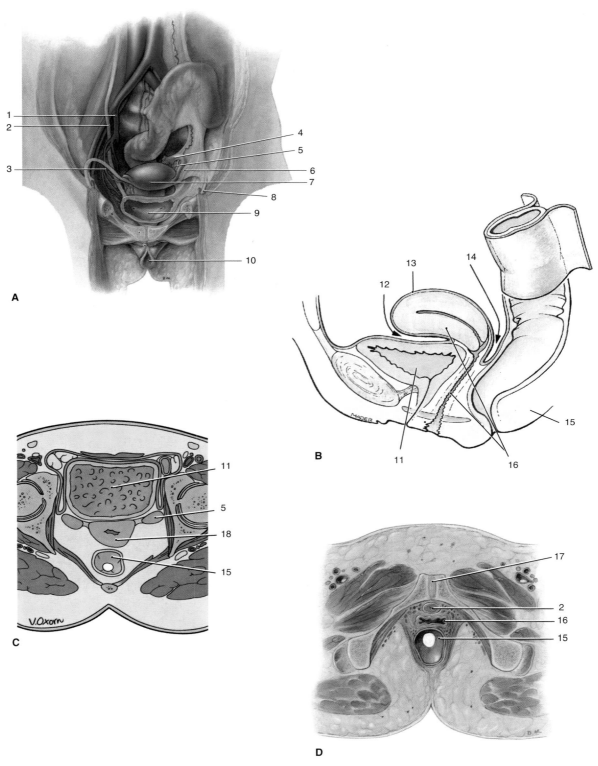

Figure 38.5 T-oncoanatomy. Female: Three-planar views. **A.** Coronal. **B.** Sagittal. **C.** Transverse superior axial (see text). **D.** Transverse inferior axial. (1) Internal iliac artery. (2) Ureter. (3) Uterine artery. (4) Uterine artery. (5) Ovary. (6) Broad ligament of uterus. (7) Fundus of uterus. (8) Round ligament of uterus. (9) Trigone of bladder. (10) Vestibule. (11) Urinary bladder. (12) Vesicouterine pouch. (13) Peritoneum on uterus. (14) Rectouterine pouch (of Douglas). (15) Rectum. (16) Vagina. (17) Pubic symphysis. (18) Uterus.

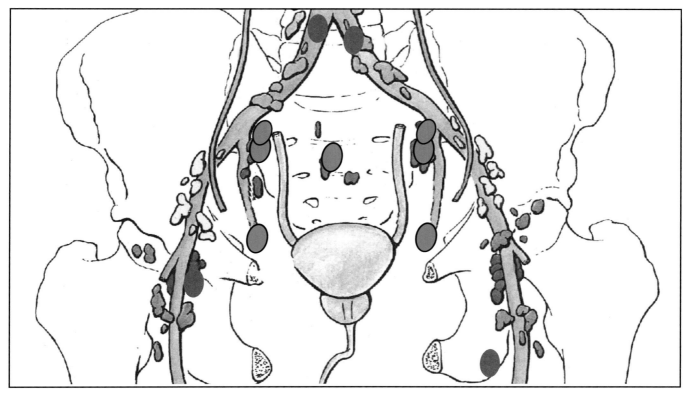

Figure 38.6 **N-oncoanatomy.** Male: Regional nodes are obturator and internal iliac nodes.

iliac and para-aortic retroperitoneal nodes occurs and drainage into the thoracic duct could naturally progress to supraclavicular node metastases; this is a rare presentation for a metastatic neck node with obscure etiology (Fig. 38.6, Table 38.2).

The regional or pelvic lymph nodes, located below the bifurcation of the common iliac arteries, include the internal iliacs, the hypogastric, the common iliac located above the pelvic basin, and the posterior, presacral, and anterior perivesical nodes. The juxtaregional lymph nodes are the inguinal nodes, the high common iliac, and the para-aortic nodes. The vessels, nerves, and lymphatics lie on

the inner wall of the true pelvis, below the pelvis basin on the obturator internus muscle.

In the female as in the male, the lymphatic drainage is to perivesical channels into the internal iliacs and to common iliac then para-aortic nodes.

M-oncoanatomy

Vascular spread, although uncommon, is usually a late event. *Dissemination follows the vesical veins into the internal iliac veins and inferior vena cava.* Tumor cells could reach the right side of the heart and then manifest themselves as pulmonary metastases. Once the left heart is

TABLE 38.2	Lymph Nodes of Urinary Bladder	
Sentinel nodes	Juxtaregional nodes
Common iliac Internal iliac nodes	Para-aortic
Regional nodes	Metastatic
Common iliac Internal iliac Anterior paravesical (obturator) External iliac Presacral	Inguinal

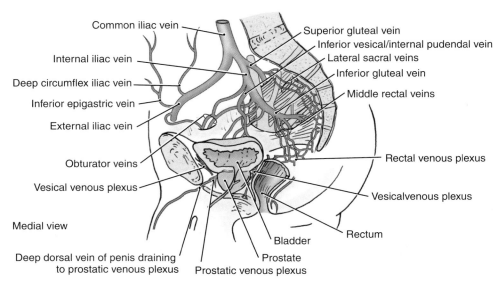

Common iliac vein
Internal iliac vein
Deep circumflex iliac vein
Inferior epigastric vein
External iliac vein
Obturator veins
Vesical venous plexus
Medial view
Deep dorsal vein of penis draining
to prostatic venous plexus
Prostatic venous plexus
Prostate
Bladder
Rectum
Vesicalvenous plexus
Rectal venous plexus
Middle rectal veins
Inferior gluteal vein
Lateral sacral veins
Inferior vesical/internal pudendal vein
Superior gluteal vein

Figure 38.7 **M-oncoanatomy.**

reached, the tumor cells could target to any other distant remote site (Fig. 38.7).

Rules of Classification and Staging

Clinical Staging and Imaging

Primary evaluation is done preferentially under anesthesia before and after endoscopic surgery providing histologic verification of depth of invasion. After transurethral resection, the bladder is palpated against the endoscope. No thickening in the wall suggests T1; some induration, T2. A thickened wall or mass suggests T3 and if fixed or massive, T4. Modern modalities or enhanced computed tomography (CT) and magnetic resonance imaging (MRI) are most useful; positron emission tomography is more investigational. Multiple biopsies are advised for field effect and presence of Tis. The entire urinary tract should be fully evaluated to exclude renal pelvis and ureters as sites of disease. Metastases workup should be considered for advanced stage bladder cancer (Table 38.3).

TABLE 38.3	Imaging Modalities for Staging Urinary Bladder Cancer	
Method	**Diagnosis and Staging Capability**	**Recommended for Use**
Primary (T) staging		
TAUS	More useful for detection than staging	No
CTe	Accurate for staging advanced T3, T4 invasion beyond bladder wall	Yes, cost effective
MRI	Provides most anatomic detail of cancer invasion into and beyond wall of urinary bladder	Yes, more accurate
Nodal (N) staging		
CTe	Valuable in assessing pelvic and para-aortic nodal enlargements	Yes, cost effective
MRI	More valuable in distinguishing adenopathy secondary to inflammation versus cancer	Yes, more cost effective
Metastases (M) staging		
Chest film	Can detect gross pulmonary or mediastinal metastases	Yes, cost effective
CT, computed tomography; CTe, CT enhanced with IV contrast; MRI, magnetic resonance imaging; TAUS, transabdominal ultrasound.		

Pathologic Staging

Following total cystectomy and pelvic node dissection, pathologic assessment of primary and nodes are feasible.

Oncoimaging Annotations

- Transabdominal ultrasonography can be used for bladder cancer surveillance, detecting 80% to 90% of tumors >5 mm in size.

- Virtual CT or MRI cystoscopy are being evaluated.

- Superficial bladder cancer (i.e., that which has not extended into the muscular layer of the bladder, stages T1 and below) is treated by transurethral resection.

- Muscle invasive bladder cancer, either alone (T2 or T3A) or with spread to the perivesical fat (T3B), to contiguous organs (T4), or to regional lymph nodes, requires radical surgical resection, often with radiotherapy.

- The critical distinction between superficial and muscle invasive bladder cancer is established by transurethral resection and not by imaging. Clinical staging is not accurate for advanced disease.

- Cross-sectional imaging using either CT or MRI aids the preoperative evaluation of locally advanced bladder cancer by demonstrating involvement of perivesical fat, invasion of contiguous organs, spread to the pelvic sidewall or anterior abdominal wall, or locoregional adenopathy.

- CT or MRI staging should be performed either before or 2 weeks after cystoscopy to minimize diagnostic errors and avoid misinterpretation.

- Both CT and MRI have a tendency to overestimate muscle and perivesical extension; both have excellent negative predictive value in excluding extravesical extension. MRI is superior to CT and transurethral ultrasonography in the evaluation of lesions located at the base or dome of the bladder.

- Differentiation of granulation tissue from persistent tumor after transurethral resection is better with MRI than CT, but limitations persist for both modalities.

Cancer Statistics and Survival

When considered together, the male genital and urinary systems are the major sites of malignancy. Prostate cancer alone accounts for 200,000 new patients annually. There are 100,000 new urinary tract cancers and 2.5-fold more of male genital cancers: 250,000 cases annually (see Table 35.5).

The dramatic gains in survival are due to multidisciplinary achievements in screening, early detection, precise diagnoses, and effective multimodal therapies. The cancer statistics are revealing of perhaps the greatest gains in survival in oncology over the past five decades. In local stage I, male genitourinary tumors, all are 90% to 100% curable according to the latest Surveillance Epidemiology and End Results data: kidney, 90%; bladder, 94%; testes, 99%; and prostate, 100%. Mortality rates are declining. The pediatric Wilms' tumor was the first malignancy in childhood to be cured, achieving >90% long-term survival and heralded the success of multimodal treatment that would be achieved in adult tumors in urology (Fig. 38.6; see also Fig. 35.7).

39
Prostate

The grading system widely adopted for tumor histology is the Gleason system of grading based on the summation of the tumor grade in the largest area and next larger area and has been incorporated into staging.

Perspective and Patterns of Spread

Prostate cancer has undergone a complete metamorphosis since the introduction of the widespread testing of males with prostate-specific antigen (PSA) blood tests in the mid 1980s. The diagnosis of prostate cancer is often made on needle biopsy transrectally guided by ultrasound. Adenocarcinomas of the prostate arise in the true gland and rarely begin in benign hyperplastic enlargements that usually occur around the prostatic urethra. Pathologically, cancers tend to be multifocal arising in the peripheral zone (90%), with only 1% from the central zone. The precursor lesion is often prostatic intraepithelial neoplasm. The grading system widely adopted for tumor histology is the Gleason system of grading based on the summation of the tumor grade in the largest area and next larger area and has been incorporated into staging. The Gleason grade ranges from 1 to 5 and sums range from 2 to 10; grades 7, 8, 9, and 10 are aggressive cancers (Table 39.1).

The patterns of spread are limited by location and by the capsule surrounding the gland (Fig. 39.1).

Most primary lesions invade the prostatic capsule first and then take the path of least resistance along the ejaculatory ducts into the space between the seminal vesicles and the bladder. The growth of the tumor outside the prostate is usually along the perivesical fascia, rather than directly into the seminal vesicles. If the local lesion has extensively invaded the seminal vesical area, then there is a 75% probability that the regional nodes are involved. Clinically, however, palpable induration in the seminal vesicle region may prove histologically to be an inflammation and not tumor extension; however, any enlargement needs to be considered neoplastic until proven otherwise. Early invasion of cancers from the prostate, directly into the bladder wall, distally into the membranous urethra, or along the vas deferens, beyond the seminal vesicles are rare. As the prostate enlarges, it elevates

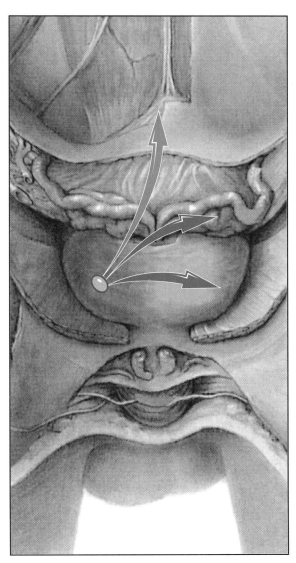

Figure 39.1 **Patterns of spread (cancer crab) of prostate cancer are color-coded for stage:** T0, yellow; T1, green; T2, blue; T3, purple; and T4, red; T1 is microscopic.

DEFINITION OF TNM

STAGE GROUPINGS

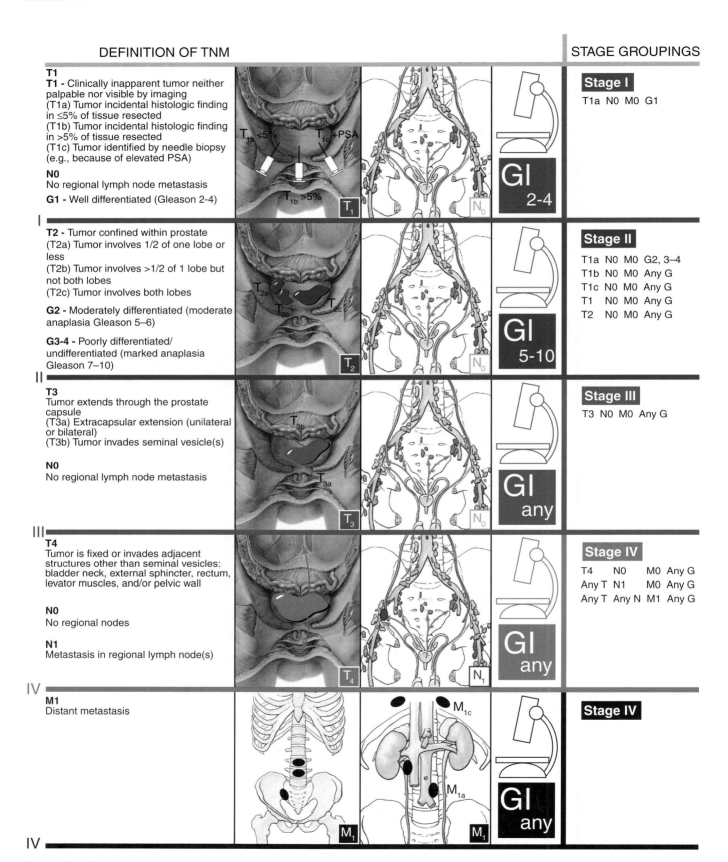

T1
T1 - Clinically inapparent tumor neither palpable nor visible by imaging
(T1a) Tumor incidental histologic finding in ≤5% of tissue resected
(T1b) Tumor incidental histologic finding in >5% of tissue resected
(T1c) Tumor identified by needle biopsy (e.g., because of elevated PSA)

N0
No regional lymph node metastasis

G1 - Well differentiated (Gleason 2-4)

Stage I
T1a N0 M0 G1

T2 - Tumor confined within prostate
(T2a) Tumor involves 1/2 of one lobe or less
(T2b) Tumor involves >1/2 of 1 lobe but not both lobes
(T2c) Tumor involves both lobes

G2 - Moderately differentiated (moderate anaplasia Gleason 5–6)

G3-4 - Poorly differentiated/ undifferentiated (marked anaplasia Gleason 7–10)

Stage II
T1a N0 M0 G2, 3–4
T1b N0 M0 Any G
T1c N0 M0 Any G
T1   N0 M0 Any G
T2   N0 M0 Any G

T3
Tumor extends through the prostate capsule
(T3a) Extracapsular extension (unilateral or bilateral)
(T3b) Tumor invades seminal vesicle(s)

N0
No regional lymph node metastasis

Stage III
T3 N0 M0 Any G

T4
Tumor is fixed or invades adjacent structures other than seminal vesicles: bladder neck, external sphincter, rectum, levator muscles, and/or pelvic wall

N0
No regional nodes

N1
Metastasis in regional lymph node(s)

Stage IV
T4   N0   M0 Any G
Any T N1   M0 Any G
Any T Any N M1 Any G

M1
Distant metastasis

Stage IV

Figure 39.2 TNM prostate cancer diagram. Vertically arranged with T definitions on left and stage groupings on right. Color bars are coded for stage: Stage I, green; II, blue; III, purple; IV, red; and metastatic, black.

TABLE 39.1	Histopathologic Type: Common Cancers of the Prostate

Type

Adenocarcinoma (>95%)
    Mucinous
    Small cell
    Papillary
    Ductal
    Neuroendocrine

Modified from Greene FL, Page DL, Fleming ID, et al., eds. *AJCC Cancer Staging Manual.* 6th ed. New York: Springer; 2002:311.

the bladder and pushes into the rectum. It seldom produces an encircling lesion that can lead to constipation. Perineural invasion is common and can lead to severe perineal and sacral pain as the sacral plexus is involved.

TNM Staging Criteria

When introduced in the first American Joint Committee on Cancer edition (1978), the system was based largely on physical examination: T1 was intracapsular, with normal gland surrounding the tumor; in T2, the capsule was invaded and gland contour deformed; in T3, tumor extended beyond the capsule into lateral sulcus; and in T4, it was fixed to neighboring structures. By the fourth edition (1992), subcategories were introduced for each stage and imaging techniques were allowed in the staging workup. In the fifth edition (1997), transrectal ultrasound (TRUS) allowed for more accurate tumor localization and guided needle biopsies. In the fifth and sixth editions, elevated PSA without identifiable or nonpalpable disease in normal glands but needle aspiration of microdeposits of cancer and was staged as T1C. Incidental microfoci, found in <5% of biopsied tissue is T1a; in T1b, >5%. T2 was subdivided by whether one or two lobes were involved. T3a was extracapsular spread, T3b was seminal vesicle involvement, and T4 was related to adjacent viscera being invaded, namely, bladder and more rarely the rectum. *The anatomic reason for either of these organ invasions or lack thereof is due to the absence of capsule where the prostate meets the urinary bladder, but the rectum is protected by a rudimentary fused cul de sac, Devonveilier fascia, between prostate and rectum, a virtually impenetrable barrier (Fig. 39.2).*

Summary of Changes

Most important is adding Gleason Grade. T2 lesions are divided into Ta unilateral, involving < one half of lobe, T2b > half of one lobe, Tc bilateral.

Orientation of Three-planar Oncoanatomy

The isocenter of the prostate is the central position in male pelvis oncoanatomy (Fig. 39.3). The prostate is positioned at the bladder neck. It is transversed by the proximal portion of the urethra, which is subject to compression and direct invasion. Once the cancer invades through the capsule, the common spread patterns are posteriorly, laterally, and/or superiorly. Lateral extension into the sulcus may lead to fixation of the gland to the lateral wall of the pelvis.

As the tumor extends superiorly, it invades into the seminal vesicle and it can block the ejaculatory ducts that transverse the substance of the gland. In its superior or anterior direction, a cancer can invade into the bladder because the capsular wall of the prostate thins and is in direct contact with its vesical muscular wall and lymphatics.

T-oncoanatomy

The prostate is both a glandular and a muscular organ that consists of four zones. It is firmly fixed in position by a dense capsule and ligamentous attachments. The urethra courses form the base of the bladder to the bulb of the penis. The cortical structure of the prostate's apex is directed below the perineum. Its flat base touches the base of the bladder. The lateral surfaces are convex, resting against the fascia of the levator ani muscles (Fig. 39.4).

- *Coronal: The prostate sits at the pelvic inlet and is surrounded by a number of distinct ligamentous structures as it rests along the levator ani muscles and on the sphincter urethrae muscle and its superior fascia.* The urogenital diaphragm along with the central tendon of the perineum (perineal body) and the deep perineal space, act as a distinct floor.

- *Sagittal*: This diaphragm separates the prostate gland from the bulb of the penis. Posteriorly, *Denonvillier fascia separates the prostate gland from the rectum* and acts as a major resistance to tumor invasion because it is composed of obliterated layers of the peritoneal cavity that extend downward.

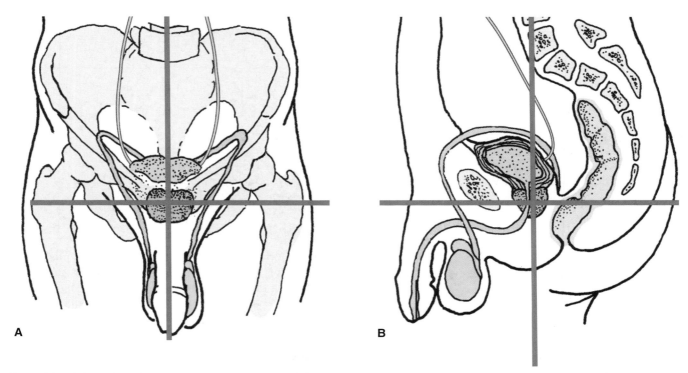

Figure 39.3 **Orientation of T-oncoanatomy.** The anatomic isocenter for three-planar anatomy of prostate is at the coccyx level. **A.** Coronal. **B.** Sagittal.

- *Transverse*: The prostate gland lies anterior to the rectum and is readily palpable. Transrectal imaging with ultrasound and biopsy is possible because of this anatomy. Note the prostatic venous plexus is rich anteriorly and communicates with the dorsal vein of the penis.

The ductus vas deferens and the seminal vesicles lie posterior to the bladder. They drain into the ejaculatory duct, which has the diameter of a lead pencil. The nerves of the prostate are derived from the pelvic sympathetic plexuses.

N-oncoanatomy

A rich lymphatic network exists with lateral drainage and posterior sacral trunk. In addition to the internal and external iliac lymph nodes, it is possible, because of the latter trunk, for prostate cancers to bypass pelvic lymph nodes and spread directly to retroperitoneal lymph nodes in the para-aortic region first. The most commonly involved lymph node is the obturator node. In addition, there is a rich network of lymphatics that drain into internal and external iliac nodes and along the superior hemorrhoidal veins and a posterior sacral trunk directly into para-aortic nodes (Fig. 39.5; Table 39.2).

M-oncoanatomy

The arteries are branches of the rectal (hemorrhoidal) and inferior vesical arteries. The thin-walled veins are

set inside and outside the prostatic capsule forming a plexus of prostatic-vesical veins. This rich plexus of veins surrounds the prostate and interconnects with the blood in the dorsal vein of the penis. These veins drain into another rich plexus of veins in addition to the internal iliac vein. *A rich anastomoses of intervertebral veins ascends from the internal iliac veins. This is referred to as the Batson's circulation.* This venous pathway accounts for the distribution and frequency of osseous metastases; it also connects with ventral venous plexus (Fig. 39.6).

Rules of Classification and Staging

Clinical Staging and Imaging

Clinical assessment before treatment includes a digital rectal examination and needle biopsy guided by TRUS. For nonpalpable disease, imaging with endorectal magnetic resonance imaging (MRI) is superior to computed tomography (CT). Enhanced CT is valuable to assess lymph nodes, but if PSA is low (<20 mg/mL) and the Gleason grade is favorable (<7), sophisticated imaging is discouraged because of a high-false positive rate with imaging. Stages T2A, 2B, and 2C of the fourth edition have returned because the recurrence-free survival rate was significantly different for definitions in the fifth edition (Table 39.3).

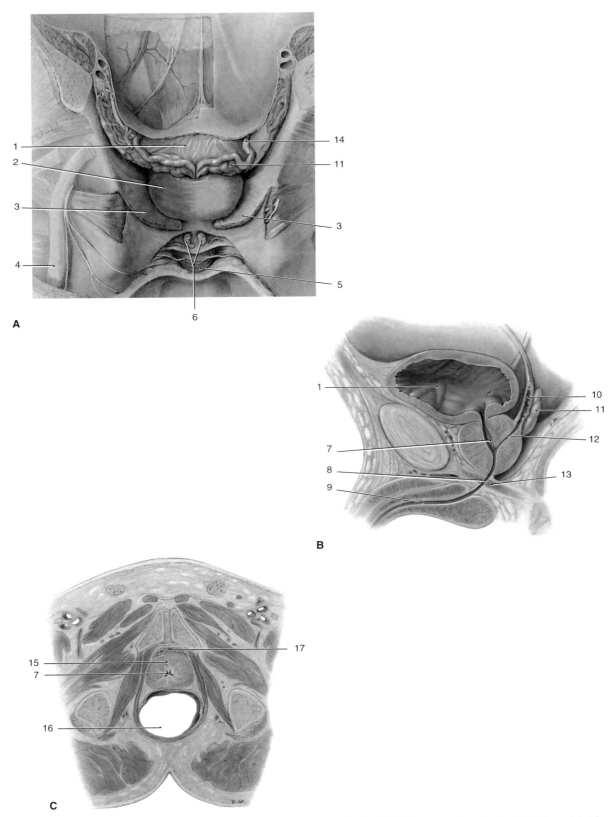

Figure 39.4 **T-oncoanatomy:** Three-planar views. **A.** Coronal. **B.** Sagittal. **C.** Transverse (see text). (1) Urinary bladder. (2) Prostate (enlarged). (3) Levator ani. (4) Sciatic nerve. (5) Bulbospongiosus. (6) Bulbourethral glands. (7) Prostatic urethra. (8) Membranous urethra. (9) Spongy urethra. (10) Ampulla of ductus deferens. (11) Seminal vesicle. (12) Ejaculatory duct. (13) Sphincter urethrae (external). (14) Ductus deferens. (15) Prostate. (16) Rectum. (17) Prostatic venous plexus.

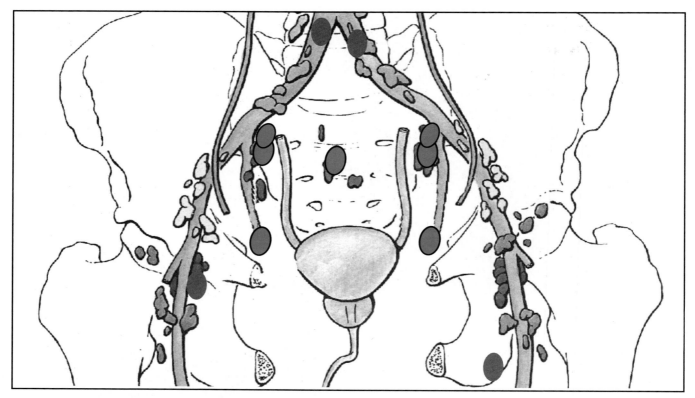

Figure 39.5 N-oncoanatomy: Obturator nodes of hypogastric or internal iliac chain.

Pathologic Staging

With a total prostatectomy seminal vesiculectomy, regional nodes are carefully examined for surgical margins by descriptors: R1, microscopic; R2, macroscopic. A positive rectal biopsy permits pT4 and a positive biopsy of extraprostatic soft tissue justifies a pT3 as does a positive biopsy of seminal vesicles.

Oncoimaging Annotations

• TRUS is recommended if either DRE or PSE is abnormal.

• The main role of TRUS is in ultrasound-guided biopsy.

• The role of CT is detection of lymph node or other distant metastases.

• Endorectal MRI (eMRI) is superior to the use of body coil.

• eMRI renders the highest detection of extracapsular extension or seminal vesicles invasion, but variations in image quality and interpretation are among the main reasons for the slow dissemination of this technique.

TABLE 39.2	Lymph Nodes of Prostate	
Sentinel nodes		Juxtaregional nodes
Internal iliac Obturator		Para-aortic
Regional nodes		Metastatic nodes
Common iliac Hypogastric External iliac Presacral Intercalating		Inguinal

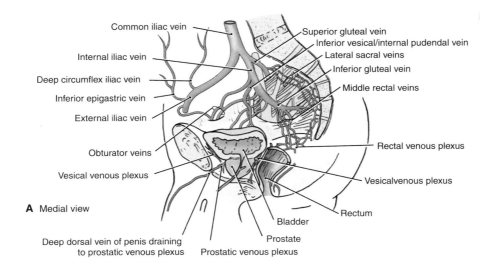

A Medial view

Common iliac vein
Internal iliac vein
Deep circumflex iliac vein
Inferior epigastric vein
External iliac vein
Obturator veins
Vesical venous plexus

Superior gluteal vein
Inferior vesical/internal pudendal vein
Lateral sacral veins
Inferior gluteal vein
Middle rectal veins
Rectal venous plexus
Vesicalvenous plexus
Rectum

Deep dorsal vein of penis draining to prostatic venous plexus
Prostatic venous plexus
Prostate
Bladder

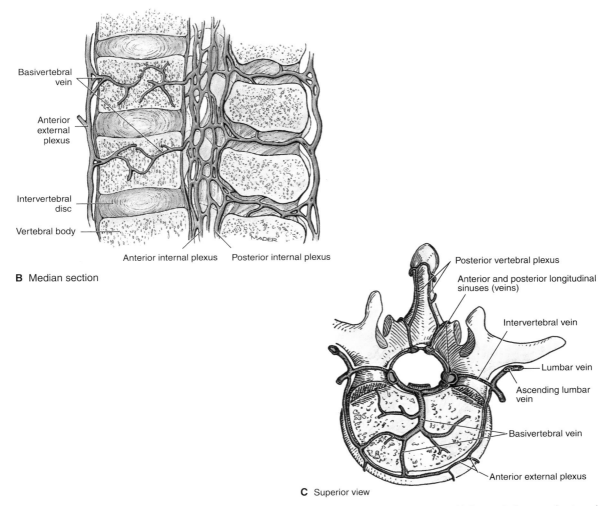

Basivertebral vein
Anterior external plexus
Intervertebral disc
Vertebral body

Anterior internal plexus   Posterior internal plexus

B Median section

Posterior vertebral plexus
Anterior and posterior longitudinal sinuses (veins)
Intervertebral vein
Lumbar vein
Ascending lumbar vein
Basivertebral vein
Anterior external plexus

C Superior view

Figure 39.6 **M-oncoanatomy. A.** Periprostatic and perivesical plexus of veins communicates with internal plexus and external plexuses of intervertebral veins. **B.** External plexus. Through the body of each vertebra come veins that form a small anterior external vertebral plexus. In the pelvic regions, the ascending lumbar, and lateral sacral veins further link segment to segment. **C.** Internal plexus. The vertebral canal contains a plexus of thin-walled, valveless veins that surround the dura mater. Anterior and posterior longitudinal channels (venous sinuses) can be discerned in this plexus (Batson's).

TABLE 39.3	**Imaging Modalities for Staging Prostate Cancer**	
Method	**Diagnosis and Staging Capability**	**Recommended for Use**
Primary (T) staging		
TRUS	Accurate for tumor localization but not for assessing T stage	Routine use for guiding biopsies of the prostate gland
CTe	Not useful for stage T1–T3 disease but for evaluation of stage T4 disease (e.g., bladder, rectum invasion)	Recommended only for patients with clinically suspected stage T3–T4 disease
MRI	Probably the most accurate technique available for assessing T stage; anatomy well shown	May be cost effective in evaluating patients at intermediate and high clinical risk of having extraprostatic disease
MRS	An adjunct to MRI for improved tumor localization and staging	Under investigation; early results useful as an adjunct to MRI
Nodal (N) staging		
CTe	Excellent for detecting enlarged nodes >1 cm versus large blood vessels	Yes, less expensive and time consuming than MRI
MRI	Excellent if node is replaced by cancer; yields positive intense signal	Yes, but more expensive and time consuming than CTe
Metastases (M) staging		
Bs-Tc	Identifies bone metastases	Recommended for patients with PSA >10 ng/mL, Gleason score >8, or clinical stage T3–T4 disease
CT-Ch	Identifies hematogenous or lymphatic metastases to chest, more sensitive than chest radiograph	May be used to confirm abnormal findings on the chest radiograph or to evaluate patients with pulmonary symptoms
CT-Ab	Identifies hematogenous metastases to liver, abdominal viscera or lymphatic metastases to para-aortic lymph nodes	Not cost effective in the evaluation of patients with PSA <20 ng/mL because of low yield of abnormal studies
CT-Pv	Identifies invasion of adjacent organs (i.e., bladder, rectum, pelvic sidewall)	Not cost effective in patients with PSA <20 ng/mL or clinical stage T1–T2 because of low yield of abnormal studies
PET	May increase the sensitivity for detecting lymph node and visceral metastases	Under investigation; early results show promise

BS-Tc, bone scintigraphy; CT, computed tomography; CTe, CT enhanced with IV contrast; CT-Ab, abdominal CT; CT-Ch, chest CT; CT-Pv, pelvic CT; MRI, magnetic resonance imaging; MRS, magnetic resonance spectroscopic imaging; PET, positron emission tomography; PSA, prostate-specific antigen; TRUS, transrectal ultrasound.
Modified from Bragg DG, Rubin P, Hricak H, eds. *Oncologic Imaging.* 2nd ed. Philadelphia: Elsevier; 2002:579.

- Early results on the use of spectroscopic MRI are promising, but the modality is still considered a research tool.
- Treatment follow-up is limited by imaging; either TRUS (with biopsy) or eMRI is most commonly used.

Cancer Statistics and Survival

When considered together, the male genital and urinary system are the major sites of malignancy. Prostate cancer alone accounts for 200,000 new patients annually. There are 100,000 new urinary tract cancers and 2.5-more of male genital cancers, or 250,000 cases annually (see Table 35.5).

Between 1988 and 1992, the incidence rates of prostate cancers tripled from 75,000 new cases annually to 225,000. Prostate cancer in men is similar to breast cancer in women, accounting for 33% of all cancers and outdistancing lung cancer (13%) and colon and rectum (11%) combined. The 5-year survival is best of all cancers at 98.5%, but still represents 30,000 deaths yearly and is the second leading cause of death in the United

States. Despite declining death rates in whites, African American men are dying at twice the rate of prostate cancer. Significant geographic variation has been observed; it is highest among blacks in the United States, followed by whites in Scandinavia and the United States. The lowest rates are in Asia.

The dramatic gains in survival are due to multidisciplinary achievements in screening, early detection, precise diagnoses, and effective multimodal therapies. The cancer statistics reveal perhaps the greatest gains in survival in oncology over the past five decades. In local stage I, male genitourinary tumors are all 90% to 100% curable according to the latest Surveillance Epidemiology and End Results data: Kidney, 90%; bladder, 94%; testes, 99%; and prostate, 100%. Mortality rates are declining. The pediatric Wilms tumor was the first malignancy in childhood to be cured, achieving >90% long-term survival, and heralded the success of multimodal treatment that would be achieved in adult tumors in urology (see Fig. 35.7 and Table 35.6).

Cross-sectional anatomy of the penis reflects the staging system of penile and urethral cancers.

Perspective and Patterns of Spread

Penile and urethral cancers are uncommon in the United States, accounting for 1% of all malignancies in men. Circumcision has been shown to be effective in decreasing and preventing such cancers in Jewish, Nigerian, and Ugandan men who practice circumcision. Phinosis and smegma correlate with penile cancers. A relationship to sexually transmitted diseases, chronic infection, and trauma has been implicated in urethral cancers. The age group most afflicted are in their 50s and 60s. Presenting symptoms are superficial nodular lesions, ulcerative sores, pain and itching, bleeding, and urinary burning. Palpable inguinal nodes are often present, but may be ignored. If ignored, adenopathy may be present in 30% to 45%; fortunately, at least half are due to associated infection rather than cancer.

The skin continues distal to the glans penis to form a smooth retractable sheath, the prepuce, which is lined by mucous membrane and has a moist stratified squamous epithelium. This is most often the site of both premalignant in situ lesions as is the glans itself. Bowen disease is squamous cell cancer in-situ that may involve the skin of the shaft. It often appears as a dull red plaque with crusting and oozing. Erythroplasia of Queyrat is an epidermoid cancer in situ that involves the mucosal or mucocutaneous junction at the prepuce or glans. The predominant cancer is squamous cell carcinoma as expected with mucous membranes. Basal cell cancers account for only 1% to 2% of penile cancers (Table 40.1). *Either the glans (60%) or the prepuce (30%) is most often the site of origin of cancer. Skin of the shaft accounts for <10%.*

The patterns of spread vary with location. Cancers of the skin and mucous membrane of the glans invade superficially and then penetrate into the corpus spongiosum and cavernosum (Fig. 40.1).

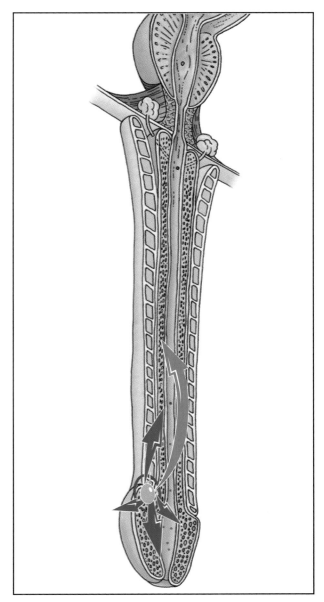

Figure 40.1 **Patterns of spread (cancer crab) of penis cancer are color coded for stage:** Tis or Ta, yellow; T1, green; T2, blue; T3, purple; and T4, red.

DEFINITION OF TNM

STAGE GROUPINGS

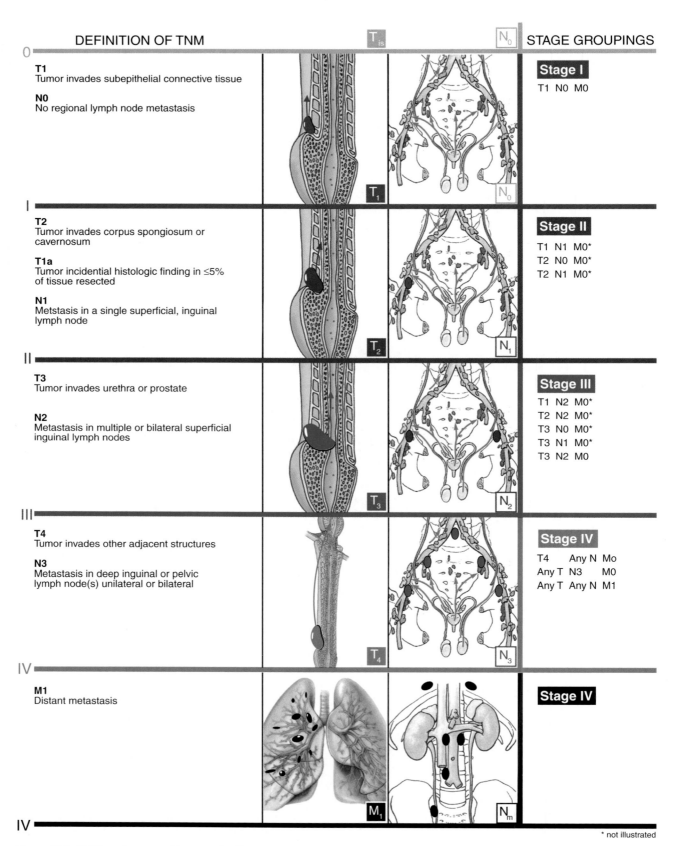

T1
Tumor invades subepithelial connective tissue

N0
No regional lymph node metastasis

Stage I
T1 N0 M0

T2
Tumor invades corpus spongiosum or cavernosum

T1a
Tumor incidential histologic finding in ≤5% of tissue resected

N1
Metstasis in a single superficial, inguinal lymph node

Stage II
T1 N1 M0*
T2 N0 M0*
T2 N1 M0*

T3
Tumor invades urethra or prostate

N2
Metastasis in multiple or bilateral superficial inguinal lymph nodes

Stage III
T1 N2 M0*
T2 N2 M0*
T3 N0 M0*
T3 N1 M0*
T3 N2 M0

T4
Tumor invades other adjacent structures

N3
Metastasis in deep inguinal or pelvic lymph node(s) unilateral or bilateral

Stage IV
T4   Any N Mo
Any T N3   M0
Any T Any N M1

M1
Distant metastasis

Stage IV

* not illustrated

Figure 40.2 TNM penis cancer diagram. Penile cancers once extensive require amputation. Vertically arranged with T definitions on left and stage groupings on right. Color bars are coded for stage: Stage 0, yellow; I, green; II, blue; III, purple; IV, red; and metastatic, black.

TABLE 40.1	Histopathologic Type: Common Cancers of the Penis
Type	
Cell types are limited to carcinomas.	

Modified from Greene FL, Page DL, Fleming ID, et al., eds. *AJCC Cancer Staging Manual.* 6th ed. New York: Springer; 2002:304.

TNM Staging Criteria

The staging of penile cancers and urethral cancers has been based on depth of invasion rather than size. In the early versions of the International Union Against Cancer classification, it was classified similarly to other skin cancers. Since the third edition, there have been no changes in penile cancer staging; urethral cancers are noted separately. Cross-sectional anatomy of the penis reflects the staging system of penile and urethral cancers.

Initial superficial stage Tis is cancer in situ and Ta is verrucal, noninvasive lesion. Subepithelial or subcutaneous spread is T1. Once invasion occurs through the deep (Buck's) fascia, the corpus spongiosum or cavernosum are invaded (stage T2). Invasion into urethra is T3 and adjacent structures T4 (Fig. 40.2).

Summary of Changes

No changes have been made from the fifth edition of the AJCC CSM.

Orientation of Three-planar Oncoanatomy

The isocenter is taken at the penile base outside the boney pelvis (Fig. 40.3).

T-oncoanatomy

- *Coronal*: The penis and urethra have an anterior projectile portion and a posterior anchoring part into the prostate in males.

- *Sagittal*: These are surrounded by a deep penile fascia (Buck's fascia), which is separated from skin by a layer of connective tissue. Penile and urethral cancers mirror image their patterns of invasion and advancement as to depth of tissue penetration.

- *Transverse*: The axial cross-section identifies its major anatomic features: *The urethra is embedded in the corpus spongiosum and the main erectile corpora cavernosum (Fig. 40.4).*

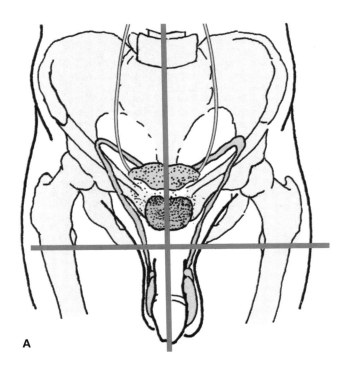
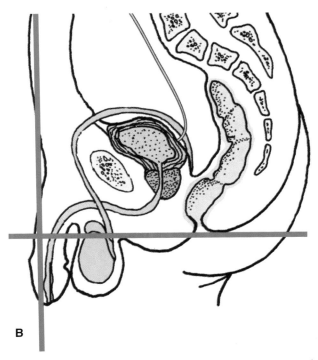

Figure 40.3 **Orientation of T-oncoanatomy.** The anatomic isocenter for three-planar anatomy of penis is below the pelvis. **A.** Coronal. **B.** Sagittal.

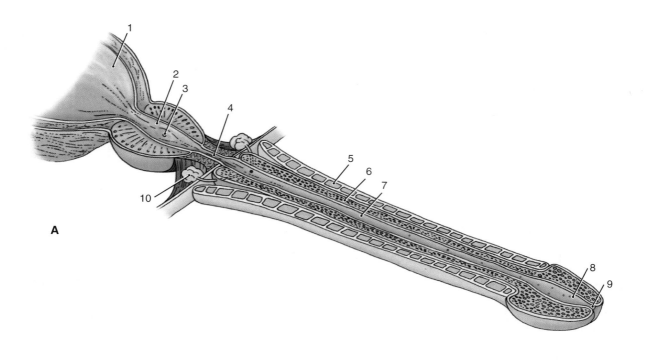

A

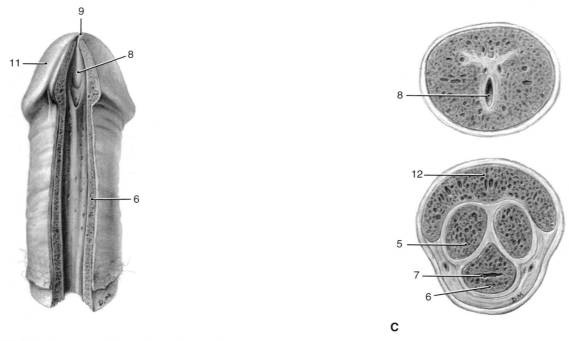

B

C

Figure 40.4 **T-oncoanatomy:** Three-planar views. **A.** Coronal. **B.** Sagittal. **C.** Transverse (see text). (1) Urinary bladder. (2) Prostatic urethra. (3) Prostatic utricle. (4) Membranous urethra. (5) Corpus cavernosus. (6) Corpus spongiosum. (7) Spongy urethra. (8) Navicular fossa. (9) External urethral orifice. (10) Bulbourethral gland. (11) Glans penis. (12) Corona of glans penis.

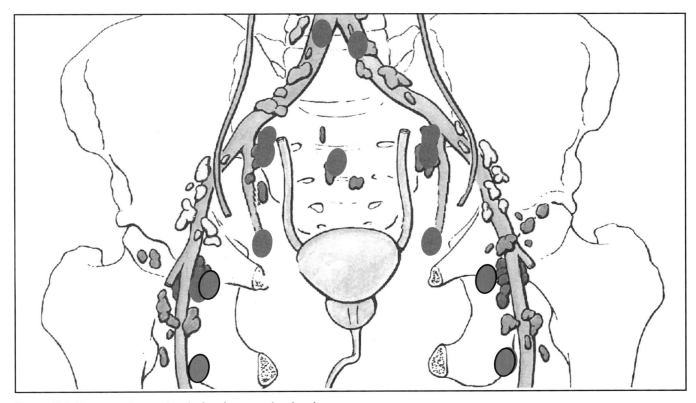

Figure 40.5 **N-oncoanatomy.** Inguinal nodes are regional nodes.

N-oncoanatomy

The lymphatic channels of the prepuce and penis are rich and the shaft skin drains into inguinal nodes. *The rich anastomoses at the base of the penis result in bilateral drainage into superficial and deep inguinal nodes.* Sentinel nodes are often located at the junction of saphenous and superficial epigastric veins. The lymphatics of the bulbomembranous and prostatic urethra follow three routes: External iliac nodes, obturator and internal iliac nodes, and presacral nodes. Pelvic external iliac nodes are seldom involved without inguinal node involvement first (Fig. 40.5; Table 40.2).

M-oncoanatomy

Distant metastases are uncommon, except in advanced disease at the base of the penis, despite the rich vascular anastomoses and penile blood supply, which

TABLE 40.2	**Lymph Nodes of Penis**	
Sentinel nodes		
Superficial inguinal Femoral		
Regional nodes		Metastatic nodes
Deep inguinal (Cloquet's Node) Bilateral inguinal		Right para-aortic Left para-aortic Mediastinal Left supraclavicular
Juxtaregional nodes		
Common iliac Internal iliac External iliac		

drains into the dorsal vein of the penis and then into the periprostatic and perivesical venous plexus (see Fig. 35.6A).

Rules of Classification and Staging

Clinical Staging and Imaging

Careful physical examination and endoscopy are adequate to determine primary extension and nodal involvement. Imaging is reserved for determining metastatic pelvic nodal involvement and remote metastases when stage is advanced. Computed tomography is preferred to magnetic resonance imaging because it is more cost effective.

Pathologic Staging

Complete resection of primary and part of penis requires determination of appropriate clearance of surgical margins. Lymphadenectomy specimens should note number, size, and extranodal extensions.

Cancer Statistics and Survival

When considered together, the male genital and urinary systems are the major sites of malignancy. Prostate cancer alone accounts for 200,000 new patients annually. There are 100,000 new urinary tract cancers and 2.5-fold more of male genital cancers, or 250,000 cases annually (see Table 35.5).

The dramatic gains in survival are due to multidisciplinary achievements in screening, early detection, precise diagnoses, and effective multimodal therapies. The cancer statistics are revealing of perhaps the greatest gains in survival in oncology over the past five decades. In local stage I, male genitourinary tumors are 90% to 100% curable according to the latest Surveillance Epidemiology and End Results data: Kidney, 90%; bladder, 94%; testes, 99%; and prostate, 100%. Death and mortality rates are declining. The pediatric Wilms tumor was the first malignancy in childhood to be cured, achieving >90% long-term survival, and heralded the success of multimodal treatment that would be achieved in adult tumors in urology.

The staging criteria are based on conceiving of the testes as an abdominal organ.

Perspective and Patterns of Spread

An enlarged or swollen testes is common in young men. It is usually due to a benign event as an epididymitis or a swelling indicative of some trauma. Despite the infrequent occurrence of testicular tumors, which only account for 1% of all cancers in males, it is the most common tumor in young men between 20 and 40 years of age. However, the benign appearance of hydroceles and varicoceles may disguise a testicular tumor. Thus, increased size of the testes, whether it is sudden or slow in onset, painless or tender, requires careful investigation and consideration before a course of treatment can be decided upon.

Testicular tumors are divided into seminomas, embryonal cancers, teratocarcinomas or teratomas, and choriocarcinomas (Table 41.1). *There are two hypotheses for the generation of this large variety of tumors; the most popular thesis is that a single germ cell gives rise to seminomas and to the multipotential cells that form the other tumor types versus the thesis that totipotent cells exist that can give rise to the nonseminomatous tumors only.*

The remarkable aspect of all testicular tumors is their high curability. Seminomas traditionally treated with radical orchidectomy followed by para-aortic radiation have yielded cure rates of ≥95%. One of the first malignancies controlled by multiagent chemotherapy are the nonseminomatous cancers (NSC) of the testes. Stage I and II NSC have 95% long-term survivals; even disseminated metastatic disease can be eradicated the majority of times (50%–60%). The best example of success is Lance Armstrong and his incredible performance as a cycling champion setting and breaking records as the seventh consecutive winner of the Tour de France.

Seminomas, embryonal tumors, and teratocarcinomas tend to be confined to the testes. Direct extension through the capsule of the testis into the fascia and muscle of the scrotal wall is an uncommon pattern of

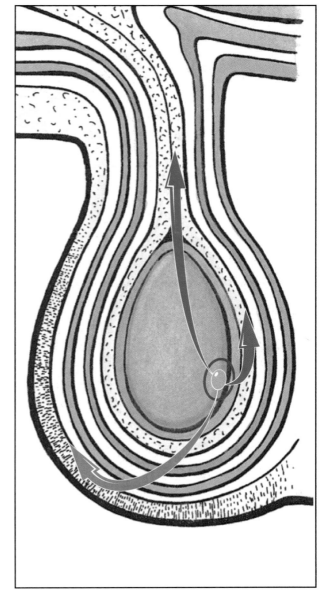

Figure 41.1 **Patterns of spread (cancer crab) of testes cancer are color coded for stage:** T0, yellow; T1, green; T2, blue; T3, purple.

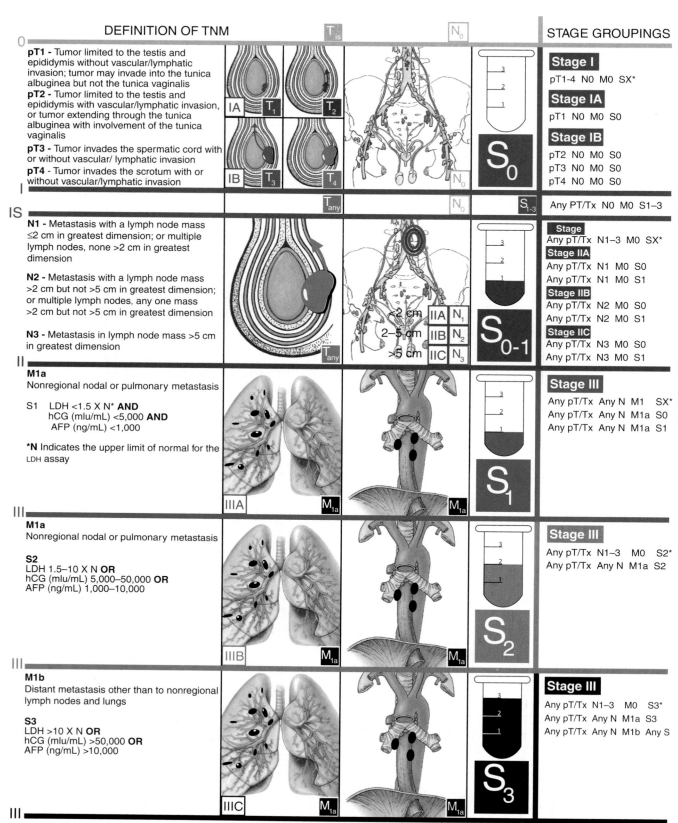

DEFINITION OF TNM

pT1 - Tumor limited to the testis and epididymis without vascular/lymphatic invasion; tumor may invade into the tunica albuginea but not the tunica vaginalis

pT2 - Tumor limited to the testis and epididymis with vascular/lymphatic invasion, or tumor extending through the tunica albuginea with involvement of the tunica vaginalis

pT3 - Tumor invades the spermatic cord with or without vascular/ lymphatic invasion

pT4 - Tumor invades the scrotum with or without vascular/lymphatic invasion

N1 - Metastasis with a lymph node mass ≤2 cm in greatest dimension; or multiple lymph nodes, none >2 cm in greatest dimension

N2 - Metastasis with a lymph node mass >2 cm but not >5 cm in greatest dimension; or multiple lymph nodes, any one mass >2 cm but not >5 cm in greatest dimension

N3 - Metastasis in lymph node mass >5 cm in greatest dimension

M1a
Nonregional nodal or pulmonary metastasis

S1   LDH <1.5 X N* **AND**
hCG (mIu/mL) <5,000 **AND**
AFP (ng/mL) <1,000

*N Indicates the upper limit of normal for the LDH assay

M1a
Nonregional nodal or pulmonary metastasis

S2
LDH 1.5–10 X N **OR**
hCG (mIu/mL) 5,000–50,000 **OR**
AFP (ng/mL) 1,000–10,000

M1b
Distant metastasis other than to nonregional lymph nodes and lungs

S3
LDH >10 X N **OR**
hCG (mIu/mL) >50,000 **OR**
AFP (ng/mL) >10,000

STAGE GROUPINGS

Stage I
pT1-4 N0 M0 SX*

Stage IA
pT1 N0 M0 S0

Stage IB
pT2 N0 M0 S0
pT3 N0 M0 S0
pT4 N0 M0 S0

Any PT/Tx N0 M0 S1–3

Stage
Any pT/Tx N1–3 M0 SX*

Stage IIA
Any pT/Tx N1 M0 S0
Any pT/Tx N1 M0 S1

Stage IIB
Any pT/Tx N2 M0 S0
Any pT/Tx N2 M0 S1

Stage IIC
Any pT/Tx N3 M0 S0
Any pT/Tx N3 M0 S1

Stage III
Any pT/Tx Any N M1   SX*
Any pT/Tx Any N M1a S0
Any pT/Tx Any N M1a S1

Stage III
Any pT/Tx N1–3   M0   S2*
Any pT/Tx Any N M1a S2

Stage III
Any pT/Tx N1–3   M0   S3*
Any pT/Tx Any N M1a S3
Any pT/Tx Any N M1b Any S

* not illustrated

Figure 41.2 TNM testes cancer diagram.   Testes cancers are unique in serum markers. They have a greater impact on Stage Groupings and Substages than anatomic extent. Vertically arranged with T definitions on left and stage groupings on right. Color bars are coded for stage: Stage 0, yellow; I, green; II, blue; III, purple; IV, red; and metastatic, black.

TABLE 41.1	World Health Organization Histologic Classification of Tumors of the Testis

Type

Seminomatous germ cell tumor
  Classic type
  With Syncytiotrophoblasts

Nonseminomatous
  Pure
    Embryonal carcinoma
    Yolk sac tumor
    Teratoma
    Choriocarcinoma

  Mixed

Modified from Greene FL, Page DL, Fleming ID, et al., eds. *AJCC Cancer Staging Manual.* 6th ed. New York: Springer; 2002:320.

spread (Fig. 41.1). Occasionally, the epididymis is invaded early. Involvement of the rete testis without evidence of further extension is considered an early lesion in behavior, if the involvement is contained within the epididymis.

TNM Staging Criteria

The staging criteria are based on conceiving of the testes as an abdominal organ. *The tunica albuginea is the equivalent of the first wrap of the serosa and once penetrated by cancer is T1. If the tunica vaginalis is penetrated it is equivalent to the peritoneum and is T2.* The tunica vaginalis has a visceral and parietal layer and both need to be penetrated for the cancer to invade the scrotal wall (T4; Fig. 41.2).

The major route for local extension is through the lymphatic channels of the testes that emerge from the mediastinum of the testis and continue along the spermatic cord. The major lymphatic drainage of the testes is different on the left and right. The lymphatics of the testes follow the spermatic vessels and are very commonly the major route of spread of testicular tumors.

Cancer from the germ cells of the testis usually develops during the years of greatest sexual activity. The undescended testis has a greater tendency to undergo carcinomatous change, even after an orchiopexy has been performed. The associated hormonal secretions and the amount of the hormone may produce endocrine effects, including gynecomastia and altered laboratory determinations (human chorionic gonadotropin). In addition, because of their embryonal origin, testicular tumors may produce tumor associated antigens alpha fetoprotein. A third serum marker is lactic acid dehydrogenase. *Collectively, these three serum biomarkers are incorporated into the staging system as S1, S2, or S3 depending on their level of elevation.* Particularly noteworthy is this is the first and only staging system that incorporates serum biomarkers into its progression.

Summary of Changes

No changes have been made from the fifth edition of the AJCC CSM.

Orientation of Three-planar Oncoanatomy

The isocenter is taken at the center of the scrotum outside the boney pelvis (Fig. 41.3).

T-oncoanatomy

The testes are composed of convoluted seminiferous tubules with a stroma containing functional endocrine interstitial cells (Fig. 41.4).

- *Coronal*: Both are encased in a dense barrier capsule, the tunica albuginea, with fibrous septa extending into and separating the testes into lobules.
- *Transverse*: The testis is surrounded by a remnant of the peritoneum, the tunica vaginalis, and explains the occurrence of hydroceles that account for approximately 10% of testicular tumors.
- *Sagittal*: The tubules converge and exit at the mediastinum of the testis into the rete testis and efferent ducts that join a single tubule. This tubule, the epididymis, is coiled outside the upper and lower pole of the testicle, then joins the muscular vas deferens conduit that accompanies the vessels and lymphatic channels of the spermatic cord.

N-oncoanatomy

The spermatic lymphatic collecting ducts on the right side tend to *follow the vascular components of the cord and*

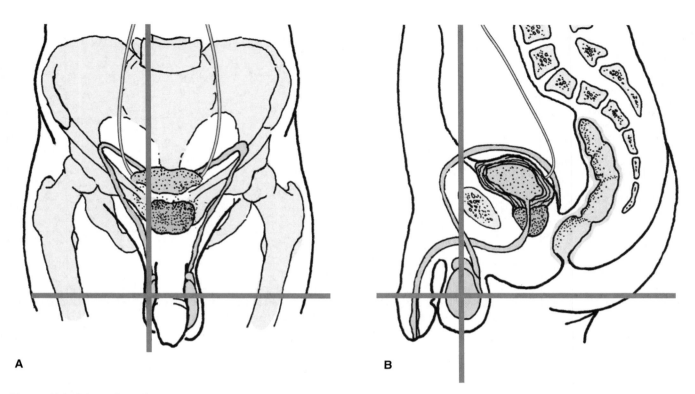

Figure 41.3 Orientation of T-oncoanatomy. The anatomic isocenter for three-planar anatomy of testes is below the pelvis. **A.** Coronal. **B.** Sagittal.

drain into the paracaval lymph nodes in the area where the spermatic vein enters the inferior vena cava and the artery arises from the aorta. The spermatic lymphatic collecting ducts on the left side also tend to *follow the vascular components of the cord and drain into the para-aortic nodes* in the region where the spermatic and the inferior mesenteric arteries arise out of the aorta and also into the nodes of the left renal hilum in the region where the left spermatic vein joins the left renal vein. Juxtaregional or second station nodes are those of the pelvis and mediastinal and supraclavicular regions (Fig. 41.5; Table 41.2).

M-oncoanatomy

The spermatic vein on the right side drains directly into the inferior vena cava. On the left side, it drains into and through the renal vein. This causes a higher pressure gradient in the left spermatic vein, which leads to slight dilatation of the pampiniform venous plexus that accounts for the lower lying position of the left testicle as compared to the right (Fig. 41.5).

Venous drainage of the spermatic veins is into the systemic circulation by way of the inferior vena cava, placing the lungs as the major metastatic target organ. The lung is the major target organ for nonseminoma testicular cancers. Seminomas tend to follow lymphatic progression giv-

ing rise to transdiaphragmatic nodes if retroperitoneal nodes are involved. Either mediastinal nodes or a left supraclavicular node can be involved if the thoracic duct is infiltrated.

Rules of Classification and Staging

Clinical Staging and Imaging

Clinical examination of primary can be enhanced by sonograms, computed tomography (CT), and magnetic resonance imaging (MRI)/coil examination. In addition, nodal assessment entails CT of abdomen and pelvis for para-aortic and renal hilar nodes and chest for mediastinal nodes and lung. Serum for marker should be collected before treatment (Table 41.3).

Pathologic Staging

Full assessment of radical orchidectomy specimen for spread, that is, intratesticular or extratesticular, is worth noting as is invasion of epididymis and for spermatic cord. Multiple tissue sections including one distant from tumor to determine whether tubular germ cell neoplasia (cancer in situ) is present. Careful evaluation for vascular invasion in multiple sections should be noted. If a retroperitoneal node is evaluated, location,

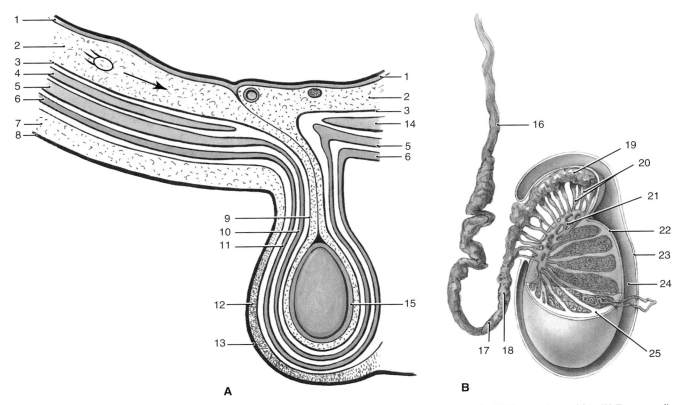

Figure 41.4 T-oncoanatomy: Three-planar views. **A.** Coronal. **B.** Sagittal. (1) Peritoneum (parietal). (2) Extraperitoneal fat. (3) Transversalis fascia. (4) Transverse abdominal muscle. (5) Internal abdominal oblique muscle. (6) External abdominal oblique aponeurosis. (7) Subcutaneous fat. (8) Skin. (9) Internal spermatic fascia. (10) Cremasteric fascia (muscle). (11) External spermatic fascia. (12) Dartos muscle. (13) Scrotal skin. (14) Rectus abdominis muscle. (15) Tunica vaginalis. (16) Ductus deferens. (17) Tail of epididymis. (18) Body of epididymis. (19) Head of epididymis. (20) Efferent ductules. (21) Rete testis. (22) Visceral tunica vaginalis. (23) Parietal tunica vaginalis. (24) Cavity of tunica vaginalis. (25) Tunica albuginea.

size, and extranodal soft tissue extension should be recorded.

Oncoimaging Annotations

- Scrotal ultrasonographic scanning is an extension of the physical examination. It should be utilized in most patients with a scrotal mass, especially when the physical examination is difficult or inconclusive.

- MRI is considered an adjunct to ultrasonography for indeterminate testicular lesions or in patients with a discrepancy between ultrasonographic findings and the physical examination.

TABLE 41.2	Lymph Nodes of Testes	
Sentinel nodes		
Left renal hilar Right paracaval nodes		
Regional nodes		Metastatic nodes

Right para-aortic
   Left para-aortic
   Left renal vein
		Mediastinal
		Left supraclavicular
		Hilar

Juxtaregional nodes		

Common iliac
   External iliac
   Inguinal		

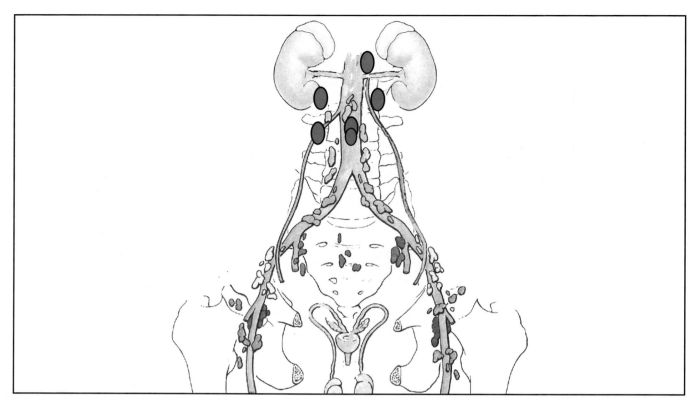

Figure 41.5 N-oncoanatomy.   Regional lymph nodes are in the para-aortic area. **Left:** Renal hilar nodes; **right:** Paracaval nodes.

TABLE 41.3	Imaging Modalities for Staging Testis Cancer	
Method	**Diagnosis and Staging Capability**	**Recommended for Use**
Primary (T) staging		
Scrotal US	More useful for differential diagnosis (tumor versus cyst)	No
Scrotal MRI	Only if physical examination and US show a discrepancy	No
Nodal (N) staging		
CTe-Abd	Most helpful detecting number and size of abdominal para-aortic lymph nodes	Yes, most cost effective
MRI	Less valuable for determining adenopathy in abdomen.	No
Metastases (M) staging		
Chest film	Can detect metastases >2 cm in size	Yes
Cte-Ch	Effective for detecting suspected pulmonary or mediastinal nodes	Yes, if chest film is suspicious
CTe-Abd	Can detect liver and visceral metastases	Yes
PET BS-Tc	Identifies bone metastases	No, investigational

CT, computed tomography; CT-Ch, chest CT; CTe, CT enhanced with IV contrast; CTe-Abd, abdominal CTe; MRI, magnetic resonance imaging; PET, positron emission tomography; TAUS, transabdominal US; US, ultrasound.
Modified from Bragg DG, Rubin P, Hricak H, eds. *Oncologic Imaging.* 2nd ed. Philadelphia: Elsevier; 2002:605.

- Cross-sectional imaging (CT preferred over MRI) is helpful in the evaluation of nodal disease and metastatic spread.
- The finding of the nodal location (regional nodes), nodal size (≥ 7 mm), and number of detected nodes all play a role in CT/MRI diagnosis of nodal disease.
- Neither CT nor MRI can differentiate benign from malignant nodal involvement, and both understage the early metastatic disease in up to 30% of patients.
- Neither CT nor MRI can differentiate between active tumor and posttreatment fibrosis.

Cancer Statistics and Survival

When considered together, the male genital and urinary systems are the major sites of malignancy. Prostate cancer alone accounts for 200,000 new patients annually. There are 100,000 new urinary tract cancers and 2.5-fold more of male genital cancers, or 250,000 cases annually (see Table 35.5).

The dramatic gains in survival are due to multidisciplinary achievements in screening, early detection, precise diagnoses, and effective multimodal therapies. The cancer statistics are revealing of perhaps the greatest gains in survival in oncology over the past five decades. In local stage I, male genitourinary tumors are 90% to 100% curable according to the latest Surveillance Epidemiology and End Results data: Kidney, 90%; bladder, 94%; testes, 99%; and prostate, 100%. Death and mortality rates are declining. The pediatric Wilms' tumor was the first malignancy in childhood to be cured, achieving >90% long-term survival, and heralded the success of multimodal treatment that would be achieved in adult tumors in urology (see Fig. 35.7 and Table 35.6).

The types of cancers vary as a function of location in both the male and female urethra.

Perspective and Patterns of Spread

Cancers of the urethra are quite uncommon, but occur more often among females. Common presentation is a structure interfering with urination in males; in females, urinary frequency, hesitancy, and a palpable urethral mass are often noted. Bleeding without a history of trauma or venereal disease should raise suspicion of an underlying malignancy. On examination, a palpable urethral mass especially in females is present in the majority of cases (75%) and can appear as papillary growths, soft fungating lesions, or ulcerations with a foul-smelling discharge. Obstructive symptoms and incomplete voiding (66%) also lead patients to seek medical evaluation as well as relief of symptoms. The types of cancers vary as a function of location in both the male and female urethra. *At the bladder neck, transitional cell cancers occur; in the central portion, pseudostratified epithelium gives rise to squamous cell cancers. Adenocarcinosarcomas occur in the prostatic portion of the male urethra and in the anterior or terminal aspect of the female urethra.* Once separated, urethroscopy, cystoscopy, and biopsy provide the diagnosis. Squamous cell cancer (60%) exceeds both transitional cell cancer (20%) and adenocarcinomas (10%) (Table 42.1).

The patterns of cancer spread relate to surrounding anatomy in males and females. *In the male, it advances and eventually may invade the penis, prostate or urinary bladder, whereas, in the female, vaginal invasion along the anterior wall of the vagina is more frequent.* The labia can be involved if it spreads inferiorly or into the bladder if it progresses superiorly (Fig. 42.1).

TNM Staging Criteria

Urethral cancers behave in an inverse fashion to penile cancers. Tis cancer is limited to the mucosa; T1, to the

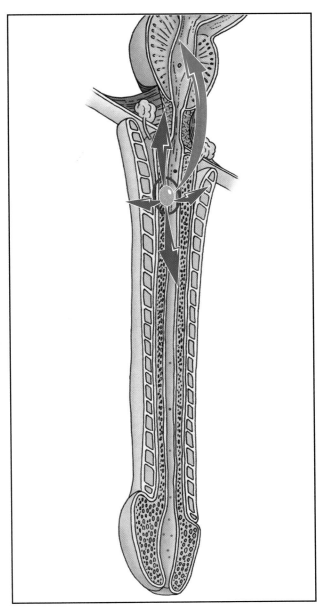

Figure 42.1 **Patterns of spread (cancer crab) of urethra cancer are color coded for stage:** Tis or Ta, yellow; T1, green; T2, blue; T3, purple; and T4, red.

DEFINITION OF TNM   T_{is}   N₀   STAGE GROUPINGS

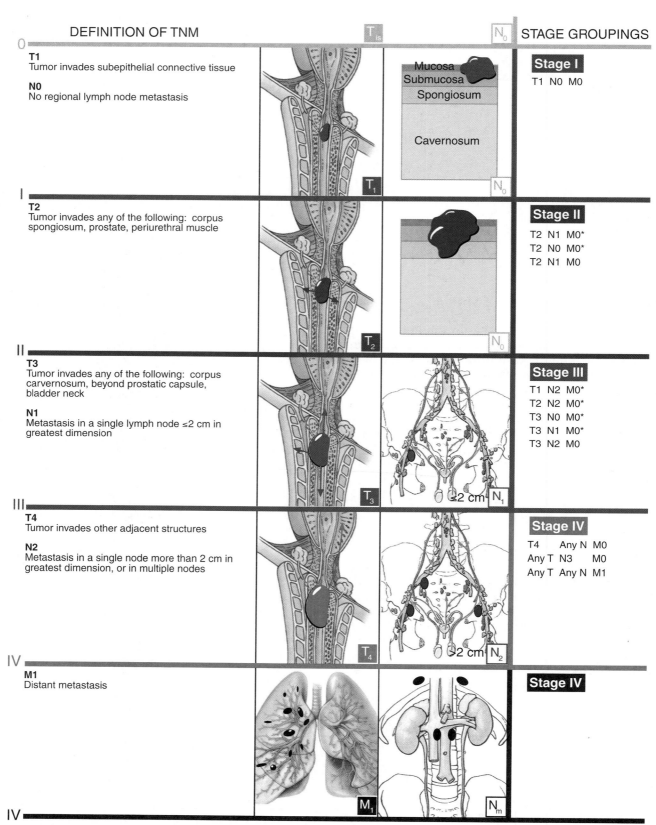

T1
Tumor invades subepithelial connective tissue

N0
No regional lymph node metastasis

Mucosa
Submucosa
Spongiosum

Cavernosum

Stage I

T1 N0 M0

T2
Tumor invades any of the following: corpus spongiosum, prostate, periurethral muscle

Stage II

T2 N1 M0*
T2 N0 M0*
T2 N1 M0

T3
Tumor invades any of the following: corpus carvernosum, beyond prostatic capsule, bladder neck

N1
Metastasis in a single lymph node ≤2 cm in greatest dimension

Stage III

T1 N2 M0*
T2 N2 M0*
T3 N0 M0*
T3 N1 M0*
T3 N2 M0

≤2 cm   N₁

T4
Tumor invades other adjacent structures

N2
Metastasis in a single node more than 2 cm in greatest dimension, or in multiple nodes

Stage IV

T4   Any N M0
Any T   N3   M0
Any T   Any N M1

>2 cm   N₂

M1
Distant metastasis

Stage IV

M₁   N_m

* not illustrated

Figure 42.2 TNM urethra cancer diagram.   Urethra cancers when extensive in males T3 may require amputation. Vertically arranged with T definitions on left and stage groupings on right. Color bars are coded for stage: Stage 0is and 0a, yellow; I, green; II, blue; III, purple; IV, red; and metastatic, black.

TABLE 42.1	Histopathologic Type for Urethra Cancer

Type

This classification applies to urothelial (transitional cell), squamous, and glandular carcinomas of the urethra and to urothelial (transitional cell) carcinomas of the prostate and prostatic urethra. There should be histologic or cytologic confirmation of the disease.

Reprinted from Greene FL, Page DL, Fleming ID, et al., eds. *AJCC Cancer Staging Manual*. 6th ed. New York: Springer; 2002:320.

subepithelial connective tissues. T2 is invasion of the corpus spongiosum; T3, corpus cavernous; and T4, adjacent organs (Fig. 42.2). Urethral cancers are more common in females and require histopathologic evidence of their spread to be accurately staged.

Summary of Changes

No changes have been made from the fifth edition of the AJCC CSM.

Orientation of Three-planar Oncoanatomy

The isocenter is taken at the base of the urethra outside the boney pelvis (Fig. 42.3).

T-oncoanatomy

The urethral cancers in the male urethra originate at the bladder neck to the external urethral meatus (see Fig. 40.4A–C).

- *Coronal*: The posterior urethra is subdivided into the membranous urethra, the portion passing through the urogenital diaphragm, and the prostatic urethra. The prostatic urethra is covered by transitional cell epithelium and gives rise to transitional cell carcinomas.
- *Sagittal*: The anterior spongy portion of the urethra is covered by stratified squamous epithelium changing to pseudostratified columnar epithelium proximally in the membranous portion. The common cancer is squamous cell cancer.
- *Transverse*: The spongy portion of the urethra lies in the spongy corpiosum of the penis.

In the female, the urethra courses from the bladder neck to an opening in the vestibule of the vagina. It is intimately related to the anterior wall of the vagina.

N-oncoanatomy

In the male, *the lymphatic channels of the prepuce and penis are rich and the shaft skin drains into inguinal nodes.* The rich anastomoses at the base of the penis result in bilateral drainage into superficial and deep inguinal nodes. Sentinal nodes are often located at the junction of saphenous and superficial epigastric veins. *The lym-phatics of the bulbomembranous and prostatic urethra follow three routes: external iliac nodes, obturator and internal iliac nodes, and presacral nodes.* Pelvic external iliac nodes are seldom involved without inguinal node involvement first (Table 42.2; Fig. 42.4A).

In the female, *lymphatics of the anterior urethra drain into the superficial and then deep inguinal nodes. The posterior urethra drains to obturator, internal iliac nodes similar to the bladder.* External iliac nodes are a sign of advancement and sentinel lymph nodes tend to be inguinal or femoral nodes (Fig. 42.4B).

M-oncoanatomy

In the male, distant metastases are uncommon except in advanced disease at the base of the penis despite the rich vascular anastomoses and penile blood supply, which drains into the dorsal vein of the penis and then into the periprostatic and perivesical venous plexus.

In the female, depending on location, hematogenous spread leads to drainage into vesical and internal iliac veins, the vena cava and right side of heart into lungs. Proximal or entire urethral cancers are more aggressive and tend to metastasize (see Fig. 35.6A).

Rules of Classification and Staging

Clinical Staging and Imaging

Imaging is reserved for determining metastatic pelvic nodal involvement and remote metastases when stage is advanced. The primary site is assessed by physical examination—inspection and palpation followed by cystourethroscopy biopsy and cytology. Contrast filling of bladder and voiding cystometrogram are worthwhile (Table 42.3).

Pathologic Staging

Complete resection of primary and part of penis requires determination of appropriate clearance of surgical margins. Lymphadenectomy specimens should note number, size, and extranodal extensions. Assignment of stage following resection allows depth of invasion be determined. In males, urethral neoplasms can arise in prostate epithelium or ducts and are classified as prostate urethral cancer.

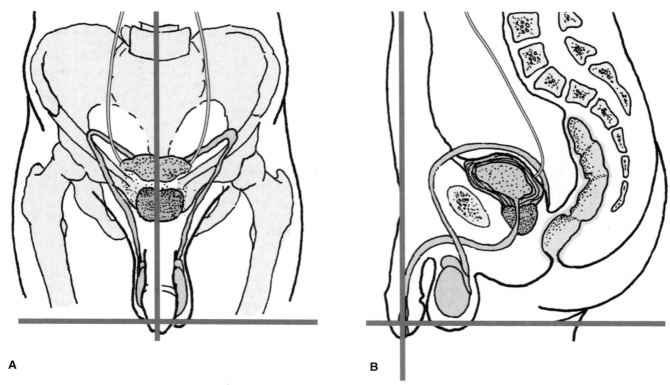

Figure 42.3 Orientation of T-oncoanatomy. The anatomic isocenter for three-planar anatomy of urethra is below the pelvis. **A.** Coronal. **B.** Sagittal.

Oncoimaging Annotations

• Diagnosis of urethral cancer is by cystoscopy and biopsy.

• Magnetic resonance imaging is superior to computed tomography in the evaluation of local tumor extent.

Cancer Statistics and Survival

When considered together, the male genital and urinary systems are the major sites of malignancy. Prostate cancer alone accounts for 200,000 new patients annually. There are 100,000 new urinary tract cancers and 2.5-fold more male genital cancers, or 250,000 cases annually (see Table 35.5).

The dramatic gains in survival are due to multidisciplinary achievements in screening, early detection, precise diagnoses, and effective multimodal therapies. The cancer statistics are revealing of perhaps the greatest gains in survival in oncology over the past five decades. In local stage I, male genitourinary tumors are 90% to

TABLE 42.2	Lymph Nodes of Urethra	
Sentinel nodes		
Proximal obturator (proximal) Superficial inguinal nodes (distal)		
Regional nodes		Metastatic nodes
External iliac Hypogastric Presacral Intercalating		Mediastinal Left supraclavicular
Juxtaregional nodes		
Common iliac Right para-aortic Left para-aortic		

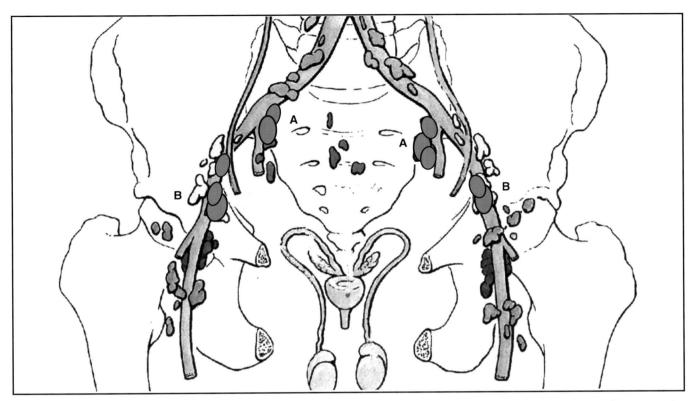

Figure 42.4 N-oncoanatomy. The regional nodes vary depending on part of urethra involved. **A.** Prostatic urethra to obturator nodes. **B.** Spongy urethra to inguinal nodes.

100% curable according to the latest Surveillance Epidemiology and End Results data: Kidney, 90%; bladder, 94%; testes, 99%; and prostate, 100%. Mortality rates are declining. The pediatric Wilms' tumor was the first malignancy in childhood to be cured, achieving >90% long-term survival, and heralded the success of multimodal treatment that would be achieved in adult tumors in urology (see Fig. 35.7).

Method	Diagnosis and Staging Capability	Recommended for Use
Primary (T) staging		
TAUS	More useful for detection than staging	No
Cte	Accurate for staging advanced T3, T4 invasion beyond bladder wall	Yes, cost effective
MRI	Provides most anatomic detail of cancer invasion into and beyond wall of urinary bladder	Yes, more accurate
Nodal (N) staging		
Cte	Valuable in assessing pelvic and para-aortic nodal enlargements	Yes, cost effective
MRI	More valuable in distinguishing adenopathy secondary to inflammation versus cancer	Yes, more cost effective
Metastases (M) staging		
Chest film	Can detect gross pulmonary or mediastinal metastases	Yes, cost effective

TABLE 42.3   Imaging Modalities for Staging Urethra Cancer

CT, computed tomography; Cte, CT enhanced with IV contrast; MRI, magnetic resonance imaging; TAUS, transabdominal ultrasound.

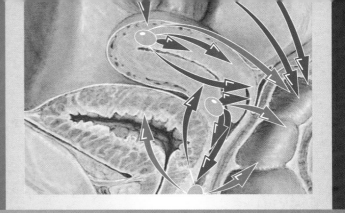

SECTION 5

GYNECOLOGIC PRIMARY SITES

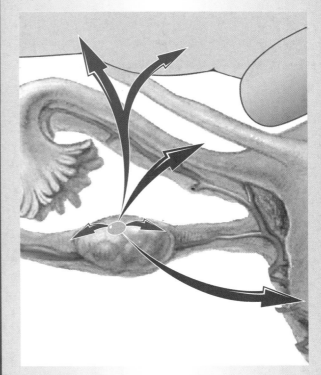

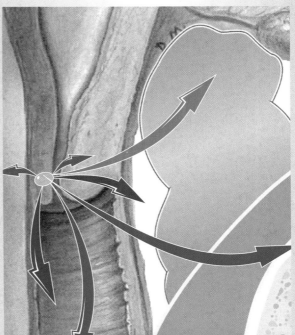

Introduction and Orientation

The staging criteria for gynecologic cancers reflect their oncoanatomy, which can be characterized as variants of both hollow and solid organs.

Perspective and Patterns of Spread

Although the incidence of gynecologic cancers is highest during the reproductive years, it does not become a significant killer until menarche. In developing countries, carcinoma of the cervix remains a leading cause of death following multiple pregnancies. By contrast, in the Western world with the introduction of the Papanicolaou smear cytology tests, the cancer can be detected in its early stages. Its incidence remains high, the third most common gynecologic cancer, largely owing to increases in sexual activity as a result of better contraception, especially among women who have begun at an early age and have multiple sexual partners. According to the most recent Surveillance Epidemiology and End Results figures, uterine cervix, uterine corpus, and ovary account for 12% of all new cases and the same percentage of deaths. This translates into approximately 90,000 diagnoses and 35,000 deaths annually.

Ovarian and uterine cancers often occur during menopause. Although death rates have dramatically declined for cervical and uterine cancers, ovarian cancer survival rates remain the same. Most ovarian cancers are advanced on detection and spread widely. In contrast, uterine cancers usually remain contained within the uterus, and are clinically more evident as they produce postmenopausal bleeding.

Three of the six sites that give rise to a large variety of neoplasms are discussed in this chapter. The ovary, the fallopian (uterine) tubes, uterus, cervix, vagina, and vulva are each afflicted with neoplastic disease. Adenocarcinomas predominate in the ovary, fallopian tube, and uterus. Squamous cell cancers occur in the cervix, vagina, and vulva. Special germ cell tumors or dysgerminomas, teratomas, and granulose cell cancers are unique to the ovary. Gestational trophoblastic neoplasms and sarcomas are aggressive malignancies that invade deeply into the uterus. The patterns of spread of each

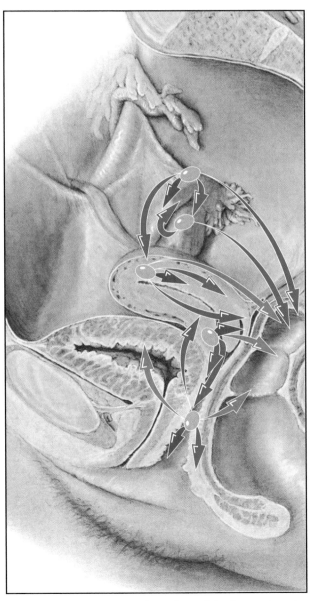

Figure 43.1 Patterns of spread. Collage of the four major primary sites are color coded to demonstrate T0 (yellow), T1 (green), T2 (blue), T3 (purple), and T4 (red).

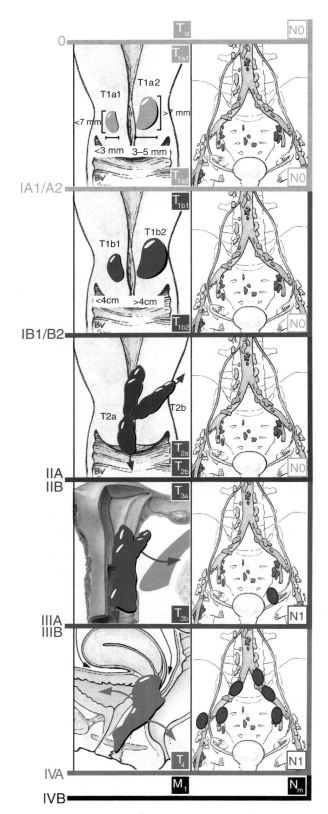

Figure 43.2 **TNM staging systems.** Vertical presentation of stages with definitions on left and stage grouping on right. Bar color coding of stage: Stage T0, yellow; I, green; II, blue; III, purple; IV, red; and metastatic, black.

malignancy determines the outcome: Some are invasive; others grow slowly. Each has a different tendency to metastasize.

TNM Patterns of Spread and Staging Criteria

The cervix uteri cancer is a good starting point for comprehension of the oncoanatomy of the female pelvis by understanding spread patterns of cancer of the cervix (Fig. 43.1). This cancer was the first staged and is both the archetype and prototype for cancer staging (Fig. 43.2). Cervical cancers are often detected by Papanicolaou smear tests when they are localized to the cervix in their in situ phase. *The concept of microinvasion was first defined as 5.0 mm depth and then 3.0 mm.* Once a cancer forms, it can spread in numerous directions as it invades deeper into the stroma, and then adjacent structures. Superficial spread involves the uterus superiorly and the vagina inferiorly. *The common infiltration pattern is laterally into the parametrial ligaments where the ureter and the uterine branches of the hypogastric or internal iliac artery and veins are present.* Surgical dissections require isolation of the uterine artery to avoid ligation of the ureter. As the tumor extends laterally into the cardinal or broad ligaments, it becomes fixed to the sidewall of the pelvis. When this occurs, the prognosis becomes grave and leg edema and pelvis pain occur (stage T3). With anteroposterior spread, the bladder and the rectum are invaded and fistula formation can occur.

Pelvic pain can have many different patterns. It can even be referred to the extremities. *As invasion occurs in the sacral and coccygeal plexus areas, zones of hyperesthesia, hypoesthesia, and even anesthesia can occur in and around the perineum, radiating into the thigh and lower limb.* Eventually, muscle invasion and bone destruction can be seen in uncontrolled, advanced, and, particularly, in recurrent tumors when standard treatment procedures have failed. The borderline between the false and true pelvis is particularly vulnerable because this is the attachment of the lateral cervical ligaments. Erosion of the medial inner cortex of the true pelvis occurs. *In the anterior direction, cervical cancer invades into the bladder and can cause bullous edema and eventually erosion of the mucosa,* which leads to urinary bleeding and fistula formation. Posteriorly, rectal invasion can lead to bleeding and fistula formation. This complication is rarely found in fundal uterine cancer.

The uterine fundus usually contains the malignant process within itself. This may relate to the fact that the uterus is normally invaded by a more naturally occurring neoplastic process, namely, the placenta of pregnancy. Thus, the first pathways of cancer spread are superficial: Inferiorly into the cervix and superiorly and laterally into the fallopian tubes. When deep invasion occurs, it is usually into the myometrium, toward the serosal surface. With cervical invasion, the spread pattern is

TABLE 43.1	Overview of Histogenesis of Primary Cancer Sites of the Gynecologic Pelvis	
Primary Site Normal Anatomic Structures	**Derivative Normal Cell Epithelium**	**Cancer Histopathologic Type Primary Site**
Ovary	Peritoneal lining Germ cells	Serous, mucinous, endometrioid adenocarcinoma Special cancers: Granulosa cell dysgerminoma
Fallopian tubes	Ciliated simple columnar cells and peg cells	Serous adenocarcinoma
Uterine fundus	Simple columnar Deep glands	Endometrioid adenocarcinoma Adenosquamous cancer mixed Note differentiation and grading
Uterine placenta	Chorionic villi	Choriocarcinoma
Uterine cervix	Stratified squamous Mucous secretory columnar epithelium	Squamous cell cancers Mucinous adenocarcinoma
Vagina	Stratified squamous cell	Squamous cell cancer
Vulva	Stratified squamous epithelium Bartholin gland	Basal cell cancer Squamous cell cancer Adenocarcinoma

similar to cervical cancer that invades laterally into the parametrium. Vaginal metastases commonly follow lymphatic channels; skip into the distal vagina, and occur as suburethral nodules. In summary, the major tumor spread patterns at this site are into the (a) myometrium, (b) serosa and peritoneal cavity, (c) cervix, (d) vagina, and (e) fallopian tube and ovary.

The ovary is as much a structure of the whole peritoneal cavity as it is of the pelvis. This is particularly true once it has become subject to malignant transformation. The ovary is positioned essentially at the bottom of the peritoneal cavity. Its blood supply reflects its abdominal origin. When cancer forms in the ovary, it invades through its capsule and forms excrescences. Tumor cells are released and seed the peritoneal surface, often invading the gynecologic tract in the manner of an ovum and/or filling the cul-de-sac. *Because there is no true separation between the pelvic and abdominal cavities, this cancer often seeds the omentum, mesentery, and intestine serosal surface.* The inferior surface of the diaphragm provides the lymphatic drainage of the abdominal cavity. Thus, the diaphragm may act as a "blotter" for these dispersed tumor cells in the peritoneal cavity. Ascites and pleural effusion are common in advanced stages. In summary, ovarian cancer spread patterns are inferiorly and medially into and onto the uterus, laterally to the pelvic wall, posteriorly into the pouch of Douglas (rectouterine), or superiorly seeding into the peritoneal cavity.

Summary of Changes

There are no changes in the sixth edition of the AJCC CSM.

Overview of the Histogenesis in the Gynecologic Pelvis

The female reproductive system consists of paired ovaries, paired uterus fallopian tubes, and a single uterus, which is pear-shaped with thick muscular walls terminating into cervix (Fig. 43.3). The cervix is at the apex of the vagina with its vestibule centered in the vulva. The specialized gonadal cells of the ovary are in sharp contrast to the epithelial surface of the fallopian tube, which are lined by simple columnar ciliated cells projecting into its lumen as folds, and the endometrial lining of the uterus, which has simple columnar cells over a spongy functionalis layer, which is shed. All of these structures give rise to adenocarcinomas. The cervix is the transitional organ, with an endocervical canal rich in mucus secretion and a surface of squamous cells that blend into the vagina as a stratified squamous cell epithelium. The vulva labia mucosa is a mucosal surface that becomes skin in the labia majora, again lined by stratified squamous cells. Squamous cell cancers are the predominant cancer in the lower female genital tract (cervix, vagina, and vulva).

Overview of Oncoanatomy

The juxtaposition of pelvic and abdominal viscera obscures the fact of their separation by the peritoneum. *The entire gynecologic tract is retroperitoneal except for the ovary; the digestive system is intraperitoneal.* The isocenters of the six primary gynecologic cancers are shown

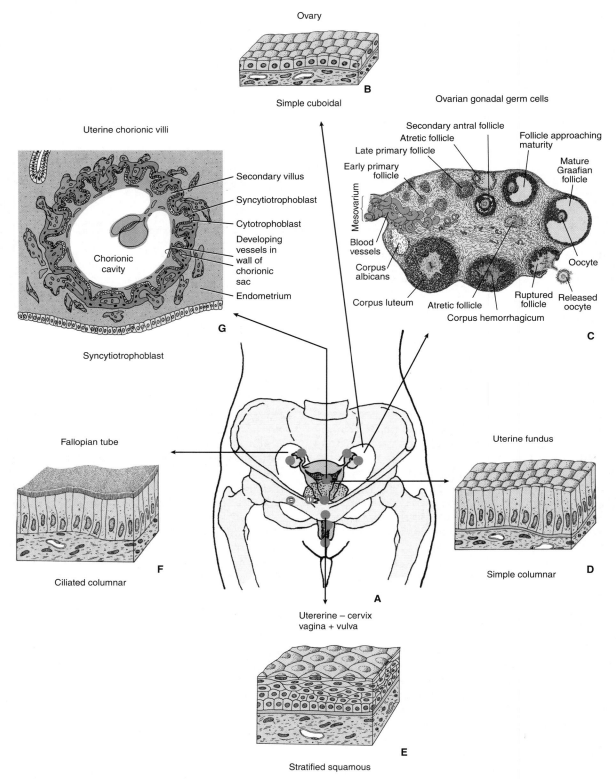

Ovary

B

Simple cuboidal

Ovarian gonadal germ cells

Uterine chorionic villi

Secondary antral follicle
Atretic follicle
Follicle approaching maturity
Late primary follicle
Early primary follicle
Mesovarium
Mature Graafian follicle

Secondary villus
Syncytiotrophoblast
Cytotrophoblast
Developing vessels in wall of chorionic sac
Endometrium

Chorionic cavity

Blood vessels
Corpus albicans
Corpus luteum
Atretic follicle
Corpus hemorrhagicum
Ruptured follicle
Oocyte
Released oocyte

G

C

Syncytiotrophoblast

Fallopian tube

Uterine fundus

A

Utererine – cervix vagina + vulva

F

Ciliated columnar

Simple columnar

D

Stratified squamous

E

Figure 43.3 Overview of oncoanatomy. There are six potential sites for gynecologic cancer, each with a distinctive anatomy and histology. The cancer can be traced to a derivative cell. **A.** Schematic of female internal sex organs. The anatomic isocenters are displayed for gynecologic primary cancer sites. **B.** Ovary epithelial neoplasms include the common varieties of adenocarcinomas (serosa, endometrioid, mucinous) and also give rise to **C.** a rich variety of germ cell neoplasms. **D.** The uterine wall undergoes dramatic proliferative change monthly in its glandular epithelium during the menstrual cycle, and gives rise to adenocarcinomas. **E.** The cervix has a simple columnar epithelium and changes to a stratified squamous epithelium, which gives rise to squamous cell cancers. **F.** The fallopian tube is lined by ciliated columnar epithelium and tends to give rise mainly to serous adenocarcinomas. **G. Syncytiotrophoblast** gives rise to choriocarcinoma, gestational trophoblast tumors.

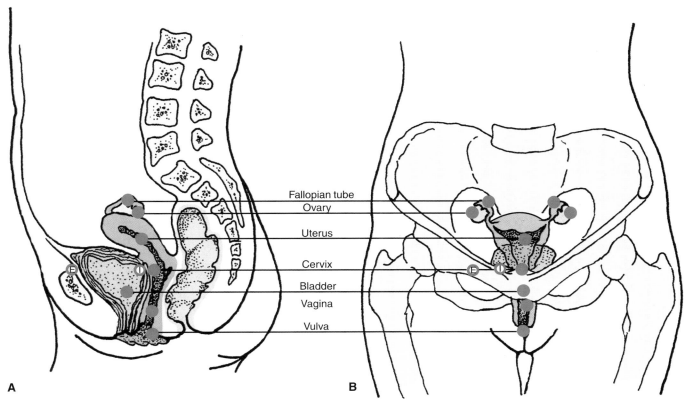

 External iliac inguinal node
 Internal iliac cbturator node

Figure 43.4 Orientation of T-oncoanatomy of the female pelvis, which houses all the internal female genital organs. From a cephalad-to-caudad fashion each is presented at a different vertebral level. **A.** Coronal and **B.** sagittal views with primary sites presented from cephalad to caudad at specific transverse levels related to vertebrae.

in their pelvic location and range from S2 to the coccyx (Fig. 43.4).

In Table 43.1, the six primary sites are tabulated with their surrounding anatomic structures and viscera, their sentinel lymph nodes, and osseous landmarks. The presentation is in a cephalad-to-caudad fashion and includes relationships to the urinary bladder, urethra, rectum, and anus, which are also extraperitoneal in the true pelvis.

Ovary

The ovaries are a pair of solid, flattened ovoids, 2.0 to 4.0 cm in diameter. They are connected by a peritoneal fold to the broad ligament and by the suspensory ligament of ovary to the lateral wall of the pelvis. Cancers arise from the mesothelial covering of the ovary rather than its germ cells.

The lymphatic drainage occurs via the ovarian and round ligament trunks and an external iliac accessory route into the

following regional nodes: The para-aortic nodes are the major regional nodes followed by the external iliac, common iliac, hypogastric, lateral sacral, and, rarely, the inguinal nodes. Although the ovary is pelvic in location, its lymphatic drainage recapitulates its abdominal or homologous origin, namely, the para-aortic lymph nodes. Its vestigial relationship via the round ligament to the labia majora reaffirms its similarity to the testes in its intimate scrotal location, which makes drainage to inguinal nodes possible. Ovarian cancers seed and invade the uterus which drain into pelvic nodes.

Uterus and Fallopian Tubes

The upper two thirds of the uterus above the level of the internal cervical os is called the "corpus uteri." The fallopian tubes enter at the upper lateral corners of its pear-shaped body. That portion of the muscular organ positioned above the line joining the tubouterine orifices is called the fundus. Cancers arise mainly from

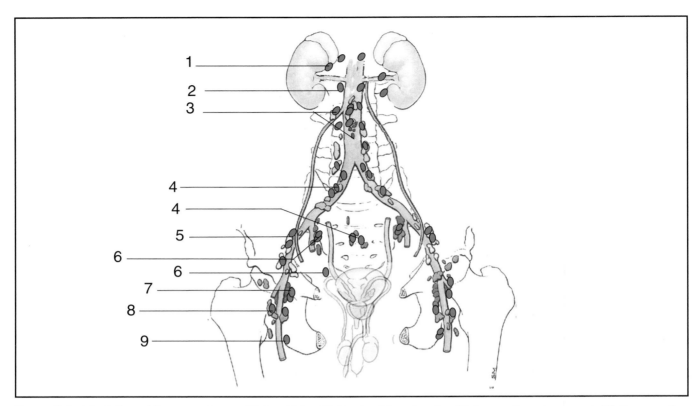

Figure 43.5 Orientation of N-oncoanatomy. (1) Renal hilar. (2) Renal pelvis and ureter. (3) Para-aortic and paracaval. (4) Common Iliac. (4') Presacral. (5) External iliac. (6) Internal iliac. (6') Obturator. (7) Deep inguinal. (8) Superficial inguinal. (9) Femoral.

its epithelial columnar lining cells. The relationship of the uterus to other pelvic tissues is important, particularly to the rectum and bladder. Cervical cancer tends to invade these structures instead of the body of the uterus; when the rectovaginal or vesicovaginal septum becomes invaded, the juxtaposition of the vaginal wall directly to the bladder and the rectum makes these organs directly accessible. *The body of the uterus sits in the peri-* *toneal cavity. Although it is juxtaposed to these structures, it is separated by the peritoneal lining, making direct invasion rare.*

Cervix

The cervix comprises the lower third of the uterus. It is roughly cylindrical in shape, projecting into the upper

TABLE 43.2	Orientation of T-Oncoanatomy of GYN Primary Sites			
Primary Site	**Coronal**	**Sagittal**	**Transverse**	**Axial Level**
Ovary	Lateral/apical parametrium	Intimacy with fallopian tubes	Positioned in both peritoneal and pelvic cavity	S3
Fallopian tube	Lateral/apical parametrium	Intimacy with fallopian tubes	Positioned in both peritoneal and pelvic cavity	S2, S3
Uterine fundus	Superior portion of uterus	Antiflexed superior to cervix	Rests on urinary bladder	S2
Cervix	Inferior portion of uterus	Intimate contact of anterior lip of cervix to urinary bladder	Urinary bladder anteriorly and rectum posteriorly	Femoral head
Vagina	Urethra in anterior wall	Urethra in anterior wall and rectum next to posterior wall	Intimate to urethra and anus	Femoral neck
Vulva	Perineum showing muscle anatomy and compartment	Relationship to urinary tract and urethra and anus	Intimate to urethral meatus and anus	Femoral trochanter

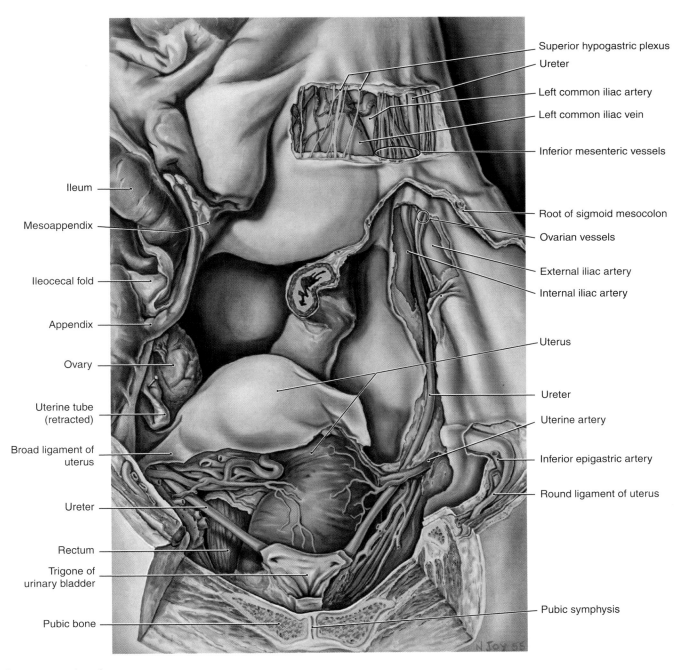

Anterosuperior view

Figure 43.6 **Orientation of M-oncoanatomy.**

anterior vaginal fornix. It communicates with the vagina through an orifice, namely, the cervical os. Cancer of the cervix may originate on the vaginal surface or in the cervical canal and be either squamous cell or adenocarcinomas. The mesometrium, or broad ligament of the uterus, contains a number of very important structures that determine the course of events in a number of oncologic presentations and complications. *The course of*

the ureter, which is the critical structure, passes from its lateral position in the abdomen to its medial location in the pelvis by moving horizontally to insert into the bladder. It is crossed superiorly and medially by the uterine artery. The long, transverse course of the ureter makes it particularly vulnerable to entrapment by cancer spread from the cervix because it lies juxtaposed to the cervix before its entry to the bladder. Along the sidewall of the pelvis,

TABLE 43.3		Orientation of Gynecologic Primary Sites and Sentinel Lymph Nodes		
Cancer Types	**Axial Level Structure/Site**	**Anatomic Adjacent Structure/Site**	**Sentinel Nodes**	
Adenocarcinoma of ovary	S3	Small intestine, mesentery omentum, uterus	Para-aortic nodes	
Adenocarcinoma of fallopian tubes	S2/3	Large intestine, mesentery omentum, uterus	Para-aortic nodes	
Adenocarcinoma of uterine fundus*	S2	Small intestine, sigmoid, bladder, rectum	Para-aortic and obturator nodes	
Squamous cell cancer of the cervix	S1	Bladder, rectum, uterus, vagina	Obturator and internal iliac nodes	
Squamous cell of the vagina	Coccyx, axial level, ischium	Cervix, bladder, rectum, pouch of Douglas	Obturator, internal and external iliac nodes	
Basaloid cancer of vulva	Femur	Anus, urethra, vagina	Inguinal and femoral nodes	

*Trophoblastic gestational cancers are uterine in location but placental in origin.

the obturator nerve and vessel enter into the obturator canal.

Vagina

The vagina is the external os, and the cervix is the internal os. *The vagina itself is a fibromuscular tube that extends from the cervix to the vestibule of the external genitalia.* It consists of numerous folds of an inner mucosa, a middle muscle layer, and an outer fibrous adventitia. The vagina has no glands and is lubricated by the cervical mucus glands. It is lined by stratified squamous epithelium, has a loose fibroelastic connective tissue and rich vasculature, which comprise the lamina propria, then a smooth muscle layer. The urethra runs anteriorly. The predominant cancer is squamous cell.

Vulva

The vestibule of the vagina is the region between the labia minora and hymen. The labia majora are external and fuse into the mons pubis. The prepuce of the clitoris is like a hood over the clitoris. The underlying musculature consists of three muscles: The bulbospongiosus, ischiocavernosus, and the transverse perineal superficialis. Deep to this is the perineal membrane and the "urogenital diaphragm" or urethral sphincter.

N-Oncoanatomy

The gynecologic organs lie in the true pelvis and are supplied by the hypogastric or internal iliac artery, which enters the broad ligament artery as the uterine artery (Fig. 43.5; Table 43.2). The venous drainage and lymphatics are parallel reentering into the internal iliac veins. *The obturator node is the sentinel node for cervix and is located in a plane posterior to the external iliac nodes*

(Table 43.3). This lymph node is in the true pelvis. Occasionally, there is an aberrant channel connecting an internal iliac node to an external iliac node. The external iliac node chain runs with the external iliac artery and vein and is well anterior to the internal iliac node chain. The obturator node, when involved, is often associated with cancer of the cervix infiltrating in the broad ligament. Once this occurs, retrograde or abnormal flow patterns alter the course of lymphatics and collateral channels can connect internal and external iliac nodes. The cervix is drained by preuteral, postuteral, and uterosacral lymphatic routes into the following first station nodes: Parametrial, hypogastric (obturator), external iliac, presacral, and common iliac. Para-aortic nodes are second station and juxtaregional.

The fundus of the uterus, fallopian tubes, and ovaries may follow lymphatic channels related to the ovarian artery and vein. The major lymphatic trunks are the uteroovarian (infundibulopelvic), parametrial, and presacral, and drain into the hypogastric, external iliac, common iliac, presacral, and para-aortic nodes. The ovary descends from their retroperitoneal para-aortic location in the fetus by the gubernaculums. Thus, ovarian cancer can spread to nonregional as well as regional nodes, that is, the para-aortic, pelvic, and even inguinal nodes owing to attachment of the round ligament. The sentinel nodes depend on location of the cancer in the vagina: In the superior portico, it is similar to the cervix; inferiorly, it is similar to the vulva. The distal vagina and vulva can drain into the inguinal and femoral nodes as well as pelvic iliac lymph nodes.

M-Oncoanatomy

The internal and external iliac veins enter the inferior vena cava and the common target organ for cervical,

TABLE 43.4	Imaging Modalities for Staging Gynecologic Cancer	
Method	Diagnosis and Staging Capability	Recommended for Use
Primary (T) staging		
CTe	Reliable for defining adnexal ovarian masses, extension to gynecologic organs, peritoneal seeding and ascites	Yes, contrast to visualize vessels and intestines
MRI	Role of MRI is emerging as criteria for malignancy defined	Yes, but supplemental to CT for soft tissues
TVUS	Excellent for screening and diagnosis	No, not reliable to define invasion
PET	High activity suggests malignancy versus benign status of solid or cystic pelvic masses	No
Nodal (N) staging		
CTe	Excellent for detecting nodal adenopathy >1 cm in size	Yes, cost effective
MRI	Available for supplementing CT	Yes, if cancer is high grade
Needle biopsy	Confirms lesions detected by radionuclide scan, CT scans, or lymphangiogram	Patients with suspicious lesions, image-guided aspirations
Metastases (M) staging		
Barium enema	Rectovaginal wall invasion	Yes, for patients with suspicious lesions
Urography	Detects ureteral obstruction, bladder invasion; screens for unsuspected renal anomaly	All operative candidates
Bone scan	Useful to assess omental and liver metastases	Yes, if suspected
CT		Yes, if suspected

CT, computed tomography; CTe, CT enhanced with IV contrast; MRI, magnetic resonance imaging; TVUS, transvaginal ultrasound.

uterine, and ovarian cancers are the lungs. The neurovascular plexus relates to the sympathetic and parasympathetic nerves, which are rarely involved. Cervical cancer, when metastatic to lymph nodes, can invade directly into adjacent vertebral bodies (Fig. 43.6) and be extremely destructive laterally excavating vertebrae and intervertebral disks.

Rules of Classification and Staging

Clinical Staging and Imaging

The importance of clinical staging by physical examination, and standard laboratory and readily available radiologic procedures as intravenous pyelography and barium enema was the essence of its universal adaptation. The International Federation of Gynecology and Obstetrics recognized the fact that alternative radiation treatment to surgery never allowed for surgical pathologic staging in cervical cancer. Clinical staging preceded any treatment and may not be changed because of subsequent findings once therapy started. The staging process, however, has been modified to allow colposcopy, endocervical curettage, hymenoscopy, cystoscopy, and

protoscopy, and requires suspected bladder and rectal cancer be confirmed by biopsy. Fine-needle aspiration of cytologically palpable nodes may be used to confirm cancer, but laparoscopy or radiologically guided biopsy is not allowed. Although encouraged, sophisticated imaging, such as computed tomography (CT), magnetic resonance imaging (MRI), positron emission tomography, and ultrasonography (US) are not allowed to alter stage because these technologies are not always available (Table 43.4).

The completely resected specimen including the primary site and regional lymph nodes must be thoroughly analyzed and are pTNM designated. Radical hysterectomy and bilateral salpingo-oophorectomy with pelvic lymph node resection is the usual procedure for pathologic evaluation.

The staging has remained unchanged at most gynecologic primary sites; in fact, the rules for classification *still do not allow* for sophisticated imaging, which includes CT, MRI, and US to alter staging. The multidisciplinary approach to decision making is truly interdisciplinary, most often involving a gynecologic oncologist and a dedicated radiation oncologist. Over the decades, diagnostic and therapeutic protocols in

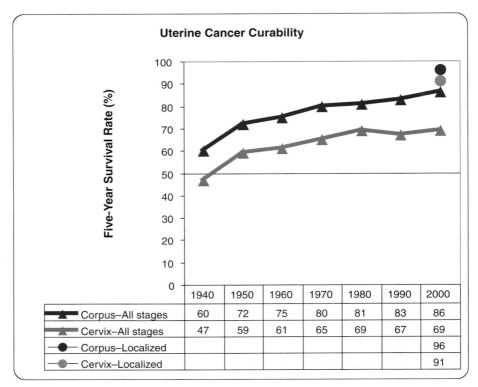

Uterine Cancer Curability

	1940	1950	1960	1970	1980	1990	2000
Corpus–All stages	60	72	75	80	81	83	86
Cervix–All stages	47	59	61	65	69	67	69
Corpus–Localized							96
Cervix–Localized							91

Figure 43.7 **Trajectory of cancer survival.**

national cooperative groups have provided a scientific basis for introducing combined modalities and introducing innovations into clinical practice.

Cancer Statistics and Survival

Female genital system cancers collectively account for 80,000 new cases annually, with uterine corpus exceeding cervix by a factor of four. Both are highly curable and deaths are relatively low. The major gynecologic killer is ovarian cancer, with 16,000 annual deaths, which exceeds the other six primary sites combined.

The survival rate gains in both cervix uteri and fundus uteri have been incremental. Recognizing that invasive cancers of the gynecologic tract have had a higher baseline, better than 50% in the 1950s, the gains for all stages are only 15% or 2% to 3% per decade. As noted, mortality rates have plummeted owing to early detection, especially of cervical cancer because it is most often detected in its noninvasive stage. Localized uterine cancers are more than 90% curable (Fig. 43.7; Table 43.5).

TABLE 43.5	**Female Genital System: Cancer Statistics**				
			Five-Year Survival Rates (%)		
Site	Incidence	Mortality	1950	2000	% Gain
Uterine cervix	10,370	3,710	59	73	+14
Uterine corpus	40,880	7,310	72	86	+14
Ovary	22,220	16,210	30	52	+22
Vulva	3,870	870	—	—	—
Vagina and associated structures	2,140	810	—	—	—

Modified from American Cancer Society. *Cancer Facts and Figures 2005*. Atlanta: American Cancer Society; 2005:4.

TABLE 43.6	Cancer Curability by Stages at Diagnosis (1995–2001)			
	Five-Year Survival Rates (%)			
Site	All Stages	Local	Regional	Distant
Uterine cervix	73	92	55	17
Uterine corpus	84	96	66	25
Ovary	45	94	68	29

Modified from Ries LAG, Eisner MP, Kosary CL, et al. eds. *SEER Cancer Statistics Review, 1975–2001.* National Cancer Institute. Bethesda, MD. Available: http://seer.cancer.gov/csr/1975_2001/,2004; Tables V, XII, XXI.

The cancer survival rates indicate the gain in survival for uterine corpus and cervix have been modest (14%) over the past five decades. However, most uterine cervix cancers are detected as cancer-in-situ, and this is not reflected in the figures. Ovarian cancer survival has improved by 22% and, as stated, remains lethal because most cases are detected late owing to its insidious onset and inaccessibility of ovarian nodules to early diagnosis. On the bright side is the high cure and 5-year survival rates for stage I patients with cervical cancer (92%), uterine corpus cancer (96%), and ovarian cancer (95%; Table 43.6).

The ovary is as much a structure of the whole peritoneal cavity as it is of the pelvis.

Perspective and Patterns of Spread

Ovarian cancer is the most lethal cancer of the female genital tract, surpassing all deaths attributed to gynecologic cancers at all other sites combined. The total loss of life annually in 2004 was 16,000, compared with 13,000 for all other gynecological sites. The estimated incidence is 25,000 new cases annually. The common symptom and sign is the insidious accumulation of ascitic fluid masquerading as weight gain and increase in abdominal girth. Unlike the other common gynecologic cancers, vaginal bleeding is rare. Clinical detection is most often due to routine physical and pelvic examination coupled with pursuit of imaging and serum markers in high-risk patients with familial histories or those testing positive for both *BRCA*-1 and -2 oncogene mutations.

The World Health Organization list of histopathologies is endorsed by the American Joint Committee on Cancer/International Union Against Cancer (Table 44.1). Between 80% and 90% are epithelial cancers; 5% to 10% are bilateral. Serous carcinomas are the most common subtype, microscopically containing papillary and glandular elements. The staging of these cancers demands surgical laparotomy exploration of both the pelvic and peritoneal cavity including the omentum, the mesentery, the liver, and diaphragm because abdominal seeding is a dominant pattern of spread (Fig. 44.1).

TNM Staging Criteria

The ovary is as much a structure of the whole peritoneal cavity as it is of the pelvis. This is particularly true once it has become subject to malignant transformation. The ovary is positioned essentially at the bottom of the peritoneal cavity. Its blood supply reflects its abdominal origin.

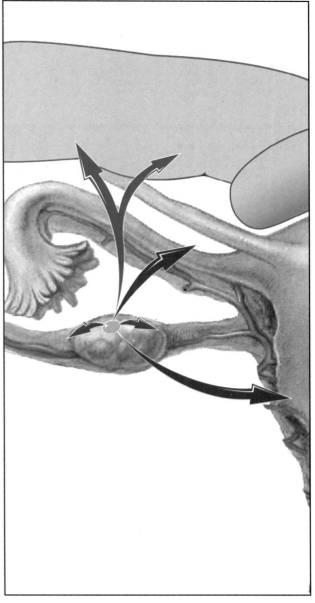

Figure 44.1 **Patterns of spread.** The cancer crab is color coded for stage: T0, yellow; T1, green; T2, blue; T3, purple; and T4, red.

DEFINITION OF TNM

STAGE GROUPINGS

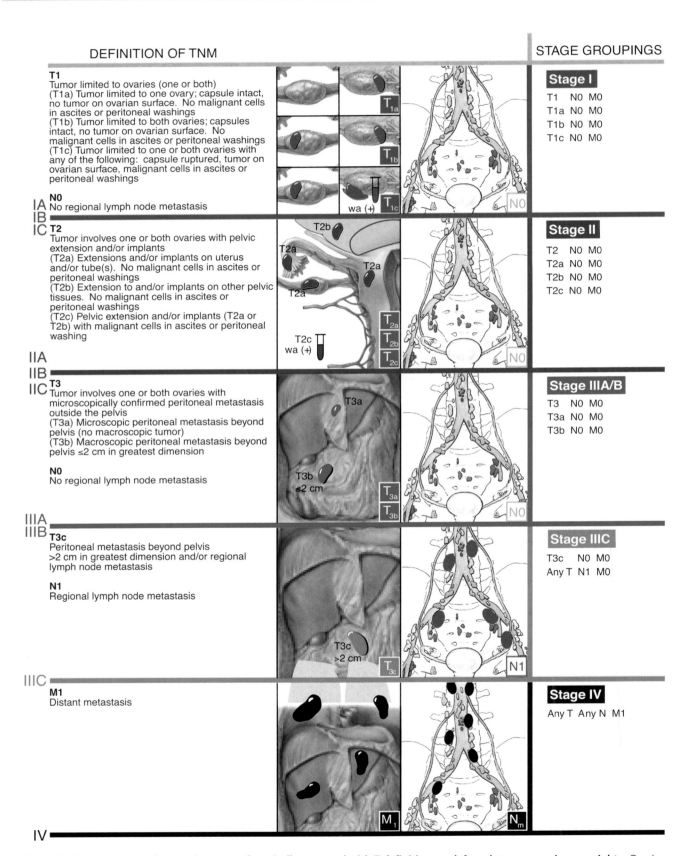

T1
Tumor limited to ovaries (one or both)
(T1a) Tumor limited to one ovary; capsule intact, no tumor on ovarian surface. No malignant cells in ascites or peritoneal washings
(T1b) Tumor limited to both ovaries; capsules intact, no tumor on ovarian surface. No malignant cells in ascites or peritoneal washings
(T1c) Tumor limited to one or both ovaries with any of the following: capsule ruptured, tumor on ovarian surface, malignant cells in ascites or peritoneal washings

N0
No regional lymph node metastasis

IA
IB
IC

T2
Tumor involves one or both ovaries with pelvic extension and/or implants
(T2a) Extensions and/or implants on uterus and/or tube(s). No malignant cells in ascites or peritoneal washings
(T2b) Extension to and/or implants on other pelvic tissues. No malignant cells in ascites or peritoneal washings
(T2c) Pelvic extension and/or implants (T2a or T2b) with malignant cells in ascites or peritoneal washing

IIA
IIB
IIC

T3
Tumor involves one or both ovaries with microscopically confirmed peritoneal metastasis outside the pelvis
(T3a) Microscopic peritoneal metastasis beyond pelvis (no macroscopic tumor)
(T3b) Macroscopic peritoneal metastasis beyond pelvis ≤2 cm in greatest dimension

N0
No regional lymph node metastasis

IIIA
IIIB

T3c
Peritoneal metastasis beyond pelvis >2 cm in greatest dimension and/or regional lymph node metastasis

N1
Regional lymph node metastasis

IIIC

M1
Distant metastasis

IV

Stage I
T1   N0 M0
T1a N0 M0
T1b N0 M0
T1c N0 M0

Stage II
T2   N0 M0
T2a N0 M0
T2b N0 M0
T2c N0 M0

Stage IIIA/B
T3   N0 M0
T3a N0 M0
T3b N0 M0

Stage IIIC
T3c   N0 M0
Any T N1 M0

Stage IV
Any T Any N M1

Figure 44.2 TNM staging diagram is arranged vertically arranged with T definitions on left and stage groupings on right. Ovarian cancers are cancers of the pelvis and peritoneal cavity. Resectability depends on number and size of peritoneal implants. Color bars are coded for stage: Stage I, green; II, blue; III, purple; IV, red; and metastatic disease to viscera and nodes, black.

TABLE 44.1	Histopathologic Type: Common Cancers of the Ovary

I. Epithelial tumors
  A. Serous tumors
    1. Benign serous cystadenoma
    2. Of borderline malignancy: Serous cystadenoma with proliferating activity of the epithelial cells and nuclear abnormalities, but with no infiltrative destructive growth (carcinomas of low potential malignancy)
    3. Serous cystadenocarcinoma
  B. Mucinous tumors
    1. Benign mucinous cystadenoma
    2. Of borderline malignancy: Mucinous cystadenoma with proliferating activity of the epithelial cells and nuclear abnormalities, but with no infiltrative destructive growth (carcinomas of low potential malignancy)
    3. Mucinous cystadenocarcinoma
  C. Endometrioid tumors
    1. Benign endometrioid cystadenoma
    2. Endometrioid tumors with proliferating activity of the epithelial cells and nuclear abnormalities, but with no infiltrative destructive growth (carcinomas of low potential malignancy)
    3. Endometrioid adenocarcinoma
  D. Clear cell tumors
    1. Benign clear cell tumors
    2. Clear cell tumors with proliferating activity of the epithelial cells and nuclear abnormalities, but with no infiltrative destructive growth (low potential malignancy)
    3. Clear cell cystadenocarcinoma
  E. Brenner (transitional cell tumor)
    1. Benign Brenner
    2. Borderline malignancy
    3. Malignant
    4. Transitional cell
  F. Squamous cell tumor
  G. Undifferentiated carcinoma
    1. A malignant tumor of epithelial structure that is too poorly differentiated to be placed in any other group
  H. Mixed epithelial tumor
    1. Tumors composed of two or more of the five major cell types of common epithelial tumors (types should be specified)

Reprinted from Greene FL, Page DL, Fleming ID, et al., eds. *AJCC Cancer Staging Manual.* 6th ed. New York: Springer; 2002:277.

When cancer forms in the ovary, it invades through its capsule and forms excrescences. *Tumor cells are released and seed the peritoneal surface, often invading* the gynecologic tract in the manner of an ovum or filling the cul-de-sac. *Because there is no true separation between the pelvic and abdominal cavities, this cancer often seeds the omentum, mesentery, and intestine.* The diaphragm may act as a "blotter" for these dispersed tumor cells in the peritoneal cavity. Ascites and pleural effusion are common in advanced stages.

The evolution of ovarian cancer staging criteria rested on careful exploratory laparotomy and gradually required multiple sampling of a variety of peritoneal sites as omentum, mesentery, liver, and the diaphragm. By the fourth edition, the three stages each have three subcategories. The pattern of spread in the earliest stages is limited to the ovary (stage T1a); if both ovaries are involved, T1b, and positive washings or ascites is T1c. Once extension occurs to pelvic organs or implants on uterus or tubes, it is T2a; onto pelvic wall or bladder, T2b; and positive washings or ascites, T2c. Once peritoneal metastatic seeding occurs into the abdominal peritoneal cavity but is microscopic tumor, it is stage T3a; macroscopic tumor <2 cm, T3b; and macroscopic tumor >2 cm, T3c (Fig. 44.2).

Important clarifications include the following: Only malignant ascites affect staging, and liver capsule metastases are T3, but liver parenchyma are M1. Pleural effusion must have positive cytology to be M1 stage. Patients with only intraperitoneal carcinoma without ovarian involvement or minimally involved should be labeled as "extraovarian" peritoneal carcinoma and by definition are stage T3 or M1.

Summary of Changes

No changes have been made since the fifth edition of the AJCC CSM.

Orientation of Three-planar Oncoanatomy

The isocenter of the ovary is at the roof of female genital system at the S2, S3 level, 5 to 10 cm lateral to midline (Fig. 44.3).

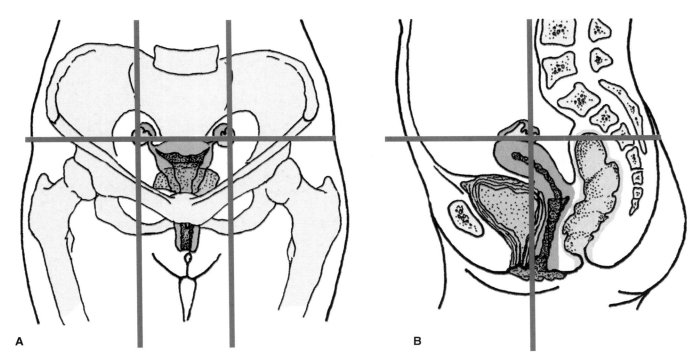

Figure 44.3 Orientation of oncoanatomy of the ovary. The anatomic isocenter is off the midline on each side at the true pelvis inlet estimated at the transverse S1 to S3 level. **A.** Coronal. **B.** Sagittal.

T-oncoanatomy

- *Coronal*: The ovaries are a pair of solid, flattened ovoids, 2.0 to 4.0 cm in diameter in the premenopausal woman. They are connected by a peritoneal fold to the broad ligament and by the suspensory ligament of the ovary to the lateral wall of the pelvis (Fig. 44.4).

- *Sagittal*: The ovary is connected also by the round ligament and the ovarian ligament to the pelvic brim. During its functioning years, the menstrual cycle is regulated by ovulation and is divided into a proliferative phase (follicular) and secretory (luteal) phase. It is in the postmenopausal state that neoplasia occurs. Rather than becoming atrophic and cystic, mitotic activity occurs.

- *Transverse*: The uterus is usually asymmetrically placed; in this example, it leans to the left. The round ligament of the female takes the same subperitoneal course as the deferent duct of the male. The free edge of the medial four fifths of the broad ligament contains the uterine tube, and that of the lateral one fifth, the ovarian vessels in the suspensory ligament of the ovary.

N-oncoanatomy

The lymphatic drainage occurs via the ovarian ligament and round ligament trunks and an external iliac accessory route into the following regional nodes: The para-aortic nodes are the major regional nodes followed by the external iliac, common iliac, hypogastric, lateral sacral, and, rarely, to the inguinal nodes (Fig. 44.5; Table 44.2). *Although the ovary is pelvic in location, its lymphatic drainage recapitulates its abdominal or homologous origin; the para-aortic lymph nodes.* Its vestigial relationship via the round ligament to the labia reaffirms its similarity to the testes in its intimate scrotal location, which makes drainage to inguinal nodes possible. Although an inguinal node can be considered a first station node, most oncologists regard an extrapelvic node as metastatic.

M-oncoanatomy

The ovarian veins drain into the inferior vena cava and target to right side of the heart and then to lungs (see Fig. 43.6). However, peritoneal seeding, as mentioned, is a predominant metastatic pattern involving the abdominal cavity, liver, and diaphragm. Malignant ascites is the predominant death pattern.

Rules of Classification and Staging

Clinical Staging

Physical and pelvic examinations are limited in their assessment. Reliance on imaging is essential, and includes transvaginal ultrasound (TVUS), magnetic resonance imaging (MRI), enhanced computed tomography (CT), and positron emission tomography (PET). All are of value or patients with advanced cancer present (see Table 43.4). Laparotomy and histologic confirmation of

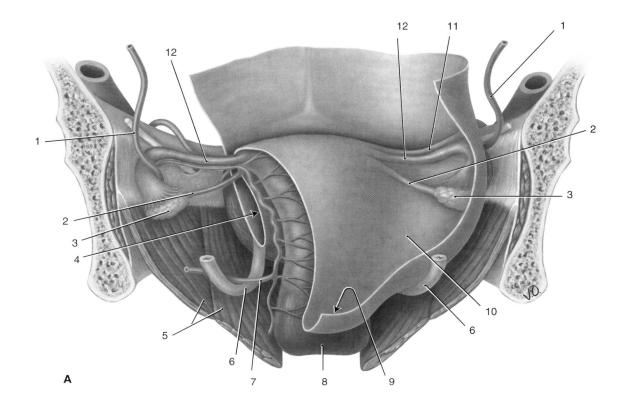

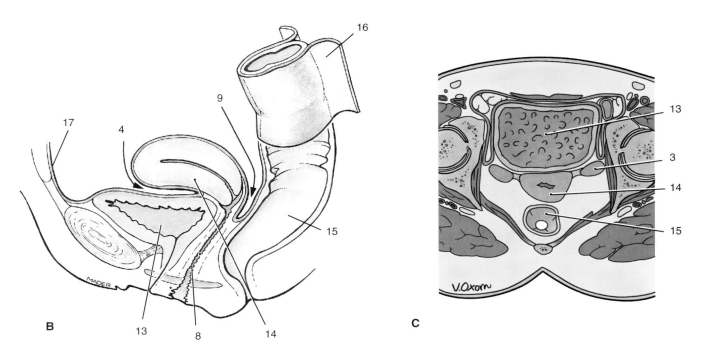

Figure 44.4 **T-oncoanatomy:** Three-planar views. **A.** Coronal. **B.** Sagittal. **C.** Transverse. (1) Ovarian artery. (2) Ligament of ovary. (3) Ovary. (4) Vesicouterine pouch. (5) Levator ani muscle. (6) Ureter. (7) Uterine artery. (8) Vagina. (9) Rectouterine pouch. (10) Broad ligament. (11) Round ligament of uterus. (12) Uterine tube. (13) Urinary bladder. (14) Uterus. (15) Rectum. (16) Peritoneum. (17) Peritoneum of abdominal wall.

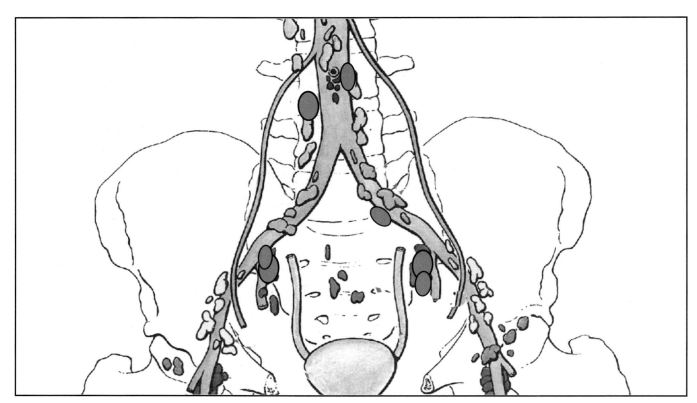

Figure 44.5 N-oncoanatomy. Although the ovary drains to the high para-aortic nodes, most ovarian cancers spread initially in the pelvis placing both the internal and external iliac nodes at risk.

spread are required for accurate staging. Imaging can guide pelvic and peritoneal areas to assess.

Surgical-pathologic Staging

Ovarian cancer is surgically/pathologically staged. Laparotomy and resection of the ovarian mass and biopsy sampling of peritoneal sites include any suspicious peritoneal nodules or implants on omentum, mesentery, diaphragm, pelvic, and para-aortic lymph nodes. Peritoneal washing with cytospins as well as for

ascites to establish positive cells. Suspicious pulmonary nodules or supraclavicular nodes require pathologic confirmation. A detailed operative report with precise measurements in centimeters for mass lesions is mandatory before any other treatment. To stage a patient IA, multiple biopsies are required to be negative as mentioned. Second-look laparotomies may be useful after chemotherapy and debulking surgery, but do not change the original staging. The value of imaging procedures to guide surgery is highly recommended.

TABLE 44.2	Lymph Nodes of Ovary	
Sentinel nodes		Juxtaregional nodes
Obturator		Common iliac
Internal iliac		Hypogastric
		Lateral sacral
Regional nodes		
Left: renal hilar		
Right: paracaval		
Para-aortic		
Inguinal		
External iliac		

Oncoimaging Annotations

- TVUS is the optimal imaging procedure for early detection and evaluation of any adnexal mass irregularities.

- Color Doppler aids in diagnosis of malignancy if active neovascularization is identified with vessels that have a characteristic wave form shift.

- MRI is preferred to CT for adnexal mass imaging for malignancy criteria with gadolinium contrast: Criteria for malignancy include mass size >4 cm, and wall and septa thickness >3 mm with heterogeneous densities.

- Fluorine-18-labeled deoxy-D-glucose PET reliably images tumors >1 cm. In pilot studies, the sensitivity of PET appears higher than that of MRI or CT (not significant), with equivalent specificity. Large-scale studies are needed to determine the role of PET in assessing ovarian cancer.

- Cross-sectional imaging is used as an alternative to second-look laparotomy, which is no longer performed routinely.

- Significant criteria of malignancy of ovarian mass include: Size >4 cm; solid more than cystic; wall thickness >3 cm; septa >3 mm; heterogeneous appearance of nodulation; and vegetations.

- Omental cakes, especially of calcified scattered deposits, indicate advanced abdominal disease.

- Bilateral symmetrical adnexal masses suggests Krukenberg tumors secondary to the gastrointestinal tract.

- Ascites especially with internal fluid–fluid level is consistent with cancer and is referred to as "complex ascites."

Cancer Statistics and Survival

Female genital system cancers collectively account for 80,000 new cases annually, with uterine corpus exceeding cervix by a factor of four. Both are highly curable and deaths are relatively low. The major gynecologic killer is ovarian cancer, with 16,000 annual deaths, which exceeds the other six primary sites combined (see Table 43.5).

Survival Rates

The survival rate gains in both cervix uteri and fundus uteri have been incremental. Recognizing that invasive cancers of the gynecologic tract have had a higher baseline, better than 50% in the 1950s, the gains for all stages are only 15% or 2% to 3% per decade. As noted, mortality rates have plummeted owing to early detection, especially of cancer of the cervix, because it is most often detected in its noninvasive stage. Localized uterine cancers are more than 90% curable (see Fig. 43.7).

The cancer survival rates indicate the gain in survival for uterine corpus and cervix have been modest (14%) over the past five decades. However, most uterine cervix cancers are detected as cancer-in-situ and this is not reflected in the figures. Ovarian cancer survival has improved by 22% and as stated remains lethal because most cases are detected late owing to its insidious onset and the inaccessibility of ovarian nodules to early diagnosis. On the bright side is the high cure and 5-year survival rates for stage I patients with cervical cancer (92%), uterine corpus cancer (96%), and ovarian cancer (95%; see Table 43.6).

45

Fallopian Tubes

The basis for staging carcinomas of the fallopian tube clearly parallels ovarian cancer.

Perspective and Patterns of Spread

Carcinoma of the fallopian tube (FT) is rare and most often simulates ovarian cancers in presentation as an adnexal mass. Often, FT cancers are associated with two symptoms: Vaginal bleeding and abdominal pelvic pain, often spasmodic in nature. This is an uncommon female malignant cancer, representing <1% of all female cancers.

Histopathologically, FT cancers are serous adenocarcinomas. The majority are identified at surgery and the basis of this staging system is surgical-pathologic. The histopathology is similar to ovarian cancers (Table 45.1).

TNM Staging Criteria

The basis for staging carcinomas of the FT clearly parallels ovarian cancer. The patterns of spread are similar with invasion into the uterus and female genital tract versus seeding into the peritoneal cavity (Fig. 45.1). The American Joint Committee on Cancer introduced the TNM staging in the fifth edition and left it unchanged in the current sixth edition (Fig. 45.2). Laparotomy and resection of tubal masses as well as hysterectomy and suspicious sites require biopsy and histology for confirmation.

Summary of Changes

No changes have been made since the fifth edition of the AJCC CSM.

Orientation of Three-planar Oncoanatomy

The isocenter of FT is similar to ovary and is at the roof of gynecologic structures (Fig. 45.3).

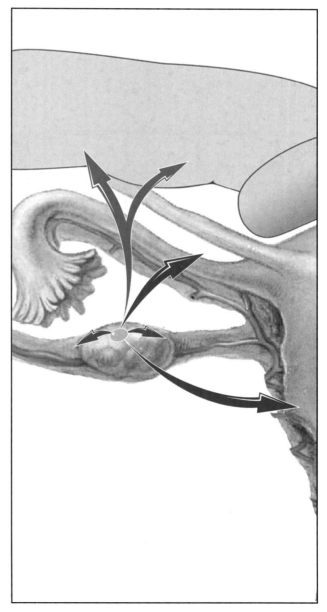

Figure 45.1 **Patterns of spread. The cancer crab is color coded for stage:** Tis, yellow; T1, green; T2, blue; T3, purple.

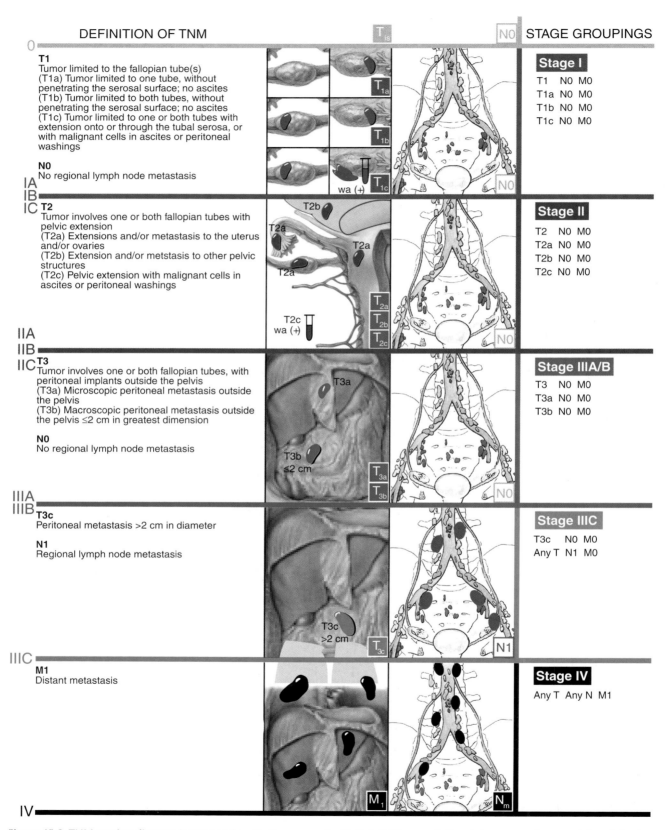

DEFINITION OF TNM

T1
Tumor limited to the fallopian tube(s)
(T1a) Tumor limited to one tube, without penetrating the serosal surface; no ascites
(T1b) Tumor limited to both tubes, without penetrating the serosal surface; no ascites
(T1c) Tumor limited to one or both tubes with extension onto or through the tubal serosa, or with malignant cells in ascites or peritoneal washings

N0
No regional lymph node metastasis

T2
Tumor involves one or both fallopian tubes with pelvic extension
(T2a) Extensions and/or metastasis to the uterus and/or ovaries
(T2b) Extension and/or metstasis to other pelvic structures
(T2c) Pelvic extension with malignant cells in ascites or peritoneal washings

T3
Tumor involves one or both fallopian tubes, with peritoneal implants outside the pelvis
(T3a) Microscopic peritoneal metastasis outside the pelvis
(T3b) Macroscopic peritoneal metastasis outside the pelvis ≤2 cm in greatest dimension

N0
No regional lymph node metastasis

T3c
Peritoneal metastasis >2 cm in diameter

N1
Regional lymph node metastasis

M1
Distant metastasis

STAGE GROUPINGS

Stage I

T1   N0 M0
T1a N0 M0
T1b N0 M0
T1c N0 M0

Stage II

T2   N0 M0
T2a N0 M0
T2b N0 M0
T2c N0 M0

Stage IIIA/B

T3   N0 M0
T3a N0 M0
T3b N0 M0

Stage IIIC

T3c   N0 M0
Any T N1 M0

Stage IV

Any T Any N M1

Figure 45.2 TNM staging diagram is arranged vertically arranged with T definitions on left and stage groupings on right. Fallopian tube cancers are quite rare and are resectable as Stage II (blue) and are borderline resectable in Stage IIIA. Color bars are coded for stage: Stage 0, yellow; I, green; II, blue; III, purple; IV, red; and metastatic disease to viscera and nodes, black.

TABLE 45.1	Histopathologic Type: Common Cancers of the Fallopian Tube

Adenocarcinoma is the most frequently seen histology.

Modified from Greene FL, Page DL, Fleming ID, et al., eds. *AJCC Cancer Staging Manual.* 6th ed. New York: Springer; 2002:286.

T-oncoanatomy

The FT is an appendage that extends from the posterior superior aspect of the uterus and opens to the peritoneal cavity and the ovary. It has a length of 10 cm (see Fig. 44.4A–C).

N-oncoanatomy

The lymphatic drainage occurs via the ovarian ligament and round ligament trunks and an external iliac accessory route into the following regional nodes: The para-aortic nodes are the major regional nodes followed by the external iliac, common iliac, hypogastric, lateral sacral, and, rarely, the inguinal nodes (Fig. 45.4; Table 45.2). Although the ovary is pelvic in location, its lymphatic drainage recapitulates its abdominal or homologous origin, the para-aortic lymph nodes. Its vestigial relationship via the round ligament to the labia reaffirms its similarity to the testes in its intimate scrotal location, which makes drainage to inguinal nodes possible. Although an inguinal node can be considered a first station node, most oncologists regard an extrapelvic node as metastatic.

M-oncoanatomy

The ovarian veins drain into the inferior vena cava and target to right side of the heart and then to lungs (see Fig. 43.6). However, peritoneal seeding, as mentioned, is a predominant metastatic pattern involving the abdominal cavity, liver, and diaphragm. Malignant ascites is the predominant death pattern.

Rules for Classification and Staging

Clinical Staging

Physical and pelvic examinations are limited in their assessment. Reliance on imaging is essential, and includes transvaginal ultrasound, magnetic resonance imaging (MRI), enhanced computed tomography (CT), and positron emission tomography. All are of value for patients with advanced cancer (Table 45.3). Laparotomy and histologic confirmation of spread are required for accurate staging. Imaging can guide pelvic and peritoneal areas to assess.

Surgical-pathologic Staging

Surgical-pathologic staging criteria apply because laparotomy with resection is necessary to distinguish tubal from ovarian masses. Laparotomy and resection of FT mass and biopsy sampling of peritoneal sites include any suspicious peritoneal nodules or implants on omentum, mesentery, diaphragm, pelvic, and para-aortic lymph nodes. Peritoneal washing with cytospins is performed as well for ascites to establish positive cells. Suspicious pulmonary nodules or supraclavicular nodes require pathologic confirmation. A detailed operative report with precise measurements in centimeters for mass lesions is mandatory before any other treatment. To stage a patient as IA, multiple biopsies are required to be negative, as mentioned. Second-look laparotomies may be useful after chemotherapy and debulking surgery, but do not change the original staging. Imaging procedures to guide surgery are highly recommended.

Oncoimaging Annotations

- Hydrosalpinx with solid nodulation suggests FT carcinoma.
- CT is the recommended imaging modality for staging. MRI is reserved for patients with contraindications to iodinated contrast media (essential for diagnostic CT study) and for questions unanswered by CT.
- CT with intravenous contrast, helical technique, provides excellent cross-sectional imaging for detecting signs of malignancy as varied morphology cystic/solid walls or internal septa, lobulated papillary mass, implants 1 to 3 cm in size, and coarse calcifications.
- MRI is highly accurate in determining the origin of an adnexal mass and in characterizing ovarian masses as benign, malignant, or non-neoplastic. Intravenous gadolinium should be used because it improves lesion characterization.
- CT is useful for detecting small or large bowel invasion, mesenteric and omental "cake" masses, adenopathy, liver involvement, and ascites.

Cancer Statistics and Survival

Female genital system cancers collectively account for 80,000 new cases, with uterine corpus exceeding cervix

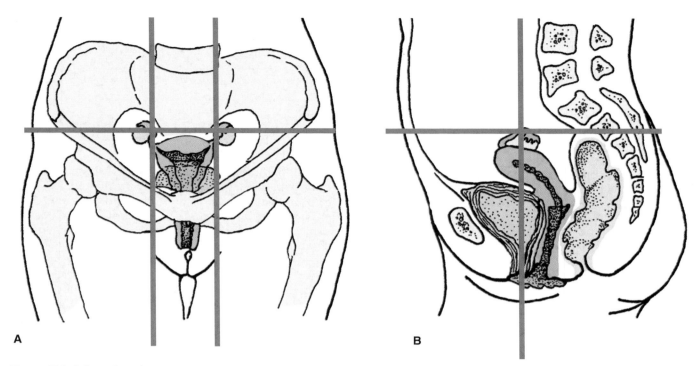

Figure 45.3 Orientation of oncoanatomy of the FT: The anatomic isocenter is off the midline on each side at the true pelvis inlet estimated at the transverse S1 to S3 level. **A.** Coronal. **B.** Sagittal.

by a factor of four. Both are highly curable and deaths are relatively low. The major gynecologic killer is ovarian cancer with 16,000 annual deaths, which exceeds the other six primary sites combined.

Survival Rates

The survival rate gains in both cervix uteri and fundus uteri have been incremental. Recognizing that invasive cancers of the gynecologic tract have had a higher baseline, better than 50% in the 1950s, the gains for all stages are only 15% or 2% to 3% per decade. As noted, mortality rates have plummeted owing to early detection, especially for cancer of the cervix, because it is most

often detected in its noninvasive stage. Localized uterine cancers are >90% curable.

The cancer survival rates indicate the gain in survival for uterine corpus and cervix have been modest (14%) over the past five decades. However, most uterine cervix cancers are detected as cancer-in-situ and this is not reflected in the figures. Ovarian cancer survival has improved by 22% and, as stated, remains lethal; most cases are detected late because of its insidious onset and inaccessibility of ovarian nodules to early diagnosis. On the bright side is the high cure and 5-year survival rates for stage I patients with cervical cancer (92%), uterine corpus cancer (96%), and ovarian cancer (95%; see Table 43.5).

TABLE 45.2	Lymph Nodes of Fallopian Tubes	
Sentinel nodes		Juxtaregional nodes
Obturator		Common iliac
Internal iliac		Hypogastric
		Lateral sacral
Regional nodes		
Left: renal hilar		
Right: paracaval		
Para-aortic		
Inguinal		
External iliac		

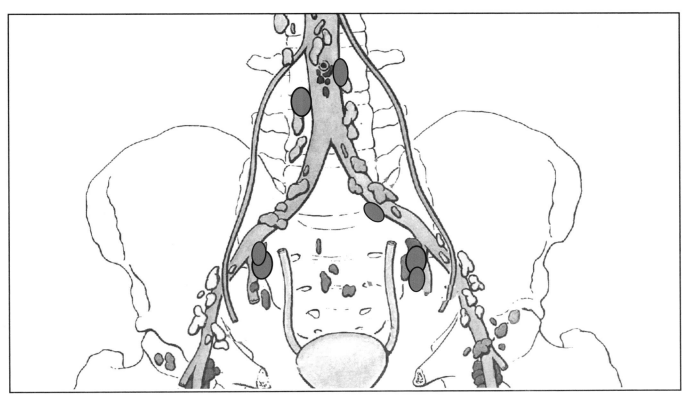

Figure 45.4 N-oncoanatomy. Although the FT drains to the high para-aortic nodes, most FT cancers spread initially in the pelvis placing both the intestinal and external iliac nodes at risk.

TABLE 45.3	Imaging Modalities for Staging Fallopian Tube Cancer	
Method	**Diagnosis and Staging Capability**	**Recommended for Use**
Primary (T) staging		
CTe	Reliable for defining adnexal ovarian masses, extension to gynecologic organs, peritoneal seeding, and ascites	Yes, contrast to visualize vessels and intestines
MRI	Role of MRI is emerging as criteria for malignancy defined	Yes, but supplemental to CT for soft tissues
TVUS	Excellent for screening and diagnosis	No, not reliable to define invasion
Nodal (N) staging		
CTe	Excellent for detecting nodal adenopathy >1 cm in size	Yes, cost effective
MRI	Available for supplementing CT	Yes, if cancer is high grade
Metastases (M) staging		
Barium enema		Yes, for patients with suspicious lesions
Bone scan	Useful to assess omental and liver metastases	Yes, if suspected
CT		Yes, if suspected

CT, computed tomography; CTe, CT enhanced with IV contrast; MRI, magnetic resonance imaging; TVUS, transvaginal ultrasound.

46

Fundus Uteri

The uterine cancers and sarcomas are related to the essential components of the uterus: A pear-shaped organ lined by simple columnar epithelium and tubular glands that extend to the myometrium.

Perspective and Patterns of Spread

Endometrial cancers are among the most curable gynecologic cancers and may relate to the capability of its normal physiologic functions of menstruation and pregnancy to shed its lining and the placenta. With the continual stimulus of hormones, it is not surprising to note it is the most common gynecologic cancer in the United States and Western Europe. With approximately 40,000 cases, deaths are limited to 10%, or 2% of all cancer deaths in women. The postmenopausal woman presenting with unexpected menstruation or vaginal bleeding allows for early referral. Diagnosis is readily made on histologic examination of the fractional dilatation and curettage. Risk factors include hosts with obesity, diabetes mellitus, and hypertension. Unopposed estrogen replacement and tamoxifen therapy have been cited as reasons to abandon such treatment for postmenopausal women owing to increased risk of inducing endometrial cancers.

The uterine cancers and sarcomas are related to the essential components of the uterus: A pear-shaped organ lined by simple columnar epithelium and tubular glands that extend to the myometrium. The endometrium consists of two layers—the functionalis, a superficial layer sloughed with menstruation, and the basalis, which is a deep narrow layer whose glands regenerate the functionalis. The types of cancers are predominantly adenocarcinomas; however, they can be serous, endometrioid, or mucinous, similar to the ovarian cancers. This reflects the embryonic mesonephros anlage (Table 46.1). The pattern of spread is reflected in the basic anatomy of the uterine fundus (Fig. 46.1), anteriorly or posteriorly into its wall, which is resisted by the serosa. Inferiorly, it invades the cervix and vagina. With further advancement, it can enter bowel and bladder.

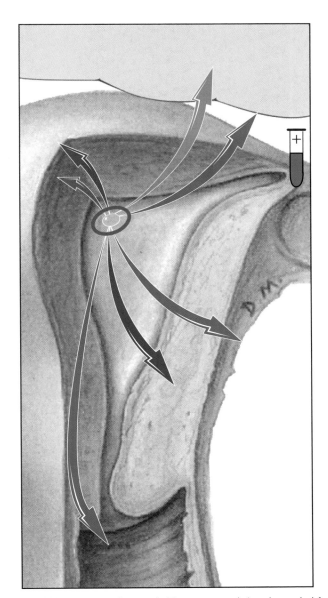

Figure 46.1 **Patterns of spread.** The cancer crab is color coded for stage: Tis, yellow; T1, green; T2, blue; T3, purple; and T4, red.

DEFINITION OF TNM

STAGE GROUPINGS

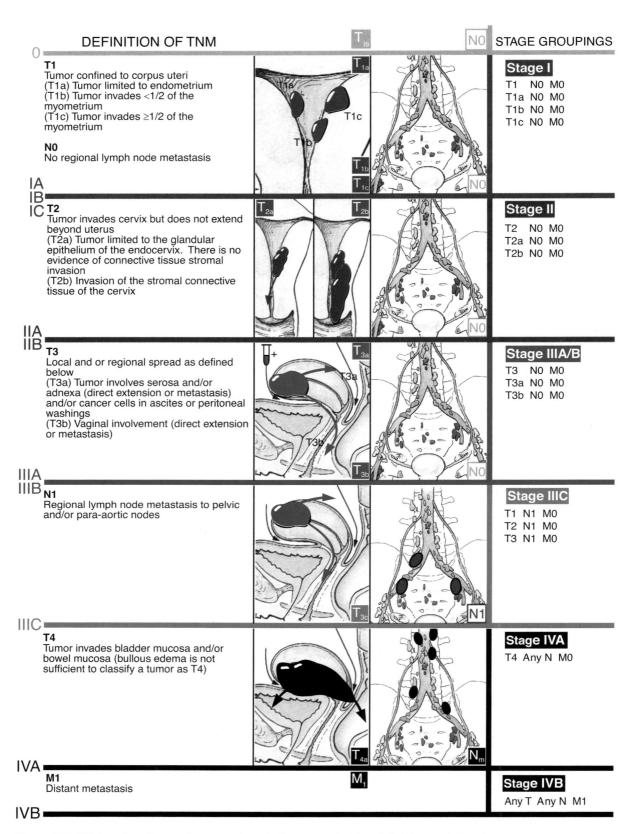

T1
Tumor confined to corpus uteri
(T1a) Tumor limited to endometrium
(T1b) Tumor invades <1/2 of the
myometrium
(T1c) Tumor invades ≥1/2 of the
myometrium

N0
No regional lymph node metastasis

Stage I

T1 N0 M0
T1a N0 M0
T1b N0 M0
T1c N0 M0

T2
Tumor invades cervix but does not extend
beyond uterus
(T2a) Tumor limited to the glandular
epithelium of the endocervix. There is no
evidence of connective tissue stromal
invasion
(T2b) Invasion of the stromal connective
tissue of the cervix

Stage II

T2 N0 M0
T2a N0 M0
T2b N0 M0

T3
Local and or regional spread as defined
below
(T3a) Tumor involves serosa and/or
adnexa (direct extension or metastasis)
and/or cancer cells in ascites or peritoneal
washings
(T3b) Vaginal involvement (direct extension
or metastasis)

Stage IIIA/B

T3 N0 M0
T3a N0 M0
T3b N0 M0

N1
Regional lymph node metastasis to pelvic
and/or para-aortic nodes

Stage IIIC

T1 N1 M0
T2 N1 M0
T3 N1 M0

T4
Tumor invades bladder mucosa and/or
bowel mucosa (bullous edema is not
sufficient to classify a tumor as T4)

Stage IVA

T4 Any N M0

M1
Distant metastasis

Stage IVB

Any T Any N M1

Figure 46.2 TNM staging diagram is arranged vertically arranged with T definitions on left and stage groupings on right.
Uterine fundus cancers are most often detected early and are readily resectable at Stage I and II with excellent cure rates. There
are four main stages, each with two or three substages. Color bars are coded for stage: Stage 0, yellow; I, green; II, blue; III,
purple; IV, red; and metastatic disease to viscera and nodes, black.

TABLE 46.1	Uterine Sarcoma Classification Proposed by the Gynecologic Oncology Group

Mesenchymal
  Leiomyosarcoma
  Endometrial stromal sarcoma: low and high grade
  Mixed differentiated sarcomas with epithelial elements
  Other uterine sarcomas

Mixed epithelial-stromal
  Adenocarcinoma with heterologous elements
  Carcinosarcoma with heterologous elements

Modified from Rubin P, Williams J, eds. *Clinical Oncology: A Multidisciplinary Approach for Physicians and Students.* 8th ed. Philadelphia: Elsevier; 2001:484.

TNM Staging Criteria

The patterns of spread are similar to a hollow organ with minor modification (Fig. 46.1). The criteria for corpus uteri have remained the same; however, the clinical examination has been supplanted by surgical pathologic assessment. In the early editions, stage I was confined to corpus and divided by its enlargement: Stage IA, ≤8 cm; IB ≥8 cm in greatest length. With the fourth edition, stage I was limited to endometrium (IA); with myometrial invasion, stage IB penetrates less than half the thickness of the myometrium, and IC, more than half the thickness (Fig. 46.2). In earlier editions, stage II was gross clinical involvement of the cervix, but was changed and now requires specific histopathologic verification. Stage IIA is surface endocervical involvement; deeper stomal invasions signify stage IIB. Stage III is extension beyond uterus, spreading into serosa or adnexa. Stage IIIA is vaginal involvement; IIIB is invasion of other genital sites but remaining in true pelvis. Stage IV was divided into IVA, which is similar to cervix with invasion of rectum and bladder, and stage IVB, metastatic spread to distant organs. These criteria have not changed in the sixth edition. Lymph node invasion has been relegated to stage III, and more recently advanced and categorized to stage IIIC.

The rules for classification were noted in the fourth edition. Uterine enlargement could be due to fibroids and other disorders, such as adenomyosis. These argued for dilation and curettage to establish the diagnosis, with emphasis on fractional curettage beginning with scraping the cervix. In the sixth edition, that fractional curettage requires histopathologic evidence of stromal invasion or hysterectomy with microscopic verification.

The importance of surgical-pathologic evaluation applies to regional lymph nodes as well as the primary sites.

Summary of Changes

No changes have been made since the fifth edition of the AJCC CSM.

Orientation of Three-planar Oncoanatomy

The isocenter for the uterus is at the S4 level but can vary from S2 to S5 depending on the degree of anteflexion or retroflexion (Fig. 46.3).

T-oncoanatomy

- *Coronal: The upper two-thirds of the uterus above the level of the internal cervical os is called the "corpus uteri."* The fallopian tubes enter at the upper lateral corners of its pear-shaped body. That portion of the muscular organ positioned above the line joining the tubouterine orifices is called the "fundus."

- *Sagittal:* The body of the uterus sits in the peritoneal cavity. Although it is juxtaposed to these structures, it is separated by the peritoneal lining, making direct invasion rare.

- *Transverse:* The relationship of the uterus to other pelvic tissues is important, particularly to the rectum and bladder. The rectouterine or the vesicouterine septum becomes invaded. Note that the juxtaposition of the vaginal wall directly to the bladder and the rectum makes these organs directly accessible (Fig. 46.4).

N-oncoanatomy

When the cervix is invaded, extension into bladder and rectum can be due to the *major lymphatic trunks—the uteroovarian, parametrial, and presacral—that drain into the hypogastric, external iliac, common iliac, presacral, and para-aortic nodes.* However, the fundus also drains via ovarian lymphatics to retroperitoneal lymph nodes. The sentinel node could be either an obturator node or a para-aortic lymph node (Fig. 46.5; Table 46.2).

M-oncoanatomy

The major venous drainage is via uterine veins or ovarian veins into the vena cava (see Fig. 43.6).

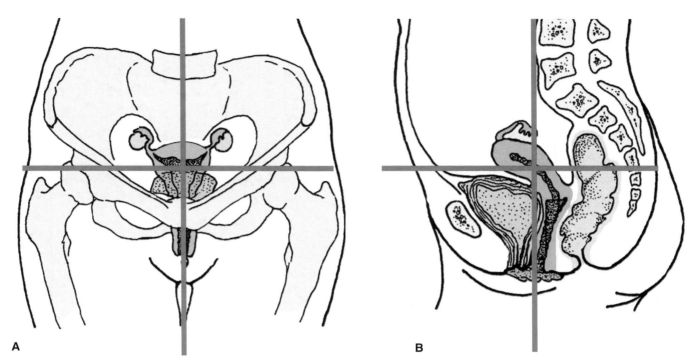

A   **B**

Figure 46.3 **Orientation of oncoanatomy of uterine fundus.** The anatomic isocenter is at the midline and at the S3 to S4 level inside the true pelvis. **A.** Coronal. **B.** Sagittal.

Rules of Classification and Staging

Clinical Staging

With few exceptions, hysterectomy and bilateral salpingo-oophorectomy are performed for both staging and diagnosis. Uterine enlargement can be assessed, but myometrial and serosal invasion is difficult to determine on pelvic examination. FIGO mandates surgical staging, cautioning that aggressive wide lymph node sampling may be too risky because pelvic and para-aortic nodes are at risk. Imaging is utilized when available, especially for high-grade cancer and enlarged uteri preoperatively (Table 46.3).

Surgical-pathologic Staging

The completely resected specimen including the primary site and regional lymph nodes, which must be thoroughly analyzed and are pTNM designated. Radical hysterectomy and bilateral salpingo-oophorectomy with pelvic lymph node resection is the usual procedure for pathologic evaluation.

Although the staging has remained unchanged at most gynecologic primary sites, the rules for classification still do not allow for sophisticated imaging, which includes computed tomography (CT), magnetic resonance imaging (MRI), and ultrasonography to alter staging. The multidisciplinary approach to decision making is truly interdisciplinary, most often involving a gynecologic oncologist and a dedicated radiation oncologist. Over the decades, diagnostic and therapeutic protocols in national cooperative groups have provided a scientific basis for introducing combined modalities and introducing innovations into clinical practice.

Oncoimaging Annotations

- MRI is preferred to detect tumors, which are hyperintense on T2-weighted and gadolinium-enhanced images, and helps to distinguish between lesions versus fluid and necrosis in heterogeneous uterine masses.

- MRI after gadolinium is best to determine myometrial invasion.

- MRI best demonstrates cervical stromal invasion on sagittal gadolinium-enhanced views, but still needs pathologic confirmation.

- MRI is a useful adjunct to clinical staging and is between 84% and 94% accurate overall.

- CT is useful for guiding needle biopsies.

- Ultrasonography has its advocates to determine depth of myometrial invasion and is recommended to screen postmenopausal bleeders: An endometrial stripe of ≤7 mm is within normal range and ≤4 mm virtually excludes carcinoma.

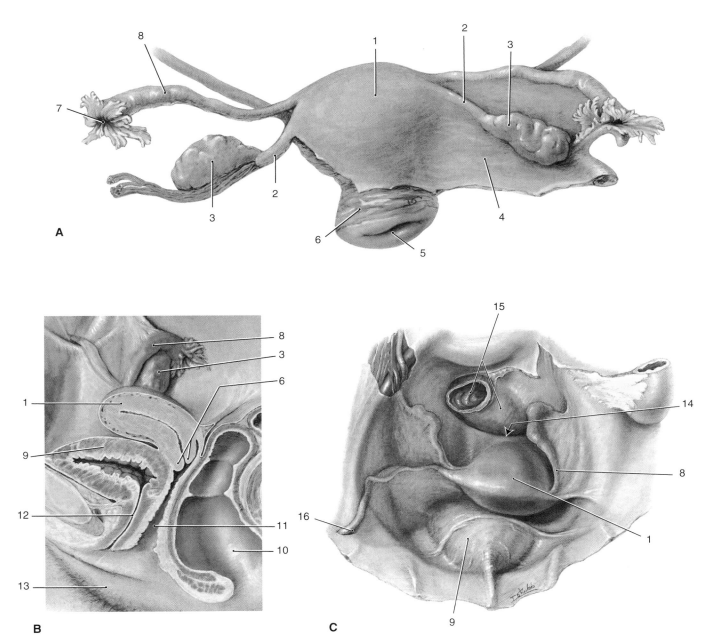

Figure 46.4 **T-oncoanatomy:** Three-planar views. **A.** Coronal. **B.** Sagittal. **C.** Transverse. (1) Uterus. (2) Ligament of ovary. (3) Ovary. (4) Broad ligament. (5) Cervical ostium. (6) Cervix of uterus. (7) Tubal abdominal ostium. (8) Fallopian tube. (9) Urinary bladder. (10) Rectum. (11) Vagina. (12) Urethra. (13) Vulva. (14) Rectouterine pouch of Douglas. (15) Sigmoid/rectal junction. (16) Round ligament of uterus.

- MRI for staging: Sagittal and axial images assess spread to uterus, bladder, rectum, and pelvic sidewall.
- Positron emission tomography with FDG can detect 1-cm nodules with 80% accuracy for peritoneal metastases.
- Ultrasonography has been used to evaluate depth of myometrial invasion.

- Gadolinium is useful to differentiate tumor infiltrate (enhanced) versus debris (nonenhanced) in enlarged uterus.

Cancer Statistics and Survival

Female genital system cancers collectively account for 80,000 new cases, with uterine corpus exceeding cervix

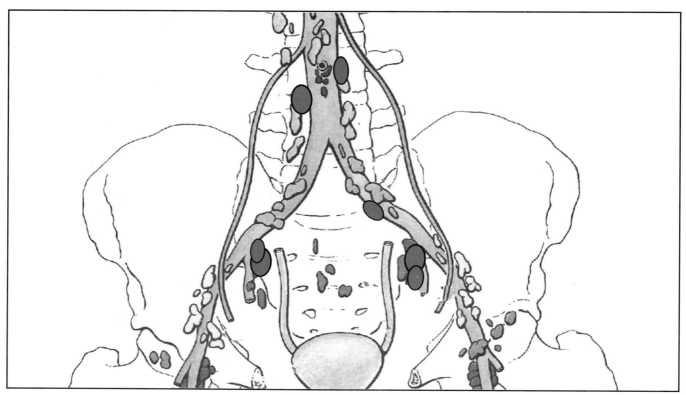

Figure 46.5 N-oncoanatomy: The sentinel nodes for confined uterine fundal (stage T1) adenocarcinomas are into the internal iliac and to para-aortic nodes. With invasion of the cervix (T2), the cancer behaves as cancer of the cervix and can spread to hypogastric or obturator nodes.

by a factor of four. Both are highly curable and deaths are relatively low. The major gynecologic killer is ovarian cancer with 16,000 annual deaths, which exceeds the other six primary sites combined (see Table 43.5).

Survival Rates

The survival rate gains in both cervix uteri and fundus uteri have been incremental. Recognizing that invasive cancers of the gynecologic tract have had a higher baseline, better than 50% in the 1950s, the gains for all stages

are only 15% or 2% to 3% per decade. As noted, mortality rates have plummeted owing to early detection, especially for cancer of the cervix, because it is most often detected in its noninvasive stage. Localized uterine cancers are >90% curable (see Fig. 43.7).

The cancer survival rates indicate the gain in survival for uterine corpus and cervix have been modest (14%) over the past five decades. However, most uterine cervix cancers are detected as cancer-in-situ and this is not reflected in the figures. Ovarian cancer survival has improved by 22% and as stated remains lethal because most cases are detected late owing to its insidious onset and

TABLE 46.2	Lymph Nodes of Fundus Uteri	
Sentinel nodes	Juxtaregional nodes
Obturator Internal iliac	Common iliac Hypogastric Lateral sacral
Regional nodes	
Para-aortic External iliac Inguinal	

TABLE 46.3	Imaging Modalities for Staging Uterine Corpus Cancer	
Method	Diagnosis and Staging Capability	Recommended for Use
Primary (T) staging		
CTe	Reliable for defining adnexal ovarian masses, extension to gynecologic organs, peritoneal seeding and ascites	Yes, contrast to visualize vessels and intestines
MRI	Role of MRI is emerging as criteria for malignancy defined	Yes, but supplemental to CT for soft tissue
TVUS	Excellent for screening and diagnosis	No, not reliable to define invasion
PET	High activity suggests malignancy versus benign status of solid or cystic pelvic masses	No
Nodal (N) staging		
CTe	Excellent for detecting nodal adenopathy >1 cm in size	Yes, cost effective
MRI	Available for supplementing CT	Yes, if cancer is high grade
Needle biopsy	Confirms lesions detected by radionuclide scan, CT scans, or lymphangiogram	Patients with suspicious lesions, image-guided aspirations
Metastases (M) staging		
Barium enema		Yes, for patients with suspicious lesions
Urography	Detects ureteral obstruction, bladder invasion; screens for unsuspected renal anomaly	All operative candidates
Bone scan	Useful to assess omental and liver metastases	Yes, if suspected
CT		Yes, if suspected

CT, computed tomography; CTe, CT enhanced with IV contrast; MRI, magnetic resonance imaging; PET, positron emission tomography; TVUS, transvaginal ultrasound.

inaccessibility of ovarian nodules to early diagnosis. On the bright side is the high cure and 5-year survival rates for stage I patients with cervical cancer (92%), uterine corpus cancer (96%), and ovarian cancer (95%).

Survival rates have been excellent for uterine fundus improving over five decades from 78% to 86%, an increase of 14%. For each stage I, the 5-year results are outstanding, rising to 96% (see Table 43.6).

Gestational Trophoblastic Tumors of the Uterus

In addition to an anatomic stage, a substage—A (low risk) or B (high risk)—is assigned based on nonanatomic factors.

Perspective and Patterns of Spread

The spectrum of gestational trophoblastic tumors (GTT) can include molar pregnancy, invasive hydatiform mole to the neoplastic placental derived trophoblastic tumor, and the very aggressive choriocarcinoma (Table 47.1; Fig. 47.1). A history of molar gestation is a major risk factor and is somewhat higher among black women. At one time these malignancies (GTT) were incurable, but with chemotherapy complete regression and ablation are readily achievable. In fact, the eradication of GTT was among the first chemotherapeutic successes and provided a major stimulus to pursue other malignancies with drug therapy. Fortunately, human chorionic gonadotropin (hCG) is a marker for persistent tumor. If hCG levels remain elevated after delivery of a molar pregnancy with dilation and curettage, then persistent disease remains to be treated. Fortunately, methotrexate is effective as single-agent therapy.

The staging system has evolved over time, recognizing that anatomic extent and histopathology were elegant but limited in their ability to prognosticate. In the 1990s, The International Federation of Gynecology and Obstetrics introduced a Prognosis Scoring Index (Table 47.2), which included age, antecedent pregnancy, interval months from index pregnancy, largest tumor size, size of metastases, number of metastases identified, and response to chemotherapy. In addition to an anatomic stage, a substage—A (low risk) or B (high risk)—is assigned based on nonanatomic factors. The prognostic scores are ≥0, 1, 2, or 4 for individual risk factors. A score ≤7 is A (low risk) and ≥8 is B (high risk).

TNM Staging Criteria

It is the highly malignant choriocarcinoma that has access to the rich vascular blood supply of a failed

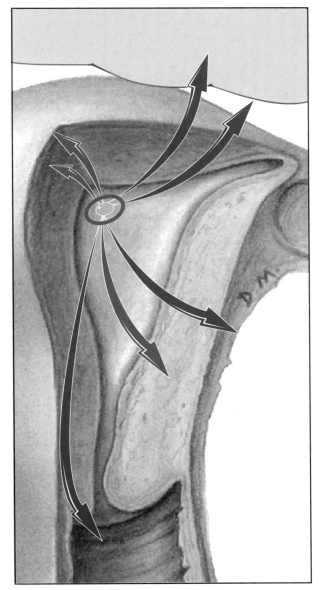

Figure 47.1 **Patterns of spread.** The cancer crab is color coded for stage: T0, yellow; T1, green; T2, blue.

DEFINITION OF TNM   STAGE GROUPINGS

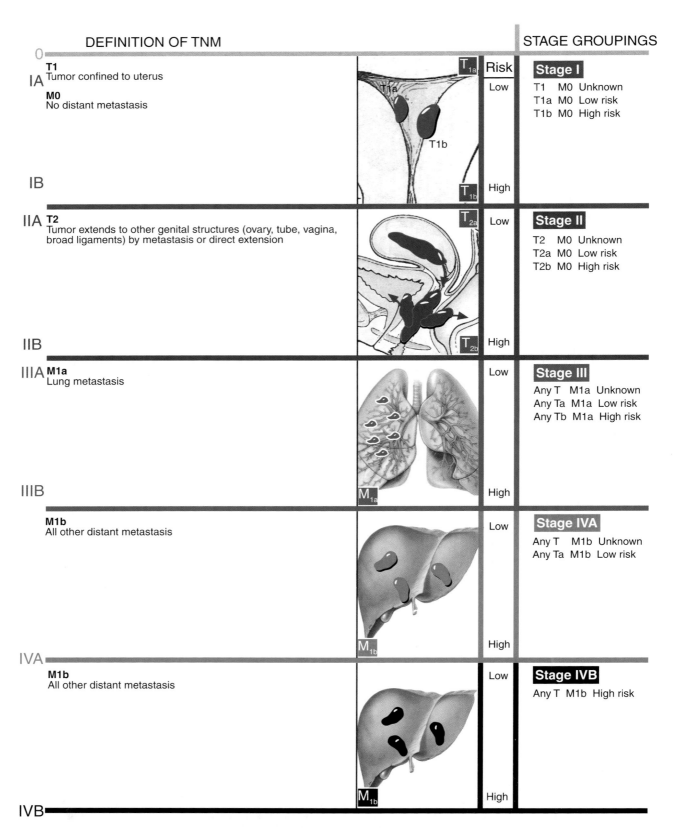

T1
Tumor confined to uterus

M0
No distant metastasis

Stage I

T1	M0	Unknown
T1a	M0	Low risk
T1b	M0	High risk

T2
Tumor extends to other genital structures (ovary, tube, vagina, broad ligaments) by metastasis or direct extension

Stage II

T2	M0	Unknown
T2a	M0	Low risk
T2b	M0	High risk

M1a
Lung metastasis

Stage III

Any T	M1a	Unknown
Any Ta	M1a	Low risk
Any Tb	M1a	High risk

M1b
All other distant metastasis

Stage IVA

| Any T | M1b | Unknown |
| Any Ta | M1b | Low risk |

M1b
All other distant metastasis

Stage IVB

| Any T | M1b | High risk |

Figure 47.2 **TNM staging diagram is arranged vertically arranged with T definitions on left and stage groupings on right.** Gestational trophoblastic tumors are highly metastatic but highly curable with chemotherapy. There are four main stages, each with two or three substages. Color bars are coded for stage: Stage 0, yellow; I, green; II, blue; III, purple; IV, red; metastatic disease to viscera and nodes, black.

TABLE 47.1	Histopathologic Type: Common Cancers of Gestational Trophoblastic

Hydatidiform mole
    Complete
    Partial	

Invasive hydatidiform mole	
Choriocarcinoma	
Placental site trophoblastic tumors	

Modified from Greene FL, Page DL, Fleming ID, et al., eds. *AJCC Cancer Staging Manual.* 6th ed. New York: Springer; 2002:294.

placenta and can rapidly invade hematogenously. Presentations of metastatic disease may be encountered before recognizing the local regional manifestations of GTT. As noted, the serum tumor marker, β-hCG, is an important diagnostic as well as a staging prognostic aid. After surgical removal by dilatation and curettage or hysterectomy, myometrial invasion may be evident (T1). *Nodal metastases are uncommon.* Local spread to cervix, ovary, or vagina (stage T2) is common and lung is a favored metastatic site. Dissemination to liver often occurs, but such remote sites as the kidney, gastrointestinal tract, spleen, bone, and brain also may be involved (Fig. 47.2).

Summary of Changes

The "Risk Factors" portion of the stage groups has been revised as Table 47.2 onto A Low Risk (score 7 or less); B Low Risk (score 8 or more).

Orientation of Three-planar Oncoanatomy

The isocenter for the uterus is at the S4 level but can vary from S2 to S5 depending on the degree of anteflexion or retroflexion (Fig. 47.3).

T-oncoanatomy

* *Coronal*: The upper two thirds of the uterus above the level of the internal cervical os is called the "corpus uteri." The fallopian tubes enter at the upper lateral corners of its pear-shaped body. That portion of the muscular organ positioned above the line joining the tubouterine orifices is called the "fundus."

* *Sagittal*: The body of the uterus sits in the peritoneal cavity. Although it is juxtaposed to these structures, it is separated by the peritoneal lining, making direct invasion rare.

* *Transverse*: The relationship of the uterus to other pelvic tissues is important, particularly to the rectum and bladder. The rectovaginal or the vesicovaginal septum can be invaded. Note that the juxtaposition of the vaginal wall directly to the bladder and the rectum makes these organs directly accessible (see Fig. 46.4 A-C).

N-oncoanatomy

When the cervix is invaded, extension into bladder and rectum can be due to the *major lymphatic trunks, the utero-ovarian (infundibulopelvic), parametrial, and presacral nodes that drain into the hypogastric, external iliac, common iliac, presacral, and para-aortic nodes.* However, the fundus also drains via ovarian lymphatics to retroperitoneal lymph nodes. The sentinel node could be either an obturator node or a para-aortic lymph node (Fig. 47.4; Table 47.3).

M-oncoanatomy

The major venous drainage is via uterine veins or ovarian veins into the vena cava (see Fig. 43.6).

Rules of Classification and Staging

The initial diagnostic procedures are the staging criteria. Both clinical and pathologic criteria establish the primary tumor anatomic extent; however, specific criteria suggest persistent and/or metastatic GTT and require chemotherapy.

Imaging recommendations apply to the metastatic workup, and are similar to uterus fundus as to primary site and pelvic nodes (Table 47.4).

Clinical Staging

With few exceptions, hysterectomy and bilateral salpingo-oophorectomy are performed for both staging and diagnosis. Uterine enlargement can be assessed but myometrial and serosal invasion is difficult to determine on pelvic examination. FIGO mandates surgical staging, cautioning that aggressive and wide lymph node sampling may be too risky because pelvic and para-aortic

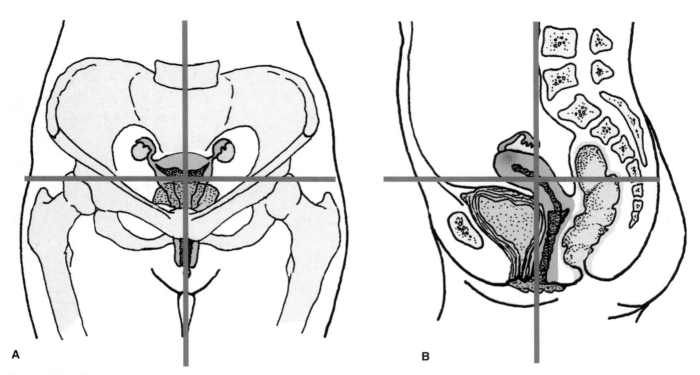

A   **B**

Figure 47.3 Orientation of oncoanatomy of GTT: The anatomic isocenter is at the midline and at the S3 to S4 level inside the true pelvis.
A. Coronal. **B.** Sagittal.

TABLE 47.2	Prognostic Scoring Index			
	Risk Score			
Prognostic Factor	**0**	**1**	**2**	**4**
Age	<40	≥40		
Antecedent Pregnancy	Hydatidiform mole	Abortion	Term Pregnancy	
Interval months from index pregnancy	<4	4–<7	7–12	>12
Pretreatment hCG (IU/ml)	$<10^3$	$\geq10^3 - <10^4$	$10^4 - <10^5$	$\geq10^5$
Largest tumor size, including uterus	<3 cm	3–<5 cm	≥5 cm	
Site of metastases	Lung	Spleen, kidney	Gastrointestinal tract	Brain, liver
Number of metastases identified		1–4	5–8	>8
Previous failed chemotherapy			Single drug	Two or more drugs
Total Score				

Low risk is a score of 7 or <. High risk is a score of 8 or >.
Reprinted from Greene FL, Page DL, Fleming ID, et al., eds. *AJCC Cancer Staging Manual.* 6th ed. New York: Springer; 2002:295.

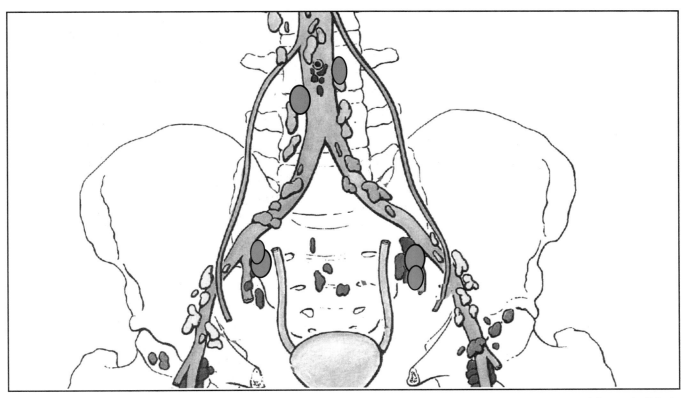

Figure 47.4 **N-oncoanatomy:**   The sentinel nodes for GTT into the internal iliac and to para-aortic nodes. With invasion of the cervix (T2) the cancer behaves as cancer of the cervix and can spread to hypogastric or obturator nodes.

nodes are at risk. Imaging is utilized when available especially for high-grade cancer and enlarged uteri preoperatively.

Surgical-pathologic Staging

The completely resected specimen including the primary site and regional lymph nodes, which must be thoroughly analyzed, are pTNM designated. Radical hysterectomy and bilateral salpingo-oophorectomy with

pelvic lymph node resection is the usual procedure for pathologic evaluation.

Although the staging has remained unchanged at most gynecologic primary sites, the rules for classification still do not allow for sophisticated imaging, which includes computed tomography (CT), magnetic resonance imaging (MRI), and ultrasonography (US) to alter staging. The multidisciplinary approach to decision making is truly interdisciplinary, most often involving a gynecologic oncologist and a dedicated radiation

TABLE 47.3	Lymph Nodes of Gestational Trophoblastic Tumors	
Sentinel nodes		Juxtaregional nodes
Internal iliac Para-aortic		Common iliac Hypogastric Lateral sacral
Regional nodes		
Renal hilar Para-aortic External iliac Inguinal		

Method	Diagnosis and Staging Capability	Recommended for Use
TABLE 47.4	**Imaging Modalities for Staging Gestational Trophoblastic Cancer**	
Primary (T) staging		
CTe	Defines cervical involvement, tumor size, and vaginal extension; myometrial invasion may suggest cervix invasion	Yes, has displaced barium enema and IVP; need histologic confirmation
MRI	Preferred for cross-sectional anatomy tumor size, depth of myometrial invasion	Yes, for high-grade cancers
EUUS	Can detect widening of echogenic endometrial stripe and myometrial invasion	No, more for detection; accuracy not high
Nodal (N) staging		
CTe	Excellent for detecting nodal adenopathy >1 cm in size	Yes, cost effective
MRI	Available for supplementing CT	Yes, if cancer is high grade
Metastases (M) staging		
Barium enema		Yes, for patients with suspicious lesions
Bone scan	Useful to assess omental and liver metastases	Yes, if suspected
CT		Yes, if suspected

CT, computed tomography; CTe, CT enhanced with IV contrast; EUUS, endouterine ultrasound; IVP, intravenous pyelography; MRI, magnetic resonance imaging.

oncologist. Over the decades, diagnostic and therapeutic protocols in national cooperative groups have provided a scientific basis for introducing combined modalities and introducing innovations into clinical practice.

Oncoimaging Annotations

*   Chest CT with helical techniques allow for detection of pulmonary metastases at the 5- to 10-mm size.
*   CT is preferred over US for detection with needling for pathologic confirmation of liver metastases.
*   MRI is superior to CT for detecting peritoneal metastases.

Cancer Statistics and Survival

Female genital system cancers collectively account for 80,000 new cases with uterine corpus exceeding cervix by a factor of four. Both are highly curable and deaths are relatively low. The major gynecologic killer is ovarian cancer with 16,000 deaths annually, which exceeds the other six primary sites combined.

Survival Rates

The survival rate gains in both cervix uteri and fundus uteri have been incremental. Recognizing that invasive cancers of the gynecologic tract have had a higher baseline, >50% in the 1950s, the gains for all stages are only 15% or 2% to 3% per decade. As noted, mortality rates have plummeted owing to early detection, especially of cancer of the cervix because it is most often detected in its noninvasive stage. Localized uterine cancers are >90% curable.

The cancer survival rates indicate the gain in survival for uterine corpus and cervix have been modest (14%) over the past five decades. However, most uterine cervix cancers are detected as cancer-in-situ and this is not reflected in the figures. Ovarian cancer survival has improved by 22% and, as stated, remains lethal because most cases are detected late owing to its insidious onset and inaccessibility of ovarian nodules to early diagnosis. On the bright side is the high cure and 5-year survival rates for stage I patients with cervical cancer (92%), uterine corpus cancer (96%), and ovarian cancer (95%).

48

Uterine Cervix

The patterns of cancer spread are determined by the anatomy and the central position of the cervix in the female genital system.

Perspective and Patters of Spread

The success of conquering cancer of the uterine cervix is due to the widespread and highly effective screening using the PAP smear of exfoliative cytology. There are 65,000 cases of noninvasive carcinoma in situ compared with 13,000 new cases of invasive cancer, usually early stages. There are fewer than 5,000 deaths annually; unfortunately, all are often elderly, postmenopausal women who are less active sexually and are not being screened, or women in low socioeconomic groups, Latinos, and African Americans. The low incidence among Jewish women suggests male circumcision may be a factor.

The cervix is the terminal end of the uterus that protrudes in the vagina and *its lumen is lined with a mucus-secreting, simple columnar epithelium; however, when the cervix protrudes into the vagina, the epithelium is stratified squamous and is nonkeratinized.* It is not surprising that of the several histopathologic types 80% to 90% are squamous cell cancers and only 5% to 10% are adenocarcinomas. Table 48.1 lists the variations and subtypes as well as the grading of cervical cancers. The patterns of cancer spread are determined by the anatomy and the central position of the cervix in the female genital system (Fig. 48.1): First, within the cervix, then (a) inferiorly into the vagina, (b) laterally into the parametrium, or (c) anteriorly into the bladder or posteriorly into the rectum.

TNM Staging Criteria

The cervix is at the anatomic isocenter of the female pelvis. The TNM staging criteria have been established and reflect cancer spread patterns. Cervical cancer is the archetype as the first cancer staged >70 years ago. Since 1937, the International Federation of Gynecology and

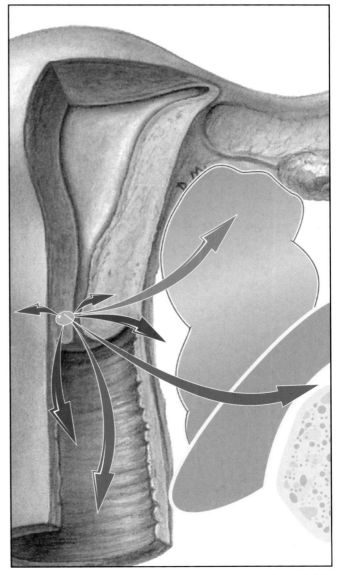

Figure 48.1 **Patterns of spread.** The cancer crab is color coded for stage: Tis, yellow; T1, green; T2, blue; T3, purple; and T4, red.

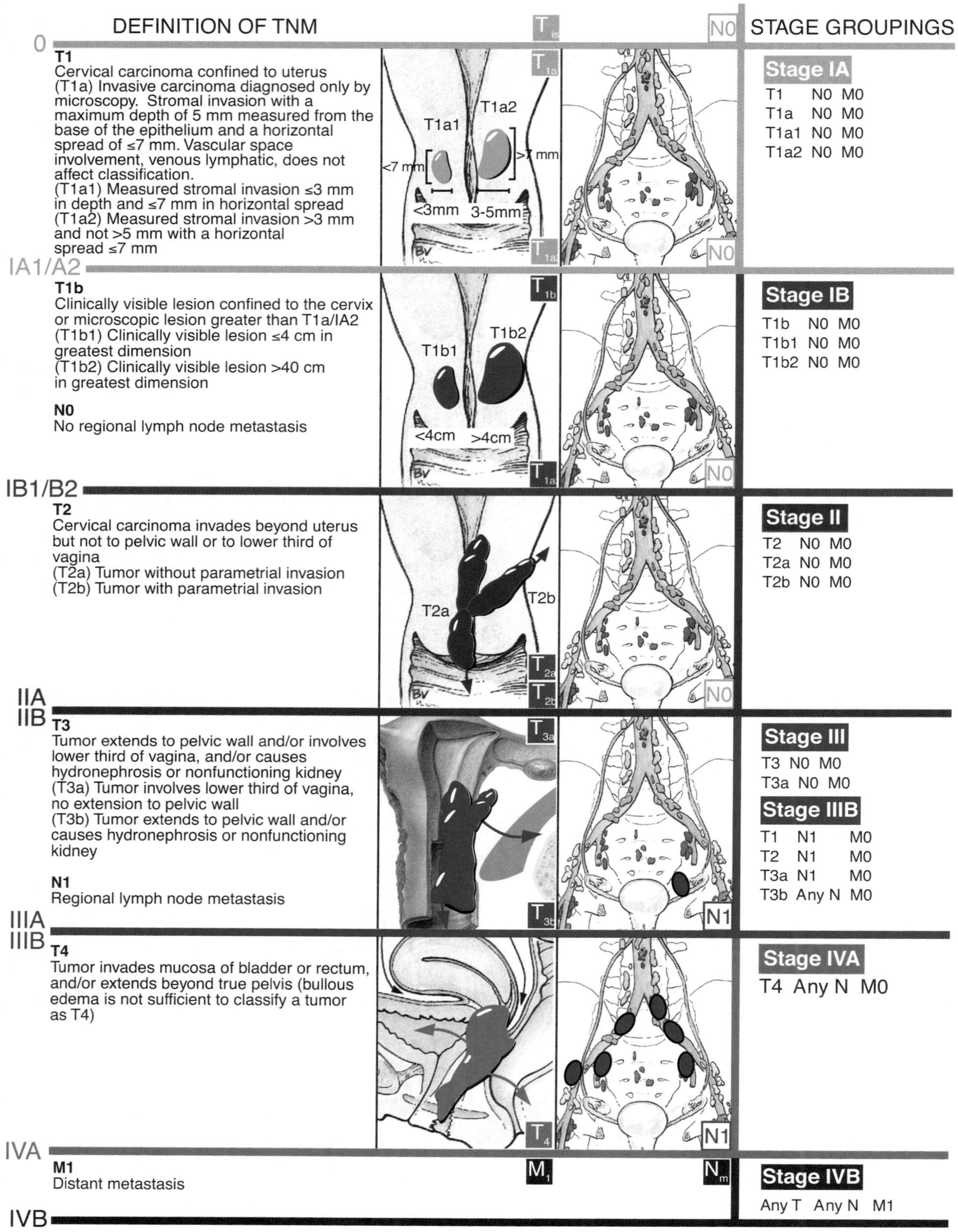

DEFINITION OF TNM

STAGE GROUPINGS

0

T1
Cervical carcinoma confined to uterus
(T1a) Invasive carcinoma diagnosed only by microscopy. Stromal invasion with a maximum depth of 5 mm measured from the base of the epithelium and a horizontal spread of ≤7 mm. Vascular space involvement, venous lymphatic, does not affect classification.
(T1a1) Measured stromal invasion ≤3 mm in depth and ≤7 mm in horizontal spread
(T1a2) Measured stromal invasion >3 mm and not >5 mm with a horizontal spread ≤7 mm

IA1/A2

T1b
Clinically visible lesion confined to the cervix or microscopic lesion greater than T1a/IA2
(T1b1) Clinically visible lesion ≤4 cm in greatest dimension
(T1b2) Clinically visible lesion >40 cm in greatest dimension

N0
No regional lymph node metastasis

IB1/B2

T2
Cervical carcinoma invades beyond uterus but not to pelvic wall or to lower third of vagina
(T2a) Tumor without parametrial invasion
(T2b) Tumor with parametrial invasion

IIA
IIB

T3
Tumor extends to pelvic wall and/or involves lower third of vagina, and/or causes hydronephrosis or nonfunctioning kidney
(T3a) Tumor involves lower third of vagina, no extension to pelvic wall
(T3b) Tumor extends to pelvic wall and/or causes hydronephrosis or nonfunctioning kidney

N1
Regional lymph node metastasis

IIIA
IIIB

T4
Tumor invades mucosa of bladder or rectum, and/or extends beyond true pelvis (bullous edema is not sufficient to classify a tumor as T4)

IVA

M1
Distant metastasis

IVB

Stage IA

T1	N0	M0
T1a	N0	M0
T1a1	N0	M0
T1a2	N0	M0

Stage IB

T1b	N0	M0
T1b1	N0	M0
T1b2	N0	M0

Stage II

T2	N0	M0
T2a	N0	M0
T2b	N0	M0

Stage III

T3	N0	M0
T3a	N0	M0

Stage IIIB

T1	N1	M0
T2	N1	M0
T3a	N1	M0
T3b	Any N	M0

Stage IVA

T4 Any N M0

Stage IVB

Any T Any N M1

Figure 48.2 TNM staging diagram is arranged vertically arranged with T definitions on left and stage groupings on right. Uterine cervix cancers are often detected in microinvasive stages and most resectable in Stage IA or IB cancers. With further invasion, chemoradiation treatment is effective. There are four main stages each with two or three substages. Color bars are coded for stage: Stage 0 and IA, yellow; IB, green; II, blue; III, purple; IV, red; and metastatic disease to viscera and nodes, black.

TABLE 48.1	Histopathologic Type: Common Cancers of the Cervix	

Squamous carcinoma
  Large cell nonkeratinizing
  Large cell keratinizing
  Small cell nonkeratinizing
		Mixed epithelial carcinoma
		  Adenosquamous
		  Glassy cell

Adenocarcinoma
  Endocervical
  Endometrioid
  Clear cell Others
		Neuroendocrine
		  Carcinoid
		  Small cell

Modified from Bragg DG, Rubin P, Hricak H, eds. *Oncologic Imaging.* 2nd ed. Philadelphia: Elsevier; 2002:465.

Obstetrics (FIGO) has collected data as to cancer of cervix survival and outcomes from numerous institutions. The pooled results became the international gold standard on reporting cancer survival results.

The TNM introduced by Denoix simply adapted their categories to fit the FIGO stages. Although the basic definitions have been stable, the increasing success of finding preinvasive cancers has lead to expanding the subcategories of stages I because of conization techniques. Thus, in early editions of the American Joint Committee on Cancer/International Union Against Cancer system, stage I was simply a cancer confined to the cervix without any size or specific measurement requirements. The staging preferably was a bimanual examination under anesthesia. With the fourth edition (1992), microscopic sizing of invasion was introduced as subcategories of IA and further defined in the fifth edition with the subcategories of IB, designating ≤4.0 cm as the divide between IB1 and ≥4.0 cm as IB2.

The stage IA microinvasive lesions are defined as a maximum depth of 5.0 mm for the favorable category, which implies that there will be few instances of lymphatic or capillary infiltration and, even if present, do not change this criteria. Stage IB are visible lesions or microinvasion beyond 5.0 mm. As noted, 4.0 cm divides stage IB1 and IB2 cancers.

Spread patterns beyond the cervix lead to stage II. *Superior invasion into the uterus is ignored for staging.* Inferior invasion into the vagina is T2a and lateral spread into the parametrium is T2b. Stage III cancers extend to the pelvic wall (T3b) or lower third of the vagina (T3a), which alters lymph nodes at risk. Stage T4a is designated for anterior spread into the bladder, which requires biopsy proof; T4b is rectal invasion, which occurs only from vaginal extension because the posterior lip of the cervix is separated from the rectum by the rectouterine pouch of Douglas.

Summary of Changes

No changes were made in the current sixth edition of the AJCC CSM (Fig. 48.2).

Orientation of Three-planar Oncoanatomy

The isocenter of the cervix is the central structure in the female pelvis. It is retropubic at the level of the coccyx and midway between the ovaries and vulva (Fig. 48.3).

T-oncoanatomy

* *Coronal:* The cervix comprises the lower third of the uterus. It is roughly cylindrical in shape, projecting through the upper vaginal wall. It communicates with the vagina through an orifice called the "external os." Cancer of the cervix may originate on the vaginal surface or in the cervical canal.

* *Sagittal:* Invasion of the bladder trigone from a cancer in the anterior lip of the cervix and fornix of the vagina. Vaginal extension into its posterior fornix and wall precedes rectal wall invasion.

* *Transverse:* The mesometrium or the broad ligament of the uterus contains a number of very important structures that determine the course of events in a number of oncologic presentations and complications. *The course of the ureter, which is a critical normal structure, passes from its lateral position in the abdomen to its medial location in the pelvis by moving horizontally to insert into the bladder.* It is crossed superiorly and medially by the uterine artery. The long transverse course of the ureter makes it particularly vulnerable to entrapment by cancer spread from the cervix because it lies juxtaposed to the cervix before its entry to the bladder. Uncontrolled stage IV cancer blocks both ureters, resulting in hydronephrosis and renal failure, leading to a uremic death. Along the sidewall of the pelvis, the obturator nerve and vessel enter into the obturator foramen (Fig. 48.4).

N-oncoanatomy

The cervix is drained by preureteral, postureteral, and uterosacral lymphatics. *Cancers confined to the cervix drain first to obturator nodes, then to hypogastric or internal iliac nodes.* These are the first station lymph nodes and are on the lateral wall of the true pelvis, where the

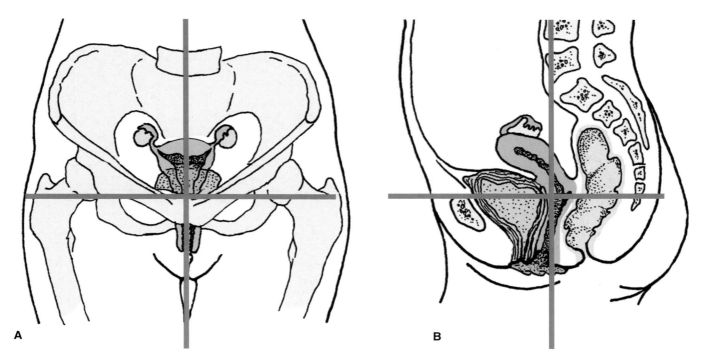

A

B

Figure 48.3 Orientation of oncoanatomy of uterine fundus. The anatomic isocenter is at the midline at the floor of the true pelvis at the S4/S5 level. **A.** Coronal. **B.** Sagittal.

internal obturator artery and vein penetrate the levator ani muscle. The lymphatics follow the uterine vein, which drains into the internal and not the external iliac (Fig. 48.5; Table 48.2).

As the cancer invades more deeply and extensively, the lymph nodes beyond the true pelvis are at risk. *When the cancer invades the parametrium and is fixed to the side wall of the pelvis, lymphatic anastomoses to the external iliac nodes may lead to their involvement.* With vaginal invasions up to its lower third, inguinal nodes are at risk. Rectal invasions may lead to the inferior mesenteric nodes being at risk.

The cervical cancer sentinel node is the obturator node placing the internal iliac chain at risk, when the cancer is stage I or II. With more extensive infiltration of the cancer, second and third station or echelons of nodes are at risk.

M-oncoanatomy

The arterial and venous blood supply and drainage are via the uterine vessels and hematogenous spread is via the internal iliac to the common iliacs and inferior vena cava. The lung is the target metastatic organ. Skeletal invasion of the lateral cortex of the true pelvis or vertebrae are due to lymphatic and lymph node metastatic cancer penetrating the nodal capsule and directly invading the juxtaposed bone. Once this occurs, the cancer spreads beyond the confines of the lymph nodes and it often savagely destroys the pelvic bone and/or vertebrae crossing and eradicating intervertebral discs (see Fig. 43.6).

Rules of Classification and Staging

Clinical Staging and Imaging

The *sine qua non* of clinical staging occurs before treatment, preferably performed by a multidisciplinary team consisting of a gynecologic oncologist and a radiation oncologist with the patient under anesthesia. Imaging is advisable, but cannot be used to alter staging; however, there is little doubt that newer modalities as computed tomography (CT), magnetic resonance imaging (MRI), ultrasonography (US), and positron emission tomography are more accurate than clinical palpation, inspection, colposcopy, endocervical curettage, hysteroscopy, or cystoscopy. Suspected bladder and rectal invasion must be confirmed on biopsy. Fine needle aspiration should be used to determine enlarged node status (Table 48.3).

Surgical-pathologic Staging

The completely resected specimen including the primary site and regional lymph nodes, which must be thoroughly analyzed, are pTNM designated. Radical hysterectomy and bilateral salpingo-oophorectomy with pelvic lymph node resection is the usual procedure for pathologic evaluation.

Although the staging has remained unchanged at most gynecologic primary sites, the rules for classification still do not allow for sophisticated imaging, which includes CT, MRI, and US, to alter staging. The

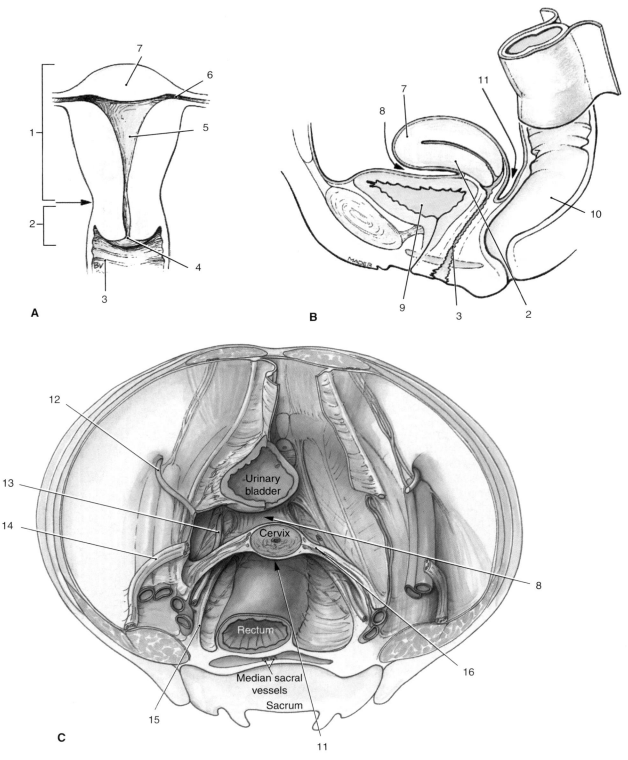

Figure 48.4 T-oncoanatomy: Three-planar views. **A.** Coronal. **B.** Sagittal. **C.** Transverse. (1) Body of uterus. (2) Cervix of uterus. (3) Vagina. (4) External ostium. (5) Uterine cavity. (6) Uterine tube. (7) Fundus of uterus. (8) Vesicouterine pouch. (9) Urinary bladder. (10) Rectum. (11) Rectouterine pouch. (12) Round ligament of uterus. (13) Ureter. (14) Suspensory ligament of ovary (contains ovarian vessels). (15) Uterosacral ligament. (16) Transverse cervical (cardinal) ligament.

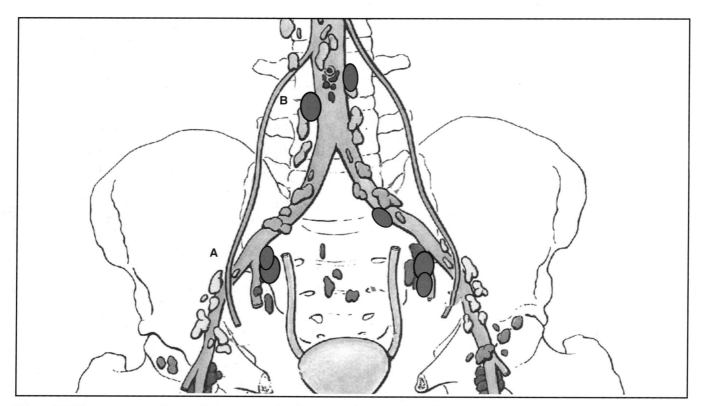

Figure 48.5 N-oncoanatomy. The sentinel nodes are the obturator nodes of the internal iliac chain. **A.** Internal iliac chain. **B.** Paraortic nodes are juxtaregional.

multidisciplinary approach to decision making is truly interdisciplinary, most often involving a gynecologic oncologist and a dedicated radiation oncologist. Over the decades, diagnostic and therapeutic protocols in national cooperative groups have provided a scientific basis for introducing combined modalities and introducing innovations into clinical practice.

Oncoimaging Annotations

- CT is most useful for advanced stages greater than stage III and is worthwhile in assessing cervix size.

Because cancers are isodense on CT, cervical cancer dimensions are not as accurate, but are excellent for staging purposes.

- CT is not reliable for early parametrial invasion, but is accurate in determining advanced disease with pelvic side wall fixation.
- CT suggests parametrial, bladder, and rectal invasion when fat planes exist between cervix and structure or they show irregular thickening.
- MRI identifies cancer on T2-weighted images as an intense signal increasing its accuracy to detect cancer size and lymph nodes involved.

TABLE 48.2	Lymph Nodes of Cervix	
Sentinel nodes	Juxtaregional nodes
Obturator nodes of the internal iliac chain	Para-aortic
Regional nodes	
Left: renal hilar Right: paracaval External iliac Hypogastric Lateral sacral Common iliac	

TABLE 48.3	Imaging Modalities for Staging Cervix Cancer	
Method	Diagnosis and Staging Capability	Recommended for Use
Primary (T) staging		
CTe	Reliable for defining adnexal ovarian masses, extension to gynecologic organs, peritoneal seeding, and ascites	Yes; contrast helps to visualize vessels and intestines
MRI	Role of MRI is emerging as criteria for malignancy defined	Yes, but supplemental to CT for soft tissues
TVUS	Excellent for screening and diagnosis	No, not reliable to define invasion
PET	High activity suggests malignancy versus benign status of solid or cystic pelvic masses	No
Nodal (N) staging		
CTe	Excellent for detecting nodal adenopathy >1 cm in size	Yes, cost effective
MRI	Available for supplementing CT	Yes, if cancer is high grade
Needle biopsy	Confirms lesions detected by radionuclide scan, CT scans, or lymphangiogram	Patients with suspicious lesions, image-guided aspirations
Metastases (M) staging		
Barium enema	Rectovaginal wall invasion	Yes, for patients with suspicious lesions
Urography	Detects ureteral obstruction, bladder invasion; screens for unsuspected renal anomaly	All operative candidates
Bone scan	Detects bone metastases	Yes, if suspected
CT	Useful to assess omental and liver metastases	Yes, if suspected

CT, computed tomography; CTe, CT enhanced with IV contrast; MRI, magnetic resonance imaging; PET, positron emission tomography; TVUS, transvaginal ultrasound.

- Gadolinium-enhanced MRI allows for identification of soft tissue invasion in vagina and parametria.
- CT: Early parametrial invasion is not as reliably predicted as advanced parametrial extension to pelvic wall.
- MRI: More accurate for assessing parametrial invasion and tumor size.
- MRI can demonstrate intact normal fibrous rim around cervix cancer and has high negative predictive value (95%) for parametrial invasion.
- MRI provides a more accurate assessment of cancer infiltration of rectum and bladder.

Cancer Statistics and Survival

Female genital system cancers collectively account for 80,000 new cases, with uterine corpus exceeding cervix by a factor of four. Both are highly curable and deaths are relatively low. The major gynecologic killer is ovarian cancer, with 16,000 deaths annually, which exceeds the other six primary sites combined.

Survival Rates

The survival rate gains in both cervix uteri and fundus uteri have been incremental. Recognizing that invasive cancers of the gynecologic tract have had a higher baseline, >50% in the 1950s, the gains for all stages are only 15% or 2% to 3% per decade. As noted, mortality rates have plummeted owing to early detection, especially of cancer of the cervix because it is most often detected in its noninvasive stage. Localized uterine cancers are >90% curable (see Table 43.5).

The cancer survival rates indicate the gain in survival for uterine corpus and cervix have been modest (14%) over the past five decades. However, most uterine cervix cancers are detected as cancer-in-situ and this is not reflected in the figures. Ovarian cancer survival has improved by 22% and, as stated, remains lethal because most cases are detected late owing to its insidious onset and inaccessibility of ovarian nodules to early diagnosis. On the bright side is the high cure and 5-year survival rates for stage I patients with cervical cancer (92%), uterine corpus cancer (96%), and ovarian cancer (95%).

Survival rates for cancer of the cervix have improved from 1950 to 2000 for all stages, rising from 59% to 67%, an increment of 18%. For stage I localized cancers, the cure rate exceeds 90% (see Table 43.6 and Fig. 43.7).

The pattern of spread relates to paravaginal invasion and in lateral soft tissues follows the same criteria of the staging system of cervix uteri.

Perspective and Patterns of Spread

The vagina is a fibromuscular tubular structure varying between 8 and 10 centimeters long, connecting the uterus to the external female genitals. It is one of the least likely sites in the female genital tract to give rise to malignancies. According to the latest Surveillance Epidemiology and End Results/American Cancer Society data, there will be approximately 2,000 new cases with a mortality rate of 30% to 40%. This is in part due to the strict criteria of the American Joint Committee on Cancer (AJCC)/International Union Against Cancer (UICC), which excludes any growth that involves the cervix or the vulva. Although, classically, squamous cell cancer arises from its stratified squamous epithelium, they are second to adenocarcinomas (Table 49.1). This is because most common isolated vaginal cancers are most often adenocarcinomas, metastatic often from endometrial malignancies. Of special interest are adenocarcinomas in young women, attributed to the administration of DES to their mothers during pregnancy, particularly in the first 18 weeks in utero. Fortunately, once suspected, these clear cell cancers have been diagnosed in early stages (I and II). A large variety of malignancies can occur and are tabulated in Table 49.1. Sarcoma botryoides occurs mainly in children <5 years and is characterized as grape-like clusters (Fig. 49.1).

TNM Staging Criteria

The pattern of spread relates to paravaginal invasion and in lateral soft tissues is stage T2, and follows the same criteria of the staging system of cervix uteri. Thus extension to the pelvic sidewall laterally (stage T3) and anteriorly into the urethra can occur or into the urinary bladder or posteriorly into the rectum (stage T4). Most cancers

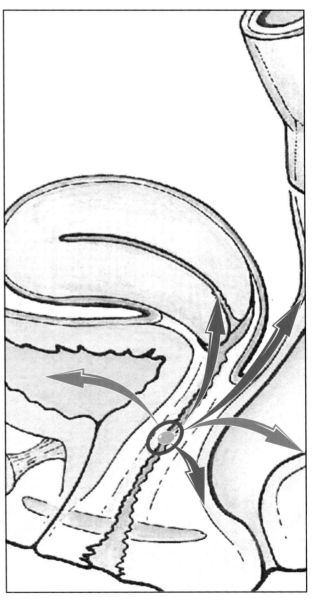

Figure 49.1 **Patterns of spread.** The cancer crab is color coded for stage: Tis, yellow; T1, green; T2, blue; T3, purple; and T4, red.

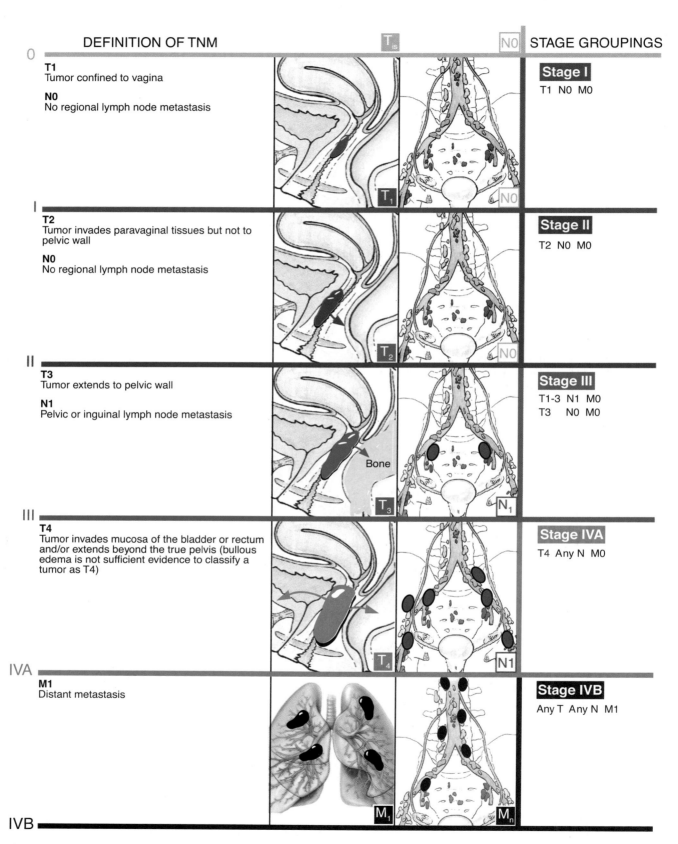

DEFINITION OF TNM

T1
Tumor confined to vagina

N0
No regional lymph node metastasis

T2
Tumor invades paravaginal tissues but not to pelvic wall

N0
No regional lymph node metastasis

T3
Tumor extends to pelvic wall

N1
Pelvic or inguinal lymph node metastasis

T4
Tumor invades mucosa of the bladder or rectum and/or extends beyond the true pelvis (bullous edema is not sufficient evidence to classify a tumor as T4)

M1
Distant metastasis

STAGE GROUPINGS

Stage I
T1 N0 M0

Stage II
T2 N0 M0

Stage III
T1-3 N1 M0
T3   N0 M0

Stage IVA
T4 Any N M0

Stage IVB
Any T Any N M1

Figure 49.2 TNM staging diagram is arranged vertically arranged with T definitions on left and stage groupings on right. Vaginal cancers are not common and if the diagnosis is adenocarcinoma, metastatic uterine cancer should be considered in older women and search for DES administration in younger women. There are four main stages, each with two or three substages. Color bars are coded for stage: Stage 0, yellow; I, green; II, blue; III, purple; IV, red; and metastatic disease to viscera and nodes, black.

TABLE 49.1	Histopathologic Type: Common Cancers of the Vagina	
Squamous cell carcinoma		Melanoma
Adenocarcinoma		Sarcoma

Modified from Greene FL, Page DL, Fleming ID, et al., eds. *AJCC Cancer Staging Manual.* 6th ed. New York: Springer; 2002:252.

are squamous cell carcinomas arising from the vaginal mucosa of stratified squamous epithelium (Fig. 49.2).

Summary of Changes

No changes have been made since the fifth edition of the AJCC CSM.

Orientation of Three-planar Oncoanatomy

The isocenter of the vagina is retropubic with inferior extension and is well below the level of the coccyx to the inferior aspect of the pubic bone (Fig. 49.3).

T-oncoanatomy

The vagina is a fibromuscular sheath is composed of three layers: mucosa, muscle, and adventitia (Fig. 49.4).

- *Coronal*: The intimate relationship of the urethra in the anterior wall of the vagina is noted.
- *Sagittal*: The muscle layer is composed of smooth muscle arranged in a circular, then longitudinal direction. The sphincter muscle urethrovaginalis composed of skeletal muscle is at its terminal end, the vestibule.
- *Transverse*: The pelvic wall is closer to the vagina than at the cervical level, and vaginal cancer becomes fixed earlier.

N-oncoanatomy

The vaginal tube lymphatics is dictated at its extremes with the upper two thirds draining into the obturator and hypogastric nodes in the true pelvis. In its lower third, it drains into inguinal nodes and then external iliac node (Fig. 49.5; Table 49.2).

M-oncoanatomy

The adventitia has a rich vascular venous plexus, which has been the attribute for attracting metastatic deposits. It is anastomosed to the vesical veins and drains into the internal iliacs similar to the cervix. However, at its inferior vestibule it follows pudendal vessels into the internal iliacs and femorals into the external iliacs (see Fig. 43.6).

Rules of Classification and Staging

Clinical Staging

Clinical staging involves careful scrutiny and inspection, palpation, and speculum evaluation for vaginal and urethral extension. (If cervix is involved, the staging is assigned and similar to cervical carcinoma.)

Surgical-pathologic Staging

Pathologic staging can be made if the resection is performed before radiation or chemotherapy. The International Federations of Gynecology and Obstetrics/AJCC/UICC vulval T1,T2 criteria are similar to other skin cancers, emphasizing 2-cm size criteria.

Oncoimaging Annotations

Imaging recommendations apply only to advanced unresectable stage III or IV presentations that involve vagina (Table 49.3).

Cancer Statistics and Survival

Female genital system cancers collectively account for 80,000 new cases, with uterine corpus exceeding cervix by a factor of four, but both are highly curable and deaths are relatively low. The major gynecologic killer is ovarian cancer, with 16,000 deaths annually, which exceeds the other six primary sites combined.

Survival Rates

The survival rate gains in both cervix uteri and fundus uteri have been incremental. Cancer of vagina survival rates are similar to cervix. Recognizing that invasive cancers of the gynecologic tract have had a higher baseline, >50% in the 1950s, the gains for all stages are only 15% or 2% to 3% per decade. As noted, mortality rates have plummeted owing to early detection, especially of cancer

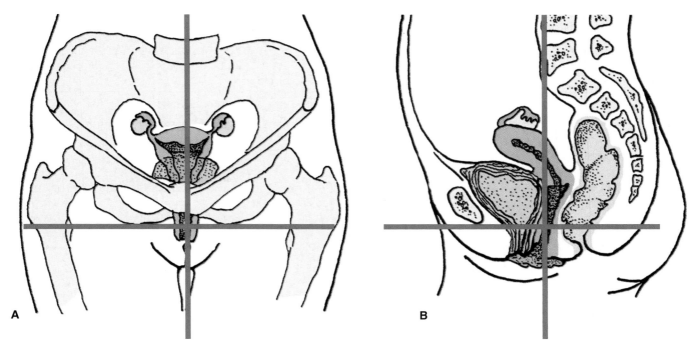

Figure 49.3 Orientation of oncoanatomy of the vagina. The anatomic isocenter is at the midline at the floor of the true pelvis at the S4/S5 level. **A.** Coronal. **B.** Sagittal.

of the cervix because it is most often detected in its non-invasive stage. Localized uterine cancers are >90% curable.

The cancer survival rates indicate the gain in survival for uterine corpus and cervix have been modest (14%) over the past five decades. However, most uterine cervix cancers are detected as cancer-in-situ and this is not reflected in the figures. Ovarian cancer survival has im-proved by 22% and as stated remains lethal because most cases are detected late because of its insidious onset and inaccessibility of ovarian nodules to early diagnosis. On the bright side is the high cure and 5-year survival rates for stage I patients with cervical cancer (92%), uterine corpus cancer (96%), and ovarian cancer (95%). Cancer of the vagina has similar survival rates to the cervix (see Table 43.5).

TABLE 49.2	Lymph Nodes of Vagina	
Sentinel nodes	Juxtaregional node
Obturator	Para-aortic
Internal iliac (proximal)	
Inguinal (distal)	
Regional nodes	
Hypogastric	
External iliac	
Deep inguinal	
Common iliac	
Lateral sacral	
Paracaval	

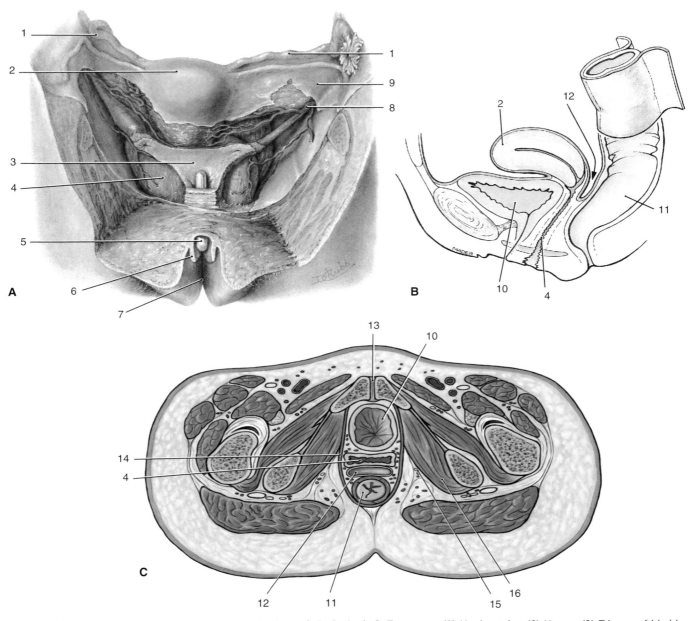

Figure 49.4 T-oncoanatomy. Three-planar views. **A.** Coronal. **B.** Sagittal. **C.** Transverse. (1) Uterine tube. (2) Uterus. (3) Trigone of bladder. (4) Vagina. (5) Rod in urethra. (6) Labia minorus. (7) Labia majorus. (8) Uterine artery. (9) Round ligament of uterus. (10) Urinary bladder. (11) Rectum. (12) Rectouterine pouch. (13) Pubic symphysis. (14) Levator ani muscle. (15) Pudendal canal. (16) Obturator internus muscle.

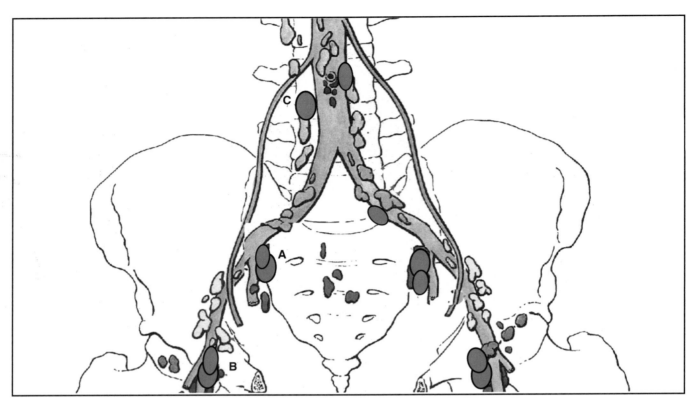

Figure 49.5 N-oncoanatomy. The sentinel nodes are: **A.** The obturator nodes of the internal iliac chain, external iliac. **B.** Juxtaregional. **C.** Paraortic nodes.

TABLE 49.3	Imaging Modalities for Staging Vagina Cancer	
Method	**Diagnosis and Staging Capability**	**Recommended for Use**
Primary (T) staging		
CTe	Defines cervical involvement and tumor size, also vaginal extension	Yes, has displaced barium enema and IVP
MRI	Preferred for cross-sectional anatomy of pelvis to assess by its high signal intensity of the cancer invasion	Yes, gadolinium enhances signal intensity of cancer. Recommended for T1b and above.
Nodal (N) staging		
CTe	Excellent for assessing adenopathy and tumor necrosis in nodes	Yes, cost effective
MRI	Comparable to CT in detecting nodal disease	Yes, both T and N can be simultaneously assessed.
Metastases (M) staging		
Barium enema		Yes, for patients with suspicious lesions
Bone scan		Yes, if suspected
CT	Useful to assess omental and liver metastases	Yes, if suspected
PET	Useful body scan for metastases	No, investigational

CT, computed tomography; CTe, CT enhanced with IV contrast; IVP, intravenous pyelography; MRI, magnetic resonance imaging; PET, positron emission tomography.

The staging is similar to most skin cancers; both size and depth of invasion are the critical criteria.

Perspective and Patterns of Spread

Cancers of external female genitalia arise in a variety of anatomic sites and are superficial but difficult to recognize and identify because of their location. A predisposing factor is human papilloma virus (HPV); HPV16 appears as the most common variety and require cofactors as herpes simplex virus to complete the induction neoplastic process. Vulval cancers are uncommon, slightly over 1% with approximately 4,000 new cases, 20% of which may result in death. The majority occurs in the labia majora and minora (70%) and 10% to 15% in the clitoris, with other sites being infrequent. The most common symptoms are vulval pruritus and bleeding or spotting, but otherwise are asymptomatic.

The spread patterns are similar to other skin cancers appearing as surface lesions (Fig. 50.1) that fail to heal and gradually spread superficially and then in depth. The rich lymphatics of the perineum result in lymph node enlargement in the groin, which can be unilateral or bilateral. The external genitalia are lined by stratified squamous epithelium and lead to squamous cell carcinomas (90%). In addition there are numerous secretory glands (Skene and Bartholin) that may give rise to adenocarcinomas. Preinvasive changes as Bowen's disease or Paget's disease with erythroplasia or leukoplasia may be the earliest sign of disease. Melanomas account for a few percent of most series (Table 50.1).

TNM Staging Criteria

The staging is similar to most skin cancers; both size and depth of invasion are the critical criteria: T1 <2 cm and T2 >2 cm with modification in stage I for depth of invasion 1a <1 mm and 1b >1 mm. T3 has superior spread into the vagina or urethra and T4 has reached more deeply to the bladder or rectum. Lymph nodes

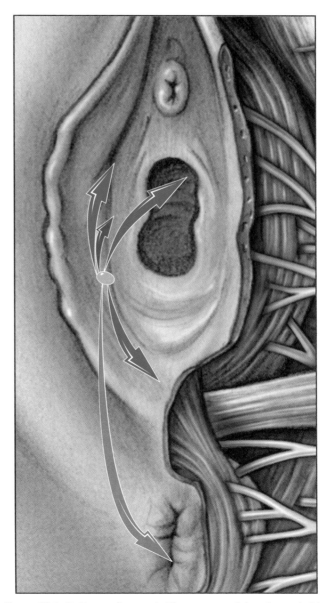

Figure 50.1 **Patterns of spread.** The cancer crab is color coded for stage: Tis and T0, yellow; T1, green; T2, blue; T3, purple; and T4, red.

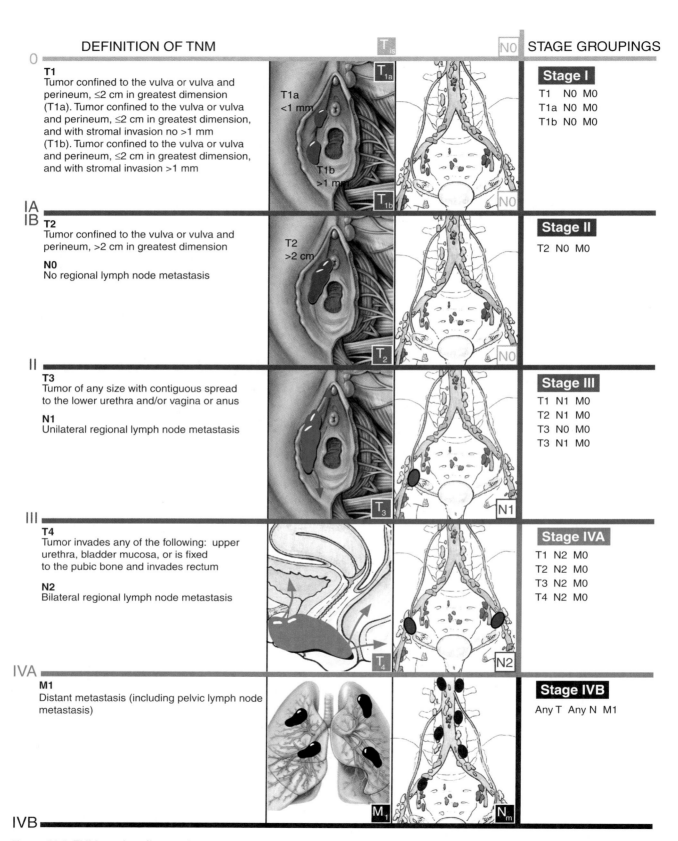

DEFINITION OF TNM

T1
Tumor confined to the vulva or vulva and perineum, ≤2 cm in greatest dimension (T1a). Tumor confined to the vulva or vulva and perineum, ≤2 cm in greatest dimension, and with stromal invasion no >1 mm (T1b). Tumor confined to the vulva or vulva and perineum, ≤2 cm in greatest dimension, and with stromal invasion >1 mm

T2
Tumor confined to the vulva or vulva and perineum, >2 cm in greatest dimension

N0
No regional lymph node metastasis

T3
Tumor of any size with contiguous spread to the lower urethra and/or vagina or anus

N1
Unilateral regional lymph node metastasis

T4
Tumor invades any of the following: upper urethra, bladder mucosa, or is fixed to the pubic bone and invades rectum

N2
Bilateral regional lymph node metastasis

M1
Distant metastasis (including pelvic lymph node metastasis)

STAGE GROUPINGS

Stage I
T1   N0 M0
T1a N0 M0
T1b N0 M0

Stage II
T2 N0 M0

Stage III
T1 N1 M0
T2 N1 M0
T3 N0 M0
T3 N1 M0

Stage IVA
T1 N2 M0
T2 N2 M0
T3 N2 M0
T4 N2 M0

Stage IVB
Any T Any N M1

Figure 50.2 TNM staging diagram is arranged vertically arranged with T definitions on left and stage groupings on right. Vulva cancers are most resectable when detected as stage I or II lesions, stage III requires radical vulvectomy with inguinal node dissection often bilaterally. There are four main stages, each with two substages for stages II and IV. Color bars are coded for stage: Stage 0, yellow; I, green; II, blue; III, purple; IV, red; and metastatic disease to viscera and nodes, black.

TABLE 50.1	Histopathologic Type: Common Cancers of the Vulva
Vulvar intraepithelial neoplasia, grade III	Paget's disease of vulva
Squamous cell carcinoma in situ	Adenocarcinoma, NOS
Squamous cell carcinoma	Basal cell carcinoma, NOS
Verrucous carcinoma	Bartholin's gland carcinoma

NOS, not otherwise specified.
Modified from Greene FL, Page DL, Fleming ID, et al., eds. *AJCC Cancer Staging Manual.* 6th ed. New York: Springer; 2002:245.

are simply categorized as N1 unilateral or N2 bilateral. When extensive cancerous infiltration of the entire perineum may occur with recurrent cancers that are incompletely treated (Fig. 50.2).

The staging criteria have remained stable.

Summary of Changes

No changes since the fifth edition of the AJCC CSM.

Orientation Three-planar Oncoanatomy

The orientation three-planar anatomy shows the vulvar isocenter is at level of perineum (Fig. 50.3).

T-oncoanatomy

- *Coronal*: The labia majora and labia minora are folds of skin with varying degrees of fat, covered by stratified squamous epithelium, covered with hair on the external surface labia majora but devoid of hair on the inner smooth surface. The homolog for labia majora is the scrotum.
- *Sagittal*: The vestibule is the space surrounded by the labia minora. The clitoris is located between the labia minora and is the homolog to the erectile bodies of the male penis containing numerous capillaries and autonomic nerve fibers.
- *Transverse*: The urethra and crus of clitoris are shown anteriorly at the vestibule of the vagina (Fig. 50.4).

N-oncoanatomy

The femoral and inguinal nodes are the first station sentinel nodes and spread into the external iliac pelvic nodes follows. If the cancer invades the vagina or bladder, the obturator and internal iliac nodes are at risk (Fig. 50.5; Table 50.2).

M-oncoanatomy

The perineal veins drain into the femoral/inguinal then external iliac veins to inferior vena cava or internal pudendal veins into internal iliac veins to inferior vena cava (Fig. 50.6).

Rules of Classification and Staging

Clinical Staging

Clinical staging involves careful scrutiny and inspection, palpation, and speculum evaluation for vaginal and urethral extension. (If the cervix is involved, the staging is assigned and similar to cervical carcinoma.)

Surgical-pathologic Staging

Staging can be made if the resection is performed before radiation or chemotherapy. The International Federations of Gynecology and Obstetrics/American Joint Committee on Cancer/International Union Against Cancer criteria are similar to other skin cancers emphasizing 2-cm size criteria.

Oncoimaging Annotations

Imaging recommendations apply only to adnexal unresectable stage III or IV presentations that involve vagina.

Cancer Statistics and Survival

Female genital system cancers collectively account for 80,000 new cases, with uterine corpus exceeding cervix by a factor of four. Both are highly curable and deaths are relatively low. The major gynecologic killer is ovarian cancer, with 16,000 deaths annually, which exceeds the other six primary sites combined.

Survival Rates

The survival rate gains in both cervix uteri and fundus uteri have been incremental. Recognizing that invasive cancers of the gynecologic tract have had a higher baseline, >50% in the 1950s, the gains for all stages are only 15% or 2% to 3% per decade. As noted, mortality rates

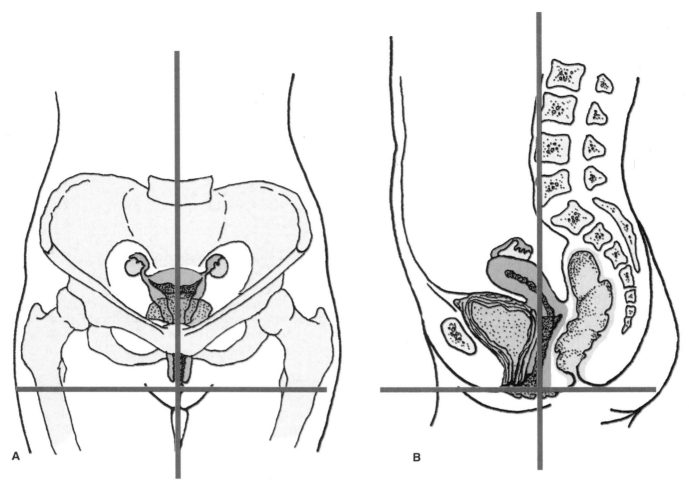

Figure 50.3 Orientation of oncoanatomy of the vulva. The anatomic isocenter is at the midline at the vestibule of the vulva and is presented in **A.** Coronal. **B.** Sagittal planes.

TABLE 50.2	Lymph Nodes of Vulva		
Sentinel nodes		Juxtaregional nodes	
Superficial femoral Inguinal		External iliac Contralateral inguinal Common iliac Para-aortic	
Regional nodes			
Superficial femoral Superficial inguinal Node of Cloquet Deep inguinal			

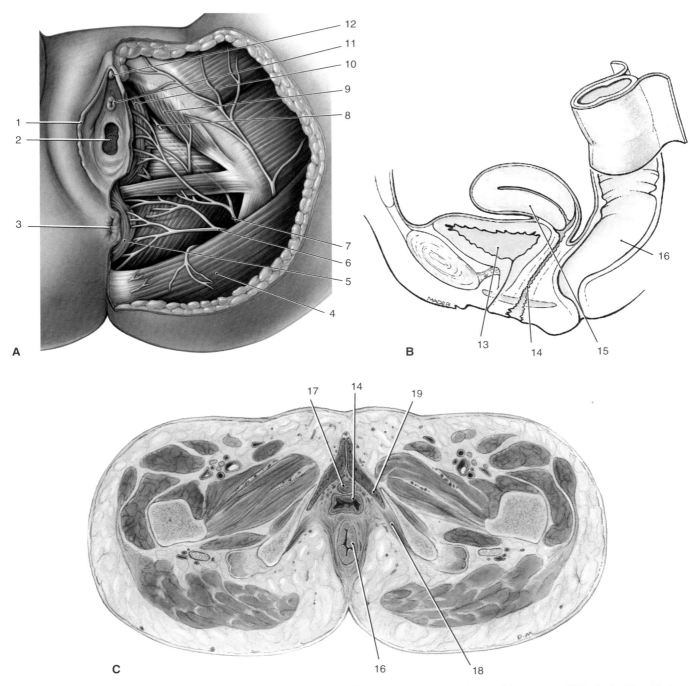

Figure 50.4 T-oncoanatomy. Three-planar views. **A.** Coronal. **B.** Sagittal. **C.** Transverse (see text). (1) Labia minorus. (2) Vaginal orifice. (3) Anus. (4) Gluteus maximus. (5) External anal sphincter. (6) Inferior rectal nerve. (7) Pudendal nerve. (8) Dorsal nerve of the clitoris. (9) Ischiocavernosus muscle. (10) Bulb of vestibule. (11) External urethral orifice. (12) Glans clitoris. (13) Urinary bladder. (14) Vagina. (15) Uterus. (16) Rectum. (17) Urethra. (18) Obturator internus muscle. (19) Crus of clitoris.

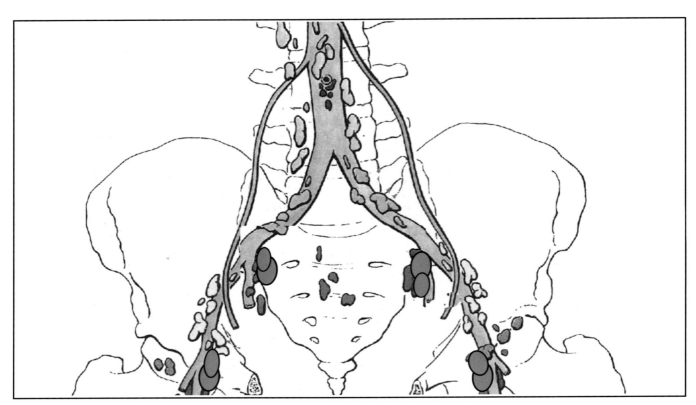

Figure 50.5 N-oncoanatomy. The sentinel nodes are the femoral and inguinal nodes; however, with deep invasion of vagina or pelvic organs, such as bladder or anus, deeper pathways are opened.

have plummeted owing to early detection, especially of cancer of the cervix, because it is most often detected in its noninvasive stage. Localized uterine cancers are >90% curable.

The cancer survival rates indicate the gain in survival for uterine corpus and cervix have been modest (14%) over the past five decades. However, most uterine cervix cancers are detected as cancer-in-situ and this is not reflected in the figures. Ovarian cancer survival has improved by 22% and, as stated, remains lethal because most cases are detected late owing to its insidious onset and inaccessibility of ovarian nodules to early diagnosis. On the bright side is the high cure and 5-year survival rates for stage I patients with cervical cancer (92%), uterine corpus cancer (96%), and ovarian cancer (95%) (see Table 43.6).

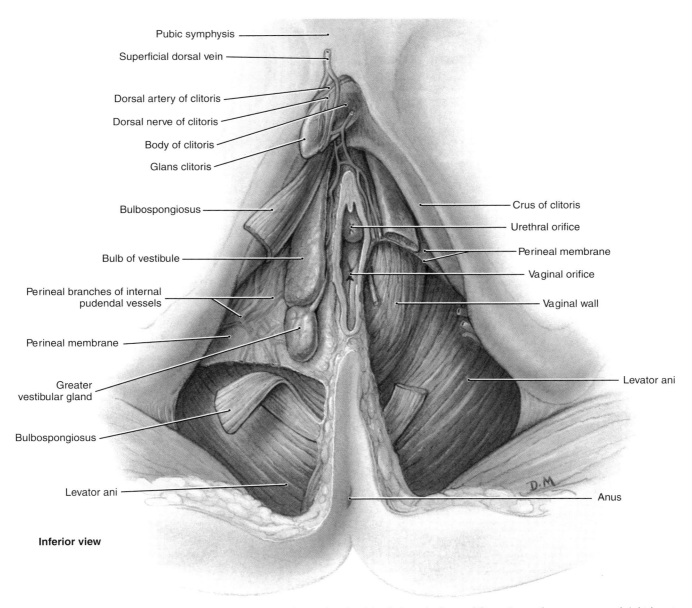

Pubic symphysis

Superficial dorsal vein

Dorsal artery of clitoris

Dorsal nerve of clitoris

Body of clitoris

Glans clitoris

Bulbospongiosus

Bulb of vestibule

Perineal branches of internal
pudendal vessels

Perineal membrane

Greater
vestibular gland

Bulbospongiosus

Levator ani

Crus of clitoris

Urethral orifice

Perineal membrane

Vaginal orifice

Vaginal wall

Levator ani

Anus

Inferior view

Figure 50.6 **M-oncoanatomy.** The venous drainage is via internal pudendal vein into the internal iliac veins to the vena cava and right heart.

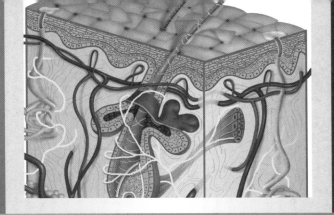

SECTION 6

GENERALIZED ANATOMIC PRIMARY SITES

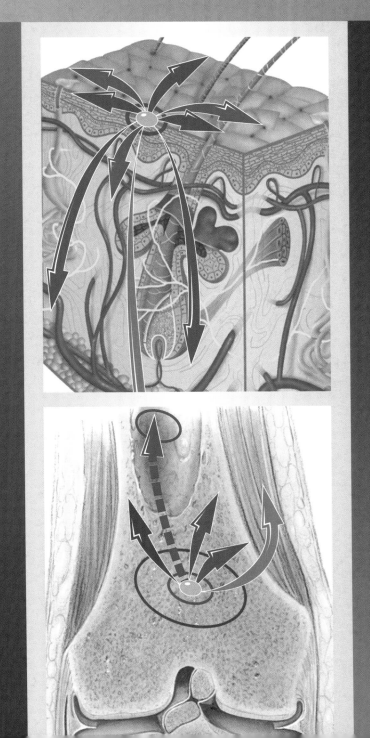

51

Introduction and Orientation

The generalized sites can give rise to primary tumors (T), sarcomas rather carcinomas, in many different anatomic sites but in addition the lymphoid system and the circulatory system are intimately related to N and M categories, respectively.

The anatomic neoplastic odyssey in addition to the 60 specific primary sites includes six generalized anatomic systems. *These are the integumentary system, the musculoskeletal systems, and the lymphoid and hematopoietic systems.* The sixth system, *the cardiovascular system,* is low in incidence for primary tumors, but is the major distribution and transport means of circulating cancer cells to distant and remote sites. Unlike specific site cancers, these malignancies can arise in a large variety of locations, making them a true challenge to diagnose, stage, and manage. The histogenesis of the generalized sites provides insight to its biologic behavior.

Perspective

The integumentary system (Fig. 51.1) is the anatomic site that results in more cancers than all the other primary sites together.

- *Skin cancers* have continued to rise rapidly over the past 30 years. Skin cancers are the most common of all cancers and among the most preventable. In the United States alone, 900,000 to 1,200,000 new cases are predicted each year. The high curability of basal and squamous cell skin cancers reduces the threat to life, but disfigurement can occur in individuals who are predisposed genetically (xeroderma pigmentosa), childhood irradiation for acne, or sun worshippers owing to the multiplicity of lesions.
- *Melanomas* are the antithesis to ordinary skin cancers in that widespread metastases can occur for these malignancies, which are measured in millimeters. Basal cell cancers rarely spread. Essential to understanding the TNM staging system is the need to study the cellular complexity of epidermal and dermal layers. There are a myriad of different cells, up to 20 to 25 in the skin, each of which can become malignant. To understand the biologic behavior of these highly

varied cellular components, an understanding of the cellular and physiologic activities of the integument is essential. The melanocyte at the epidermal/dermal interface is a cell with long dendritic processes that extends between cells into the basal stratum.

Musculoskeletal systems consist of three important components, soft tissue tissues as connective tissue (Fig. 51.2), muscle (Fig. 51.3), and skeletal bone (Fig. 51.4), each giving rise to malignancies that are referred to as sarcomas rather than carcinomas.

- *Soft tissue sarcomas* are a unique class of tumors, distinct from skin cancers. As a class, soft tissue tumors are highly varied despite their origin from the omnipresent mesenchymal cell. *The mesenchymal cell through a de-repression process can proliferate and dedifferentiate yielding multiple histopathologic subtypes (Fig. 51.3).* The degree of malignancy is based more on the tumor grade than on the tissue type and in fact dominates in TNM staging and classification over anatomic extent of the malignant infiltration. There are many nuances and clinical challenges for *the same tumor types in different parts of the anatomy.* Soft tissue tumors arising in the extremity are more manageable and favorable than those in truncal and axial locations. Of particular note is the predominance of soft tissue sarcomas in children and relative rarity of epithelial cancers, which is the reverse of adult malignancies. Muscle per se can give rise to a variety of sarcomas reflecting the type of muscle cell (Fig. 51.4). Most rhabdosarcomas are embryonal and occur in childhood. An element of gene deletions and overexpression is often associated, with both benign and malignant growth abnormalities being present in pediatric populations. Proto-oncogenes can be expressed in these circumstances providing genetic and chromosomal biomarkers which may be useful in the future for staging.

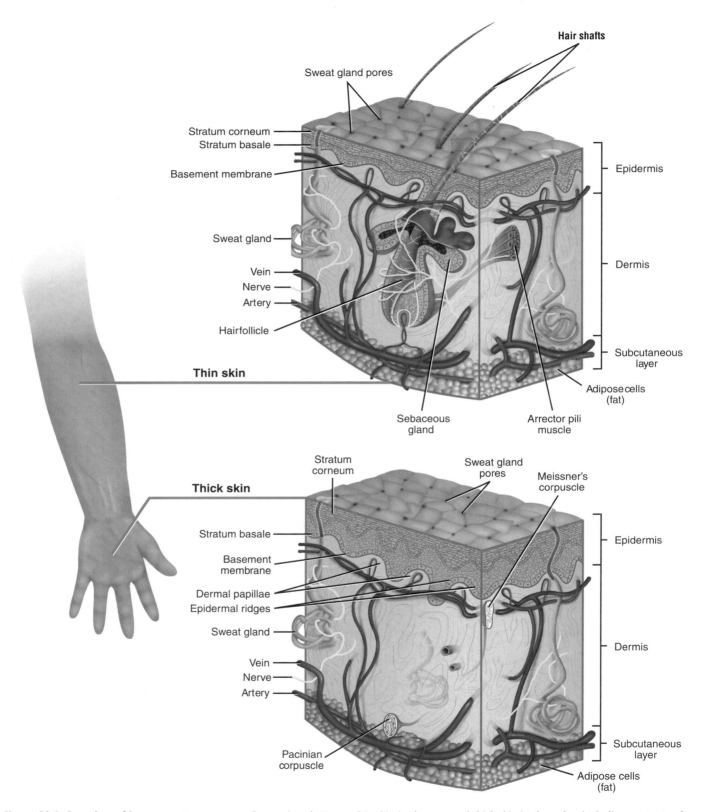

Figure 51.1 Overview of integumentary system. Comparison between thin skin in the arm and thick skin in the palm, including contents of the connective tissue dermis.

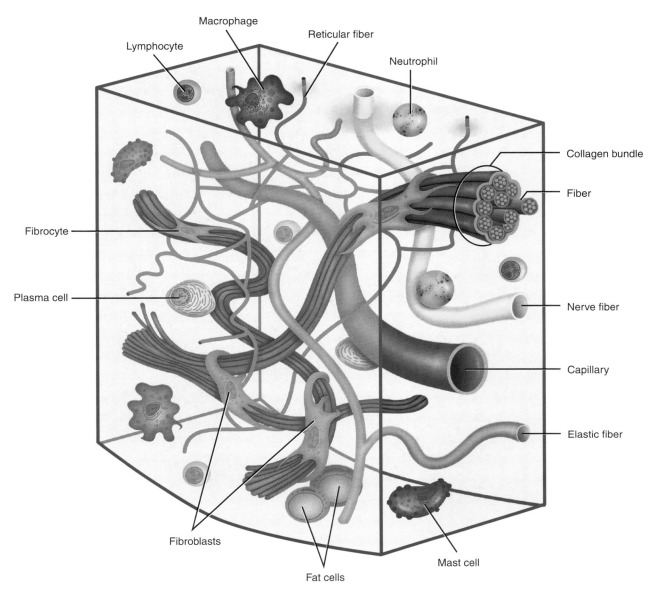

Figure 51.2 **Overview of mesenchymal soft tissue.** Composite illustration of loose connective tissue with its predominant cells and fibers.

- *Bone tumors*: The classification and staging of bone tumors has been as varied as their malignant histopathologic typing which often require supplementary radiographic images to ascertain its location and origin. Again, as in other sarcomas, the grade impacts staging, as does anatomic extent, but to a lesser degree than anatomic size. Rules for classification allow for of imaging technologies ranging from magnetic resonance imaging (MRI) to computed tomography (CT) and, to some extent radioisotope ^{99m}Tc scanning. Biopsy is an essential aspect of staging and needs to be thoughtfully located to allow for subsequent en bloc bone tumor resection for more accurate histopathology typing and grading.

The anatomic aspects of skeletal growth are essential to understanding biologic behavior and patterns of spread of osseous malignancies (Fig. 51.4). The fundamental organization of bone formation as endochrondral or intramembranous is the key to appreciating how the skeleton grows, models, and remodels into compact and cancellous bone. Each bone—long, short, cuboid, and flat—is organized and grows differently as a function of age. Malignant tumors tend to occur in sites of major growth activity, that is, the distal rather than proximal physis of long bone, i.e., the distal femur rather than a short bone as a metacarpal. Neoplasms are more likely to occur at puberty and in young, growing adults than the elderly, because of the loss of mitotic potential with age.

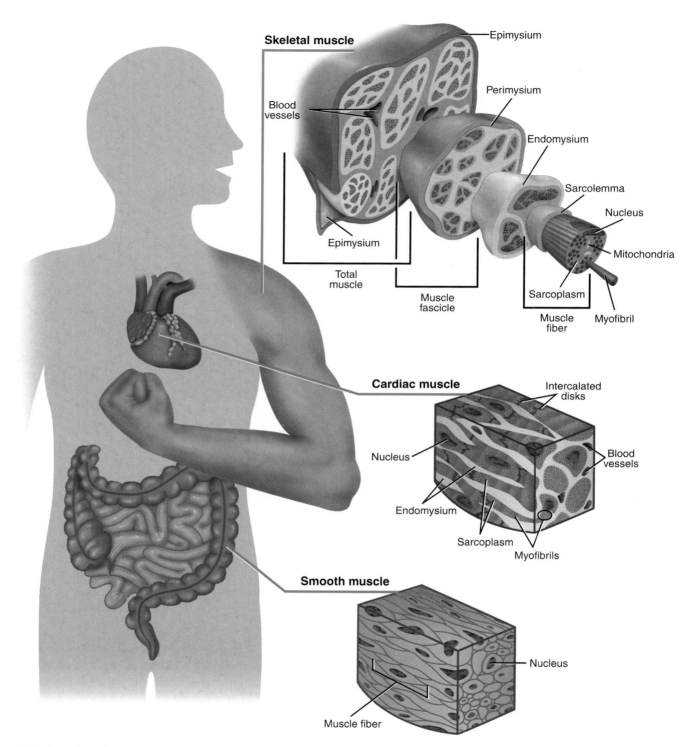

Figure 51.3 **Overview of muscular tissue.** Microscopic illustrations of the three types of muscles, namely, skeletal, cardiac, and smooth.

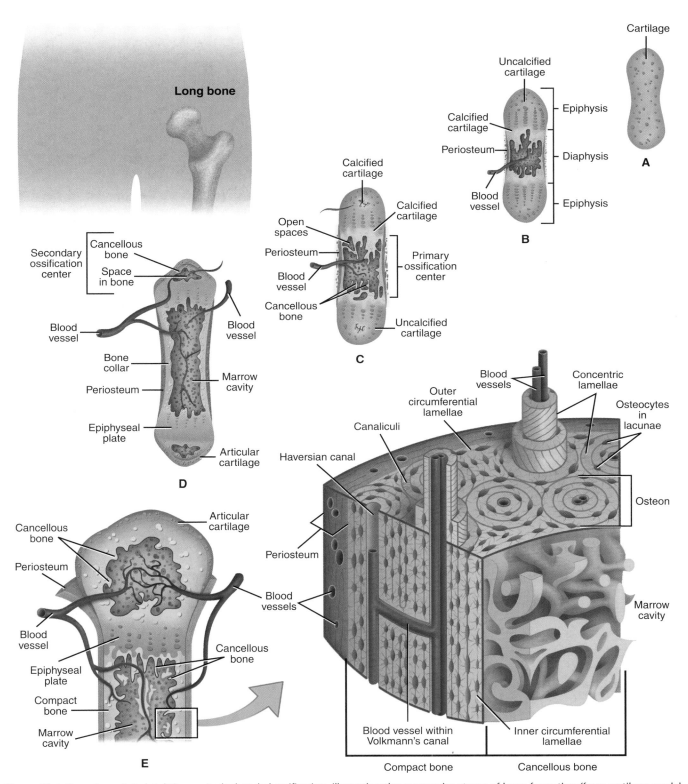

Figure 51.4 **Overview of skeletal tissue.** Endochondral ossification, illustrating the progressive stages of bone formation (from cartilage model to bone) and including the histology of a section of formed bone.

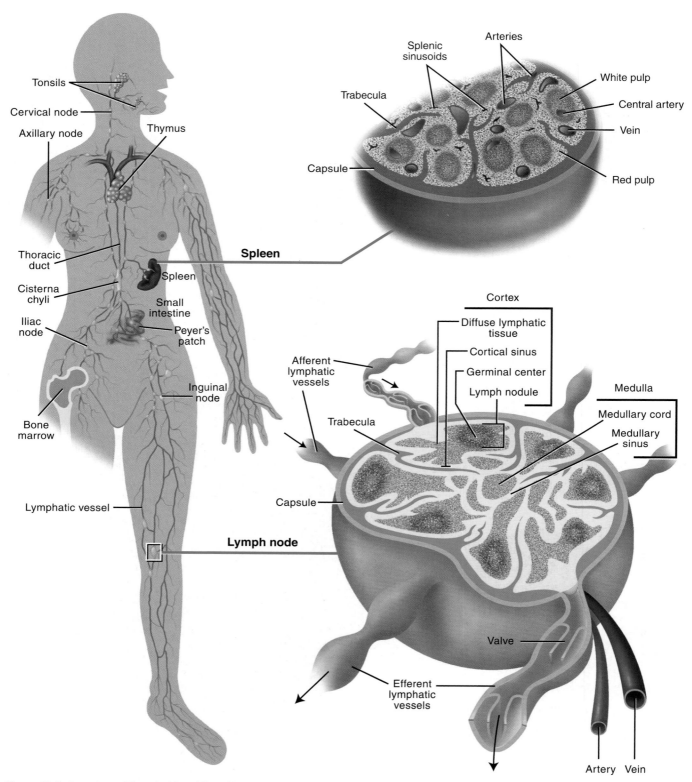

Figure 51.5 Overview of lymphoid and lymphatics system. Location and distribution of the lymphoid organs and lymphatic channels in the body. Internal contents of the lymph node and spleen are illustrated in greater detail.

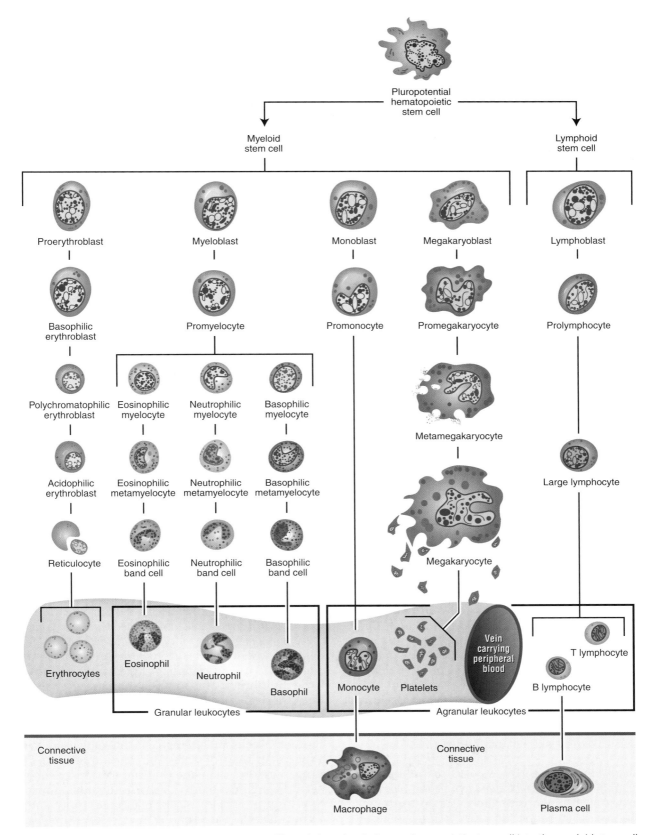

Figure 51.6 Overview of hematopoietic system. Differentiation of a pluripotent hemopoietic stem cell into the myeloid stem cell line and lymphoid stem cell line during hemopoiesis.

The lymphoid system (Fig. 51.5) is ubiquitously distributed and lymphomas affect all age groups. The lymphoid system consists of an elaborate fine network of channels that drain into lymphatic chain of nodes eventually emptying into the thoracic duct. In addition to regional lymph nodes, there are numerous extranodal collections of lymphoid tissue.

- *Hodgkin disease*: The staging of anatomic extent in both Hodgkin disease and lymphoma lead to the term "lymph node regions" (LNR) defined in 1965 at Rye, New York. Although they are not based on any physiologic or natural anatomic boundaries, LNR have become accepted by clinical consensus. The diaphragm acts as the great divide with the cisterna chyli located inferior to the right diaphragmatic leaf and giving rise to the thoracic duct, which courses through the thorax where it crosses over to the left side at T4 and terminates in the left neck. *"Lymph node-bearing region" anatomy of lymphomas needs to be reconciled with "regional first-station nodes" of normal anatomic structures that constitute organ primary sites that give rise to cancer.* Extranodal sites are "E," although in some sense are equivalent to the "T" of cancer. The concept of retrograde spread from a lymph node to a structure as Waldeyer's ring or lung may be treated as a subgroup of stage, namely, IIE, whereas bone marrow, liver, pleura, or cerebrospinal fluid requires a stage IV disseminated designation.
- *Lymphomas* are a heterogeneous group of malignancies that present as either limited or diffuse adenopathy. The evaluation of classification of lymphoid malignancies has been mutated to its present diversity because of the continual progress of immunobiology, which is superimposed on descriptive histopathology. Immunophenotyping and genetic features have resulted in 25 different categories of lymphoma, including Hodgkin disease. The Revised European–American Classification is now the standard adopted by the World Health Organization tabulation, which has B-cell and the T-cell/natural killer cells as the great divide. The staging workup to determine anatomic extent is demanding since numerous ancillary procedures include sophisticated imaging, exploratory procedures and biopsy proof of involvement.
- *Mycosis fungoides* is a primary cutaneous T-cell lymphoma that involves soft tissues and regional lymph nodes, and has a TNM classification that is clinically used and deserves to be maintained.

Hematopoietic system (Fig. 51.6) is constituted by the bone marrow and its cellular products in the blood. The bone marrow although intimately related to the lymphoid system in a neoplastic sense is integrated with bone anatomically. Fetal bone marrow at birth occupies the shaft of all long bones in their medullary cavity and then recedes at puberty and adolescence to proximal portions of the humerus and femur.

- *Multiple myelomas*: Multiple myeloma is a neoplastic disorder characterized by a single clone of plasma cells, believed to be derived from B cells. Diffuse, small, lytic bone lesions are more common than solitary plasmacytomas that are highly curable. For the diagnosis of multiple myeloma, 10% of bone marrow cells on aspiration need to be plasma cells; the production of monoclonal (M) protein encountered in serum and urine are characteristics of this disease.
- The *leukemias* have not been included in TNM classification and are considered disseminated diseases; anatomic staging per se may not be relevant. However, these diseases of white blood cells are either myeloid or lymphoid neoplasms and provide a view of the future in that molecular biology technology has enabled the identification of leukemia-specific cytogenetic and molecular signatures. The correlation of clinicopathologic courses and a specific cytogenetic marker can lead to the development and use of specific targeted therapy to molecular events. The ability to detect minimal residual disease provides a sharper end point to terminate aggressive cyclic chemotherapy and/or radiation regimens. Generally, leukemias are divided into acute or chronic depending on whether the clonal hematopoietic stem cell disorder is characterized by arrested differentiation of stem cells leading to immature blast cells. This block in differentiation may occur in hematopoietic lineages, before lineage commitment, or during developmental stages within a lineage.

The cardiovascular system (Fig. 51.7) is the major means of circulation of blood cells, nutrients and electrolytes to all normal tissues and organs in the body. The main components are the heart and an elaborate vascular tree consisting of arteries carrying oxygenated blood, veins returning deoxygenated blood, and a vast mesh of microvascularization, which is the microcirculation of capillaries in all normal tissues and organs. *Although neoplastic disease rarely affects the heart as a primary site, it is the major means of distributing neoplastic cancer and sarcoma cells to remote sites resulting in disseminated metastases.* The venous system is of greater interest to explain the distribution of metastases than the arterial system. *The concept of oligometastases as the first stage of a more disseminated process is defined as a limited number or a few foci of cancer cells in one organ system.* Although there are numerous circulating cells, oligometastases may be the initial phase of metastatic cancer residing in another organ system than the one the cancer cell originated in. The argument as to a genetically programmed "seed versus soil" as the basis for metastases is not addressed. The anatomic basis for oligometastases is hypothesized on the venous drainage of the primary site and the target metastatic organ is the first to receive the released cancer

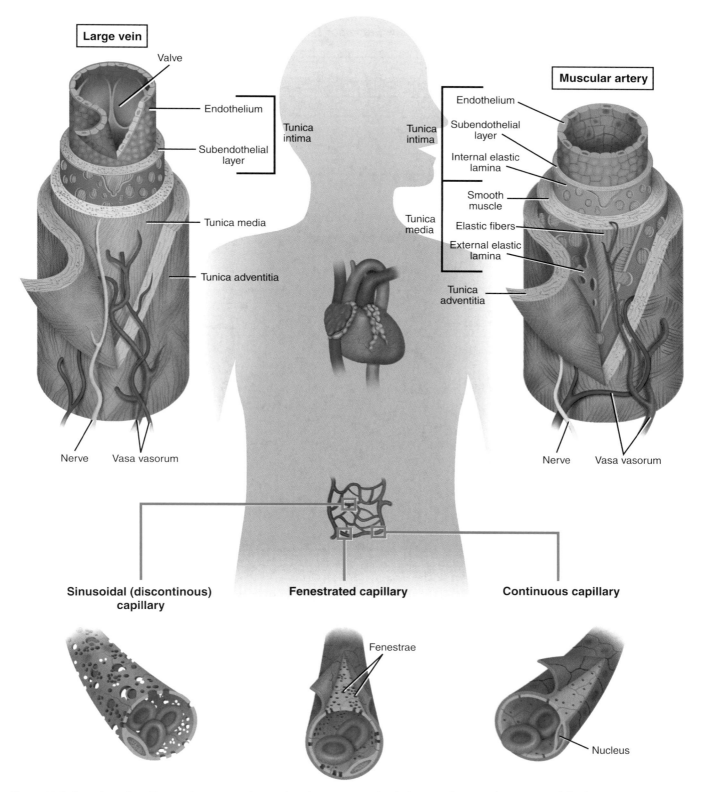

Large vein

Valve

Endothelium

Subendothelial layer

Tunica intima

Tunica media

Tunica adventitia

Nerve   Vasa vasorum

Muscular artery

Endothelium

Subendothelial layer

Internal elastic lamina

Tunica intima

Smooth muscle

Elastic fibers

External elastic lamina

Tunica media

Tunica adventitia

Nerve   Vasa vasorum

Sinusoidal (discontinous) capillary

Fenestrated capillary

Fenestrae

Continuous capillary

Nucleus

Figure 51.7 **Overview of cardiovascular system.** Comparison (transverse sections) of a muscular artery, large vein, and the three types of capillaries.

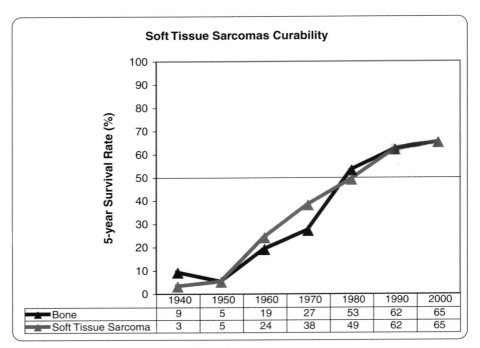

Figure 51.8 Trajectory of soft tissue sarcoma curability.

cells. The four most common sites for remote metastases are lung, liver, bone, and lymphoid.

- *Lung*: Pulmonary metastases are the most common because the entire venous hypoxic blood is returned to the heart via the superior and inferior vena cava. Primary cancer sites as head and neck, lung itself, breast, male genitourinary, and female gynecologic cancers tend to appear initially as lung metastases. Bone and soft tissue sarcomas tend to appear in lung first as the target metastatic organ.
- *Liver*: The digestive system from the distal esophagus to the rectum drains into portal circulation; solitary or oligometastases to the liver are frequently present for gastrointestinal tract cancers.
- *Bone's* medullary cavity consists of sinusoidal sites that attracts metastatic cells. Thus, the bone marrow is an optimal site to initiate metastases in bone, with the vertebrae as the most common osseous metastases, as well as the proximal portion of the femur and pelvis. The prostate is the most common primary cancer site, followed by breast and lung. The Batson circulation is a rich network of intervertebral veins that interconnects with the periprostatic plexus, the hemiazygos, and azygos veins so that a retrospread from primary sites can float malignant cells into vertebrae.
- *Lymphoid*: Because lymph node involvement is so common, one needs to note all lymphatics drain into the cisterna chili and then into the thoracic duct, which drains into the left neck at the junction of the internal jugular and subclavian veins. The first sign

of a hidden primary is often a left supraclavicular node, so-called, *Virchow's node*.

TNM Patterns of Spread and Staging Criteria

Each of the generalized systems has classification and staging criteria that are unique and idiosyncratic to that tissue/organ. As such, each system and its associated malignancies are presented separately.

Overview of the Oncoanatomy

The oncoanatomy of each generalized system is concisely described with a more thorough presentation offered in the chapter dealing with the staging of its malignant tumors.

Orientation of Three-planar Oncoanatomy

Because major regional sectors—head and neck, thorax, abdomen, male and female pelvis—have been thoroughly covered in the presentation of the 50 primary cancer sites, the focus of the oncoanatomy is the appendicular anatomy, that is, lower and upper limbs.

Rules for Classification and Staging

The value and importance of cross-sectional imaging is well demonstrated and recognized when determining anatomic extent of the malignancy involving a generalized site. CT, MRI, single-photon emission computed tomography, and positron emission tomography each have a role in both the initial staging and follow-up evaluation. Detailed oncoimaging recommendations are offered at each site.

Cancer Statistics and Survival

Skin cancers are the most preventable and most curable. Hodgkin disease was the first lymphoma to become highly curable; the other lymphomas followed because of continued gains in survival with combination chemotherapy and biologic response modifiers. The leukemias are being controlled with aggressive supralethal chemoradiation therapy and bone marrow transplantation. Acute lymphoblastic leukemia in children is currently at a very high survival rate. Soft tissue and bone sarcoma remain challenging as to cure; equally important is limb preservation. Detailed statistics and survival are presented in each chapter devoted to a generalized site. Figure 51.8 illustrates the dramatic gains in survival over the five past decades and is the trajectory of pediatric malignancies rising from incurability to curability as testimony to the multidisciplinary approach to gains in a variety of sarcomas of these generalized anatomic systems.

52

Skin Integumentary System

The T-zone around the eyes, nose, and mouth demand an outcome that preserves cosmesis and function.

Perspective and Patterns of Spread

Cancers of the skin are the most common of all malignancies, with approximately 1 million new cancers annually in the Unites States. *Worldwide, its overall incidence approaches all noncutaneous malignancies combined.* Fortunately, these lesions are readily recognized and treatment is effective, resulting in high curability. With only 1,000 deaths annually, a fraction of 1% are dying (0.001%), often in reclusive or neglected patients. Skin cancer is largely due to actinic exposure and the majority of neoplastic lesions arise in preexisting lesions. Premalignant lesions include solar keratosis, epithelial hyperplasia, leukoplakia, nevi, and burn scars.

Although the predominant cancers are basal cell or squamous cell, virtually every component cell or adnexal structure can give rise to a malignancy. The list is long (Table 52.1). The common etiology is mainly chronic exposure to ultraviolet, especially when coupled with a genetic predisposition (fair skin). Albinism, xeroderma pigmentosa, and basal cell nevus syndrome are hereditary and individuals with these syndromes are vulnerable. Immunosuppressed patients are prone to squamous cell cancer. Papillomavirus, an oncovirus, has been implicated as causes for keratoacanthomas. Chronic irritation or inflammation, as with burn scars, can give rise to squamous cell cancer and contribute to their more aggressive behavior. Radiation induction of skin cancer is common, particularly in adolescent and young adults treated with moderate doses for acne. In blacks, mortality rates are disproportionately high and may be due to their more advanced stage at diagnosis. Facial cosmetic destruction is due to recurrent basal cell cancer and death follows when this superficial cancer gains access to lymph nodes and then becomes metastatic, most often to lung.

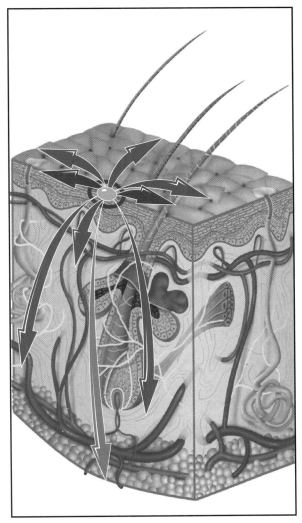

Figure 52.1 **Patterns of spread.** The spread pattern in skin is both horizontal and vertical and is color coded for stage: Tis, yellow; T1, green; T2, blue; T3, purple; and T4, red.

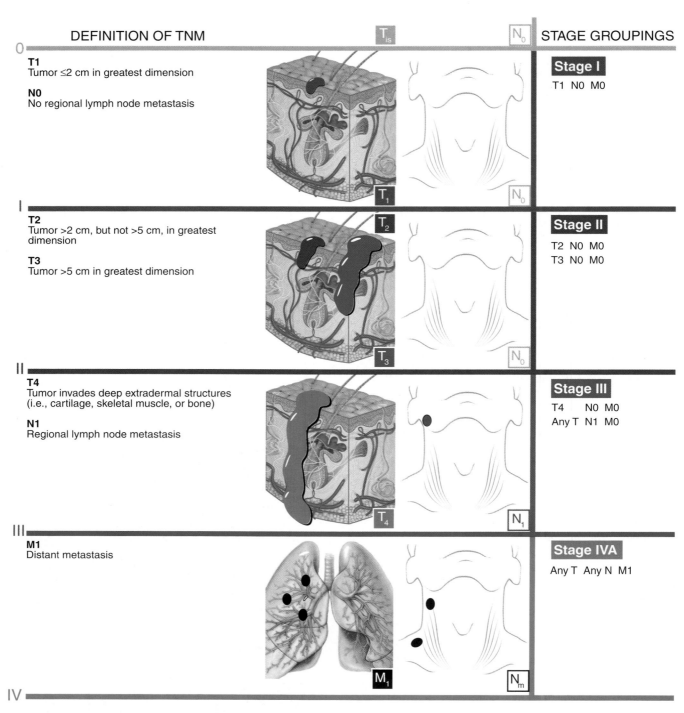

DEFINITION OF TNM   STAGE GROUPINGS

T1
Tumor ≤2 cm in greatest dimension

N0
No regional lymph node metastasis

Stage I
T1 N0 M0

T2
Tumor >2 cm, but not >5 cm, in greatest
dimension

T3
Tumor >5 cm in greatest dimension

Stage II
T2 N0 M0
T3 N0 M0

T4
Tumor invades deep extradermal structures
(i.e., cartilage, skeletal muscle, or bone)

N1
Regional lymph node metastasis

Stage III
T4   N0 M0
Any T N1 M0

M1
Distant metastasis

Stage IVA
Any T Any N M1

Figure 52.2 TNM staging diagram is arranged vertically arranged with TN definitions on left and stage groupings on right. Skin cancers are the most common curable cancers when detected early (T1, T2) and even when advanced (T3) but resectability decreases with T4 cancers due to deep invasion of cartilage, muscle and bone (purple lane). Color bars are coded for stage: Stage T0, yellow; I, green; II, blue; III, purple; IV, red; and metastatic disease to viscera and nodes, black.

TNM Staging Criteria

Cancers of the skin are very superficial tumors by virtue of location. The patterns of spread initially may be horizontal or vertical (Fig. 52.1). Once deeper inva-sion occurs, the exact anatomic site provides many nuances to management because the head and neck is the prime site. *The T-zone around the eyes, nose, and mouth demand an outcome for deeper invasion of skin cancers that preserves cosmesis and function.* If the

TABLE 52.1	Histopathology of Different Skin Cancers
Normal Cell	**Cancer Derivative**
Stratum basal	Basal cell cancer
Keratinocyte	Squamous cell cancer
Stratum spinosum	Intraepithelial cancer (Bowen disease)
Stratum granulosum	Kerotoacanthoma
Merkel cell	Merkel cell cancer
Melanocyte	Melanoma
Adnexal merocrine gland	Adenocarcinoma
Langerhans cell	Histiocytosis X
T cell	Mycosi fungoides
B cell	Cutaneous lymphomas
Endothelial cell	Kaposi sarcoma
Fibroblast	Fibrosarcoma

underlying structures—muscle, bone, or cartilage—are involved, they play an important role in success or failure. Clinical detection is often by an annual systematic examination of the integumentary system by a dermatologist. Excisional biopsy or Mohs technique of microscopic analyses of skin shavings are commonly used for diagnosis and staging. Careful palpation is essential in identifying the indurated cancer infiltrated skin from normal skin and whether the lesion is fixed or freely mobile. Lymph node regions require careful clinical assessment with biopsy of suspicious nodes.

The staging system for skin cancer has been stable (Fig. 52.2). The main criterion has been size: T1, 2 cm; T2, <5 cm; T3 >5 cm; and T4, invades deep underlying extradermal structures as cartilage, bone, and skeletal muscle. The nodal categorization is simply N1 for nodal involvement. The reason for this rather simple staging system is the vast majority of skin cancers fall into the T1N0 stage I. On the face or head and neck region, a 2-cm cancer is a relatively large area, particularly if negative margins are required. It is not only the margin around the cancer, but the depth of excision that matters. The major concern and reason for failure is the recurrent cancer that invades perineurally or into bone. These cancers can become very erosive and destructive. Distant metastases are rare and tend to be mainly pulmonary with squamous cell cancers. Basal cancers virtually never metastasize unless neglected and allowed to advance. The staging generally reflects the T stage progression.

Summary of Changes

No changes have been made since the fifth edition of the AJCC CSM.

Orientation of Oncoanatomy of Three-planar Oncoanatomy

The integumentary system encompasses the entire skin surface including its folds, openings, adnexae, derivatives, and appendages. In humans, it is the largest organ and its derivatives include nails, hair, and sweat and sebaceous glands. The skin consists of two layers, the epidermis and the dermis. *The superficial epidermis is nonvascular and consists of a stratified squamous epithelium with distinct cell types and layers referred to as stratums (Fig. 52.3A).* The *dermis* is the vascular zone and the epidermis is avascular. The majority of the dermis is a dense irregular tangle of connective tissue and below this is the *hypodermis* or *subcutaneous tissue,* which is mainly a mixture of fat and connective tissue that forms the fascial layers. The epidermis can be thick or thin in different regions of the body. Thick skin is largely keratinized and devoid of hair and glands, whereas thin skin contains hair and sweat and sebaceous glands, and tends to be the sites for malignancy.

The dermis consists of a papillary and reticular layer. The *papillary layer* is at the junction of epidermis and dermis and is irregular owing to raised projections of dermal papillae that interdigitate with epidermal ridges.

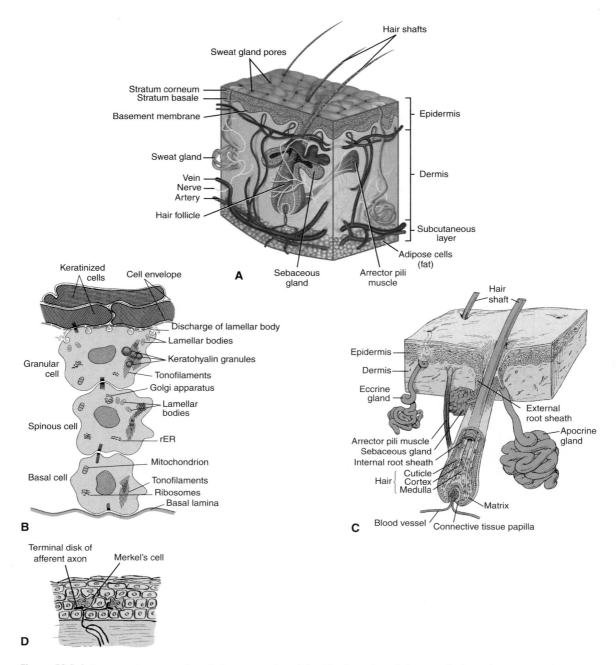

Figure 52.3 Integumentary overview. A. A cross-section of the skin shows its cellular complexity and structures. There is the epidermis epithelial cover from which most skin cancers arise. This epidermal avascular layer rests on a base of subcutaneous tissue of fat and connective tissue which is divided into a dermis of a papillary and reticular layer. **B.** Schematic diagram of keratinocytes in the epidermis consists of four layers of cells: Basal cell, spinous cells, granular cells, and keratinized cells. rER, rough endoplasmic reticulum. **C.** Appendages as eccrine gland and apocrine gland can give rise to adenocarcinomas. **D.** Merkel cells are located in basal stratum and are characterized by neurosecretory granules that give rise to aggressive Merkel cell cancers.

This layer is loose connective tissue that has capillary loops, fibroblasts, and macrophages. The *reticular layer* is thicker, denser, and has connective tissue without distinct boundaries. The hypodermis blends inferiorly and contains superficial fascia and fat tissues. This layer contains Pacinian corpuscles, whereas Meisner's corpuscles are at the dermal papillary level. Both provide the sensory receptors for skin. *The skin appendages lie in the reticular layer, extend into the hypodermis, and include hair follicles, merocrine sweat glands, and apocrine sebaceous glands.*

The layers that constitute the epidermis begin with germinal stem cells, *stratum basale* (Fig. 52.3B). The next layer is the *stratum spinosum,* which is four or five cells thick. The *stratum granulosum* is filled with granules of keratohyalin. When the cell loses its nucleus, it becomes the *stratum lucidum.* Finally, the piling of cells in the stratum corneum consists of flat, dead cells that provide the thickness to skin and account for its desquamation. There are numerous ancillary cells for different functions, such as sensory nerve endings into Merkel cells.

T-oncoanatomy

The skin can be divided into its surface sectors and the lymph node region that drains a sector.

- The *head and neck* includes the face and scalp. The vast majority of cancers arise on the skin of the face. Therefore, it is the face and scalp that demand careful attention clinically because of the complex functions, cosmesis, and special senses. All need to be preserved when resecting the cancer. The lymph node drainage of the integumentary surface differs from the upper aerorespiratory and digestive passages.
- *Anterior chest* wall from the clavicles to the navel in males tends to be hirsute. Lesions on the skin of the anterior thoracic wall drain to the anterior axillary nodes.
- *Posterior chest* wall to the same level tends to be less hirsute, is exposed more often to the sun, and subject to forming cancers. The regional nodes are along the posterior wall of the axilla although all axillary nodes are at risk.
- *Upper extremity* is an infrequent sector involved with skin cancer, but can be a site for burn and chronic inflammation. It is notorious for radiation-induced cancer in dentists who finger-held dental films during their practice. Endless resections occur with loss of fingers, then the hand, then the forearm. Involvement of epitrochlear node, then axillary nodes invariably leads to demise from pulmonary metastases.
- *Anterior abdominal wall* drains into the femoral and inguinal nodes but this sector of skin is rarely involved with skin cancers.
- *Posterior abdominal wall* or skin of the lower back is an infrequent site of malignancy and also drains to femoral and inguinal nodes anteriorly.
- *Lower extremity* is not a common site for skin cancers. Burns or chronic inflammation may cause lesions to evolve from hyperplasia to dysplasia and on to neoplasia. Popliteal nodes drain the foot and leg and ultimately drain into superficial femoral lymph nodes, which also drain the thigh.

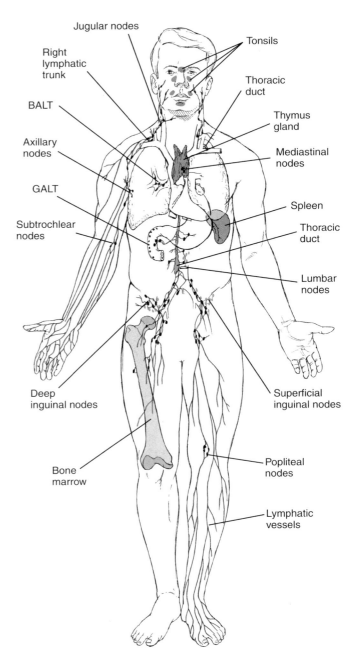

Figure 52.4 **Overview of the structures constituting the lymphatic system.** Because lymphatic tissue is the main component of some organs, they are regarded as organs of the lymphatic system (spleen, thymus, and lymph nodes). Ultimately, the lymphatic vessels empty into the bloodstream by joining the large veins at the base of the neck. The thoracic duct is the largest lymphatic vessel. BALT, bronchus-associated lymphoid tissue; GALT, gut-associated lymphoid tissue.

N-oncoanatomy

N-oncoanatomy of the skin surfaces emphasizes the *anterior* location for most if not all lymph node stations (Fig. 52.4).

- The face and scalp drain into the *superficial ring of high neck nodes* at the junction of the mandible and

TABLE 52.2	Imaging Modalities for Staging Skin Cancer	
Method	**Diagnosis and Staging Capability**	**Recommended for Use**
Primary (T) staging		
STUS	Mainly useful for recurrent deeply invading cancers	No, unless advanced
Nodal (N) staging		
CT	Searching for adenopathy in regional lymph node station	Yes, for recurrent disease
Metastases (M) staging		
CT-Ch	Evaluation for pulmonary and mediastinal disease	Yes, for advanced T3, T4 invasive disease
CT-Abd	Evaluation of liver for defects compatible with metastases	Yes, for advanced T3, T4 invasive disease
Bone scan Tc	Assessment of bone for activity followed by regular radiographs if positive	Yes, for advanced T3, T4 invasive disease or symptomatic lesions
PET	Ability to find occult foci in total body scan, especially with CT	No, investigational mainly

CT, computed tomography; CT-Abd; abdominal CT; CT-Ch, chest CT; STUS, soft tissue ultrasound.

neck: Submental, submandibular, preauricular, mastoid, and occipital nodes. Once involved, the rest of the deep lymph nodes in the neck along the carotid sheath and internal jugular vein are at risk.

- The *axillary nodes* are the recipient of lymphatics of the upper extremity and upper half of the body, both anterior and posterior skin surfaces.
- The *femoral and inguinal nodes* drain the lower extremity and the lower half of the body, both the anterior and posterior skin surfaces.

M-oncoanatomy

There is a rich network of venous channels beneath all skin surfaces that allows for venous hematogenous spread once the dermal and hypodermal layers are penetrated by invading cancers. These venous collateral channels and plexus are rich and appear once obstruction occurs.

Rules of Classification and Staging

The clinical and pathologic classifications are identical; excisional biopsy is often performed (Table 52.2). *Clinical staging* is based on physical examination, inspection and palpation of primary sites, and draining regional nodes. Imaging with regular radiographs is adequate and skull films may include facial bones and mandible for

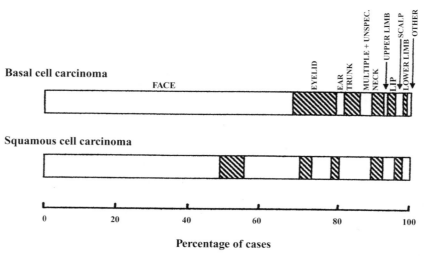

Figure 52.5 Incidence rate for basal cell carcinoma and squamous cell carcinoma.

deeply invading or fixed cancers beyond T1 in size. Computed tomography may be desirable for deeper invasion and to detect subtle cortical erosions and sclerosis.

Pathologic Staging

Complete resection of the entire site is most often performed and must provide adequate margins to determine whether there is any residuum. An immediate frozen section is essential to assure complete excision and negative margins. Mohs microsurgery provides free margins, but is a time-consuming meticulous surgical excision technique. The major advantage is being able to know a clean, deep margin has been obtained. Cancer grading is advised as well as determining histopathologic type.

Cancer Statistics and Survival

New cases of skin cancers are in the 1 million range annually and are highly curable when excised completely in their first early stage, namely, precancerous keratosis or lesions <1 cm. Fortunately, heightened awareness by the medical profession and patients has resulted in high curability rates (>95%). Once skin cancers recur in excisional scars or are neglected and invade deeply into muscle, cartilage, or bone, disfigurement and death can and do occur with local control failing to <75%.

Incidence is shown as a bar graph to indicate anatomic distribution. Note the face in the T-zone area is the most prevalent site for basal cell cancers with small percentages for trunk and limbs (Fig. 52.5).

53

The origin of melanoma can be as de novo lesions versus arising from nevi. It is due to the melanocyte, an ectodermal junctional cell located between the epidermal basale stratum and dermal papillary zone.

Perspective and Patterns of Spread

Malignant melanoma has been rising in incidence with approximately 50,000 new cases annually; the increase is at an alarming rate of 6% per year. The risk factors remain excessive sun exposure, change in a nevus, and family history of melanoma. Melanomas occur particularly in white, fair-skinned persons and are rare in blacks. Emphasis on early diagnosis has been able to lower mortality rates to 20% or 10,000 deaths annually. The **ABC** rule of the New York University Melanoma Cooperative Group is presented with **DEF** modification and alerts physicians when to be suspicious of a pigmented skin lesion:

* **A**symmetry of the lesion
* **B**order irregularity (or indistinctiveness)
* **C**olor variation
* **D**iameter >6 mm
* **E**xisting melanocytic nevi with recent change in color, size, shape
* **F**inding a new pigmented lesion, especially in persons >40 years

The histopathology categorizes four major subtypes with their patterns of spread (Table 53.1). They are lentigo malignant melanoma, superficial spreading melanoma, nodular melanoma, and acral lentiginous melanoma.

The lentigo variety is associated with sun exposure, whereas the others are characterized by an initial lesion with indolent enlargement of a primarily flat area with radial horizontal growth, followed by a vertical growth phase that signals aggressiveness and increases likelihood of nodal and hematogenous spread (Fig. 53.1).

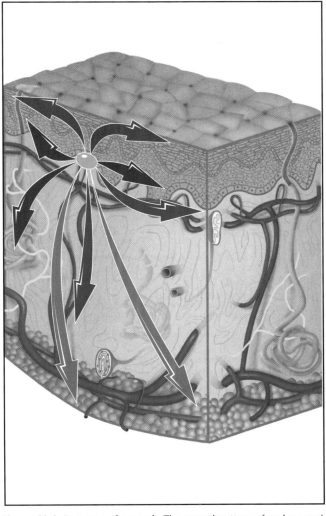

Figure 53.1 **Patterns of spread.** The spread pattern of melanoma is both horizontal and vertical and is color coded for stage: Tis, yellow; T1, green; T2, blue; T3, purple; and T4, red.

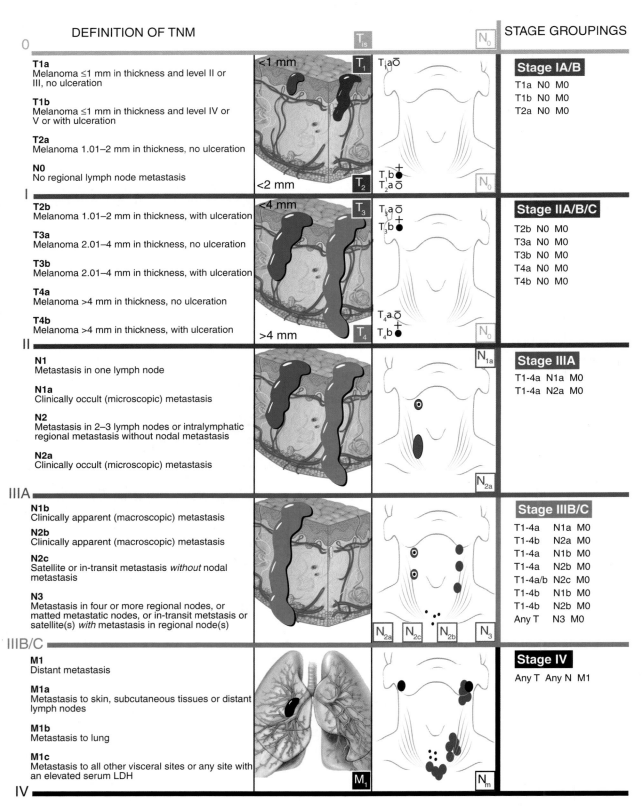

Figure 53.2 TNM staging diagram is arranged vertically arranged with T definitions on left and stage groupings on right. Melanoma with regard to size is one of the most virulent malignancies and spreads insiduously into lymph nodes. Ulcerations of a primary lesion (symbolically without ō or with ●) and in transit metastastes (∵) are ominous signs prognostically. Occult lymph nodes are microscopically positive ones. Color bars are coded for stage: Stage 0, yellow; I, green; II, blue; IIIA, purple; IIIB/C, red; and IV, metastatic disease to viscera and nodes, black.

TABLE 53.1	Histopathologic Type: Common Cancers of Melanomas of the Skin
Type	
Melanoma *in situ*	Desmoplastic melanoma
Malignant melanoma, NOS	Epithelioid cell melanoma
Superficial spreading melanoma	Spindle cell melanoma
Nodular melanoma	Balloon cell melanoma
Lentigo maligna melanoma	Blue nevus, malignant
Acral lentiginous melanoma	Malignant melanoma in giant pigmented nevus

NOS, not otherwise specified.
Modified from Greene FL, Page DL, Fleming ID, et al., eds. *AJCC Cancer Staging Manual.* 6th ed. New York: Springer; 2002:213.

TNM Staging Criteria

The origin of melanoma can be as de novo lesions versus arising from nevi. It is due to the melanocyte, an ectodermal junctional cell located between the epidermal basale stratum and dermal papillary zone. A completely revised melanoma staging system is described in the seventh edition, based on a major data analyses of numerous prognostic factors derived from a 17,000-patient data base from 13 centers. The major differences between the new version and the previous criteria are listed in Table 53.2.

The biologic aggressiveness is noted in the change of only a millimeter in size, which singles this malignancy out. Rather than measuring the cancer in centimeters, the stage and/or substage in melanomas advances by 1 mm. The T categories of melanoma are currently defined in whole integers: T1, 1 mm; T2, 2 mm; and T3, 4 mm. Subcategories such as ulceration or loss of overlying epidermis, assessed by histopathology, advances the stage. Regional nodes (N) are defined by radiogold injection at the site and dissection of the radioactive sentinel node. The number of nodes involved defines the N category. Stage grouping has many gradations of both primary and nodes. Collectively the current staging system is subcategorized into 20 subgroupings. The scientific survival data analysis is exemplary and perhaps one of the most thorough in the American Joint Committee on Cancer (AJCC) manual to justify the new subgroups (Fig. 53.4). Table 53.2 compares the difference between the previous and current staging criteria and provides a basis for subgroupings.

Summary of Changes

Melanoma thickness rather than depth of invasion or Clark levels are the new features.

- *Melanoma thickness and ulceration, but not level of invasion, are used in the T category (except for T1 melanomas).*
- *The number of metastatic lymph nodes, rather than their gross dimensions and the delineation of clinical occult (i.e., "microscopic") vs. clinically apparent (i.e., "macroscopic") nodal metastases, are used in the N category.*
- *The site of distant metastases and the presence of elevated serum lactic dehydrogenase (LDH) are used in the M category.*
- *All patients with Stage I, II, or III disease are upstaged when a primary melanoma is ulcerated.*
- *Satellite metastases around a primary melanoma and in-transit metastases have been merged into a single staging entity that is grouped into Stage IIIc disease.*
- *A new convention for defining clinical and pathologic staging has been developed that takes into account the new staging information gained from intraoperative lymphatic mapping and sentinel node excision.*

Overview of Oncoanatomy

The melanocyte is a junctional cell usually located at the interface between the dermis and the epidermis. The integumentary system encompasses the entire skin surface, including its folds, openings, adnexae, derivatives, and appendages. In humans, it is the largest organ and its derivatives include nails, hair, and sweat and sebaceous glands. The skin consists of two layers, the epidermis and the dermis (Fig. 53.3A). The superficial *epidermis* is nonvascular and consists of a stratified squamous epithelium with distinct cell types and layers referred to be strata. The *dermis* is the vascular zone and the epidermis is avascular. The majority of the dermis is a dense, irregular connective tissue and below this is the *hypodermis* or *subcutaneous tissue,* which is mainly a mixture of connective tissue and fat that forms the fascial layers (Fig. 53.3B). The epidermis can be thick or thin in

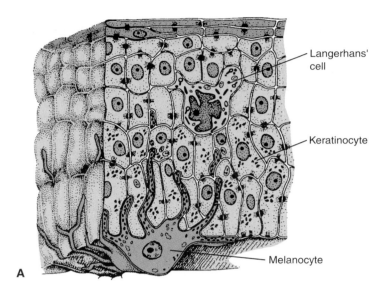

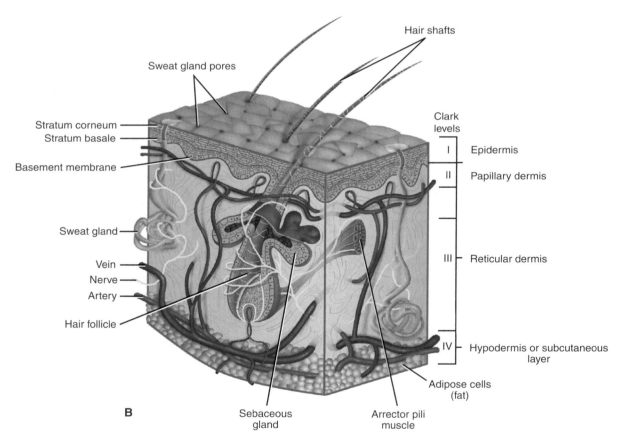

Figure 53.3 **Orientation of integumentary system. A.** The melanocyte interacts with several cells of the stratum basale and the stratum spinosum. **B.** Epidermis showing Clark levels. I. Epidermis. II. Dermis papillary. III. Reticular dermis. IV. Hypodermis or subcutaneous layer.

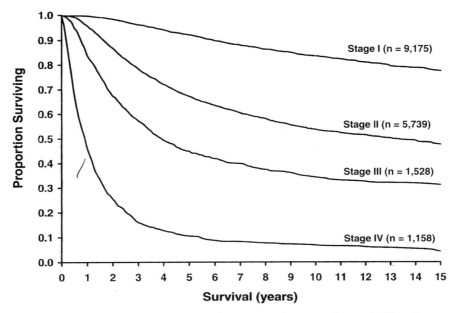

Figure 53.4 **Survival curves based on melanoma staging according to AJCC melanoma staging database.**

different regions of the body. Thick skin is largely keratinized and devoid of hair and glands, whereas thin skin is contains hair, and sweat and sebaceous glands, and tends to be the sites for malignancy.

The dermis consists of a papillary and reticular layer. The *papillary layer* is at the junction of epidermis and dermis and is irregular owing to projections of dermal papillae that interdigitate with epidermal ridges. This layer is loose connective tissue, which has capillary loops, fibroblasts, and macrophages. The reticular layer is thicker and denser; it has connective tissue without distinct boundaries. The hypodermis blends inferiorly and contains superficial fascia and fat tissues. This layer contains Pacinian corpuscles; Meisner's corpuscles are at the dermal papillary level. Both provide sensory receptors for skin. The skin appendages lie in the reticular layer, extend into the hypodermis, and include hair follicles, merocrine sweat glands, and apocrine sebaceous glands.

The layers that constitute the epidermis have a germinal stem cells, stratum basale. The next layer is the stratum spinosum, which is four or five cell thick. The stratum granulosum is filled with granules of keratonilin. When the cell loses its nucleus, it becomes the stratum lucidum. Finally, the piling of cells in the stratum corneum consists of flat, dead cells that provide the thickness to skin and account for desquamation.

T-oncoanatomy

The skin can be divided into its surface sectors and the lymph node region that drains a sector.

- The *head and neck* includes the face and scalp. It is the face and scalp that demand careful attention

clinically because of the complex functions, cosmesis, and special senses. All need to be preserved. The lymph node drainage of the integumentary surface differs from the upper aerorespiratory and digestive passages. The first station or echelon draining the skin of the face and scalp are a ring of superficial nodes: submental, submaxillary, facial, preauricular, parotid, mastoid, and occipital.

- *Anterior chest* wall from the clavicles to the navel in males tends to be hirsute. Lesions on the anterior thoracic wall skin drain to the anterior axillary nodes.
- *Posterior chest* wall to the same level tends to be less hirsute, is exposed more often to the sun, and subject to forming cancers. The regional nodes are along the posterior wall of the axilla although all axillary nodes are at risk.
- *Upper extremity* is an infrequent sector involved with skin cancer, but can be a site for burn and chronic inflammation. It is notorious for radiation-induced cancer in dentists who finger-held dental films during their practice. Endless resections occur with loss of fingers, then the hand, then the forearm. Involvement of epitrochlear node, then axillary nodes invariably leads to the patients demise from pulmonary metastases.
- *Anterior abdominal wall* draws into the femoral and inguinal nodes but this sector of skin is rarely involved with skin cancers.
- *Posterior abdominal wall* or skin of the lower back is an infrequent site of malignancy and drains to femoral and inguinal nodes.
- *Lower extremity* is not a common site for skin cancers. Burns or chronic inflammation may cause lesions to

TABLE 53.2	Differences Between the Previous (1997) Version and the Present (2002) Version of the Melanoma Staging System		
Factor	**Old System**	**New System**	**Comments**
Thickness	Secondary prognosis factor; thresholds of 0.75, 1.50, and 4 mm	Primary determinant of T staging; thresholds of 1, 2, and 4 mm	Correlation of metastatic risk is a continuous variable
Level of invasion	Primary determinant of T staging	Used only for defining T1 melanomas	Correlation only significant for thin lesions; variability in interpretation
Ulceration	Not included	Included as a second determinant of T and N staging	Signifies a locally advanced lesion; dominant prognostic factor for grouping stages I, II, and III
Satellite metastases	In T category	In N category	Merged with in transit lesions
Thick melanomas (>4.0 mm)	Stage III	Stage IIC	Stage III defined as regional metastases
Dimensions of nodal metastases	Dominant determinant of N staging	Not used	No evidence of significant prognostic correlation
Number of nodal metastases	Not included	Primary determinant of N staging	Thresholds of 1 vs. 2–3 vs. ≥4 nodes
Metastatic tumor burden	Not included	Included as a second determinant of N staging	Clinically occult ("microscopic") vs. clinically apparent ("macroscopic") nodal volume
Lung metastases	Merged with all other visceral metastases	Separate category as M1b	Has a somewhat better prognosis than other visceral metastases
Elevated serum LDH	Not included	Included as a second determinant of M staging	
Clinical vs. pathologic staging	Did not account for sentinel node technology	Sentinel node results incorporated into definition of pathologic staging	Large variability in outcome between clinical and pathologic staging; pathologic staging encouraged before entry into clinical trials

Modified from Greene FL, Page DL, Fleming ID, et al., eds. *AJCC Cancer Staging Manual.* 6th ed. New York: Springer; 2002:210.

evolve from hyperplasia to dysplasia and on to neoplasia. Popliteal nodes drain the foot and leg and ultimately drain into superficial femoral lymph nodes, which also drain the thigh.

N-oncoanatomy

N-oncoanatomy of the skin surfaces emphasizes the *anterior* location for most if not all lymph node stations (see Fig. 52.4).

- The *face* and *scalp* drain into the *superficial ring of nodes* at the junction of the mandible and neck: Submental, submandibular, preauricular, mastoid, and occipital nodes. Once involved, the rest of the

deep lymph nodes in the neck along the carotid sheath and internal jugular vein are at risk.
- The *axillary nodes* are the recipient of lymphatics of the upper extremity and upper half body both anterior and posterior skin surfaces.
- The *femoral* and *inguinal nodes* drain the lower extremity and the lower half of the body, both the anterior and posterior skin surfaces.

M-oncoanatomy

There is a rich network of venous channels beneath all skin surfaces that allows for venous hematogenous spread once the dermal and hypodermal layers are penetrated by invading cancers. These venous collateral

TABLE 53.3	Imaging Modalities for Staging Skin Melanoma	
Method	Diagnosis and Staging Capability	Recommended for Use
Primary (T) staging		
STUS	Mainly useful for recurrent deeply invading melanomas	No, unless advanced
Nodal (N) staging		
CT	Searching for adenopathy in regional lymph node station	Yes, for recurrent disease
Metastases (M) staging		
CT-Ch	Evaluation for pulmonary and mediastinal disease	Yes, for advanced T3, T4 invasive disease
CT-Abd	Evaluation of liver for defects compatible with metastases	Yes, for advanced T3, T4 invasive disease
Bone Scan Tc	Assessment of bone for activity followed by regular radiographs if positive	Yes, for advanced T3, T4 invasive disease or symptomatics
PET	Ability to find occult foci in total body scan, especially with CT	No, investigational mainly

CT, computed tomography; CT-Abd, abdominal CT; CT-Ch, chest CT; STUS, soft tissue ultrasound.

channels and plexus are rich and appear once obstruction occurs.

Rules of Classification and Staging

The clinical and pathological classifications are identified. *Clinical staging* is based on physical examination, inspection, and palpation of primary sites and draining regional nodes. Imaging with regular radiographs is adequate and includes skull films, facial bones, and mandible for deeply invading or fixed tumors beyond T1 in size. Computed tomography may be desirable for deeper invasion. Because of the high proclivity to metastasize all advanced stage melanoma must be thoroughly assessed with enhanced computed tomography and magnetic resonance imaging, especially if symptomatic (Table 53.3).

Pathologic Staging

Complete resection of the entire site is often performed with wide margins and the need to determine if there is any residuum. Skin grafting may be required to close the defect. Orientation of the section is critical to be sure the microsection is at a right angle to the skin surface. Any obliquity may increase the size of the melanoma depth of invasion. Ulceration advances the stage and must be determined on histopathology.

Cancer Statistics and Survival

Without exception, the cancer facts, findings, and statistics have been meticulously compiled (Fig. 53.4; Table 53.3). The analysis of data in melanoma in the sixth edition of the AJCC manual is very detailed and supports splitting four stages into 20 subgroupings as to outcomes. There are 55,000 new cases annually, 8,000 of whom will die. The 5-year survival rates of pathologically staged patients by Balch et al demonstrate that ulceration and nodal involvement decrease survival. The differences in 15-year survival by stage are shown for localized stages I and II (>50%) versus stage III (30%) for nodal involvement and <10% survival at 5 years for stage IV metastasis based on the AJCC database of 17,000 patients with complete clinical and pathologic data.

54

Musculoskeletal Soft Tissue Sarcoma

Anatomic extent of soft tissue sarcoma requires an understanding of compartmental anatomy by investing fascia, which applies mainly but not exclusively to limbs.

Perspective and Patterns of Spread

Soft tissues sarcomas are thought to be exclusively in their origin from mesenchyme, which is also the origin of connective tissue. The mesenchyme is an embryonic stem cell that can have a variety of connective tissue elements, any and all of which can undergo malignant transformation. Soft tissue sarcomas are not common and represent <1% of all malignancies. Because of their rarity and their slow onset, they are often identified secondary to incidental trauma. Therefore, any suspicious soft tissue mass that increases in size or has associated pain should not be dismissed but investigated. The challenge is to achieve local control without sacrifice of a limb or vital axial part and yet early enough to avoid metastatic dissemination. Exciting advances in understanding the genetic determinants of this disease have allowed for new insights in their management. The incidence of musculoskeletal tumors is estimated at <10,000 new patients annually; only 25% occur in bone (2,500 cases). For every malignant soft tissue sarcoma, there are 100 benign neoplasms. Their ratio is slightly higher in males than females. By far, the most common sites are in lower and upper extremities, followed by axial and head and neck locations, with other sites as retroperitoneum and pelvis being least common.

The histopathologic types are highly varied and include malignant fibrous histiocytoma (40%), liposarcoma, synovial sarcoma, and neurofibrosarcoma as common types (each >10%); other varieties are infrequent (each <10%; Table 54.1). Accurate assignment of histopathologic grade is the central component in staging of the patient's sarcoma. The essential features of establishing grade are nuclear, cellular morphology, and pleomorphism. The number of mitoses per high-powered field, the presence of necrosis, and the degree of cellularity all impinge on establishing grade by a

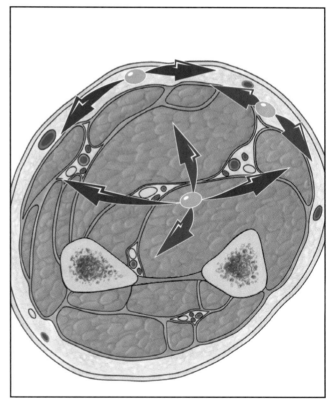

Figure 54.1 **Patterns of spread.** The spread pattern of sarcoma is both horizontal and vertical and is color coded for stage: T0, yellow; T1, green; T2, blue; T3, purple; and T4, red.

pathologist with familiarity of soft tissue sarcomas. With modern molecular biology technology, cytogenetics and molecular genetics have been added to cytochemistry, immunohistochemistry, electron microscopy, and flow cytometry supplementing, supplanting routine hematoxylin and eosin staining microscopy. Grade has

DEFINITION OF TNM

STAGE GROUPINGS

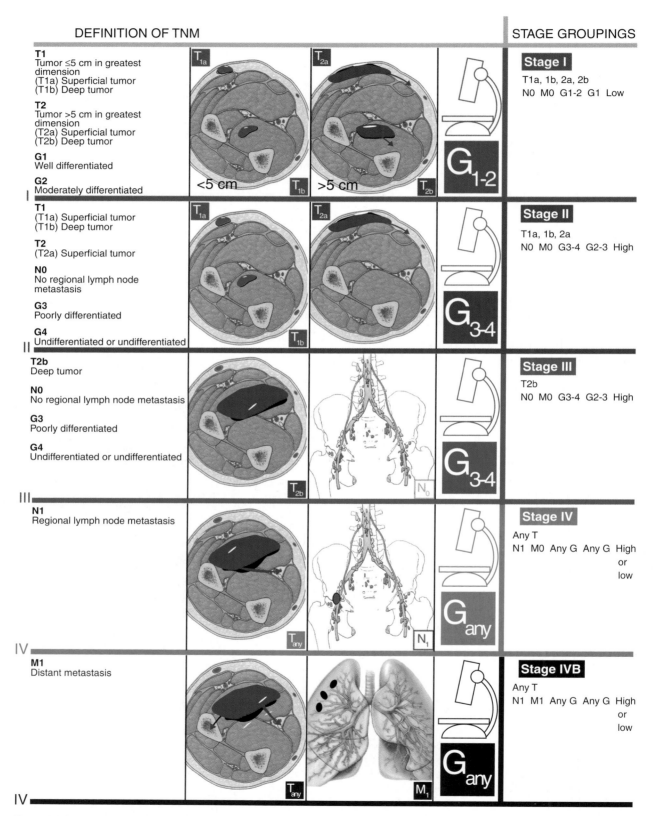

T1
Tumor ≤5 cm in greatest dimension
(T1a) Superficial tumor
(T1b) Deep tumor

T2
Tumor >5 cm in greatest dimension
(T2a) Superficial tumor
(T2b) Deep tumor

G1
Well differentiated

G2
Moderately differentiated

T1
(T1a) Superficial tumor
(T1b) Deep tumor

T2
(T2a) Superficial tumor

N0
No regional lymph node metastasis

G3
Poorly differentiated

G4
Undifferentiated or undifferentiated

T2b
Deep tumor

N0
No regional lymph node metastasis

G3
Poorly differentiated

G4
Undifferentiated or undifferentiated

N1
Regional lymph node metastasis

M1
Distant metastasis

Stage I
T1a, 1b, 2a, 2b
N0 M0 G1-2 G1 Low

Stage II
T1a, 1b, 2a
N0 M0 G3-4 G2-3 High

Stage III
T2b
N0 M0 G3-4 G2-3 High

Stage IV
Any T
N1 M0 Any G Any G High
or
low

Stage IVB
Any T
N1 M1 Any G Any G High
or
low

Figure 54.2 TNM staging diagram. Soft tissue sarcomas are resected with the goal of limb preservation and is defined by compartmental anatomy. There are four stages when histologic grade is added to the T stage. N1 is equivalent to distant metastases. Color bars are coded for stage: Stage I, green; II, blue; III, purple; IV, red; and metastatic disease to viscera and nodes, black. Note the importance of tumor grade in addition to anatomic extent.

TABLE 54.1	Histopathologic Types of Soft Tissue Sarcomas	
Type		**Derivative Normal Cell**
Alveolar soft-part sarcoma		Neuromyogenic cell
Desmoplastic small round cell tumor		Epithelioid endothelial
Epithelioid sarcoma		Fascial tendon fibrocyte
Clear cell sarcoma		Primitive mesenchymal
Chondrosarcoma, extraskeletal		Chondroblast
Osteosarcoma, extraskeletal		Osteoblast
Gastrointestinal stromal tumor		Leiomyoblast
Ewing's sarcoma/primitive neuroectodermal tumor		Primitive mesenchymal
Fibrosarcoma		Fibroblast
Leiomyosarcoma		Smooth myocyte
Liposarcoma		Adipolyte
Malignant fibrous histiocytoma		Fibroblast/histiocyte
Malignant hemangiopericytoma		Pericytes
Malignant peripheral nerve sheath tumor		Neurolemmol (Schwann)
Rhabdomyosarcoma		Myofibroblast
Synovial sarcoma		Biphasis synovial epithelial cell
Sarcoma, not otherwise specified		Mesenchymal cell

typically been assigned in four grades and the American Joint Committee on Cancer (AJCC) recommendation is into two tiers: low and high grade. From perusing the stage grouping it is evident that pathologic grade dominates the anatomic extent.

TNM Staging Criteria

Anatomic extent of soft tissue sarcoma requires an understanding of compartmental anatomy, which applies mainly, but not exclusively, to the limbs. *The depth of invasion of soft tissue sarcomas in limbs and the trunk is more important than size (Fig. 54.1).* The hypodermis is deep to the dermis and is the common location. *The term "superficial" is defined as lack of involvement of the investing fascia, whereas deep implies deep to or involving the investing fascia.* The relationship of the investing fascia is readily apparent in limbs. All intraperitoneal, retroperitoneal, intrathoracic truncal soft tissue sarcomas are considered deep. Head and neck tumors may be designated superficial or deep. There are two T stages based on size: T1, <5 cm, and T2, >5 cm. Each can be superficial (T1A or T2A) or deep (T1B or T2B) related to investing fas-

cia. Grades I and II are low, and grades III and IV are high. Nodal invasion is less common than hematogenous spread and N1 is equivalent to M1 or stage IV (Fig. 54.2).

Summary of Changes

- *G 1-2, T2b, N0 M0 tumors have been reclassified as stage I rather than stage II disease.*
- *Angiosarcoma and malignant mesenchymoma are no longer included in the list of histologic types for this site.*
- *Gastrointestinal stromal tumor and Ewing's sarcoma/ primitive neuroectodermal tumor have been added to the list of histologic types for this site.*
- *Fibrosarcoma grade I has been replaced by fibromatosis (desmoid tumor) in the list of histologic types not included in this site.*

Overview of the Oncoanatomy

The connective tissues are the derivatives of the mesenchymal stem cell. The composite illustration of loose connective

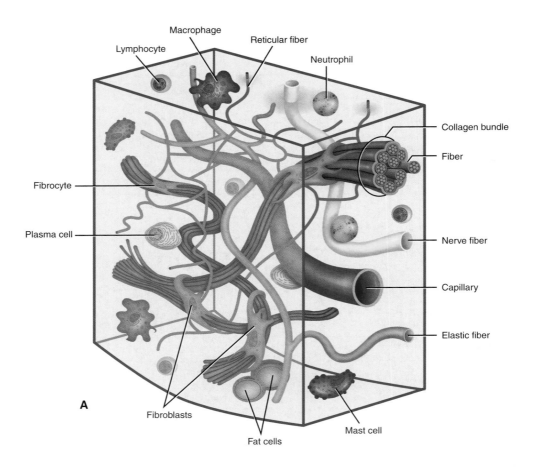

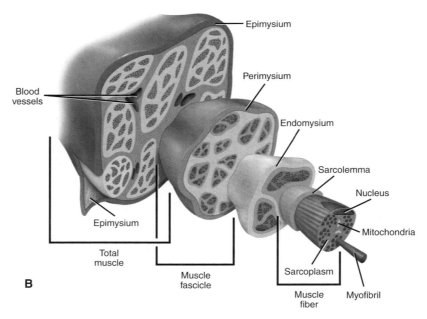

Figure 54.3 **Overview of oncoanatomy.** The mesenchymal cells give rise to **(A)** a variety of LCT elements and include fibrocytes, fibroblasts, adipocyte, macrophages, and mast cells include both collagen and reticular and elastic fibers. **(B)** Muscle compartments are composed of muscle cells and, in addition, cardiac muscle. Muscle cells are multinucleated and tend to hypertrophy rather than undergoing hyperplasia.

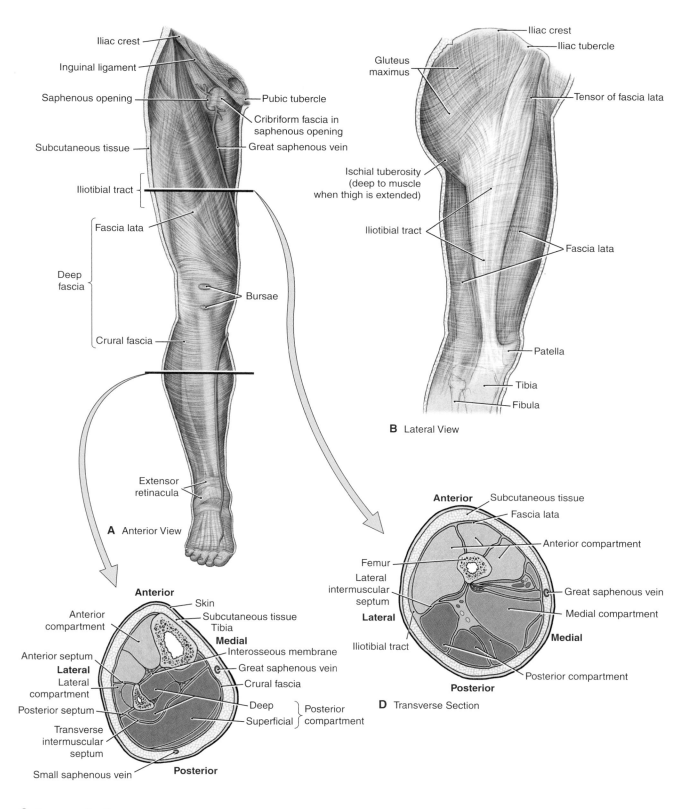

Figure 54.4 Orientation of T-oncoanatomy of the lower limb. A. Investing superficial fascia. **B.** Lateral view of investing fascia. **C.** Transverse thigh. **D.** Transverse leg showing superficial and deep compartments.

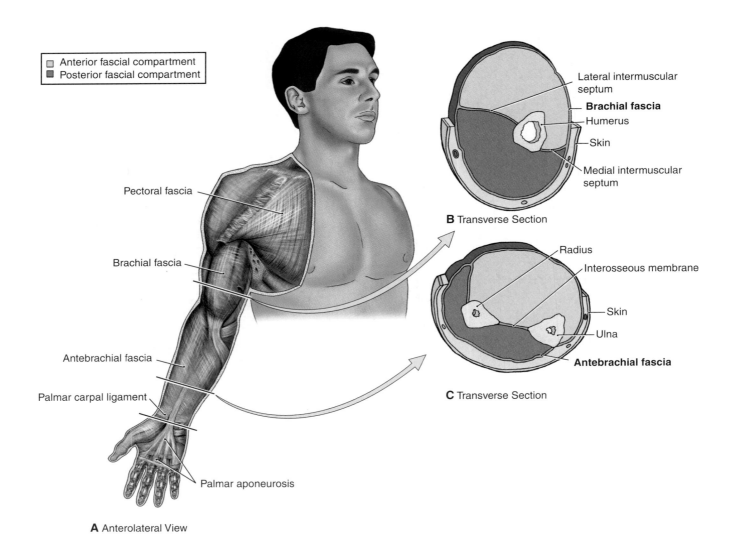

Pectoral fascia

Brachial fascia

Antebrachial fascia

Palmar carpal ligament

Palmar aponeurosis

A Anterolateral View

Lateral intermuscular septum

Brachial fascia

Humerus

Skin

Medial intermuscular septum

B Transverse Section

Radius

Interosseous membrane

Skin

Ulna

Antebrachial fascia

C Transverse Section

Figure 54.5 Orientation of T-oncoanatomy of the upper limb. A. Anterior view of investing fascia. **B.** Transverse through arm. **C.** Transverse through forearm.

TABLE 54.2	Imaging Modalities for Staging Soft Tissue Sarcomas	
Method	**Diagnosis and Staging Capability**	**Recommended for Use**
Primary (T) staging		
MRI	MRI provides optimal cross-sectional 3planar views of both axial and appendicular anatomy	Yes, superior for soft tissue extensions
CTe	CT preferably helical is complementary since it is superior in showing boney erosion and destruction by soft tissue sarcoma	Yes, advantage if bone is invaded
US	US may be of value in initial localizing of a mass or guiding needle biopsies of primary sites or nodes	No, not detailed
Nodal (N) Staging and Metastases (M) Staging		
PET	Using FDG as a total body scan, searching for disseminated disease	No, unless metastases are highly suspected

CTe, computed tomography enhanced with IV contrast; MRI, magnetic resonance imaging; PET, positron emission tomography; US, ultrasound.

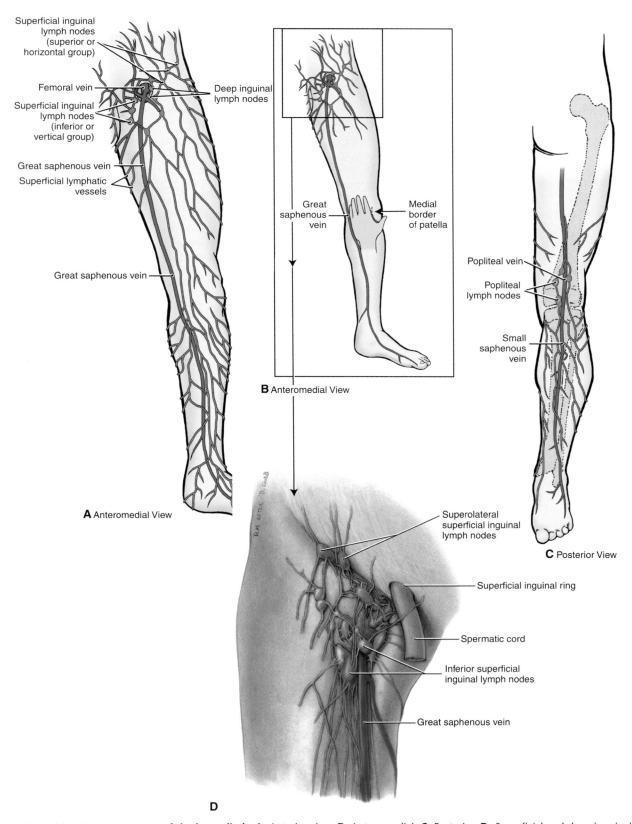

Figure 54.6 N-oncoanatomy of the lower limb. A. Anterior view. **B.** Anteromedial. **C.** Posterior. **D.** Superficial and deep inguinal nodes and superficial veins.

tissue (LCT; Fig. 54.3A) vividly illustrates the rich variety of cells and types of connective tissue fibers. LCT is constituted by the fibroblast, the fibrocyte, fat cells, mast cells, and macrophages in a rich matrix of extracellular materials as collagen bundles, reticular fibers, elastic fibers, along with abundant ground substance. This LCT constitutes the hypodermis and is the intermediate layer between the skin epidermis and dermis and the investing fascia, which is the initial tight wrapping around the musculature and neurovascular bundle and bone. *This investing fascia is the dense connective tissue, which has more collagen bundles packed together with fewer cells and less ground substance.* The "dense irregular connective tissue" defines the deep muscle compartment of limbs, the head and neck and trunk. The "dense regular connective tissue" constitutes the ligaments of muscles and joints. In dense connective tissue, fibroblasts and fibrocytes are the dominant cells.

The fusiform-shaped fibroblast synthesizes collagen fiber and ground substance. The fibrocyte is a resting cell and the adipose cells' presence or absence determines whether the connective tissue is loose or dense, respectively. Macrophages and histiocytes are numerous in LCTs, but are difficult to distinguish from fibrocytes unless they are phagocytic. It is for this reason that the malignant fibrous histiocytoma is the dominant soft tissue sarcoma. Most cells, plasma cells and lymphocytes permeate LCTs and occasional leukocytes owing to the rich network of capillaries and small vessels in the hypodermis. The collagen fibers are tough, thick proteinaceous bundles; the elastic fibers are fine, resilient, and when stretched return to their initial position; reticular fibers form delicate, netlike meshworks. Collagen is abundant in soft tissues, muscle compartments, and fascial layer tendons. Elastic fibers are abundant in blood vessels, especially arteries, lungs, urinary bladder, and Cooper's ligaments in breasts. They enable return to original shape after stretching. Reticular fibers are the network mesh in liver, lymph nodes, spleen, bone marrow, and generally in lymphatic and hematopoietic organs.

To complete the story of soft tissues, the largest bulk of soft tissue—muscle mass—needs to be presented. *There are three types of muscle tissues: skeletal, striated muscle, and to a lesser degree smooth, nonstriated muscle, and cardiac muscle (Fig. 54.3B).* Muscle cells are inactive mitotically, largely consisting of sarcoplasm, surrounded by sarcolemma membrane. Muscle contains numerous myofibrils which contain two types of contractile proteins, actin and myosin. Skeletal muscle fibers are multinucleated cells with cross-striations. *They tend to hypertrophy rather than undergo hyperplasia to increase muscle mass, which may account for the rarity of adult rhabdomyosarcoma.* In children, embryonal rhabdomyosarcoma is more common. The smooth muscle layer lines the wall of hollow viscera such as the digestive organ,

ureter, urinary bladder, and blood vessels. They tend to form benign leiomyomas more than leiomyosarcomas. Cardiac myocytes rarely give rise to any tumefaction and, in blood vessels, proliferation of myofibroblast cause restenosis rather than angiosarcomas, which account for <1% of all soft tissue sarcomas.

The last soft tissue element is nerve fibers of the peripheral nervous system, which consists of neurons, nerves, and axons. The peripheral nervous system is composed of various size axons, surrounded by layers of connective tissue that partition several nerve bundles (axons) into fascicles. The epineurium is the thicker outer layer whereas the perineurium is the thinner inner layer of nerve fibers. The supportive cell is the myelin forming neurolemmocyte (Schwann cells) and satellite cells surround the neuronal cells in paravertebral and peripheral ganglia. Neurofibrosarcoma are among the more common soft tissue malignancies and constitute 12% of soft tissue sarcomas.

Orientation of Three-planar Anatomy

The ubiquitous distribution of connective tissue and muscle presents a challenge to define this compartment anatomically. The major anatomic sectors are explored as functions of the frequency of soft tissue malignancies. The logical emphasis in oncoanatomy is on the limbs. The three-dimensional and three-planar oncoanatomies are presented for each site starting with the superficial investing fascia located deep to the skin in the hypodermis.

T-oncoanatomy

The upper and lower limbs are presented in this chapter because of the high frequency of soft tissue sarcomas in these locations. Because compartmental anatomy is the key concept, the axial or transverse planes of limbs are the focus of the primary site anatomy more than coronal or sagittal planes.

- *Lower limb* (Fig. 54.4A–D): The investing fascia is the superficial fascia. Soft tissue sarcomas arising in the LCT of the hypodermis above the investing fascia are considered superficial. The superficial fascia contains the muscle compartments that are divided by the deep fascia on the thigh, the fascia lata, and the leg crural fascia. The basic design of muscle compartments is related to limb motion: anterior (flexion), posterior (extension), medial (adduction), and lateral (abduction). All of the compartments are not present in all parts of the limb, being more common proximally than distally, where rotation becomes more important.
  1. A cross-section of the thigh identifies the superficial compartment in subcutaneous tissues as yellow and muscle compartments as beige to brown. The thigh is divided into a large anterior

compartment of the quadriceps, consisting of the vastus lateralis, medialis, intermedius, and the rectus femoris; a smaller posterior compartment of hamstring muscles; and a medial compartment that contains the neurovascular bundle.

2. The axial cross-section of the leg has the superficial hypodermis in yellow and again the muscle compartments in beige to brown. The posterior compartment predominates with the gastrocnemius muscle, and a smaller anterior and lateral compartment with the neurovascular bundle in its curvaceous descent twisting into a central position in the posterior compartment in the popliteal fossa. The deeper compartments are divided by the lateral intermuscular septum in the thigh and the interosseous membrane in the leg.

3. The neurovascular bundle first identified in the anterior thigh include from lateral to medial contains a femoral nerve, artery, vein, empty or fat, lymph nodes. NAVEL is a helpful acronym for physical examination: *n*erve, *a*rtery, *v*ein, *e*mpty or fat, *l*ymph nodes. Note that lymph nodes tend to be medial and anterior and are intimately placed with the vessels, especially veins.

- *Upper limb* (Fig. 54.5 A–C): The investing fascia is the superficial fascia and consists of the brachial fascia in the arm and the antebrachial fascia in the forearm. The brachial fascia is also the deep fascia of the arm and divides the muscle compartments into anterior (biceps) and posterior (triceps) compartments by its extensions, namely, the lateral and medial intermuscular septa. In the forearm, the antebrachial fascia is the superficial fascia and its extension in the interosseous membrane divides the anterior from the posterior compartments, which is the deep aspect of the staging system for soft tissue sarcoma.

- *Head and neck*: The superficial investing fascia is continuous superiorly and inferiorly with cranial and thoracic fascia. The superficial zone is the hypodermis. The deep zone refers to the concentric layers of fascia that encompass the anterior compartment particularly the neurovascular bundle of the carotid artery and internal jugular vein. The prevertebral fascia encompasses muscles of the posterior neck. Note that "NAVEL" is posterior to anterior; spinal cord, carotid artery, internal jugular vein, and cervical lymph nodes are medial and anterior.

- *Thoracic wall*: The superficial hypodermis overlies the deep compartment which consists of three musculomembranous layers: The external intercostals muscle and membrane, the innermost intercostals, and transversus thoracis muscle and membrane. The investing fascia is the external intercostal membrane overlying the internal intercostal muscle. Note in the axilla the NAVEL order of the brachial plexus, the axillary artery and vein with lymph nodes are mainly located anteriorly and medially beneath the pectoralis minor muscle.

- *Abdominal wall*: The investing fascia is the anterior layer of the rectum sheath. In the axial sections, the hypodermis and superficial fascia define the superficial zone of LCT and adipose tissue. The deep muscle compartment has a three muscle layer: External and internal obliques, the deepest transversus abdominis muscle—all fusing into their aponeurosis, which fuse into the anterior layer of the rectum sheath.

- *Back wall*: The thoracolumbar fascia is its posterior layer, which is the superficial investing fascia. The transverse section of the back has the various compartments: Superficial hypodermis, the posterior layer of the TLF that divides the deeper compartments—long muscles posterior to the vertebrae and the psoas muscle lateral to the spine.

- *Visceral sites* include the gastrointestinal, genitourinary, gynecologic, lung, and mediastinum. The smooth muscle layer gives rise to more benign leiomyomas than leiomyosarcomas.

- Neurovascular bundles are the sites for ganglioneuromas, neurofibrosarcomas, schwannomas, and malignant schwannomas.

N-oncoanatomy

N-oncoanatomy of the soft tissues beneath the skin surfaces emphasizes the anterior location for most if not all lymph node stations (Figs. 54.6 and 54.7).

- The axillary nodes are the recipient for lymphatics of the upper extremity and upper half body, including both anterior and posterior thoracic abdominal walls.

- The femoral and inguinal nodes drain the lower extremity and the lower half of the body on their anterior and posterior surfaces.

- The face and scalp drain into the superficial ring of nodes at the junction of the mandible and neck: Submental, submandibular, preauricular, mastoid, and occipital nodes. Once involved, the rest of the lymph nodes in the neck along the carotid arterial sheath and internal jugular vein are at risk.

M-oncoanatomy

There is a rich network of venous channels in the hypodermis of all skin surfaces that allows for hematogenous spread once the dermal and hypodermal layers are invaded by soft tissue sarcoma. Collateral venous channels and plexus are rich and rapidly appear once obstruction occurs (Fig. 54.8).

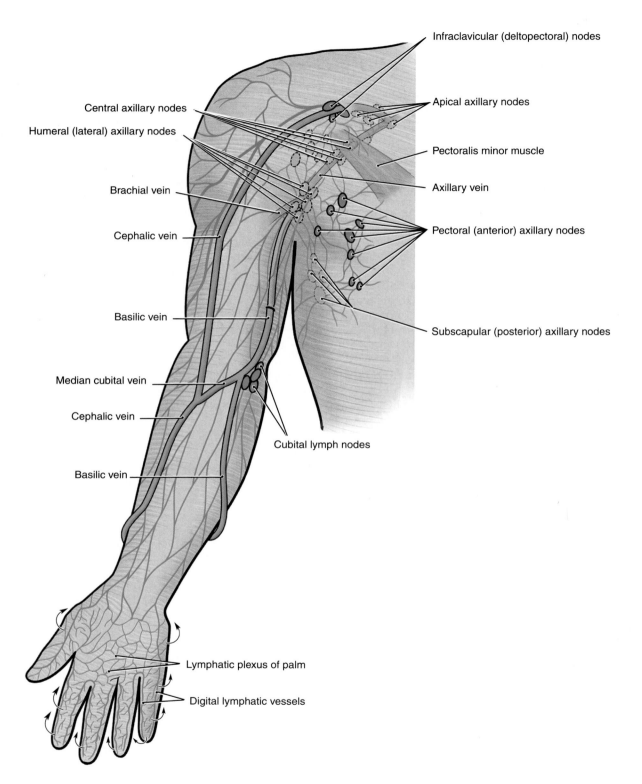

Anterior View

Figure 54.7 **N- and M-oncoanatomy of the upper limb.**

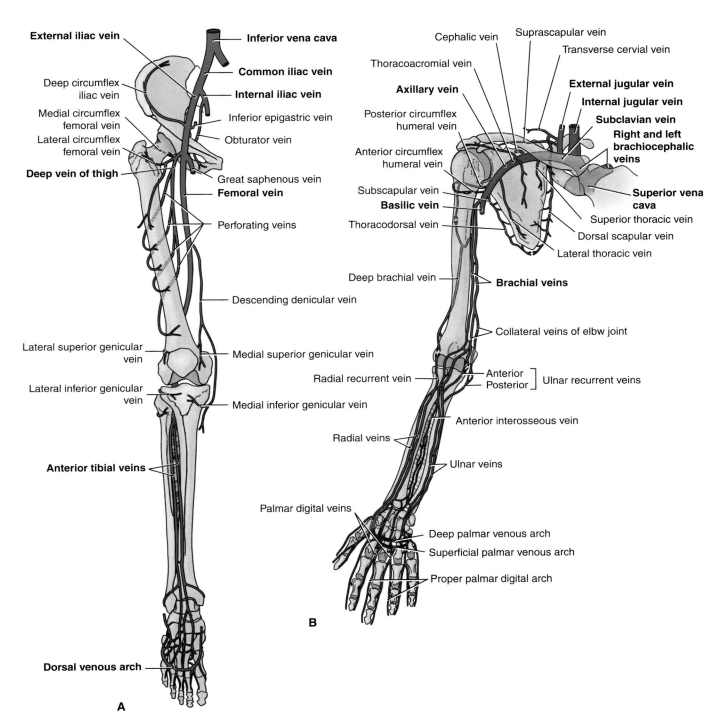

External iliac vein

Deep circumflex iliac vein

Medial circumflex femoral vein

Lateral circumflex femoral vein

Deep vein of thigh

Lateral superior genicular vein

Lateral inferior genicular vein

Anterior tibial veins

Dorsal venous arch

A

Inferior vena cava

Common iliac vein

Internal iliac vein

Inferior epigastric vein

Obturator vein

Great saphenous vein

Femoral vein

Perforating veins

Descending denicular vein

Medial superior genicular vein

Medial inferior genicular vein

Cephalic vein   Suprascapular vein

Transverse cervial vein

Thoracoacromial vein

Axillary vein

Posterior circumflex humeral vein

Anterior circumflex humeral vein

Subscapular vein

Basilic vein

Thoracodorsal vein

External jugular vein

Internal jugular vein

Subclavian vein

Right and left brachiocephalic veins

Superior vena cava

Superior thoracic vein

Dorsal scapular vein

Lateral thoracic vein

Deep brachial vein

Brachial veins

Collateral veins of elbw joint

Radial recurrent vein

Anterior
Posterior } Ulnar recurrent veins

Anterior interosseous vein

Radial veins

Ulnar veins

Palmar digital veins

Deep palmar venous arch

Superficial palmar venous arch

Proper palmar digital arch

B

Figure 54.8 **M-oncoanatomy of the limbs. A.** Lower. **B.** Upper venous.

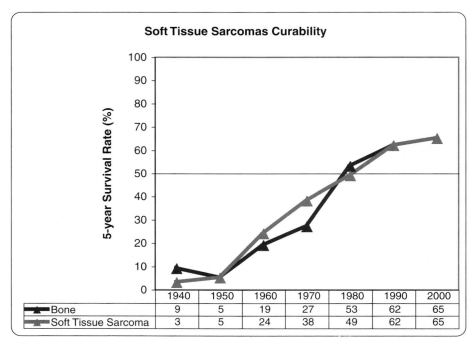

Figure 54.9 **Trajectory of soft tissue sarcoma curability.**

	1940	1950	1960	1970	1980	1990	2000
Bone	9	5	19	27	53	62	65
Soft Tissue Sarcoma	3	5	24	38	49	62	65

Rules of Classification and Staging

Clinical Staging and Imaging

Whenever feasible, physical examination in conjunction with imaging should establish size of the tumor: T1, <5 cm or T2, >5 cm. Modern cross-sectional imaging is essential and spiral computed tomography (CT) and magnetic resonance imaging (MRI) are of value and are complementary (Table 54.2).

Pathologic Staging

Pathologic staging is an essential aspect of staging; histopathologic grading is critical. Imaging is valuable for orientation of surgical margins (ink markings), particularly for conservation surgery with reliance on post-operative radiation to ablate any residuum of tumor. Immunohistochemical staining and cytogenetics may be helpful for subtyping tumors.

- *Accurate measurement of tumor size* is important because it is regarded as a continuous variable, with 5 cm as an arbitrary dividing line between T1 and T2.
- *Depth* is very important to staging; superficial is designated A and deep is designated B for each T category and stage. *Superficial* soft tissue sarcomas are in the hypodermis and do not involve the superficial investing fascia, which is the dividing line between the hypodermis and the deep muscle compartments. Note that all visceral soft tissue sarcoma are considered deep as are retroperitoneal or intraperitoneal soft tissue sarcomas.

- *Grade* is critical to stage and is referred to as low or high. Low refers to grades I and II. High refers to grades III and IV.
- *Recurrent* soft tissue sarcomas are restaged following the same rules as the primary soft tissue sarcoma.
- *Nodes* when enlarged need histopathologic confirmation because they are so uncommon.

Oncoimaging Annotations

- Ultrasonography cannot discriminate between benign and malignant soft tissue tumors and is not recommended for their classification.
- Ultrasonography is useful in guiding percutaneous biopsy and may be useful in answering specific concerns in posttreatment follow-up.
- CT tends not to add value to the workup of the primary soft tissue tumor site compared with MRI.
- MRI is the primary modality in the pretreatment assessment of these tumors. Surface coils are necessary, and axial images are required. The utility of gadolinium enhancement is controversial.
- Hemorrhage, hematoma, and inflammatory changes can be confused with tumor on MRI.
- MRI has disappointing accuracy in assigning benign or malignant tumor status and even less reliability in predicting histology in most cases.
- MRI is the dominant imaging modality for determining intracompartmental and extracompartmental

extent of an soft tissue sarcoma and its relationship to critical neurovascular structures.

- Sarcomas treated before limb salvage surgery with chemotherapy should be restaged with MRI before operation.
- The role of positron emission tomography in evaluating tumor response to neoadjuvant chemotherapy is still being explored.
- Systemic metastatic disease, usually to the lungs, and local recurrence have their maximum hazard rates within the first 2 years, defining the most frequent follow-up intervals for the first 2 years and tapering over a total of 5 years for osseous sarcomas.

Cancer Statistics and Survival

Soft tissue sarcomas account for 8,600 cases annually; bone sarcomas occurred in only 2,440 patients. Together, musculoskeletal tumors reached an incidence of 11,000 patients; <50% die. When compared with primary cancer sites, the current gains in survival over five decades dramatize the reversal of incurability of musculoskeletal sarcomas (<10%) in the 1940s and 1950s to its present 60% to 70% survival. This is a 700% increase in survival with limb preservation. The majority of these patients are pediatric and adolescent patients (Fig. 54.9).

Knowledge of the relationship of the bone growth, its polarity, and amplification, particularly the amplification at each physis growth plate, and the modeling process is essential to understanding the classification and behavior of bone tumors.

Perspective and Patterns of Spread

Primary malignant tumors of bone have been challenging for the multidisciplinary American Joint Committee on Cancer (AJCC)/International Union Against Cancer committees to develop a coherent classification and staging system. Although bone cancer is not common, it peaks in incidence in children, particularly in adolescence at the time of growth spurts. Because of therapeutic specter of amputation, there is an emotional aspect in the management of both the patient, most often pediatric, and her or his family. There are approximately 2,500 new malignant bone and joint tumors annually in the United States. Although a virtual death warrant for most children afflicted in the 1950s and 1960s, bone cancers have with the multidisciplinary approach become curable with limb preservation. Despite the high incidence in teenagers, bone malignancies are only 5% to 6% of pediatric tumors.

From the first edition of the AJCC staging manual, the focus has been on histopathologic typing and grade. The determination traditionally of the bone tumor type has allowed for bone imaging to be an intrinsic part of bone tumor pathology analysis. The relationship of the bone growth and the modeling process to the classification of bone tumors had been advocated by Lent Johnson of the AFIP (Fig. 55.1). The histopathologic types are tabulated in Table 55.1. Cytogenetic alterations and aberrations are being uncovered, but have not been formally included in staging. However, bone sarcoma grade as in soft tissue sarcomas plays an important part in staging and substaging. Clinical detection is usually stimulated by persistence of bone pain in the area of the lesion, often initially being attributed to trauma playing sports. Swelling and mass are signs of tumor progression, as are pathologic fractures. If the lesion is near a joint, unexplained sympathetic effusions and stiffness may be a presenting sign.

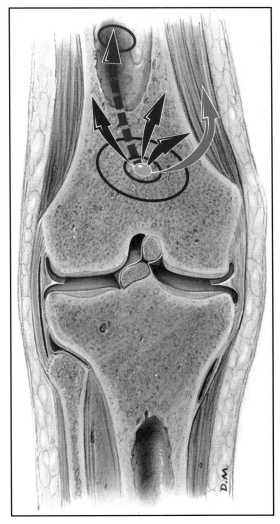

Figure 55.1 **Patterns of spread.** Bone and skeletal sarcomas spread in various bone compartments are color coded: T0, yellow; T1, green; T2, blue; T3, purple; and T4, red (into soft tissue).

DEFINITION OF TNM

STAGE GROUPINGS

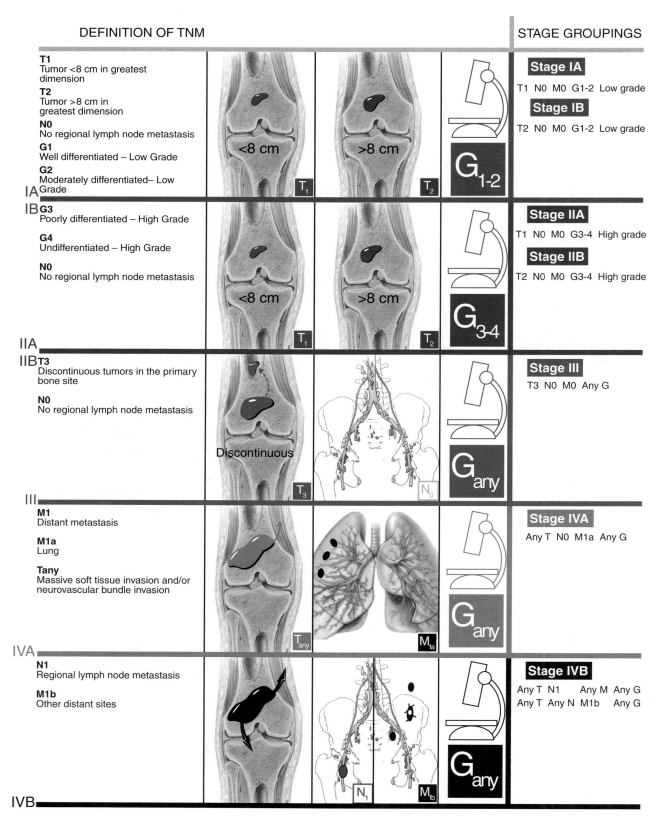

T1
Tumor <8 cm in greatest dimension

T2
Tumor >8 cm in greatest dimension

N0
No regional lymph node metastasis

G1
Well differentiated – Low Grade

G2
Moderately differentiated– Low Grade

IA

IB **G3**
Poorly differentiated – High Grade

G4
Undifferentiated – High Grade

N0
No regional lymph node metastasis

IIA

IIB **T3**
Discontinuous tumors in the primary bone site

N0
No regional lymph node metastasis

III

M1
Distant metastasis

M1a
Lung

Tany
Massive soft tissue invasion and/or neurovascular bundle invasion

IVA

N1
Regional lymph node metastasis

M1b
Other distant sites

IVB

Stage IA

T1 N0 M0 G1-2 Low grade

Stage IB

T2 N0 M0 G1-2 Low grade

Stage IIA

T1 N0 M0 G3-4 High grade

Stage IIB

T2 N0 M0 G3-4 High grade

Stage III

T3 N0 M0 Any G

Stage IVA

Any T N0 M1a Any G

Stage IVB

Any T N1   Any M Any G
Any T Any N M1b   Any G

Figure 55.2 TNM stage criteria are color-coded bars and note the importance of tumor grade in addition to anatomic extent.
Bone sarcomas are characterized by early invasion of bone marrow sinuses in cancellous bone with rapid dissemination hematogenously to lung. Early detection of M1 lung nodules can be resected with long term survival. Note lymph node metastasis (N1) carries a poorer prognosis and worse stage than lung metastasis (M1). Stage I, green; II, blue; III, purple; IV, red; and metastatic, black.

TABLE 55.1	Histopathologic Types of Bone Tumors

I. Osteosarcoma
  A. Intramedullary high grade
    1. Osteoblastic
    2. Chondroblastic
    3. Fibroblastic
    4. Mixed
    5. Small cell
    6. Other (telangiectactic, epithelioid, chondromyxoid fibroma-like,
       chodroblastoma-like, osteoblastoma-like, giant cell rich)
  B. Intramedullary low grade
  C. Juxtacortical high grade (high-grade surface osteosarcoma)
  D. Juxtacortical intermediate grade chondroblastic (periosteal osteosarcoma)
  E. Juxtacortical low grade (parosteal osteosarcoma)

II. Chondrosarcoma
  A. Intramedullary
    1. Conventional (hyaline/myxoid)
    2. Clear cell
    3. Dedifferentiated
    4. Mesenchymal
  B. Juxtacortical

III. Primitive neuroectodermal tumor/Ewing sarcoma

IV. Angiosarcoma
  A. Conventional
  B. Epithelioid hemangioendothelioma

V. Fibrosarcoma/malignant fibrous histiocytoma

VI. Chordoma
  A. Conventional
  B. Dedifferentiated

VII. Adamantinoma
  A. Conventional
  B. Well-differentiated osteofibrous dysplasia like

VIII. Other
  A. Liposarcoma
  B. Leiomyosarcoma
  C. Malignant peripheral nerve sheath tumor
  D. Rhabdomyosarcoma
  E. Malignant mesenchymoma
  F. Malignant hemangiopericytoma
  G. Sarcoma, NOS; primary malignant lymphoma; and multiple myeloma are
     not included

NOS, not otherwise specified.
Reprinted from Greene FL, Page DL, Fleming ID, et al., eds. *AJCC Cancer Staging Manual.* 6th ed. New York: Springer; 2002:188.

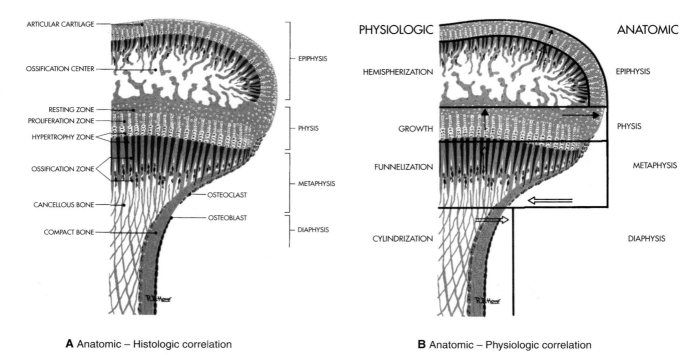

A Anatomic – Histologic correlation

B Anatomic – Physiologic correlation

Figure 55.3 **Overview of oncoanatomy. A.** Anatomic–histologic correlation of the end of a growing long bone: Epiphysis, physis, metaphysis, and diaphysis. **B.** Bone modeling at same end of a growing long bone.

The initial staging criteria were influenced by tumor location and whether the osseous mass on film was confined to bone, within its cortex, or extended beyond the cortex. Tumefaction size has recently been added. Location in epiphysis, physis, metaphysis, or diaphysis is noteworthy. Patterns of spread were within bone or beyond into soft tissues. The major concern is whether the neurovascular bundle is compromised in the lower extremity as the femoral artery wraps around the femoral shaft. Sites of rapid growth, such as the distal end of the femur and the proximal end of the tibia, are common sites of malignancies (Fig. 55.2).

TNM Staging Criteria

The staging criteria have remained simple with a major recent modification in the sixth edition of the AJCC manual. T1 changed from confined within cortex and T2 beyond the cortex to tumors that are T1 (<8 cm) and T2 (>8 cm). T3 was added as a discontinuous primary tumor, that is, two separate anatomic sites in the same bone as metaphysis and diaphysis of the shaft. Stage III, previously undefined, is currently T3. Curiously, MIa lung metastases are regarded as more favorable than regional nodes N1, translating into stages IVA and IVB, respectively. Pathologic grade impacts the TNM anatomic stage, depending on whether the tumor grade is I or II (low grade) or III or IV (high grade). The substage desig-

nation of A or B depends on low or high grade, respectively, for stages I and II (Fig. 55.2).

Summary of Changes

- *T1 has changed from "Tumor confined within the cortex" to "Tumor 8 cm or less in greatest dimension."*
- *T2 has changed from "Tumor invades beyond the cortex" to "Tumor more than 8 cm in greatest dimension."*
- *T3 designation of skip metastasis is defined as "Discontinuous tumors in the primary bone site." This designation is a stage III tumor that was not previously defined.*
- *M1 lesions have been divided into M1a and M1b.*
- *M1a is lung-only metastases.*
- *M1b is metastases to other distant sites, including lymph nodes.*
- *In the stage grouping, stage IVA is M1a, and stage IVB is M1b.*

Overview of Oncoanatomy

There is a logic to bone growth and modeling that can be applied to the classification of bone tumors. Skeletal growth is the critical factor in determining the probably location of the bone tumor. Borrowing from the concepts that were developed from research of the *Dynamic Classification of Bone Dysplasias*, the anatomy of bone and

CLINICAL MODELING

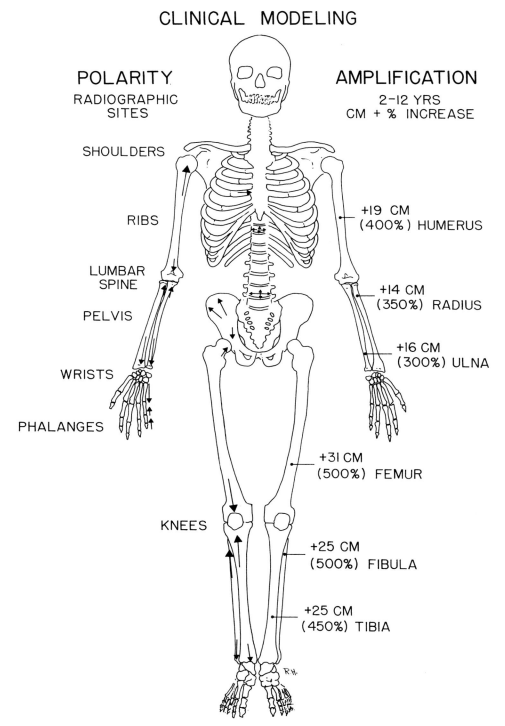

POLARITY
RADIOGRAPHIC
SITES

AMPLIFICATION
2–12 YRS
CM + % INCREASE

SHOULDERS

+19 CM
(400%) HUMERUS

RIBS

LUMBAR
SPINE

+14 CM
(350%) RADIUS

PELVIS

+16 CM
(300%) ULNA

WRISTS

PHALANGES

+31 CM
(500%) FEMUR

KNEES

+25 CM
(500%) FIBULA

+25 CM
(450%) TIBIA

Figure 55.4 Polarity and amplification of skeletal growth and modeling.

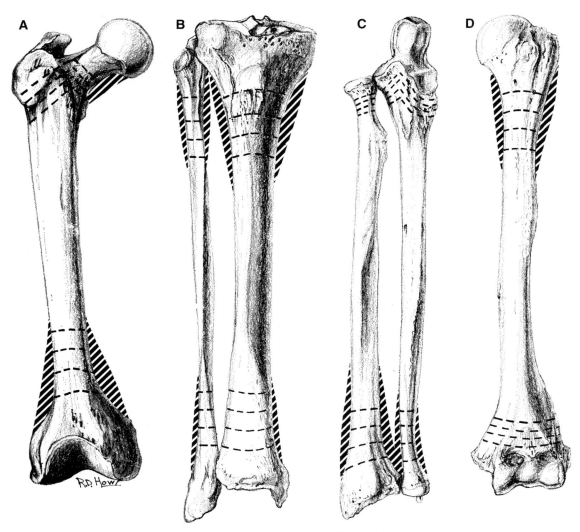

Figure 55.5 Bone modeling as a dynamic process. A. Femur. **B.** Tibia and fibula. **C.** Radius and ulna. **D.** Humerus. Striated black/white areas are reabsorbed by osteoclasts. Dash lines indicate growth by apposition. Bone cancers arise in sites of more active growth and modeling.

TABLE 55.2	Imaging Modalities for Staging Bone Cancer	
Method	**Diagnosis and Staging Capability**	**Recommended for Use**
Primary (T) staging		
MRI	MRI provides optimal cross-sectional three-planar views of both axial and appendicular anatomy	Yes, superior for soft tissue extensions and neurovascular invasion
CTe	CT (preferably helical) is complementary; it is superior in showing boney erosion and destruction by osseous sarcoma	Yes, advantage if bone is invaded
US	US may be of value in initial localizing of a mass or guiding needle biopsies of primary sites or nodes	No, not detailed
Nodal (N) and metastases (M) staging		
PET	Using FDG as a total body scan, searching for disseminated disease	No, unless metastases are highly suspected

CTe, computed tomography enhanced with IV contrast; FDG, fluorodeoxyglucose; MRI, magnetic resonance imaging; PET, positron emission tomography; US, ultrasound.

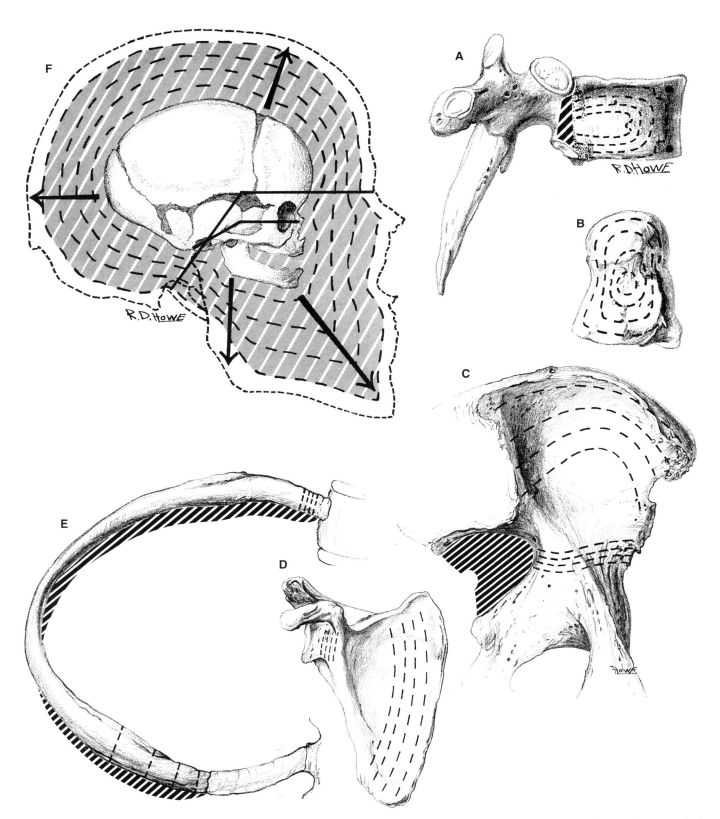

Figure 55.6 **Modeling in bones. A.** Vertebra. **B.** Carpal. **C.** Pelvis. **D.** Scapula. **E.** Rib. **F.** Skull. Striated black/white is resorbtion of bone. Dashed line indicates bone opposition.

proposed terminology are presented to provide a broader basis for *understanding the modeling and remodeling process of bone shaping in skeletal growth. Anatomic physiologic correlation is shown histologically with the vectors of bone growth and modeling in an idealized growing end of bone (Fig. 55.3A; see also Fig. 55.7).*

- *Epiphyseal segment or epiphysis*: The epiphysis grows in the form of a hemisphere from the subarticular cartilage zone; thus the term hemispherization is proffered. It is recognized that the ultimate shape of any epiphysis is rarely a true hemisphere, but nevertheless the term allows us to visualize its growth pattern.
- *Physeal segment or growth plate*: By cellular division, the cartilage disk increases its length interstitially and increases in diameter by apposition. Thus, the normal tendency is toward expansion in this segment. The simplest and most appropriate term for this segment is growth.
- *Metaphyseal segment*: The normal tendency in this zone is toward a reduction in shaft caliber by internal and external absorption. The term "constriction" is deeply entrenched in the literature, but is not descriptively accurate. The vascular erosion and osteoclastic absorption are not constrictive, but reductive in caliber. If one were to select a new term for these processes, "funnelization," borrowed from Leblond, would be preferred. It preserves the image of these absorptive activities at the ends of the shaft, which allow for progressive narrowing of caliber and the resultant concave-curve shape of the metaphysis as one passes from the end toward the middle of the shaft (Fig. 55.3B; see also Fig. 55.7).
- *Diaphyseal segment*: There is a tendency in the middle of the shaft to maintain a certain structural balance between the flaring, growing ends. To maintain this balance, the diameter of the diaphysis increases in width as the tubular bone grows in length. Proliferation of osteoblasts on the periosteal surface exceeds osteoclastic endosteal absorption, in that the cortex thickens and the marrow cavity widens as the tubular bone matures.

Although the term "tubulation" seemed appropriate in that the cortical shaft may be compared to a hollow tube, it is not exact; the spongiosa and trabeculation of the marrow space can hardly be compared to a void. The term "cylindrization," once again borrowed from Leblond, seems ideal. The vectors of diaphyseal growth are such as to ensure a cylindrical shape to the shaft. The concept of the periosteum acting as a shaping force to narrow diaphyseal caliber has no functional basis. Similarly, a lax periosteum does not lead to widening of the shaft.

- *Hemispherization*: Growth in the epiphysis at first extends in all directions, but for most of its development the epiphysis grows as a hemisphere from the subarticular zone.
- *Growth*: The zone of resting cartilage grows by apposition, increasing the transverse diameter at the shaft.
- *Funnelization*: The metaphysis is shaped like a funnel, the shape being due to active bone resorption by osteoclasis which results in a progressive reduction in shaft caliber.
- *Cylindrization*: The shaft of the bone increases in diameter by thickening of the cortex and expansion of the marrow by appositional periosteal growth.

Orientation of Oncoanatomy

To more fully *understand normal skeletal growth, there are three basic considerations: (i) Amplification or actual increases in size of bone, (ii) polarity or direction of growth, and (iii) time or scale of measurement (Fig. 55.4).*

- *Amplification* is the concept that the bone showing the greatest growth potential shows the greatest change, because it magnifies the same defect to a greater degree.
- *Polarity* is the concept that tubular bones grow in a differential pattern, with one end predominating over the other. The maximal direction of longitudinal growth is its polarity.
- *Time*: With regard to bone tumors, the expression of oncogenes overexpression or deletion is at the maximal growth, which is in the first 5 to 6 years of life, when skeletal growth is persistent, then slows over the next 5 to 6 years. With puberty, there is a maximal growth spurt over the next 5 to 6 years. Malignancy in bone appears at those sites that grow the most, namely, the distal femur and proximal tibia and proximal humeri in adolescence.

Traditionally, in classifying skeletal bone anatomy the orientation is regional. There are eight regions—head, neck, thorax, abdomen, back, pelvis, and upper and lower extremities.

- *Head*: Skull, facial bones, and mandible
- *Neck*: Cervical vertebrae (C1–C7), hyoid bone, and clavicle
- *Thorax*: Ribs, thoracic vertebrae (T1–T12), sternum manubrium, and pectoral girdle
- *Abdomen*: Lumbar vertebrae (L1–L5) and pelvic girdle (false pelvis)
- *Back*: Vertebrae composing the spine—cervical (C4–C7), thoracic (T1–T12), lumbar (L1–L5), and sacral (S5–S1)
- *Pelvis*: Sacrum (S1–S5), coccyx, and true pelvis
- *Upper limb*: Pectoral girdle, arm, forearm, and hand
- *Lower limb*: Pelvic girdle, thigh, leg, and foot

Bone typing (Figs. 55.5A–D and 55.6A–F) is based on size, shape, and modeling, and provides an insight as to normal growth, which is a dynamic balance between appositional growth of endochondral bone and the resorption and regeneration of intramembranous bone. Each bone grows and models differently. Tumefactions are the sites of most active growth and resorption activities. The five types of bone shapes are long, short, irregular, flat, and special bones.

- *Long*: Upper—humerus, radius, ulna
      Lower—femur, tibia, fibula
- *Short*: Metacarpal, metatarsal, and phalanges
- *Irregular*: Vertebrae
- *Flat*: Ribs, scapula, and pelvis
- *Special*: Skull, face, and mandible

T-oncoanatomy

The skeletal anatomic sites can be divided into five basic bone types for the purposes of presentation. Each site is presented diagrammatically to indicate sites of maximal bone growth and modeling as a correlate as to the most likely sites for bone tumors.

Femur   The femur (Fig. 55.5A) is the longest bone and, as expected, grows more in actual length from birth to age 12 years than any other bone in the body. By measurement, approximately 75% of its length is achieved at the distal growth plate. Appositional growth is greatest here and, because it is the widest growth plate, it is logically the site for tumefaction and for studying modeling errors. The proximal growth plate of the femur adds the other 25% to the shaft length, with growth occurring mainly from the cartilage disk juxtaposed to the femoral head.

Tibia   The tibia (Fig. 55.5B) grows with even polarity at both ends, with a slight margin favoring the proximal growth plate. The appositional growth is slightly greater at the knee (60%), but not so great as in the femur. In the lateral projection, most of the growth is in the anterior direction at the knee region rather than posteriorly as in the femur.

Radius and Ulna   Most of the growth is at the wrist with very modest activity at the elbow (Fig. 55.5C).

Humerus   Virtually all the appositional growth is proximal in the humeral neck (Fig. 55.5D). The distal elbow end has only modest growth. Humeral growth exceeds the radius and ulna.

Short Tubular Bones   Practically all short tubular bones are characterized by unipolarity of growth. That is, each bone usually has only one growth plate, and appositional and vertical growth take place at one end of the bone or the other. Consequently, errors in bone modeling are very much skewed. Primary tumors of short bone

are, as expected, extremely rare. The only exception to this rule is the first metacarpal.

Flat Bone

- A flat bone (e.g., the pelvis; Fig. 55.6C) can be thought of similar to tubular bones with differential growth patterns. The iliac crest has a curved apophyseal growth plate (nonarticulating) and increases in its length by interstitial growth at right angles to the apophysis. Appositional growth adds to its perimeter. Thus, 74% of its vertical length occurs at the crest. The distal growth plate located at the acetabulum is in juxtaposition to the articular cartilage of the joint and the synchondrosis between the iliac and pubic bones. The periosteal intramembranous growth in the pelvis reveals the eccentric modeling of these bones. Bone is also apposed laterally and absorbed medially, widening the sacrosciatic notch into a graceful curve.

Cuboid Bones   The vertebrae (Fig. 55.6A) at birth consist of three ossification centers, one in the body and two nuclei in the neural arch, one in each pedicle. Once again, comparing the vertebral body to a tubular bone, growth in length occurs exclusively from the proliferating cartilage plates at the cephalad and caudal surfaces. Vertebral bodies grow as a series of congruous rectangles in the first years and growth is much greater along the anterior and lateral borders than posteriorly. The amount of growth in height and width is comparable, and funnelization processes as recognized in the long bones are nil. Growth in width is a function of periosteal or intramembranous bone formation as it is in long bones.

Carpal Bone   Carpal bone (Fig. 55.6B) is organized as an ossification center.

Scapula   Scapula (Fig. 55.6D) is most active on its free margin.

Ribs   Ribs (Fig. 55.6E) are modeled more posteriorly than anteriorly.

Skull   Skull (Fig. 55.6F) grows by endochondral bone at its base and intramembraneous in its vault.

N-oncoanatomy

Bone and bone marrow are richly supplied with blood and lymphatics are intimately related to regional veins that also drain surrounding soft tissue, which so often are invaded owing to penetration of cortex. Only the major regional nodes are presented (see Fig. 52.4).

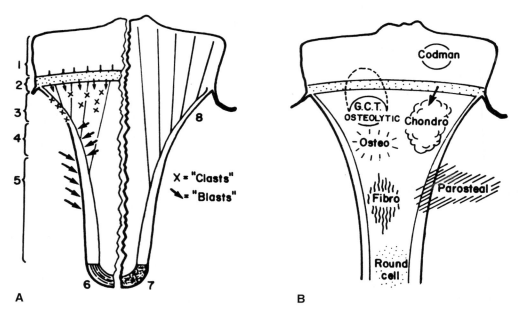

Figure 55.7 **The relationship of modeling processes to bone tumors.**

- *Femoral nodes*: Lower limb and lower half of the truncal skeleton
- *Axillary*: Upper limb and upper half of the truncal skeleton
- *Neck nodes*: Skull and facial bones

M-oncoanatomy

The venous drainage surrounding the skeletal anatomy is a rich network and accounts for both skip lesions in the same bone and the propensity of bone tumors to metastasize to other bones. The rich axial intervertebral venous network readily explains why once one vertebra is involved, others are at risk.

Rules of Classification and Staging

Clinical Staging and Imaging

Clinical staging and imaging includes physical examination, modern cross-sectional imaging, and image-guided biopsies (Fig. 55.7; Table 55.2; see also Fig. 55.3). Standard bone radiographs identify the osseous malignancy, but need to be supplemented with magnetic resonance imaging (MRI) and enhanced computed tomography (CT). MRI is superior for soft tissue and bone marrow invasion and enhanced CT for bone cortex erosion. Tumor size is estimated for staging: <8 cm or >8 cm. The entire skeleton deserves to be overviewed for metastases using ^{99m}Tc colloid. Chest CT is essential for surveying lungs for pulmonary metastases.

Image-guided biopsy is essential, but a note of caution is warranted. The biopsy site needs to be carefully planned to allow for eventual en bloc resection of the entire biopsy tract with excision of the malignant bone tumor.

Pathologic Staging

Pathologic staging incorporates the clinical findings, the complete imaging file, and the completely resected specimen. Histopathologic analyses for sarcoma grade impacts cancer staging more than tumor type. Resected regional lymph nodes need to be included. Suspicious metastatic lesions in long or other bone should be needled and confirmed by histopathology.

Oncoimaging Annotations

- MRI is the dominant imaging modality for determining intracompartmental and extracompartmental extent of an intraosseous tumor and its relationship to critical neurovascular structures.
- The routine radiograph remains the most reliable predictor of the histologic nature of a bone lesion.
- Metastases account for 65% of all malignant bone tumors in adults.
- All suspected sarcomas of bone should be staged with MRI before rather than after biopsy. As a consequence of post-biopsy edema and hemorrhage, MRI often overestimates the size and extent of tumor.
- With osteosarcoma and Ewing sarcoma, which are known to produce skip lesions, it is important to examine the entire long bone with MRI.
- Systemic metastatic disease, usually to the lungs, and local recurrence have their maximum hazard rates

within the first 2 years, defining the most frequent follow-up intervals for the first 2 years and tapering over a total of 5 years for osseous sarcomas.

Cancer Statistics and Survival

Soft tissue sarcomas account for 8,600 cases annually, whereas bone sarcomas occurred in only 2,440 pa-tients. Together, musculoskeletal tumors reached an incidence of 11,000 patients; <50% will die. When compared with primary cancer sites, the current gains in survival over five decades dramatize the reversal of incurability of musculoskeletal sarcomas (<10%) in the 1940s and 1950s to its 60% to 70% survival. This is 700% increase in survival with limb preservation (see Fig. 54.9).

56

Lymphoid Neoplasms: Hodgkin Lymphoma and Non-Hodgkin Lymphoma

The lymphoid neoplasms include an ever-increasing spectrum of disorders defined by a combination of morphology, immunophenotype and genetic features.

Perspective and Patterns of Spread

The first case described by Thomas Hodgkin, entitled "On some morbid appearances of the absorbent glands and spleen," dramatically demonstrates the concept of contiguous spread of this lymphoid disorder (Fig. 56.1). This concept of "contiguous spread" was promulgated by Kaplan, who argued for a unicentric origin, along with other pioneer radiation oncologists who advocated for prophylactically treating the uninvolved contiguous nodal regions. *Hodgkin lymphoma (HL), which usually starts in a cervical lymph node, is believed to spread in an orderly fashion. Each contiguous nodal area is believed to be the next most likely site to be involved.*

Each node, depending on its location, would involve the juxtaposed neighboring site (Fig. 56.2). Three illustrations of cervical node involvement portray advancing stages: stage I, high cervical node (Fig. 56.2A); stage II, cervical node with mediastinal mass (Fig. 56.2B); and stage III, supraclavicular node with para-aortic node spread via thoracic duct (Fig. 56.2C). For the clinician, the patterns of spread of HL highlight the regional node-bearing areas, and emphasize the need to know the location of the lymph nodes. HL can originate in any one of the different lymph node regions in the body and spread through adjacent normal lymphatic pathways. The more likely contiguous site of involvement is the one that is "upstream," because lymph flows in prograde and centrifugal fashion from the peripheral limbs to the central core. Lymphatic trunks gather the lymph and allow flow from different viscera and anatomic sites in to lymph nodes. *Once obstruction occurs, retrograde flow takes place in lymphatics and contiguous sites may be the "downstream" lymph nodes.*

Anatomic Staging System

In 1971, the Ann Arbor staging system was introduced and with minor modification in Cotswold, England, was internationally adopted in the earliest joint editions of American Joint Committee on Cancer/International Union Against Cancer (Fig. 56.3). This classification has remained stable with minor modifications and is applicable to both HL and non-Hodgkin lymphoma (NHL). *Most classifications rate an extranodal site as "localized" which deserves an "E" designation as part of the staging process.* Briefly, stage I is one node-bearing region (Fig. 56.3A), stage II is two or more node-bearing regions on one side of the diaphragm (Fig. 56.3B), stage III is node-bearing region on both sides of the diaphragm (Fig. 56.3C), and stage IV is dissemination to extranodal visceral sites (Fig. 56.3D). This anatomic classification was based on two new definitions: (1) a node-bearing region and (2) extranodal site of involvement.

- *Node-bearing regions:* There are six major and five minor regions, but they do not have a foundation anatomically and have been assigned by consensus.
- The *diaphragm* is a critical landmark in the staging process and supradiaphragmatic presentations carry a better prognosis than infradiaphragmatic. The diaphragm again is an anatomic but not a physiologic divide of the lymphoid system.
- *Extranodal sites* include Waldeyer's ring of pharyngeal lymphoid tissue, the spleen, Peyer's patches in the intestine and bone. In immunosuppressed patients, when visceral sites are involved, such as brain, liver, lung, or bone marrow, these are considered to be disseminated sites similar to metastases.

For lymphomas, the TNM system could be visualized (similar to cancer) if "extranodal (E) sites" were the origin of the malignant lymphoid process, then spreading to regional nodes. However, this parallel is not a common occurrence. Noncontiguous spread, which is less predictable and less orderly, occurs in non-Hodgkin lymphoma (NHL). The malignant lymphocyte is like the normal lymphocyte; it tends to enter the general circulation, but homes back to lymphoid tissue and accounts for the random general spread pattern of lymphomas. The normal cellular migration streams have been diagrammed by Yoffey and are referred to as "the fourth circulation." The therapeutic and diagnostic implications in treating lymphomas require a thorough evaluation of all lymphoid sites.

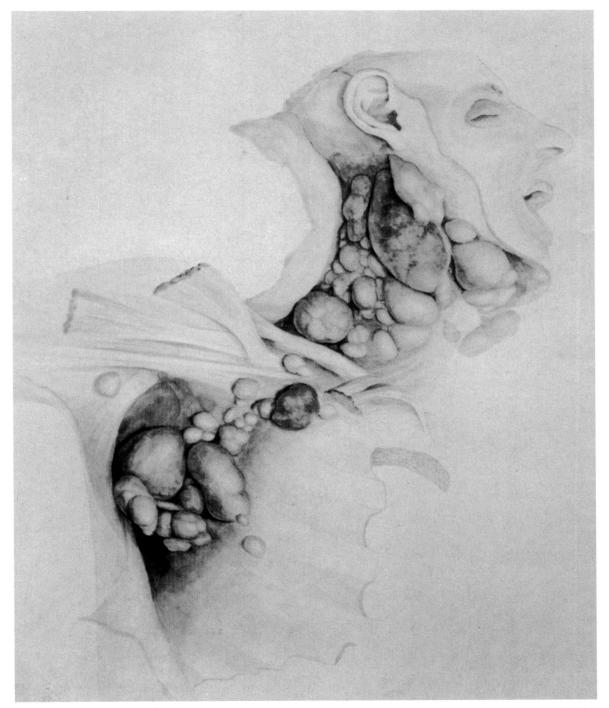

Figure 56.1 **Water color painting by Robert Carswell (1793–1857) of a patient seen by him at postmortem examination in 1828; this case was seventh described in Hodgkin's paper.** Carswell's five magnificent water color paintings are the property of University College Medical School, University of London, and were rediscovered by Dr Peter J. Dawson, who published three of them in an article in the *Archives of Internal Medicine* (1968;121:288–290). (Permission to reproduce Dawson's Figure 1 was given by the Dean of University College Hospital Medical School, by Dr. Dawson, and by the editor of the *Journal of the American Medical Association* and affiliated publications.)

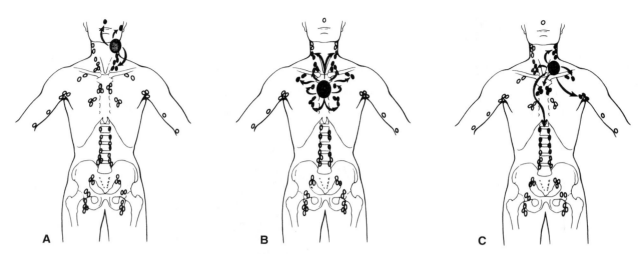

Figure 56.2 Patterns of spread in HL is due to contiguous involvement of adjacent node-bearing regions. A. High cervical node could retrograde to involve parotid lymph node or Waldeyer's Ring or prograde to supraclavicular area. **B.** Mediastinal lymph nodes could spread to supraclavicular, infraclavicular or cervical lymph nodes or involve hilar nodes as a gateway to pulmonary infiltration. **C.** Supraclavicular node retrograde spread to epigastric and celiac para-aortic lymph nodes, as well as ipsilateral axillary, cervical nodes, and contralateral supraclavicular nodes.

TABLE 56.1	WHO Classification of Lymphoid Neoplasms—REAL

B-cell Neoplasms

Precursor B-cell neoplasm
  Precursor B-lymphoblastic leukemia/lymphoma (precursor B-cell acute lymphoblastic leukemia

Mature (peripheral) B-cell neoplasms
  B-cell chronic lymphocytic leukemia/small lymphocytic lymphoma
  B-cell prolymphocytic leukemia
  Lymphoplasmacytic lymphoma
  Splenic marginal zone B-cell lymphoma of MALT type
  Nodal marginal zone B-cell lymphoma (with or without monocytoid B cells)
  Follicular lymphoma
  Mantle cell lymphoma
  Diffuse large B-cell lymphoma
  Burkitt lymphoma/Burkitt cell leukemia

T-cell and NK-cell Neoplasms

Precursor T-cell neoplasm
  Precursor T-lymphoblastic lymphoma/leukemia (precursor T-cell acute lymphoblastic leukemia)

Mature (peripheral) T/NK-cell neoplasms
  T-cell prolymphocytic leukemia
  T-cell granular lymphocytic leukemia
  Aggressive NK-cell leukemia
  Adult T-cell lymphoma/leukemia (HTLV1+)
  Extranodal NK-/T-cell lymphoma, nasal type
  Enteropathy-type T-cell lymphoma
  Hepatosplenic $\gamma\delta$ T-cell lymphoma
  Subcutaneous panniculitislike T-cell lymphoma
  Mycosis fungoides/Sezary syndrome
  Anaplastic large cell lymphoma, T-/null-cell, primary cutaneous type
  Peripheral T-cell lymphoma, not otherwise characterized
  Angioimmunoblastic T-cell lymphoma
  Anaplastic large cell lymphoma, T-/-null cell, primary systemic type

NK, natural killer; REAL, Revised European American Classification of Lymphoid Neoplasms.
Used with permission from Greene FL, Page DL, Fleming ID, et al., eds. *AJCC Cancer Staging Manual.* 6th ed. New York: Springer; 2002:394.

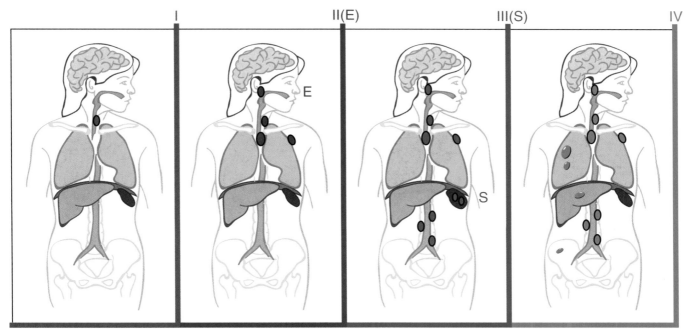

Figure 56.3 **TNM anatomic staging.** Bars are color coded: Stage I, green; II, blue; III, purple; and IV, red.

The lymphocyte is a highly mobile cell both when healthy and diseased. It can enter rapidly into the general circulation in the lymph nodes, which have rich beds of postcapillary venules, or move in a more orderly fashion from one nodal station to the next through lymphatic channels, eventually returning to the blood via the thoracic duct. Patterns of spread in lymphomas and HL are as follows.

1. An early phase involves only lymphoid tissue and lymph nodes.
2. In HL, the spread is more predictable using lymphatic channels between contiguous sites.
3. In lymphomas, the spread is random, confined to nodal and extranodal lymphoid tissues and organs.
4. The involvement of virtually all lymphoid tissues.
5. Dissemination via hematogenous channels often is a late event and transformation of lymphoma into a leukemic phase can be the terminal event.

Some clarification regarding extranodal sites:

- Spleen involvement is established if there is splenomegaly along with imaging of multiple focal defects.
- Liver involvement is due to hepatomegaly with multiple focal defects.
- Lung and bone involvement can be found as single infiltrates or multiple lesions. Both can be considered extranodal sites (E) if contiguous to a node. They need to be the only anatomic site involved to be considered focal (E)xtranodal sites. If both or more sites are involved, the patient is stage IV.

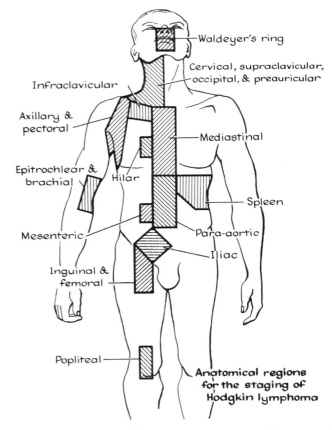

Figure 56.4 **Lymph node-bearing regions.** Diagram of the anatomic definition of separate lymph node regions adopted for staging purposes at the Rye (1965) symposium on Hodgkin's Lymphoma (HL).

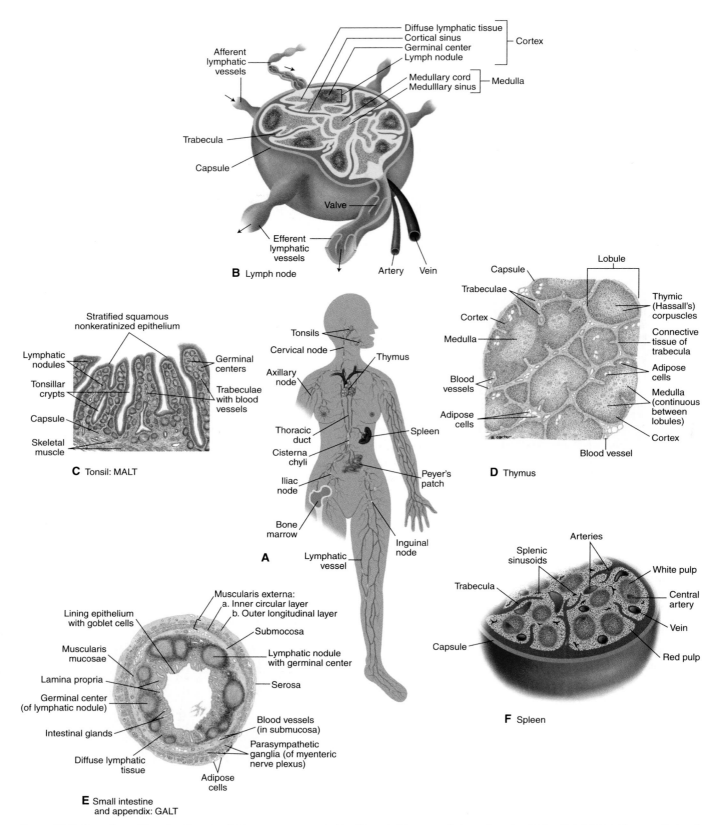

B Lymph node

- Afferent lymphatic vessels
- Diffuse lymphatic tissue
- Cortical sinus
- Germinal center
- Lymph nodule
- Cortex
- Medullary cord
- Medulllary sinus
- Medulla
- Trabecula
- Capsule
- Valve
- Efferent lymphatic vessels
- Artery
- Vein

C Tonsil: MALT

- Stratified squamous nonkeratinized epithelium
- Lymphatic nodules
- Tonsillar crypts
- Capsule
- Skeletal muscle
- Germinal centers
- Trabeculae with blood vessels

A

- Tonsils
- Cervical node
- Axillary node
- Thoracic duct
- Cisterna chyli
- Iliac node
- Bone marrow
- Lymphatic vessel
- Thymus
- Spleen
- Peyer's patch
- Inguinal node

D Thymus

- Capsule
- Trabeculae
- Cortex
- Medulla
- Blood vessels
- Adipose cells
- Lobule
- Thymic (Hassall's) corpuscles
- Connective tissue of trabecula
- Adipose cells
- Medulla (continuous between lobules)
- Cortex
- Blood vessel

E Small intestine and appendix: GALT

- Lining epithelium with goblet cells
- Muscularis mucosae
- Lamina propria
- Germinal center (of lymphatic nodule)
- Intestinal glands
- Diffuse lymphatic tissue
- Muscularis externa:
  a. Inner circular layer
  b. Outer longitudinal layer
- Submocosa
- Lymphatic nodule with germinal center
- Serosa
- Blood vessels (in submucosa)
- Parasympathetic ganglia (of myenteric nerve plexus)
- Adipose cells

F Spleen

- Splenic sinusoids
- Trabecula
- Capsule
- Arteries
- White pulp
- Central artery
- Vein
- Red pulp

Figure 56.5 Overview of lymphoid system's N-oncoanatomy. A. Total lymphoid system. **B.** Lymph node. **C.** Tonsil: MALT. **D.** Thymus. **E.** Small intestine and appendix: GALT. **F.** Spleen.

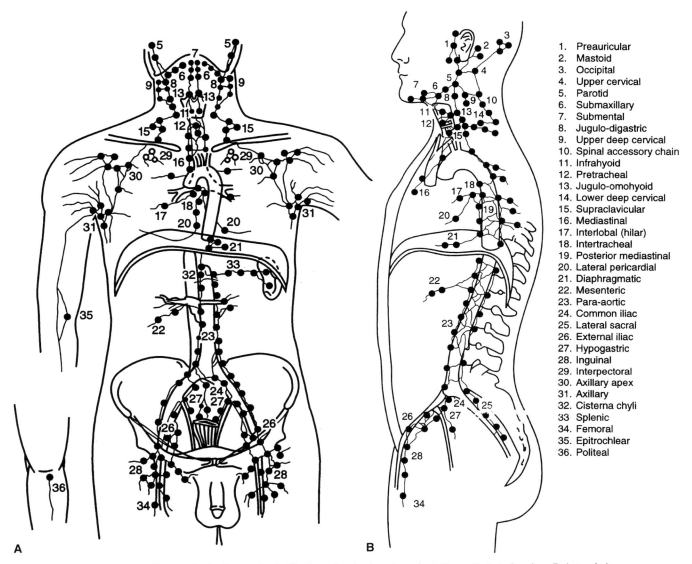

1. Preauricular
2. Mastoid
3. Occipital
4. Upper cervical
5. Parotid
6. Submaxillary
7. Submental
8. Jugulo-digastric
9. Upper deep cervical
10. Spinal accessory chain
11. Infrahyoid
12. Pretracheal
13. Jugulo-omohyoid
14. Lower deep cervical
15. Supraclavicular
16. Mediastinal
17. Interlobal (hilar)
18. Intertracheal
19. Posterior mediastinal
20. Lateral pericardial
21. Diaphragmatic
22. Mesenteric
23. Para-aortic
24. Common iliac
25. Lateral sacral
26. External iliac
27. Hypogastric
28. Inguinal
29. Interpectoral
30. Axillary apex
31. Axillary
32. Cisterna chyli
33. Splenic
34. Femoral
35. Epitrochlear
36. Politeal

Figure 56.6 N-oncoanatomy: Human body. Anatomic distribution of major lymph node stations. **A.** Anterior view. **B.** Lateral view.

TABLE 56.2	Histopathologic Types of Hodgkin Lymphoma

Type

Nodular lymphocyte predominance Hodgkin lymphoma (NLPHL)
Classic Hodgkin lymphoma (CHL)
   Nodular sclerosis Hodgkin lymphoma (NSHL)
   Mixed cellularity Hodgkin lymphoma (MCHL)
   Lymphocyte-rich classic Hodgkin lymphoma (LRCHL)
   Lymphocyte-depletion Hodgkin lymphoma (LDHL)

- Neurologic involvement is considered disseminated disease and is common in advanced stages and/or immunosuppressed patients.
- Bone marrow involvement is distinguished from bone involvement and is always considered to be disseminated disease (stage IV).

Overview of the Lymphoid System

Anatomically, the lymphoid system is ubiquitous in design and provides the immunologic function throughout the body, consisting of lymphatic channels, lymph node stations, and lymphoid extranodal sites. Lymphocytes can circulate in blood and lymphoid tissues, and are characterized by preferentially homing to and from lymph nodes (Fig. 56.4A). Each lymph node has an outer cortex and inner medulla, and aggregations of lymphocytes in lymphoid nodules, which exhibit a lighter central area, called the germinal center. The medulla consists of cords and sinuses that are filled with lymphocytes, plasma cells, and macrophages. Lymph enters from afferent channels through the medullary sinuses in the node and exits from the hilus with the arteriole and vein into efferent channels (Fig. 56.4B). Lymphatic tissue in extranodal sites is part of other organs as:

- *GALT*: Gut-associated lymphoid tissue in small intestine, appendix (Fig. 56.4D).
- *BALT*: Bronchus-associated lymphoid tissue in the respiratory system.
- *MALT*: Mucosal-associated lymphoid tissue in mucous membranes of digestive septa or tonsil (Fig. 56.4C).

In the embryo and newborn, lymphocytes are generated as T cells in the thymus gland (Fig. 56.5E) and B cells in the bursa of Fabricius (as in the appendix; Fig. 56.5D) which populate bone marrow and peripheral nodal sites. The *spleen* can be viewed as a large node or an extranodal site with a more elaborate vascular supply. A connective tissue capsule with its fibrous septa divides the interior into incomplete compartments, that is, white and red pulp. The red pulp consists of splenic cords and sinuses, which interconnect and eventually these blood channels exit via its vein. Perhaps the largest accumulation of lymphocytes are in peripheral lymph nodes and the central bone marrow with rapid exchange amongst lymphoid sites.

Overview of Lymphoid System

The lymphoid system is represented diagramatically in Figure 56.5 with more explicit anatomic identification of lymph node stations and sites (Fig. 56.5 and 56.6).

Overview of Lymphoid N-oncoanatomy

The lymphoid and lymphatic system is diverse. The organization of this system is akin to a separate circulation, which allows lymphocytes, interstitial fluid, and plasma proteins from every tissue and organ system to be collected through lymphatic channels, at regional lymph node stations. Depending on the anatomic location of the organ, the collected lymph then passes through an array of distant lymph nodes and channels, coalescing first into the cisterna chyli below the diaphragm, into the thoracic duct, and finally into the blood stream. Malignant lymphocytes follow the pathway of normal lymphocytes. An understanding of this normal pathway makes the concepts of both contiguous spread and random spread of lymphoid malignancies more readily appreciated.

The classic book on the anatomy of the lymphoid system is *Anatomy of Human Lymphatics* by H. Rouviere (1832). The drawings have been modified largely from his renderings of lymphatics and lymph nodes for each site. The lymphoid system has been of interest to many other anatomists and pathologists. Such sources as Cruikshank's *The Anatomy of the Absorbing Vessels of the Human Body* (1786), Kampmeier's *Developmental Anatomy* (1919), and Yoffey's *Lymphatics, Lymph and Lymphomyeloid Complex* (1970) are excellent historical references, which still apply today. Excellent renderings of regional node-bearing areas and anatomy exist in surgical dissection and resection diagrams for cancers of specific organs. The classic "en bloc" or "radical" operation of cancer surgery is the removal of first station or regional lymph nodes with the primary tumor. For example, a radical mastectomy is the removal of primary breast cancer, the breast and axillary lymph nodes, as compared with a simple mastectomy, which usually does not remove lymph nodes. Simple hysterectomy versus radical hysterectomy emphasizes the removal of lymph nodes in addition to the cervix and uterus in the latter operation. Concisely summarized below are some key anatomic factors.

1. There are approximately 36 major lymph node-bearing stations (Fig. 56.6).
2. Specific major lymphatic trunks drain each structure, site, and viscera, and generally coalesce in two major sites on either side of the diaphragm—the cisterna chyli or the thoracic duct. The cisterna chyli drains the abdomen and pelvis and empties into the thoracic duct which drains the lungs, mediastinum, heart, breast, and head and neck.
3. The first station (echelon) of lymph nodes comprises the "regional" lymph nodes that first receive the lymph from the major lymphatic trunks draining a structure, site, or viscera.
4. The second station (echelon) of lymph nodes is referred to as "juxtaregional." It is the next region to receive lymph from first station nodes.
5. Although bypass mechanisms and collateral channels exist, lymph generally flows from organs in a prograde fashion to their first station regional nodes.

TABLE 56.3	Staging of Hodgkin Lymphomas

Stage

I	Involvement of a single lymph node region (I); or localized involvement of a single extralymphatic organ or site in the absence of any lymph node involvement (IE) (rare in Hodgkin lymphoma).
II	Involvement of ≥ 2 lymph node regions on the same side of the diaphragm (II); or localized involvement of a single extralymphatic organ or site in association with regional lymph node involvement with or without involvement of other lymph node regions on the same side of the diaphragm (IIE). The number of regions involved may be indicated by a subscript, as in, for example, II_3.
III	Involvement of lymph node regions on both sides of the diaphragm (III), which also may be accompanied by extralymphatic extension in association with adjacent lymph node involvement (IIIE) or by involvement of the spleen (IIIS) or both (IIIE,S).
IV	Diffuse or disseminated involvement of ≥ 1 extralymphatic organs, with or without associated lymph node involvement; or isolated extralymphatic organ involvement in the absence of adjacent regional lymph node involvement, but in conjunction with disease in distant site(s). Any involvement of the liver or bone marrow, or nodular involvement of the lung(s). The location of stage IV disease is identified further by specifying the site according to the notations listed on page 400. Although anatomic disease extent is one prognostic factor in non-Hodgkin lymphoma, the prognostic factors that form the IPI for non-Hodgkin lymphoma should be used for treatment decisions along with histologic subtype of lymphoma. Additional factors that have been reported to affect the outcome in preliminary studies include tumor bulk, β-2 microglobulin, and S-phase fraction.

Used with permission from Greene FL, Page DL, Fleming ID, et al., eds. *AJCC Cancer Staging Manual.* 6th ed. New York: Springer; 2002:400.

TABLE 56.4	Imaging Modalities for Detection and Diagnosis of Hodgkin Lymphoma and Lymphomas

Method	Diagnosis and Staging Capability	Recommended for Use

CT
CT-Ch
	Intrathoracic disease if frequently assessed
	Provide additional evidence of intrathoracic disease; CT is the preferred study when the following situations are being addressed:
	  Evaluation of a suspicious or equivocal mediastinum
	  Evaluation of the "normal" mediastinum (may contain enlarged lymph nodes demonstrable by CT)
	  Evaluation of chest wall involvement in the presence of bulky mediastinal disease
	  Evaluation for pulmonary parenchymal lesions
	  Evaluation for pleural or pericardial disease
	  Anatomic extent of disease for treatment planning
		Always
		Yes

CT-Abd and CT-plv	Delineates extent of bulky lymph node disease; however, normal-sized lymph nodes that contain tumor deposits, at times readily demonstrable by lymphography, are not detected by CT. Mesenteric lymphadenopathy is relatively reliably shown by CT in NHLs.	Yes
MRI and GD	Shows promise in delineating extent of disease; pericardial involvement is well demonstrated.	Yes
Bipedal lymphography	Most accurate imaging test for evaluating retroperitoneal lymph nodes; provides convenient means for follow-up regarding response to treatment or relapse.	Yes
US	Exclusion of urinary tract obstruction with bulky lymphadenopathy.	Selected
Gallium citrate radionuclide studies	Supradiaphragmatic disease; proper technique is important for quality images.	Selected

CT, computed tomography; CT-Abd, abdominal CT; CT-Ch, chest CT; CT-plv, pelvic CT; Gd, gadolinium; MRI, magnetic resonance imaging; STUS, soft tissue ultrasound; US, ultrasonography.

6. The thoracic duct drains into the junction of the left subclavian vein and the internal jugular vein.
7. The diaphragm is rich in lymphatics and drains the peritoneal cavity. The lymphatics, located on its undersurface, are greater on the right than on the left.

Lymph from the right side of the head, right upper extremities, and right upper thorax drain into the right subclavian duct, which empties into the venous circulation at the junction of the right subclavian and internal jugular veins. Lymph from the rest of the body drains alternately to the thoracic duct, which empties on the left side at the junction of left subclavian and internal jugular vein.

The staging of HL depends on biopsy of major lymph nodal sites below the diaphragm. One needs to identify the sites that commonly are sampled. These include any enlarged para-aortic or pelvic lymph nodes and the splenic hilar nodes and spleen (which are removed). The liver and the bone marrow are biopsied, the porta hepatis is explored, and the mesentery is biopsied, particularly in NHL.

Rules for Classification and Staging

Histopathology

The lymphoid neoplasms include an ever-increasing spectrum of disorders. The large variety of sites affected and the systemic distribution of lymphomas reflects the ubiquitous distribution of the lymphocyte. The array of lymphomas and lymphoproliferative conditions has undergone a metamorphosis over the past five decades and has made their classification more accurate and perhaps more confusing. Morphologic criteria based on both the macro- and micropathology of the lymph node have been supplemented by immunotyping and genetic features of the lymphocyte. These lymphoid neoplasms have a common ancestry with either B cells, T cells, or natural killer cells. Accordingly, the NHLs collectively include the neoplastic versions of these cells and in addition include HL and lymphoid leukemias. Currently, the *R*evised *E*uropean *A*merican Classification of *L*ymphoid Neoplasms (REAL) has incorporated the histopathology of the original Working Formulation of the International Lymphoma Study Group with the newer immunomolecular markers to define 25 different categories of lymphoid neoplasm (Tables 56.1 and 56.2). HL has four varieties histopathologically (Table 56.3).

Clinical Staging and Imaging

Careful inspection and clinical palpation of all peripheral sites is mandatory: Head and neck, upper limb (epitrochlear node) and axilla, inguinal/femoral area, and lower limb (popliteal and femoral nodes). Thoracic and abdominal nodes require imaging. Liver and spleen should be palpable if enlarged. Spiral computed to-

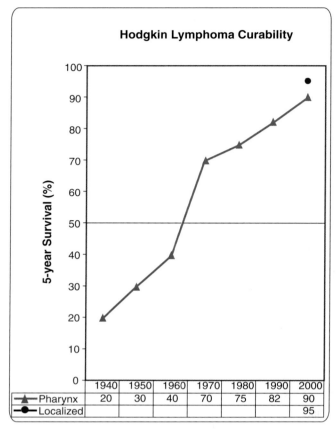

Figure 56.7 **Trajectory of the curability of HL, 1950 to 2000 (gain in survival +65%, decrease in mortality −65%).** The curability of HL rose, with dramatic doubling in survival in the decade between 1960 and 1970 and was due to the introduction of megavoltage linear accelerator technology and advances in multiagent chemotherapy.

mography (CT) and magnetic resonance imaging (MRI) can provide cross-sectional anatomy. Suspicious nodes are defined with different size thresholds. Most nodes ≥ 1 cm and certainly 1.5- to 2-cm rounded nodes are considered positive and, if possible, deserve needle aspiration or excisional biopsy to confirm. Retrocrural nodes >0.5 cm are considered highly suspicious. Imaging can establish organ invasion of liver, spleen, lung, bone, and central nervous system. MRI is excellent to show bone marrow invasion, but aspiration biopsy is advised for confirmation (Table 56.3).

Pathologic Staging

Laparotomy, once routine in HL, allowed for histopathologic verification of lymphomatous invasion of liver, spleen, bowel, mesentery, omentum, accessible bone, and bone marrow. Currently, imaging and selected image-guided biopsy of suspicious areas can provide histopathologic verification for more accurate staging. Needle biopsy is limited in HL because aspiration of a Reed Sternberg cell is essential for the diagnosis. An excisional biopsy of an enlarged node is preferred.

TABLE 56.5	TNM Classification for Mycosis Fungoides	
T1	Limited patch/plaque	(<10% of skin surface involved)
T2	Generalized patch/plaque	(≥10% of skin surface involved)
T3	Cutaneous tumors	(one or more)
T4	Generalized erythroderma	(with or without patches, plaques, or tumors)
N0		Lymph nodes clinically uninvolved
N1		Lymph nodes clinically enlarged, histologically uninvolved
N2		Lymph nodes clinically unenlarged, histologically involved
N3		Lymph nodes enlarged and histologically involved
M0		No visceral disease
M1		Visceral disease present
B0		No circulating atypical cells (<1,000 Sezary cells [CD4 + CD7 −]/ml)
B1		Circulating atypical cells (≥1,000 Sezary cells [CD4 + CD7 −]/ml)

Stage Classification of Mycosis Fungoides

IA	T1	N0	M0
IB	T2	N0	M0
IIA	T1–2	N1	M0
IIB	T3	N0–1	M0
IIIA	T4	N0	M0
IIIB	T4	N0	M0
IVA	T1–4	N2–3	M0
IVB	T1–4	N0–3	M1

Used with permission from Greene FL, Page DL, Fleming ID, et al., eds. *AJCC Cancer Staging Manual.* 6th ed. New York: Springer; 2002:397.

Oncoimaging Annotations

Hodgkin Lymphoma

- Generally, tumor is detected in cervical nodes when they are enlarged (≤10 mm), become more round, or increase in number.
- Lymphomas usually show homogeneous nodal enhancement. Central nodal necrosis is exceedingly rare.
- In the patient with low mediastinal or hilar abnormalities, CT is critical in verifying disease and better defining the contiguous lung parenchyma for unsuspected involvement.
- Nodal size criterion is reduced to 6 mm for prevascular, internal mammary, posterior mediastinal, and anterior diaphragmatic nodes.

- HL primarily involves the upper abdominal and retroperitoneal nodes, whereas NHL may involve any of the nodes, including the mesenteric nodes. Retroperitoneal lymph nodes involved with HL rarely become grossly enlarged, detracting from the accuracy of CT.

Non-Hodgkin Lymphoma

- On both ultrasonography and CT, a relatively specific finding of mesenteric NHL is the "sandwich" sign, in which tumor infiltrating the mesenteric leaves or nodes encases the mesenteric vessels.
- Waldeyer's ring is the most common head and neck site for extranodal NHL.
- Single or multiple submucosal nodules or masses are common in bowel lymphoma, and as the lesion

outgrows its blood supply, mucosal necrosis may occur, leading to ulceration and cavitation.

- Diffuse infiltration of the submucosa causes wall thickening and enlargement of the folds.
- One of the unusual features of small bowel lymphoma occurs after transmural extension of the lymphoma, resulting in aneurysmal dilation of the involved bowel.
- Lymphomatous involvement of the spleen occurs in three patterns: Diffuse infiltration, small nodules <1 cm in diameter, and macronodules. Imaging typically detects only the macronodular form.
- Lymphomatous renal masses are frequently bilateral, and often significant retroperitoneal lymphadenopathy is absent.
- MRI is exquisitely sensitive to bone marrow involvement, and in select patients, it may serve to guide biopsies.

Special Staging Features for Lymphoid Neoplasms

Non-Hodgkin Lymphoma (Table 56.4)

The International NHL Prognostic Index Factors Project (IPI) has established risk factors to develop a predictive model for outcome for aggressive forms of NHL. The five pretreatment factors listed were found to be independent statistically significant. IPI risk is defined as: Low (0–1), low intermediate (2), high intermediate (3), and high (4 or 5). Correlation with outcomes following doxorubicin combination chemotherapy was found.

Hodgkin Lymphoma

- Extranodal sites are added to stage as II "E."
- Detached site information can be noted with letters and addition of (+) positive and (−) negative signs.
- Systemic classification of symptoms: A or B to stage if (−) or (+).
  1. Fevers—unexplained, >38°C, especially recurrent.
  2. Night sweats—require change of pajamas.
  3. Unexplained >10% of body weight, 6 month before diagnosis.
  4. Not used: Pruritus, fatigue, or alcohol intolerance.

Bulky mediastinal adenopathy is defined on routine standing chest film as the ratio between maximal single width of chest versus maximum intrathoracic diameter of the mediastinal mass on same radiograph.

$$\frac{\text{Ratio of Width of Mass}}{\text{Width of Chest}} \geq 1/3 = \text{Bulky}$$

- *Mycoses fungoides* is a primary cutaneous T-cell lymphoma with its own staging system, based on physical examination as to skin surface involvement: T1, <10%; T2, >10%; T3, tumefaction as nodules; T4,

TABLE 56.6	Criteria for Staging Multiple Myeloma	
Stage*	**Criteria**	**Myeloma Cell Mass (cells × 10^{12}/m^2)**

I	All of the following:
	• Hemoglobin >10 g/dL
	• Normal serum calcium
	• Normal bone structure
	• Low M-protein production as shown by:
	  IgG <5 g/dL
	  IgA <3 g/dL
	  Urinary κ or λ <4 g/24 h
		<0.6 (low burden)

II	Fitting neither stage I nor III	0.6–1.2 (intermediate burden)

III	One or more of the following:
	• Hemoglobin <8.5 g/dL
	• Serum calcium >12 mg/dL
	• >3 lytic bone lesions
	• High M-protein production as shown by:
	  IgG >7 g/dL
	  IgA >5 g/dL
	  Urinary κ or λ >12 g/24 h
		>1.2 (high burden)

*Subclassification of stages: A, creatinine <2 mg/dL; B, creatinine ≥2 mg/dL.

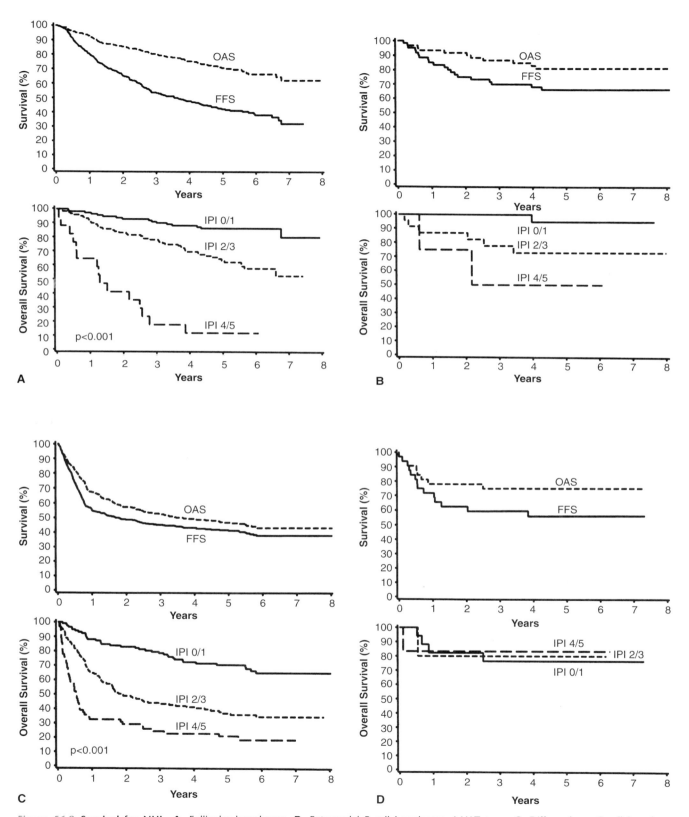

Figure 56.8 **Survival for NHL. A.** Follicular lymphoma. **B.** Extranodal B-cell lymphoma, MALT type. **C.** Diffuse, large B-cell lymphoma. **D.** Anaplastic large T-cell lymphoma. IPI, International NHL Prognostic Index Factors Project; FFS, Freedom from Relapse; OAS, Overall Actuarial Survival.

generalized. Nodes need histopathology verification for N2 or N3 criteria. Blood findings are noted as B0 or B1, circulating atypical Sezany cells (Table 56.5, Fig. 56.7).

- Multiple myeloma is a neoplastic disorder characterized by a single clone of plasma cells, believed to be derived from B cells. Diffuse small lytic bone lesions are more common than solitary plasmacytomas, which are highly curable. For the diagnosis of multiple myeloma, 10% of bone marrow cells on aspiration need to be plasma cells, the production of M protein encountered in serum and urine are characteristics of this disease (Table 56.6).

Cancer Statistics and Survival

The NHL collective dominate the incidence of lymphoid neoplasms with an estimated 65,000 new cases annually and increasing at an alarming rate perhaps due to the increase in our aging population. This compares with a relatively stable population of approximately 8,000 new HL patients annually, which has been decreasing in the older age groups, again due to more accurate immunotyping. HL has a bimodal peak incidence of 15 to 35 years and a smaller peak between 40 and 60 years. NHL increases after age 45 with each decade of age. HL was considered incurable 50 years ago and is now highly curable, particularly in the earliest stages of evolution. Fortunately, the advances in multimodal treatment, especially in multiagent chemotherapy added to shaped large radiation fields have improved survival dramatically. Although NHL is considered to be a generalized condition, HL is thought to be unicentric in origin.

The mortality rate is dramatically different; HL is highly curable, with only 1,000 deaths, compared with NHL where 20,000 (>30%) die annually. The dramatic gain in survival is shown over five decades as the first evidence of advances in all modalities when combined could conquer cancer (Fig. 56.8). This was especially true for megavoltage irradiation and extended fields techniques pioneered by Kaplan and combination chemotherapy (MOPP) by DeVita and Carbone. Numerous survival curves are presented by the International Non-Hodgkin's Lymphoma Prognostic Factors Project. The outcomes for low-risk patients are contrasted with high-risk disease: CR rates are 87% versus 44% and overall survival rates at 5-year are 73% versus 26%, respectively. Patients with low-grade follicular B-cell lymphomas live with their disease, gradually dying over a decade, whereas high-grade B-cell diffuse lymphoma patients tend to respond to therapy, as do anaplastic large T-cell, and reach a plateau and remain disease free.

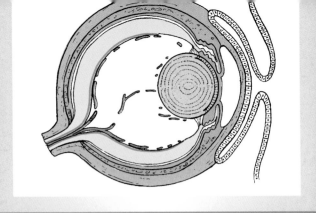

SECTION 7

OPHTHALMIC PRIMARY SITES

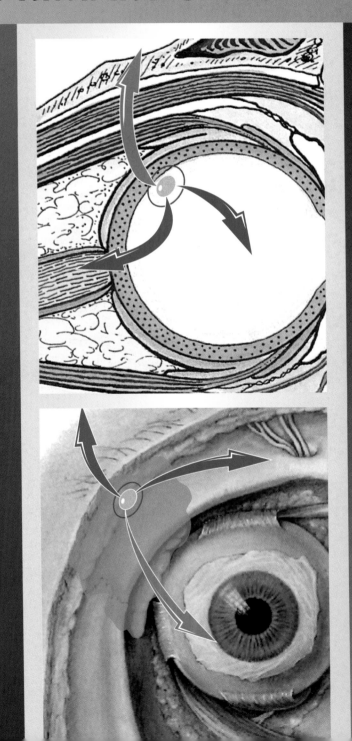

57

Introduction and Orientation

The eye is a palindrome of three letters and its on-coanatomy is characterized by being tripartite, reflecting its embryonic origin.

Perspective and Patterns of Spread

Loss of vision is frightening under any circumstances, but when coupled with malignancy, it is alarming and life threatening as well. The eye is one of our most critical sensory organs. It is our window through which we view the world. Although it is uncommon, malignancies afflict virtually every age group from the newborn to the aged. Many different primary tumors are possible, beginning with special congenital tumors, such as retinoblastomas and embryonal rhabdomyosarcomas; in the adult, common variety neoplasms are carcinomas, lymphomas, and melanomas. Many malignancies metastasize to the eye and orbit. Diagnostic and therapeutic decision making is complex and multidisciplinary.

The tissues of the eye in their embryogenic development are derived from neuroectoderm, surface ectoderm, and mesoderm (Table 57.1). Each source is a derivative of specific structural sites and in turn can lead to tumefactions that are unique. (Fig. 57.1). There are many different tumors that can arise around the orbit and in the eye due to the large variety of tissues that constitute this organ and its anatomic environment. The eye is composed of three different layers, each with its unique structures. The neoplasms are different for adults and children (Table 57.2). Each structure gives rise to a characteristic tumor that can only occur in that layer; that is, in the retina, retinoblastomas; in the pigmented choroids, the pigmented melanoma; or the sclera and conjunctiva squamous cell cancers. Each tumor spreads in a specific pattern depending on the layers involved; however, each can advance and invade into other layers and structures of the eye and orbit (Fig. 57.2).

An exact understanding of three-dimensional anatomy is essential in radiation oncology, where precision proton beams with sharp and limited Bragg peaks or strategically placed radioisotopic plaques have success-

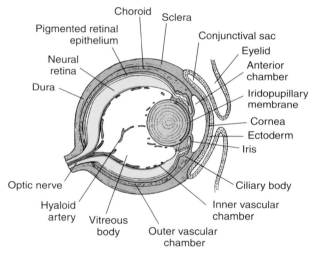

Figure 57.1 **The eye as seen in a 15-week fetus.** All the layers of the eye are established, and the hyaloid artery traverses the vitreous body from the optic disc to the posterior surface of the lens.

fully eradicated choroidal melanomas and preserved vision. In a similar fashion, carefully shaped photon beams with appropriate shielding can save an eye in children with retinoblastomas and embryonal rhabdomyosarcomas.

Preservation of vision with tumor ablation is the essential goal for both the ophthalmologic surgeon and the radiation oncologist. Precise surgical ablative procedures match accurate proton beams and have allowed for high cure rates with eye and vision conservation. Enucleation and exenteration are reserved for very advanced and recurrent sarcomas and cancers.

TNM Staging Criteria

For all intents and purposes, the T category determines the stage. The TNM stage grouping is not utilized to stage

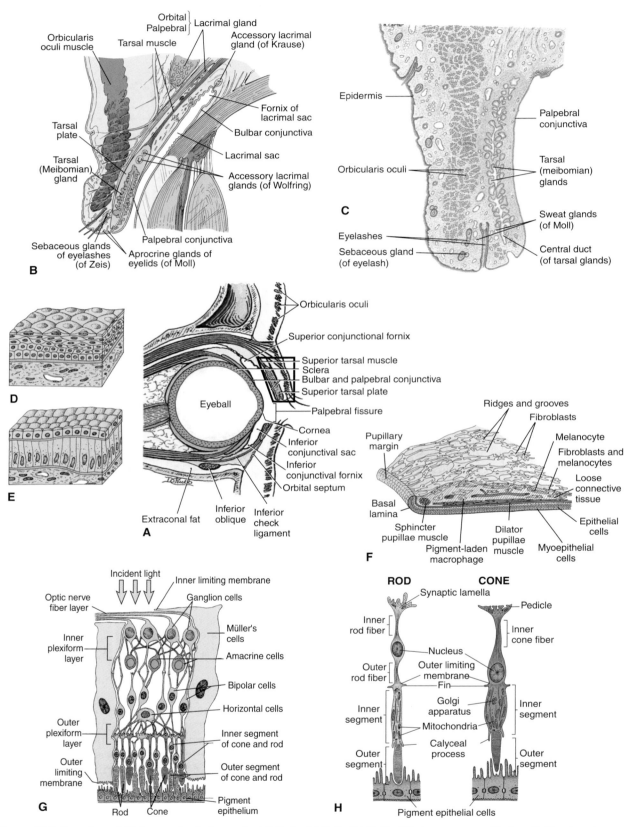

Figure 57.2 **Overview of Histogenesis. A.** Eye and orbit **B.** Eyelid **C.** Eyelid **D.** Stratified squamous epithelium **E.** Simple columnar epithelium **F.** Iris **G.** Retina **H.** Rod and cone cells.

TABLE 57.1	Embryonic Origins of the Individual Structure of the Eye	
Source	**Derivative**
Surface ectoderm	Lens Epithelium of the cornea, conjunctiva, and lacrimal gland and its drainage system
Neural ectoderm	Vitreous body (derived partly from neural ectoderm of the optic cup and partly from mesenchyme) Epithelium of the retina, iris, and ciliary body Sphincter pupillae and dilator pupillae muscles Optic nerve
Mesoderm	Sclera Stroma of the cornea, ciliary body, iris, and choroid Extraocular muscles Eyelids (except epithelium and conjunctiva) Hyaloid system (most of which degenerates before birth) Coverings of the optic nerve Connective tissue and blood vessels of the eye, bony orbit, and vitreous body

Used with permission from Ross MH, Kaye GI, Pawlina W, eds. *Histology: A Text and Atlas.* 4th ed. Philadelphia: Lippincott Williams & Wilkins; 2003:837.

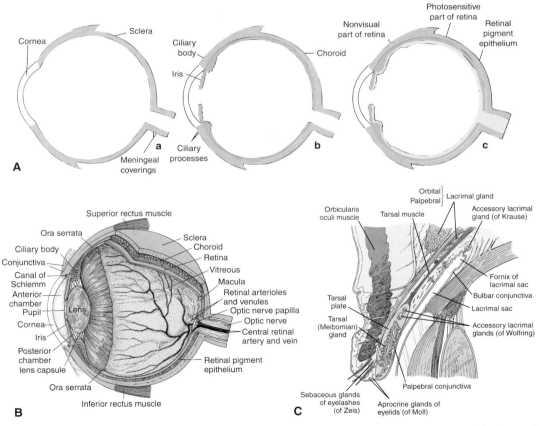

Figure 57.3 **Overview of oncoanatomy: Tripartite. A.** Three layers of eye. Schematic diagram of the layers of the eye. The wall of eyeball is organized in three separate concentric layers: (a) an outer supporting layer, the corneoscleral coat (*clear* and *blue*); (b) a middle vascular coat or uvea (*pink*); and (c) an inner photosensitive layer, the retina (*yellow*). **B.** Three chambers of eye. Schematic diagram illustrating the internal structures of the human eye. The retina consists of photosensitive and nonphotosensitive regions that differ in their function. Note that the photosensitive region of the retina occupies the posterior part of the eye and terminates anteriorly along the ora serrata. The nonphotosensitive region of the retina is located anterior to the ora serrata and lines the inner aspect of the ciliary body and the posterior surface of the iris. The other layers of the eyeball as well as the attachment of two of the extraocular muscles to the sclera are also shown. **C.** Three sectors of eyelid. Structure of the eyelid. The schematic drawing of the eyelid shows the skin, associated skin appendages, muscles, tendons, connective tissue, and conjunctiva. Note the distribution of multiple small glands associated with the eyelid and observe the reflection of the palpebral conjunctiva in the fornix of the lacrimal sac to become the bulbar conjunctiva (*continued*).

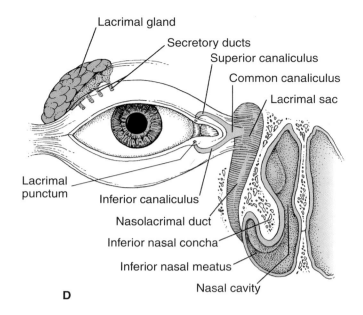

D

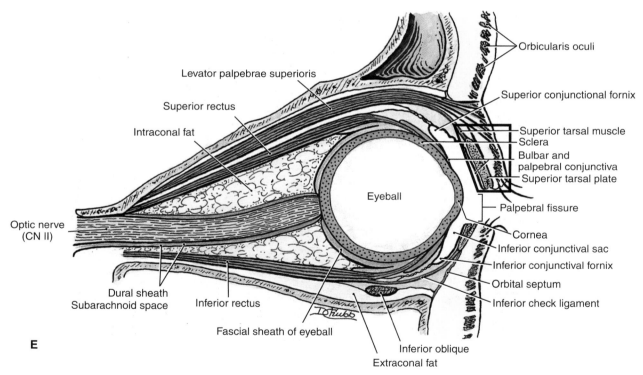

E

Figure 57.3 (*Continued*) **D.** Three aspects of lacrimal apparatus. Schematic diagram of the eye and lacrimal apparatus. This drawing shows the location of the lacrimal gland and components of the lacrimal apparatus, which drains the lacrimal fluid into the nasal cavity. **E.** Three zones of orbit. Sagittal section of orbit and eyelid.

from them (Fig. 57.2A). The eyelid (Fig. 57.2B) forms the external covers of the eye, which are composed of epidermis and dermal glandular appendages (Fig. 57.2C) that are special and specific to this site. Basal cell cancers are most common and most uncommon squamous cell cancers of the skin; adenocarcinomas arising from Meibomian, sebaceous (Zeis), or apocrine (Moll) glands are rare (Table 57.4). Squamous cell cancers of the conjunctiva arise from (Fig. 57.2D) stratified squamous epithelium. Adenocarcinomas of the lacrimal gland (Fig. 57.2E) parallel salivary gland neoplasms histopathologically and both tend to be involved by lymphoma, which can be present in the conjunctiva and/or orbit, often as isolated sites of disease. Melanomas can arise from the pigmented uveal or choroids layer of the eye globe (Fig. 57.2F), very uncommonly on the iris, and even less so in the conjunctiva. The common pediatric tumors arising from the retina (Fig. 57.2G, H) are retinoblastomas and embryonal cancers from the orbital recti muscles.

Orientation of Primary T-oncoanatomy

To appreciate the eye oncoanatomy, one needs to be aware of the tripartite segmentation, beginning with the globe of the eye (Fig. 57.3). A brief odyssey of primary sites follows:

- Globe layers (Fig. 57.3A) are organized in three concentric coats: (i) Outer corneoscleral; (ii) middle vascular uvea/choroid; and (iii) inner photosensitive retina.
- Chambers of the eye (Fig. 57.3B) consist of (i) the anterior chamber, between the cornea and iris, (ii) the posterior chamber is between the posterior surface of the iris and anterior surface and equator of the lens, and (iii) the vitreous chamber, the space between the lens and retina. The vitreous is filled with a gelatinous substance.
- Eyelid of the eye (Fig. 57.3C) consists of three layers: (i) Skin with eyelashes, (ii) Meibomian glands, sebaceous glands of Zeis, and apocrine glands of Moll, and (iii) tarsal muscle and conjunctiva cover.
- Lacrimal apparatus (Fig. 57.3D) consists of three parts, as do the tears: (i) The lacrimal gland secretions are watery, the glands of the tarsal plate provide a waxy sebaceous secretion (Meibomian) and an oily film (Zeis and Moll), which is collected by (ii) canaliculi at the inner canthus into a lacrimal sac, and (iii) a lacrimal canal that vertically descends into the nares below the inferior turbinate.
- Orbit (Fig. 57.3E) contains the globe and consists of three compartments, each of which gives rise to retro-orbital tumors, that is, by adipose tissue in which the recti muscles (medial, lateral, superior and inferior) and oblique (superior and inferior) muscles are innervated by three cranial nerves (III, IV, and

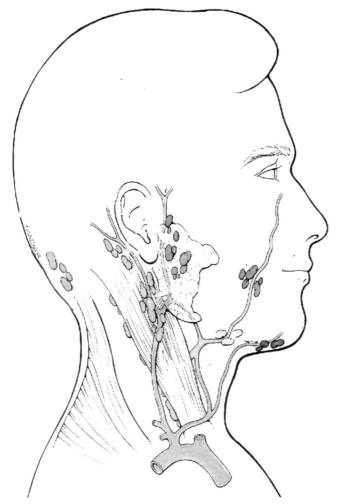

Figure 57.4 **N-oncoanatomy of eye is applicable only to the eyelid and orbital content because the eye is immunologically privileged.**

eye malignancies, with the exception of uveal melanomas. Usually, malignancies of the eye are diagnosed and staged when they are millimeters in size rather than centimeters (Table 57.3). Most often, T1 to T3 in all sites are measured in millimeters, not centimeters, for tumor progression. Careful mapping of tumor depth or height by width is often utilized. T4 lesions that invade into the orbit soft tissues tend to spread to preauricular, submandibular, and cervical nodes. The globe of the eye is immunologically privileged and without a lymphatic system. N1 is noted, but does not affect stage grouping. M1 is noted, but does not affect or modify stage IV.

Overview of Histogenesis of Eye Primary Sites

The overview begins with the sagittal section of the eye, which provides a framework for presenting the derivative normal cells and consequential tumors that arise

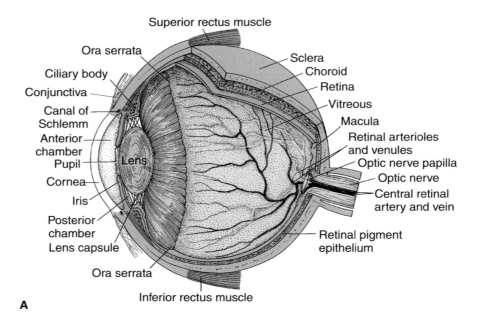

A

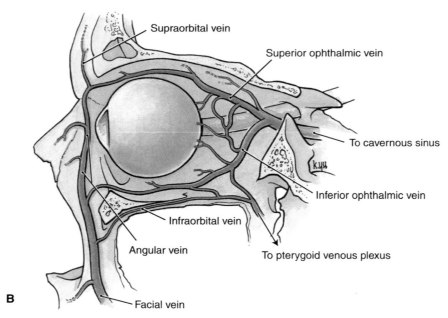

B

Figure 57.5 M-oncoanatomy of eye. A. Retinal vein. Schematic diagram illustrating the internal structures of the human eye. The retina consists of photosensitive and nonphotosensitive regions that differ in their function. Note that the photosensitive region of the retina occupies the posterior part of the eye and terminates anteriorly along the ora serrata. The nonphotosensitive region of the retina is located anterior to the ora serrata and lines the inner aspect of the ciliary body and the posterior surface of the iris. The other layers of the eyeball as well as the attachment of two of the extraocular muscles to the sclera are also shown. **B.** Orbital veins. The superior and inferior ophthalmic veins receive the vorticose veins from the eyeball (not shown) and empty into the cavernous sinus posteriorly and the pterygoid plexus inferiorly and communicate with the facial and supraorbital veins anteriorly.

TABLE 57.2	Most Common Tumors of the Eye					
	Adult			**Children**		
Site	Tumor Type	Sign	Visual Loss	Tumor Type	Sign	Visual Loss
Lid	Basal cell carcinoma	Scabbing ulcer	None	Hemangioma	Red Strawberry mass	Closed eyelid
Conjunctiva	Squamous cell carcinoma	Fleshy lesion	None	Leukemia	Raised, infiltrative mass	None
Intraocular	Melanoma	Black to brownish elevated area in choroids	Scotoma	Retinoblastoma	White reflex	Blindness
Intraorbital	Lymphoma	Mass, displacement of globe	Diplopia	Embryonal rhab-domyosarcoma	Mass, displacement of globe	Diplopia
Metastatic	Breast (lung)	Raised area in retina	Scotoma	Neuroblastoma	Proptosis, ecchymosis, pain, orbit mass	Diplopia

Used with permission from Rubin P. *Clinical Oncology.* 7th ed. Philadelphia: WB Saunders; 1993:300.

VI), and surrounded by the bony orbit. The bony orbits are like inverted pyramids tipped medially, with four walls, an apex where the optic nerve enters, and the orbital opening surrounded by the eyelids that forms the base. It is approximately 4 cm at its base and 5 cm on its axis. The optic canal is <1 cm long. The superior and inferior orbital fissure and foramen allow for nerves, arteries, and veins to enter and exit.

N-oncoanatomy

The eye globe is immunologically privileged in that it is free of lymphatics and is similar to the central nervous system. However, the eyelids and orbital contents can be involved with infiltrations of inflammatory lymphocytes, pseudolymphomas, and true lymphomas. A unique feature is direct lymphatic channels between lacrimal and parotid glands. The orbit and eyelids drain to preauricular or parotid nodes. Lesions at the inner canthus and lacrimal apparatus drain to facial and submandibular nodes (Fig. 57.4).

M-oncoanatomy

The venous supply is presented to alert us as the pathway for the metastatic spread of cancers and/or sarcomas that occur with relative frequency in the orbit and the globe of the eye in both children and adults (Fig. 57.5).

- *Orbital:* Neuroblastoma metastasis in children produce proptosis and ecchymosis (Hutchinson syndrome), whereas lymphomas and pseudolymphomas are more common in adults.

TABLE 57.3	TNM Staging Criteria for the Eye			
	T1	T2	T3	N
Eyelid*	<5 mm	>5–10 mm	>10 mm	
Conjunctiva*	≤5 mm	>5 mm		
Conjunctival melanoma*	—	≤0.8	>0.8 mm	N1
Melanoma uvea*	—	<10 mm	>10–16 mm	N1
Retinoblastoma*	—	≤3 mm		
Lacrimal gland*	≤2.5 mm	25–50 mm	>50 mm	N1
Sarcoma orbit*	<15 mm	>15 mm		N1

*No stage grouping recommended at any site except uveal melanomas of choroids.

TABLE 57.4	Histogenesis of Eye Primary Sites and Derivative Tumors	
Normal Structure	**Derivative Cell**	**Malignancy**
Eyelid, skin, glands	Germinal basal keratinocyte Simple columnar cells	Basal cell cancers Adenocarcinomas
Conjunctiva	Stratified squamous cell	Squamous cell cancer
Uvea, choroids	Melanocyte in pigmented epithelial layer	Melanomas of choroid, uvea
Retina	Retinoblast, precursor cell to inner and outer nuclear cells	Retinoblastoma
Lacrimal gland	Columnar cell	Adenocarcinoma
Recti muscles	Striated muscle cell Lymphocyte	Embryonal rhabdomyosarcoma Lymphoma

TABLE 57.5	Imaging Modalities of the Eye and Orbit	
Method	**Diagnosis and Staging Capability**	**Recommended for Use**
CT	Provides excellent anatomic detail of globe, orbital content and bony orbit. Can distinguish smooth, round cysts from infiltrative tumors versus pseudotumors and detect bone destruction and sinus invasion.	Yes
Primary tumor ultrasonography and fine needle aspiration biopsy	A scan and B scan can be used to screen intraocular and orbital tumors and cysts, especially melanomas	No
MRI	Provides excellent 3D view, orbital fat hyperintense and vitreous hypointense in tumor (T1) and reverse in T2. Can detect tumors versus pseudotumors and cysts. May be superior for diagnosis of vascular lesions, demyelinating disease	Yes
Endoscopy	Orbital endoscopy with fiber optic lights is used in conjunction with CT and/or MRI for obtaining core biopsy	Yes, when indicated
Standard orbital view	Useful for assessing optic nerve foramen and supraorbital fissure, but supplanted by CT; can detect intraocular calcification	No
Orbital phlebography	Venography particularly useful for detecting orbital varices, but is less efficient and more invasive than CT	No
Carotid angiography	Useful in diagnosis of vascularized tumors and aneurysms, but replaced by CT, MRI	No
Fluorescein angiography	Sometimes used in diagnosis of ocular melanoma	No
Biopsy	Usually an incisional or excisional biopsy is indicated to confirm malignant versus pseudotumors. Directed stereotactically by CT/MRI. Contraindicated for melanomas due to high risk of seeding.	Yes, if indicated

CT, computed tomography; MRI, magnetic resonance imaging.
Used with permission from Rubin P. *Clinical Oncology*. 7th ed. Philadelphia: WB Saunders; 1993:300.

- *Global*: Metastatic choroidal deposits from the common adult cancers of the lung and the eye cause scotomas.

The venous drainage of the eye and orbit are more the recipient of metastatic cancer than viaducts for dissemination. The eye is relatively avascular, except for the choroidal layer, which has a rich venous network. The optic nerve is surrounded by all the meningeal layers of the brain; the optic disc is a direct window into the central nervous system. Once the optic nerve is invaded by malignancy, a tumor can disseminate in the central nervous system via the subarachnoid space.

Rules for Classification and Staging

In general, clinical and pathologic assessment is essential to diagnosis and to staging with surgical resection or biopsy to establish the histopathology of the lesion. Imaging plays an important role in the evaluation.

Clinical Staging

The assessment of the tumor is based on physical examination, including careful inspection and palpation of eyelids and conjunctiva, followed by slit-lamp examination and direct and indirect ophthalmoscopy. Additional imaging techniques such as ultrasonography, computed tomography (CT), magnetic resonance imaging (MRI), fluorescein angiography. and isotopic studies may be indicated (Table 57.5).

Pathologic Staging

Resection of primary site and careful assessment of tumor size, extent, and both dimensions—height or depth plus width—is important. Margins of the resected specimen are noted when wedge resection or enucleation of the globe is done. Histopathologic type and tumor grade apply to all sites and R1 is for microscopic and R2 macroscopic residual tumor. Venous invasion V1 microscopic and V2 macroscopic also should be noted.

Cancer Statistics and Survival

The eye and orbit only account for 2,090 new diagnoses, excluding carcinomas of the eyelids. Deaths attributed to ocular malignancy are <10% of the entire group (<200 patients/year). Some of the most elegant proton and three-dimensional conformal radiation stereotactic techniques allow for cure of choroidal melanomas and retinoblastoma with preservation of vision.

Survival results remain impressive, with virtually all eye tumors when properly treated reach 90% long-term survival.

- Basal cell cancers of the eyelids are >95% curable.
- Posterior uveal/choroidal melanomas demonstrated that both radiation isotopic plaque and enucleation were found to be comparable in the Collaborative Ocular Melanoma Study group, consisting of 1,300 patients over 11.5 years. Recurrence rates with radiation range from about 15% to <5% with surgery. Cure rates range from 85% to 95%.
- Retinoblastomas are highly curable, with radiation yielding >90% local tumor control, most often with vision conservation. Those patients that relapse can still be cured by enucleation.
- Optic nerve gliomas are extremely curable by stereotactic radiation therapy. The University of Pittsburgh group reports 96%, 90%, and 90% survival at 5, 10 and 15 years, respectively, with 86% retaining vision.
- Orbital and conjunctival lymphomas, when isolated, are 100% locally controlled with chemoradiation and virtually all patients are long-term survivors.
- Embryonal rhabdomyosarcomas are the highest survivors compared with all other sites ranging >90% long-term outcomes.

58

Eyelid, Adnexa, and Conjunctiva

Eyelid of eye consists of 3 layers: skin, glands and conjunctiva.

Perspective and Patterns of Spread

Benign eyelid tumors, such as papillomas, nevi, hemangiomas, and xanthomas, occur with great frequency. Carcinoma (epithelioma) of the eyelids is the most common malignant tumor in ophthalmology (Table 58.1). Basal cell carcinomas (BCC) in the eyelids outnumber squamous cell carcinomas (SCC) 40 to 1. In the conjunctiva, SCC occurs 10 times more often than BCC. The general behavior of both these tumors is similar to that of skin carcinomas of other sites. They show a predilection for the junction of skin and conjunctiva at the margin of the eyelid. BCC is often only locally invasive, and does not metastasize. SCCs, like the cancers elsewhere, do metastasize, particularly when they recur or invade regional lymph nodes (Fig. 58.1).

Pigmented tumors of the lids, and especially of the conjunctiva, are rare. They are often difficult to manage because of the onset or degree of malignancy is not always apparent on clinical examination. Primary acquired melanosis can be particularly difficult to manage because of its widespread involvement of the conjunctiva and eyelids. Because histopathologic examination of the involved tissue can differentiate melanosis from melanomas of low malignant potential, repeat biopsy of suspicious areas is indicated. In some cases, because of extensive involvement of the ocular surface, surgical excision is impractical. In these cases, controlled cryotherapy of the involved epithelial surfaces is effective in eradicating malignant cells with minimal destruction of ocular tissues. Pterygium is a common benign condition characterized by an elevated fleshy tissue medial or lateral to the cornea. They have a neovascularization that can spread to the cornea.

A special type of cancer involving the eyelids or caruncle is sebaceous carcinoma; it is one of the "great masqueraders" and can resemble chronic inflammation or a benign mass lesion known as chalazion.

TNM Staging Criteria

Because of the fineness and thin character of the layers of the eyelid and conjunctiva size is the key criterion for localized stages measured in millimeters (Fig. 58.2).

- Skin cancer of the eyelid: T1, <5 mm; T2, >5 to <10 mm; T3,>10 mm.
- Conjunctival carcinoma: T1, >5 mm; T2, >5 mm.
- Conjunctival melanoma: T1, 0 mm; T2, <0.8 mm; T3, >0.8 mm.

T4 in most of these sites is invasion into eyelid, globe, or orbit.

Overview of Eyelid

Eyelid of the eye (Fig. 58.3) consists of three layers: (i) Skin with eyelashes, (ii) Meibomian glands, sebaceous glands of Zeis, and apocrine glands of Moll, and (iii) tarsal muscle and conjunctiva cover. Lacrimal apparatus consists of three parts, as do the tears: (i) The lacrimal gland secretions are watery, the glands of the tarsal plate provide a waxy sebaceous secretion (Meibomian) and an oily film (Zeis and Moll), which is collected by (ii) canaliculi, the inner canthus into a lacrimal sac, and (iii) a lacrimal canal that vertically descends into the nares below the inferior turbinate.

T-oncoanatomy

The eyelid is the anterior protective layer of skin and mucosa that can rapidly close when needed to avoid harm to the globe. The intricate anatomy is rarely appreciated until tumefaction occurs and benign conditions need to be distinguished from cancers. The three-planar views are most revealing if the oncoanatomy is related to specific tumors (Fig. 58.4).

- *Coronal*: The important features to note are at the inner canthus of the eye where two fine lacrimal puncta and canaliculi drain into a hidden sac, which drains into the lacrimal duct into the inferior meatus of the nose.
- *Sagittal*: The true complexity and the rich variety of tissues are noted as to lesion formation. The infected eyelash can give rise to a *sty* or *hordeolum* (a plugged tarsal gland to a *chalazion*), not to be confused with the variety of cancers that occur as adenocarcinomas of tarsal glands of Zeiss or ciliary glands at the edge of the lids and squamous cell cancer of the conjunctiva.

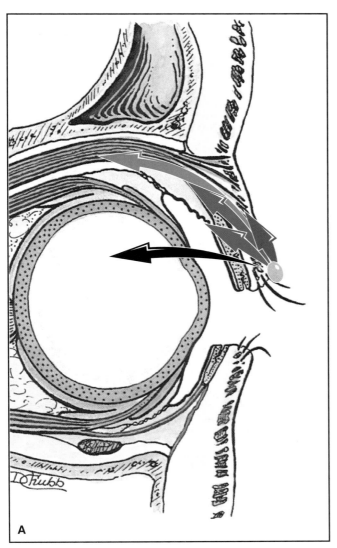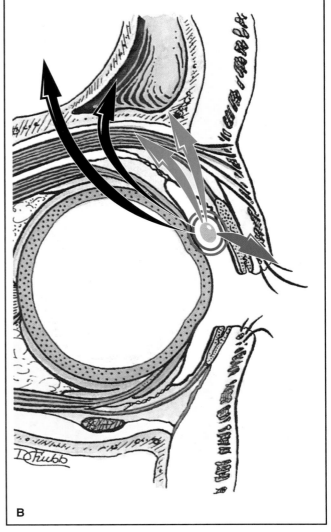

Figure 58.1 **Patterns of spread. A.** Eyelid. Primary cancers of eyelids are essentially skin cancers and are coded for progression: Tis, yellow; T1, green; T2, blue; T3, purple; T4, red. **B.** Conjunctiva. Primary cancers are coded for progression: Tis, yellow; T1, green; T2, blue; T3, purple; T4a, red; and T4b,c,d, black.

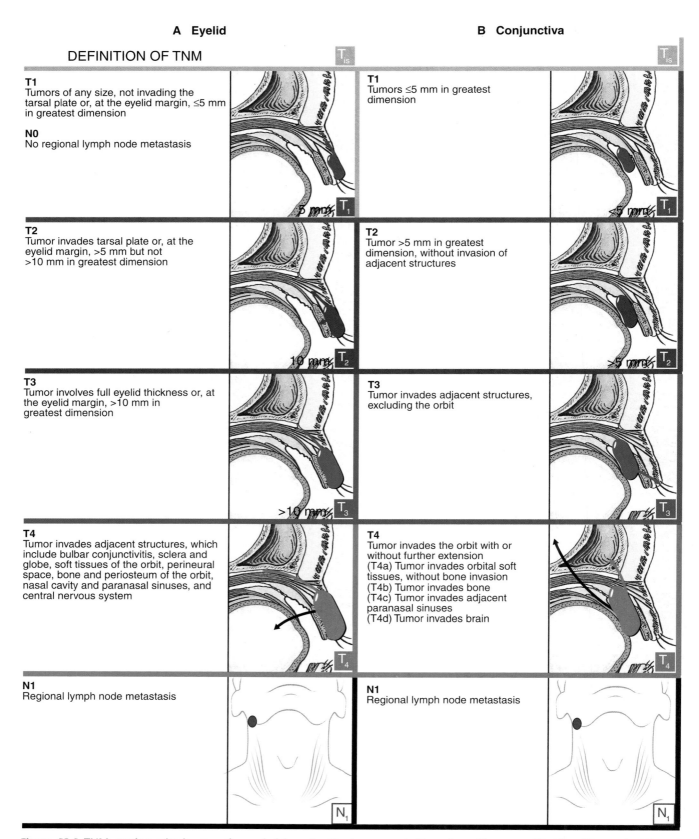

A   Eyelid

B   Conjunctiva

DEFINITION OF TNM

T_{is}

T_{is}

T1
Tumors of any size, not invading the tarsal plate or, at the eyelid margin, ≤5 mm in greatest dimension

N0
No regional lymph node metastasis

5 mm T_1

T1
Tumors ≤5 mm in greatest dimension

≤5 mm T_1

T2
Tumor invades tarsal plate or, at the eyelid margin, >5 mm but not >10 mm in greatest dimension

10 mm T_2

T2
Tumor >5 mm in greatest dimension, without invasion of adjacent structures

>5 mm T_2

T3
Tumor involves full eyelid thickness or, at the eyelid margin, >10 mm in greatest dimension

>10 mm T_3

T3
Tumor invades adjacent structures, excluding the orbit

T_3

T4
Tumor invades adjacent structures, which include bulbar conjunctivitis, sclera and globe, soft tissues of the orbit, perineural space, bone and periosteum of the orbit, nasal cavity and paranasal sinuses, and central nervous system

T_4

T4
Tumor invades the orbit with or without further extension
(T4a) Tumor invades orbital soft tissues, without bone invasion
(T4b) Tumor invades bone
(T4c) Tumor invades adjacent paranasal sinuses
(T4d) Tumor invades brain

T_4

N1
Regional lymph node metastasis

N_1

N1
Regional lymph node metastasis

N_1

Figure 58.2 TNM staging criteria are color coded bars for T advancement: Tis, yellow; T1, green; T2, blue; T3, purple; T4, red. **A.** Eyelid. **B.** Conjunctiva.

TABLE 58.1	Histopathologic Types of Eyelid Cancers and Carcinomas of the Conjunctiva
Eyelid	**Conjunctiva**
Basal cell carcinoma	Conjunctival intraepithelial neoplasia including in situ squamous cell carcinoma
Squamous cell carcinoma	Squamous cell carcinoma
Sebaceous carcinoma	Mucoepidermoid carcinoma
Merkel cell tumor	Basal cell carcinoma
Skin appendage carcinoma	
Sarcoma	

Used with permission from Agur A, Dalley A, eds. *Grant's Atlas of Anatomy*. 11th ed. Philadelphia: Lippincott Williams & Wilkins; 2005:350, 356.

- *Axial*: The magnified sagittal view provides the intricate organization of layers. Note the insertion of the levator palpebrae muscle in the upper lid. The conjunctiva covers the globe and lid meeting at the fornix.

N-oncoanatomy

The eyelids and conjunctiva drain predominantly into the preauricular nodes except for its medial margin, which follow medial lymphatics into the submandibular nodes (Fig. 58.5).

M-oncoanatomy

The pterygoid plexus of veins drain the fine veins of the eyelids into the internal jugular vein (Fig. 58.6).

Rules for Classification and Staging

Clinical Staging

Clinical staging begins with histopathologic identification of cancer type and grade and then involves careful inspection, palpation, and slit-lamp biomicroscopy. Entire conjunctival surface needs viewing with upper lid eversion. If the cancer is deeply invading T3, T4 imaging procedures are highly recommended to determine anatomic extent. Conjunctival melanoma needs to be distinguished from acquired melanosis, junctional and compound nevi, and melanoma in situ (Table 58.2).

Pathologic Staging

Pathologic staging is appropriate for total excision of cancers and exenterations. Deeply invading malignancies require notation of margins of conjunctiva and if globe is included optic nerves. Depth of lesions suspected as melanomas need to be perpendicular to skin. Sentinel node biopsy is encouraged.

Cancer Statistics and Survival

The eye and orbit only account for 2,090 new diagnoses excluding carcinomas of the eyelids. Deaths attributed to ocular malignancy are <10% of the entire group (<200 patients/year). Some of the most elegant proton and three-dimensional conformal radiation stereotactic techniques allow for cure of choroidal melanomas and retinoblastoma with preservation of vision.

Survival remains impressive; 90% survive long term. Most skin cancers about the eyelids are detected early and are readily controlled by excision and/or radiation. Only recurrent cancers that deeply invade can lead to deformity, loss of eye, and death.

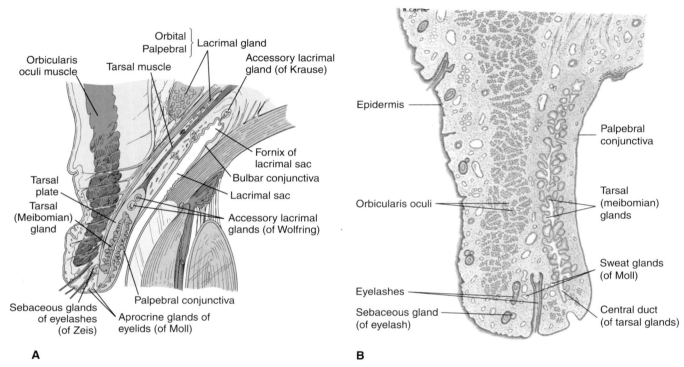

A

B

Figure 58.3 **Overview. A.** Structure of eyelid. This schematic drawing of the eyelid shows the skin, associated skin appendages, muscles, tendons, connective tissue, and conjunctiva. Note the distribution of multiple small glands associated with the eyelid and observe the reflection of the palpebral conjunctiva in the fornix of the lacrimal sac to become the bulbar conjunctiva. **B.** Photomicrograph of a sagittal section of the eyelid stained with picric acid for better visualization of epithelial components of the skin and the numerous glands. In this preparation, muscle tissue (i.e., orbicularis oculi muscle) stains yellow, and the epithelial cells of skin, conjunctiva, and glandular epithelium are green. Note the presence of the numerous glands within the eyelid. The tarsal (Meibomian) gland is the largest gland, and it is located within the dense connective tissue of the tarsal plates. This sebaceous gland secretes into ducts opening onto the eyelids. Original magnification, ×20. Inset. Higher magnification of a tarsal gland from the *boxed area,* showing the typical structure of a holocrine gland. Original magnification, ×20.

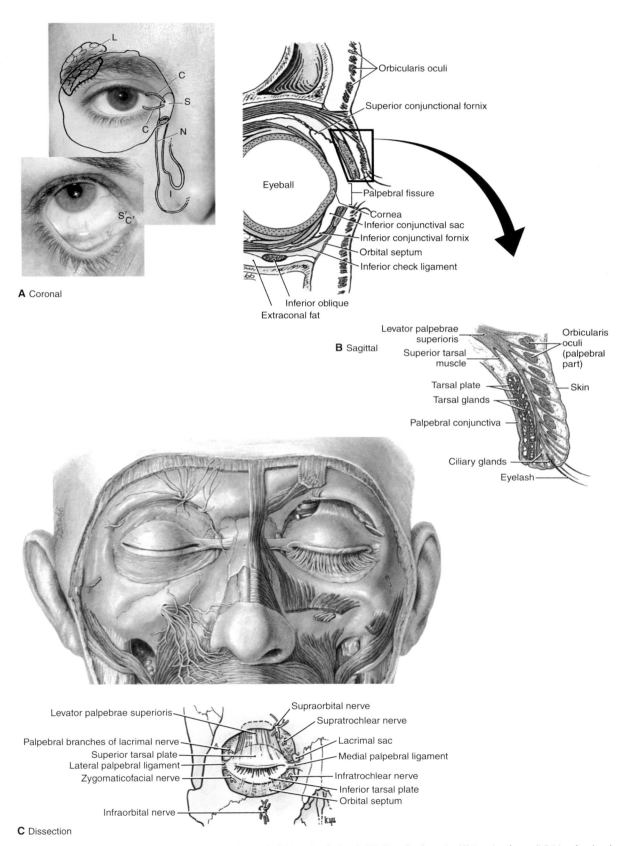

Figure 58.4 **Three-planar T-oncoanatomy. A.** Coronal. (L) Lacrimal gland; (C) Caniculunaris; (S) Lacrimal sac; (N) Nasalacrimal duct. (S′) Plica semilu; (C′) Lacrimal caruncle. **B.** Sagittal. **C.** Transverse.

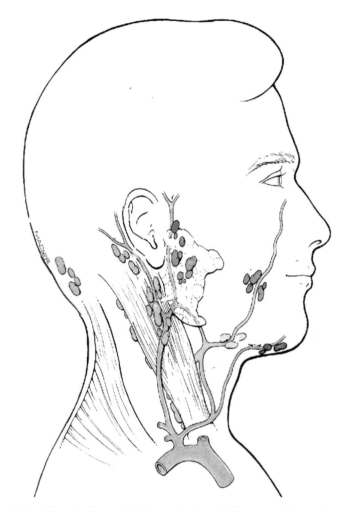

Figure 58.5 **N-oncoanatomy.** Lateral view. Preauricular node is the sentinel node. The preauricular node is the sentinel node.

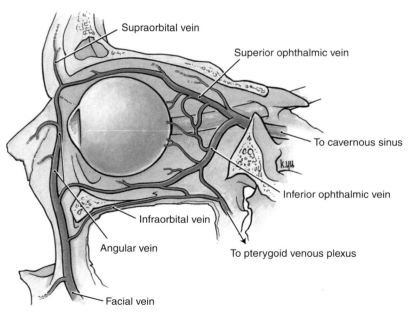

Supraorbital vein

Superior ophthalmic vein

To cavernous sinus

Inferior ophthalmic vein

Infraorbital vein

To pterygoid venous plexus

Angular vein

Facial vein

Figure 58.6 **M-oncoanatomy of the eye.** Venous drainage of eyelid.

TABLE 58.2	Imaging Modalities: Eye and Orbit	
Method	**Diagnosis and Staging Capability**	**Recommended for Use**
CT	Provides excellent anatomic detail of globe, orbital content and bony orbit. Can distinguish smooth, round cysts from infiltrative tumors versus pseudotumors and detect bone destruction and sinus invasion.	Yes
Primary tumor ultrasonography and fine-needle aspiration biopsy	A scan and B scan can be used to sreen intraocular and orbital tumors and cysts, especially melanomas	No
MRI	Provides excellent 3D view, orbital fat hyperintense and vitreous hypointense in tumor (T1) and reverse in T2; can detect tumors versus pseudotumors and cysts. May be superior for diagnosis of vascular lesions, demyelinating disease	Yes
Endoscopy	Orbital Endoscopy with fiber optic lights is used in conjunction with CT and/or MRI for obtaining core biopsy	Yes, when indicated
Standard orbital view	Useful for assessing optic nerve foramen and supraorbital fissure, but supplanted by CT; can detect intraocular calcification	No
Orbital phlebography	Venography particularly useful for detecting orbital varices, but is less efficient and more invasive than CT	No
Carotid angiography	Useful in diagnosis of vascularized tumors and aneurysms, but replaced by CT/MRI	No
Fluorescein angiography	Sometimes used in diagnosis of ocular melanoma	No
Biopsy	Usually an incisional or excisional biopsy is indicated to confirm malignant versus pseudotumors; directed stereotactically by CT/MRI; contraindicated for melanomas owing to high risk of seeding	Yes, if indicated

CT, computed tomography; MRI, magnetic resonance imaging.
Used with permission from Rubin P. *Clinical Oncology*. 7th ed. Philadelphia: WB Saunders; 1993:300.

59

Uvea

The uveal layer consists of 3 parts: the iris, ciliary body and choroid.

Perspective and Patterns of Spread

A nevus of the uveal tract may occur in the iris, ciliary body, or choroids. It can be recognized by its clinical appearance and course. The principle concern about a nevus of the eye is that it must be distinguished from a melanoma. This usually is possible because of its unchanging size, the absence of much elevation, and the fact that it interferes little with the function of the overlying retina when it occurs in the choroidal layer. However, differentiation of a large nevus from a small, dormant melanoma can be virtually impossible. In this case, routine, continued observation is mandatory. Hemangiomas of the uveal tract can be more troublesome and can show some signs of growth over a period of many years. It is usually possible to identify these tumors by use of intravenous fluorescein combined with examination of the fundus with cobalt blue light. Under these circumstances, hemangiomas fluoresce brightly.

Intraocular malignant melanoma is estimated to occur in about 0.05% of the eye-patient population. It is a tumor of adults; the average age is 50 years old. It is rare in blacks. Intraocular melanoma is the most common primary intraocular malignancy in countries with mainly white populations. Metastatic disease is the most common intraocular malignancy. There is no difference in distribution between the genders, nor is there any significant genetic relation except for the tumors predilection for whites. It is rarely associated with other melanomas, such as those of the skin. Conversely, cutaneous malignant melanomas do not commonly metastasize to the eye; however, 10 such cases were collected by Font et al.

The derivation of melanomas of the uvea has been the subject of a great deal of study and theory. It is possible that the stromal melanocytes of the uvea are the precursors of malignant melanoma. The pigmented epithelium of the retina, or of other neural crest–derived cells, is also implicated by some observers. Another hypothesis is that most melanomas arise in preexisting nevi.

Typical presentation depends on ophthalmoscopic examination. However, the term "intraocular

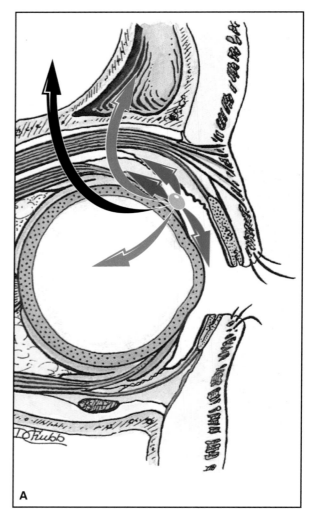

Figure 59.1 **Patterns of spread.** Primary cancers of the uvea include iris, uvea and choroid. Cancers are color coded for progression: Tis, yellow; T1, green; T2, blue; T3, purple; T4, red. **A.** Ciliary body *(continued)*

melanoma" may refer to a tumor appearing in any part of the uveal tract; this may include the iris, in which case the tumor may be visible on direct inspection. Iris melanomas may be diffuse rather than discrete nodules, presenting as heterochromia, or darkening of the iris. Acquired heterochromia in the presence of elevated intraocular pressure is particularly suspicious.

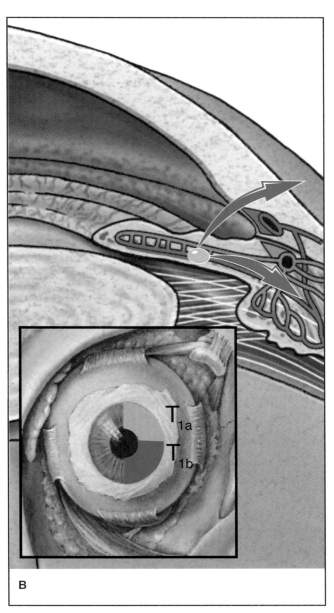

B

Figure 59.1 (*Continued*) **B.** Ciliary body.

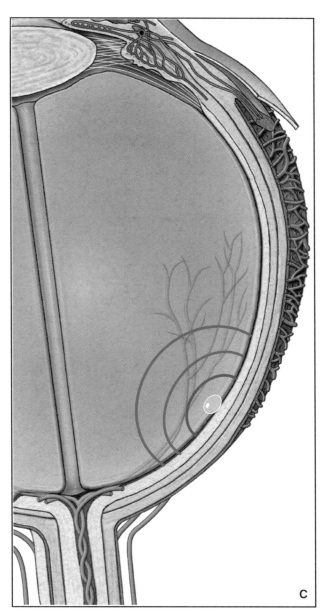

C

Figure 59.1 (*Continued*) **C.** Choroid

A Iris

DEFINITION OF TNM

B Choroid

STAGE GROUPINGS

T1
Tumor is limited to iris
(T1a) Tumor limited to the iris
not >3 clock hours in size
(T1b) Tumor limited to the iris
>3 clock hours in size
(T1c) Tumor limited to the iris
with melanomalytic glaucoma

N0
No regional lymph node
metastasis

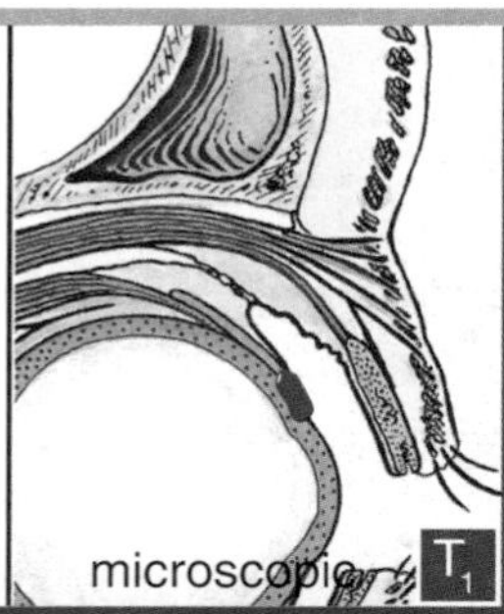

T1
Tumors ≤10 mm in greatest
diameter and ≤2.5 mm or less
in greatest height (thickness)
(T1a) without microscopic EOE
(T1b) with microscopic EOE
(T1c) without macroscopic EOE

N0
No regional lymph node
metastasis

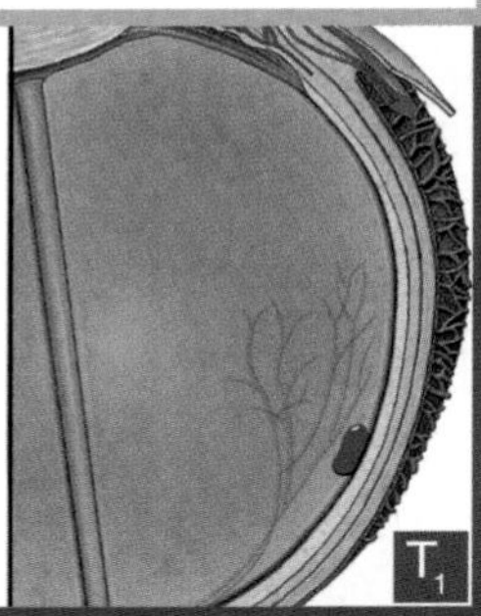

Stage I
T1   N0 M0
T1a N0 M0
T1b N0 M0
T1c N0 M0

I

T2
Tumor confluent with or
extending into the ciliary body
and/or choroid
(T2a) Tumor confluent with or
extending into the ciliary body
and/or choroid with
melanomalytic glaucoma

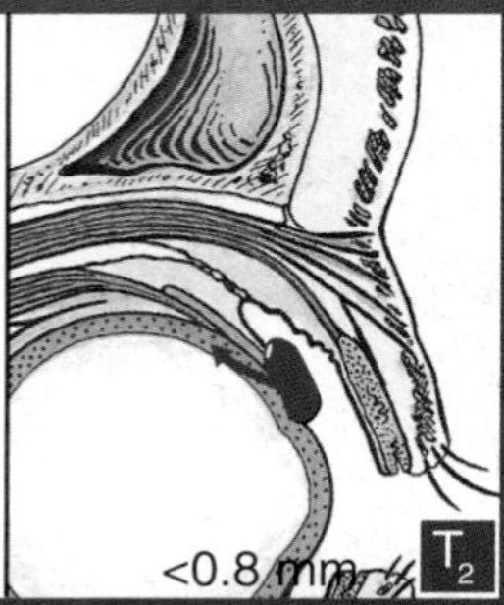

T2
Tumor 10–16 mm in greatest
basal diameter, 2.5–10 mm in
max. height
(T2a) without microscopic EOE
(T2b) with microscopic EOE
(T2c) with macroscopic EOE

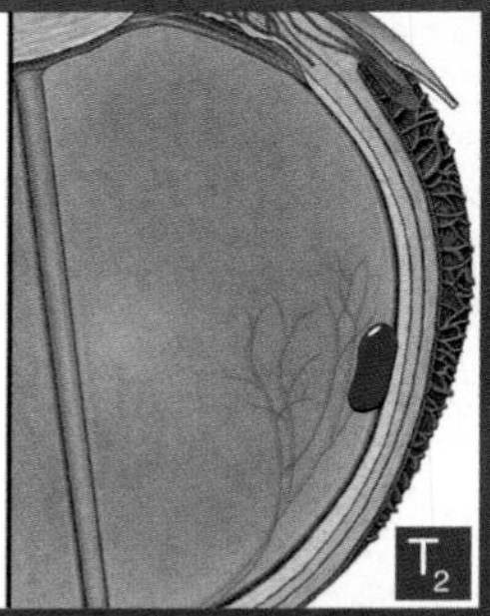

Stage II
T2   N0 M0
T2a N0 M0
T2b N0 M0
T2c N0 M0

II

T3
Tumor confluent with or
extending into the ciliary body
and/or choroid with scleral
extension
(T3a) Tumor confluent with or
extending into the ciliary body
with scleral extension and
melanomalytic glaucoma

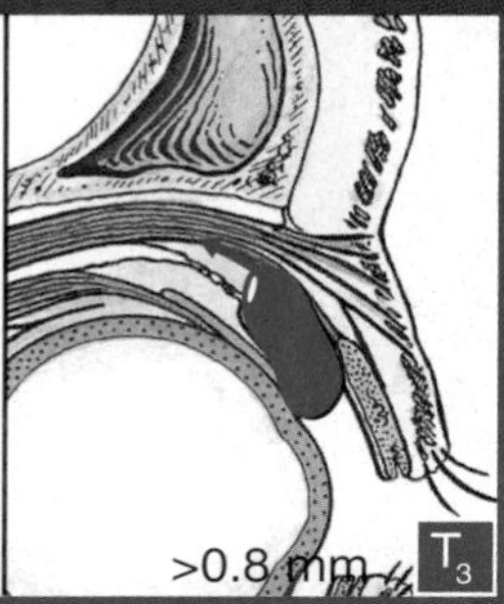

T3
Tumor >16 mm in greatest
basal diameter and/or >10 mm
in maximum height (thickness)
without EOE

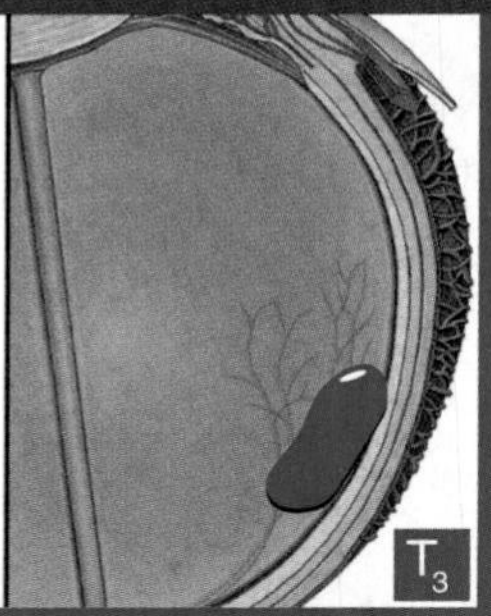

Stage III
T3 N0 M0

III

T4
Tumor with extraocular
extension

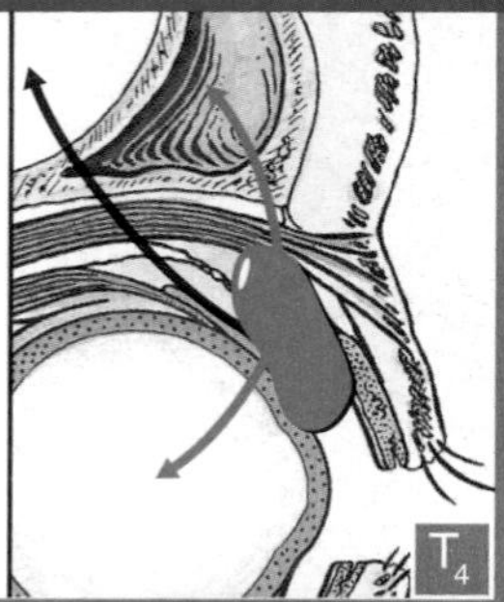

T4
Tumor more than 16 mm in
greatest diameter and/or
greater than 10 mm in
maximum height
(thickness) with extraocular
extension

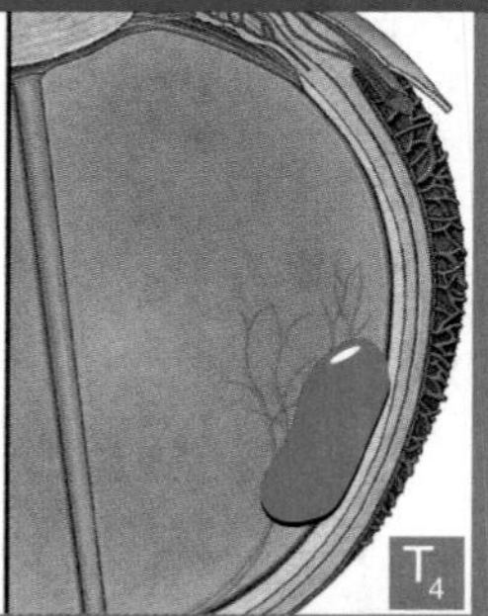

Stage III
T4 N0 M0

III

N1
Regional lymph node
metastasis

M1
Distant metastasis

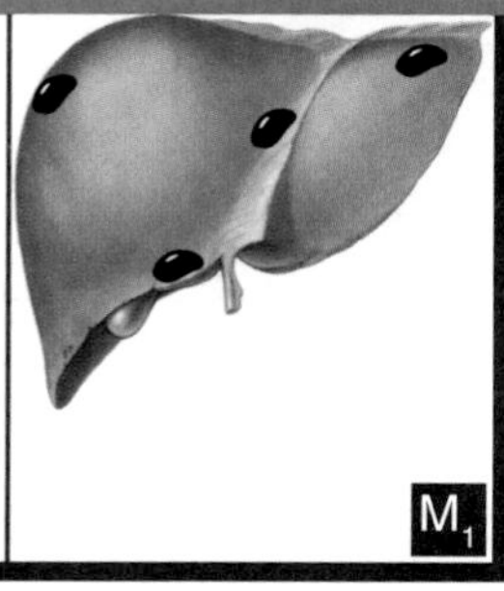

N1
Regional lymph node
metastasis

M1
Distant metastasis

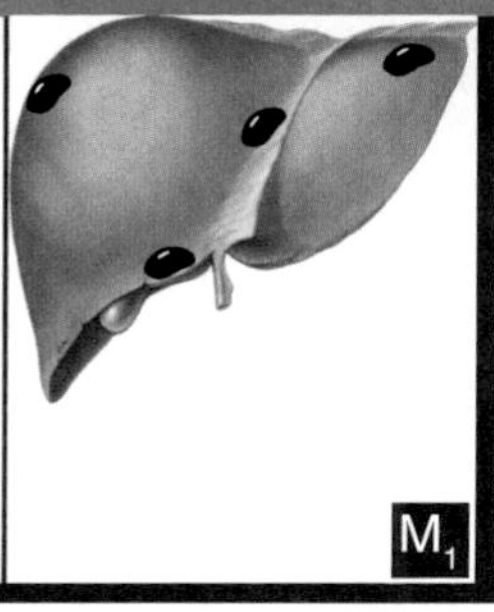

Stage IV
Any T N1   M0
Any T Any N M1

IV

Figure 59.2 **TNM staging criteria are color coded bars for stage advancement:** Stage I, green; II, blue; III, purple; III, red; and IV, black (metastatic).

TABLE 59.1	Histopathologic Types of Melanoma of the Uvea
Spindle cell melanoma	
Mixed cell melanoma	
Epithelioid cell melanoma	

Used with permission from Greene FL, Page DL, Fleming ID, et al., eds. *AJCC Cancer Staging Manual*. 6th ed. New York: Springer; 2002:367.

When it occurs in the choroid, the tumor most characteristically appears in an equatorial position within the eye. It is possible for the tumor to reach a relatively large size before it produces symptoms, such as loss of side vision or a sensation of floating spots. Therefore, the investigation of minor visual symptoms may be important. Tumor growth produces deterioration of vision as the retina overlying the tumor loses its function. The tumor frequently produces secondary changes within the eye, such as the induction of cataract, secondary glaucoma, iridocyclitis, and retinal detachment.

Histopathology has relied on Callender's classification (Table 59.1): Small, spindle-shaped cells with small condensed nuclei, referred to as spindle A, are the most benign. The 5-year mortality rate is <5%. Spindle melanoma type B is characterized by larger, more loosely packed spindle cells with prominent nucleoli. It is also relatively benign and has a 14% 5-year mortality rate. The pure epithelioid cell type occurs least commonly. This type is large and polygonal and has round nuclei, prominent cytoplasm, and resembles epithelial tumors. The mortality rate is 69%. Half of the melanomas of the eye have a mixture of cell types. The dangerous epithelioid cell types exhibit a 51% 5-year mortality rate.

Necrosis is rare in melanomas and occurs in only 7% of tumors. When it occurs, it may create severe inflammatory signs and secondary glaucoma. Pigmentation of the tumor varies from intense to amelanotic. The degree of pigmentation correlates only slightly with the degree of malignancy. Reticulin fibers are frequent and heavy in some tumors, and light in others. Reticulin content is only slightly correlated with prognosis. Newer prognostic parameters include number of mitotic figures per high-power field, and inverse standard deviation of tumor cell nucleolar area.

TNM Patterns of Spread and Staging Criteria

According to Reese, the distribution of melanomas were predominantly in the choroid (78%), then the iris (12%), and the ciliary body (10%). It is for this reason that only true choroidal melanoma is illustrated. The most common patterns of spread are intraocular via the choroidal venous network and then through the sclera extraocularly into the orbit (Fig. 59.1). Distant spread is possible since melanomas of the choroid exit via retinal veins into the internal jugular vein. Remarkably, liver is the target organ rather than lung. In fact, severe hepatomegaly due to extensive metastatic disease without an obvious gastro-intestinal tract cancer, should suggest a search for an intraocular choroidal melanoma.

Summary of Changes

The staging criteria have been modified but essentially are based on size again, measured in millimeters, both width and height: T1, <1 × 2.5 mm; T2, >10–16 × 2.5–10 mm; T3, >16 × >10 mm; and T4, extraocular extension (Fig. 59.2).

Orientation

The isocenter is anteriorly at the uvea, which is at the junction of anterior and posterior chamber (Fig. 59.3).

T-oncoanatomy

The middle layer of the globe is best appreciated in an axial view through the isocenter of globe at the pupil of the eye through to the optic nerve. The uvea is the rich vascular layer of the eye (Fig. 59.4).

- *Axial*: As most eye structures, this layer consists of three parts: (i) the iris, (ii) a ciliary body (pupil), (iii) and the choroid. The eye also contains three chambers: (i) anterior between cornea and iris, (ii) posterior between the iris and lens, and (iii) the vitreous body, which fills the globe with a gelatinous substance between lens and retina. Because this layer is pigmented, it can give rise to melanoma at any site. The major anatomic feature is the extensive vascular mesh and one can appreciate the access melanomas have to venous drainage via the vorticose vein.

- *Sagittal*: The pupil is surrounded by the iris and is the window of the eye. It is under control of the sympathetic and oculomotor nerves. Hoerner syndrome results in a small pupil and lidlag or ptosis. The pupil of the eye often can provide a major insight into numerous systemic disorders. Dilation of conjunctival capillaries is often benign and due to irritation, allergy, or infection. Ciliary injections as small capillaries surrounding a dilated pupil is an emergency

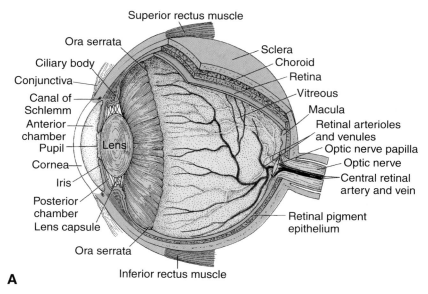

A

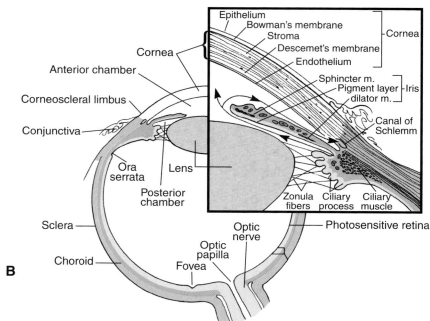

B

Figure 59.3 **Overview.** **A.** Schematic diagram illustrating the internal structures of the human eye. The retina consists of photosensitive and nonphotosensitive regions that differ in their function. Note that the photosensitive region of the retina occupies the posterior part of the eye and terminates anteriorly along the ora serrata. The nonphotosensitive region of the retina is located anterior to the ora serrata and lines the inner aspect of the ciliary body and the posterior surface of the iris. The other layers of the eyeball as well as the attachment of two of the extraocular muscles to the sclera are also shown. **B.** Schematic diagram of the structure of the eye. This drawing shows a horizontal section of the eyeball with color-coded layers of its wall. Upper inset. Enlargement of the anterior and posterior chambers shown in more detail. Note the direction of the flow of aqueous humor (arrows), which is drained by the scleral venous sinus (canal of Schlemm) at the iridocorneal angle.

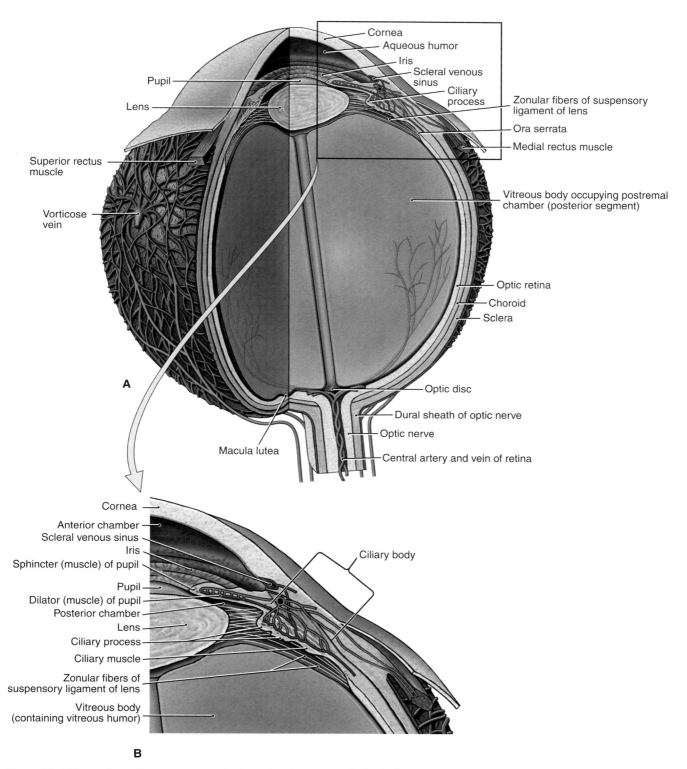

Figure 59.4 **Three-planar T-oncoanatomy. A.** Coronal and transverse. **B.** Sagittal.

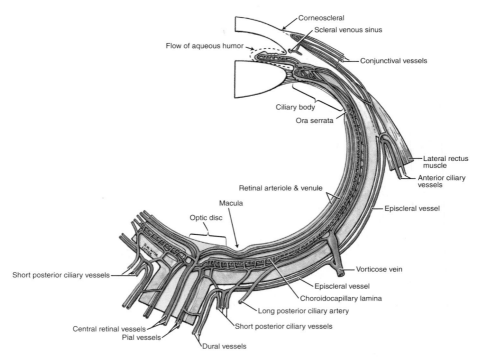

Figure 59.5 **M-oncoanatomy of the eye.** The choroid is drained by posterior ciliary veins, and four to five vorticose veins drain into the ophthalmic veins.

TABLE 59.2	Imaging Modalities: Eye and Orbit	
Method	**Diagnosis and Staging Capability**	**Recommended for Use**
CT	Provides excellent anatomic detail of globe, orbital content and bony orbit. Can distinguish smooth, round cysts from infiltrative tumors versus pseudotumors and detect bone destruction and sinus invasion.	Yes
Primary tumor ultrasonography and fine-needle aspiration biopsy	A scan and B scan can be used to screen intraocular and orbital tumors and cysts, especially melanomas	No
MRI	Provides excellent 3D view, orbital fat hyperintense and vitreous hypointense in tumor (T1) and reverse in T2; can detect tumors versus pseudotumors and cysts. May be superior for diagnosis of vascular lesions, demyelinating disease	Yes
Endoscopy	Orbital Endoscopy with fiber optic lights is used in conjunction with CT and/or MRI for obtaining core biopsy	Yes, when indicated
Standard orbital view	Useful for assessing optic nerve foramen and supraorbital fissure, but supplanted by CT; can detect intraocular calcification	No
Orbital phlebography	Venography particularly useful for detecting orbital varices, but is less efficient and more invasive than CT	No
Carotid angiography	Useful in diagnosis of vascularized tumors and aneurysms, but replaced by CT/MRI	No
Fluorescein angiography	Sometimes used in diagnosis of ocular melanoma	No
Biopsy	Usually an incisional or excisional biopsy is indicated to confirm malignant versus pseudotumors; directed stereotactically by CT/MRI; contraindicated for melanomas owing to high risk of seeding	Yes, if indicated

CT, computed tomography; MRI, magnetic resonanceimaging; 3D, three-dimensional.
Used with permission from Rubin P. *Clinical Oncology.* 7th ed. Philadelphia: WB Saunders; 1993:300.

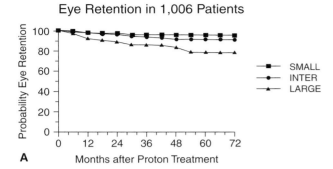

A

B

Figure 59.6 **Survival and eye retention probability. A.** Kaplan-Meier plot of eye retention probability after proton therapy in 1,006 patients with small (<3 mm high and <10 mm in diameter), intermediate (3.1–8 mm high and/or 10.1–16 mm in diameter), and large (>8 mm high and >16 mm in diameter) uveal melanomas; **B.** Kaplan-Meier plot of the probability of retaining useful vision in patients with tumors, 3 mm from the optic disc (D) and fovea (F) and >3 mm from the optic disc and/or fovea in 562 eyes with initial visual acuity 20/200 (6/60) or better.

suggesting glaucoma. The lens of the eye, the site of potential cataract formation, completes the middle layer of the eye and iris.

N-oncoanatomy

The eye globe is immunologically privileged and has no lymphatics or regional lymph nodes.

M-oncoanatomy

The pterygoid plexus of veins drain the fine veins of the eyelids into the internal jugular vein (Fig. 59.5).

Rules for Classification and Staging

Clinical Staging and Imaging

The clinical assessment requires inspection by slit-lamp examination and ophthalmoscopy. Imaging is highly desirable, especially computed tomography (CT) and fluorescein angiography (Table 59.2). If retinal detachment raises suspicion of choroidal metastases, films or CT of chest should be considered. In women, mammography is worthwhile.

Pathologic Staging

Resection of primary site with margins is essential and may include iridectomy to eyewall resection to enucleation of globe. Measurements should include size (height and depth) of choroidal lesion, measurements of iris uveal lesion in clock hours of involvement, and margin of resection. Sentinel and/or palpable regional nodes include size and location.

Cancer Statistics and Survival

The eye and orbit only account for 2,090 new diagnoses annually, excluding carcinomas of the eyelids. Deaths attributed to ocular malignancy are <10% of the entire group (<200 patients/year). Some of the most elegant proton and three-dimensional conformal radiation stereotactic techniques allow for cure of choroidal melanomas and retinoblastoma with preservation of vision. Results from ocular melanomas are presented in Figure 59.6. Survival remains impressive, with 90% long-term survival.

- Posterior uveal/choroidal melanomas demonstrated that radiation isotopic plaque and enucleation were found to be comparable in the Collaborative Ocular Melanoma Study group consisting of 1,300 patients over 11.5 years. Recurrence rates with radiation range about 15%, and <5% with surgery.
- The probability of choroids melanoma control by the Harvard proton beam control is 96.3%. The absolute local recurrence rate after helium ion therapy is <3%. Custom plaque irradiation appears to be an effective method for treating iris melanomas as well.

Trilateral neuroblastoma occurs when both eyes are involved and there is a pinealblastoma in the pineal gland.

Perspective and Patterns of Spread

Retinoblastoma is a hereditary malignancy and occurs in approximately 1 in 20,000 live births. There is no known difference in the incidence between whites and blacks, males and females, or in children in various parts of the world. Thirty percent of retinoblastomas are bilateral and all bilateral tumors are germinal. Forty percent of all retinoblastomas are germinal (i.e., 25% of all unilateral tumors are germinal). In these cases, there is a 100% chance of an autosomal-dominant pattern of hereditary transmission to the next generation as well as a life-long significant risk of development of a second nonocular malignancy (85%). More than 90% of retinoblastoma cases are diagnosed before age 5 years. The median age at diagnosis is 14 months for bilateral cases and 23 months for unilateral tumors. There is a 5% association with other congenital defects, of which mental retardation is the most common. In the syndrome designated Dq-1, half of the patients have retinoblastoma, as well as a high incidence of other defects, including psychomotor retardation, skeletal abnormalities, congenital heart disease, and other eye defects. Spontaneous regression occurs in 1% of all retinoblastoma patients. This has been attributed to the tumor's outgrowing its vascular supply and becoming infarcted and necrotic.

Retinoblastoma has been documented to result from a genetic mutation. Retinoblastoma behaves like an autosomal-dominant syndrome with a >90% penetrance, but the abnormal tumor-producing mutant allele is recessive. Seventy percent of retinoblastomas present as unilateral tumors. In all the bilateral and in 25% of the unilateral presentations, a germinal mutation affecting all cells in the body has occurred. Despite the high occurrence rate of germinal mutations (40% of cases), only 12% of patients have a positive family history; the other 88% represent the first germinal mutation in the family.

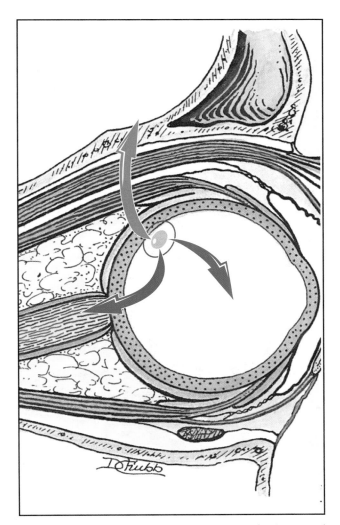

Figure 60.1 **Patterns of spread.** Primary cancers of retina are color coded for progression: T0, yellow; T1, green; T2, blue; T3, purple; T4, red.

DEFINITION OF TNM

T1
Tumor confined to the retina (no vitreous seeding or significant retinal detachment). No retinal detachment or subretinal fluid > 5 mm from the base of the tumor
(T1a) Any eye in which the largest tumor is ≤3 mm in height **and** no tumor is located closer than 1 DD (1.5 mm) to the optic nerve or fovea
(T1b) All other eyes in which the tumor(s) are confined to the retina regardless of location or size (up to half the volume of the eye). No vitreous seeding. No retinal detachment or subretinal fluid >5 mm from the base of the tumor

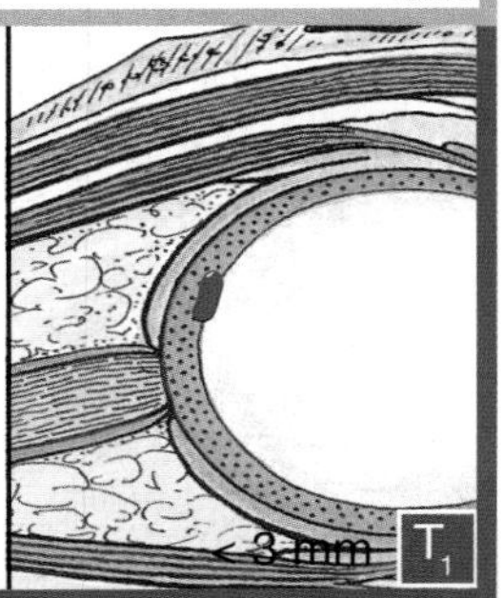

T2
Tumor with contiguous spread to adjacent tissues or spaces (vitreous or subretinal space)
(T2a) *Minimal tumor spread to vitreous and/or subretinal space.* Fine local or diffuse vitreous seeding and/or serous retinal detachment up to total detachment may be present, but **no** clumps, lumps, snowballs, or avascular masses **are allowed** in the vitreous or subretinal space. Calcium flecks in the vitreous or subretinal space are allowed. The tumor may fill up to 2/3 the volume of the eye.
(T2b) *Massive tumor spread to the vitreous and/or subretinal space.* Vitreous seeding and/or subretinal implantation may consist of lumps, clumps, snowballs, or avascular tumor masses. Retinal detachment may be total. Tumor may fill up to 2/3 the volume of the eye.
(T2c) Unsalvageable intraocular disease. Tumor fills >2/3 the eye or there is no possibility of visual rehabilitation or one or more of the following are present:
• Tumor-associated glaucoma, either neovascular or angle closure
• Anterior segment extension of tumor
• Ciliary body extension of tumor
• Hyphema (significant)
• Massive vitreous hemorrhage
• Tumor in contact with lens
• Orbital cellulites-like clinical presentation (massive tumor necrosis)

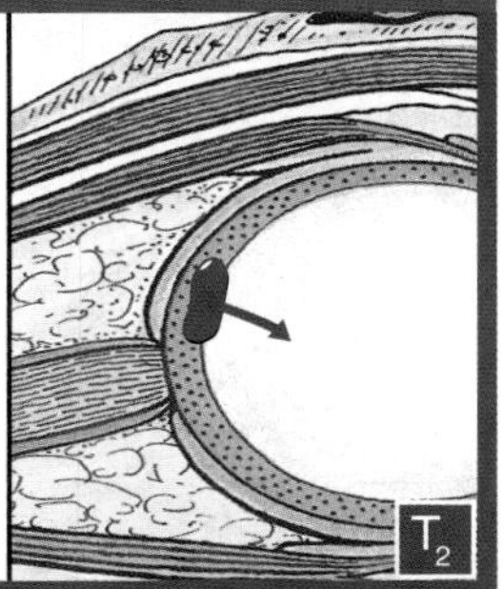

T3
Invasion of the optic nerve and/or optic coats

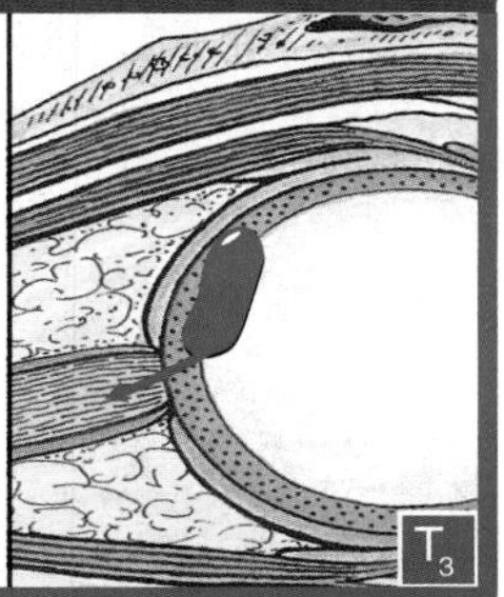

T4
Extraocular tumor

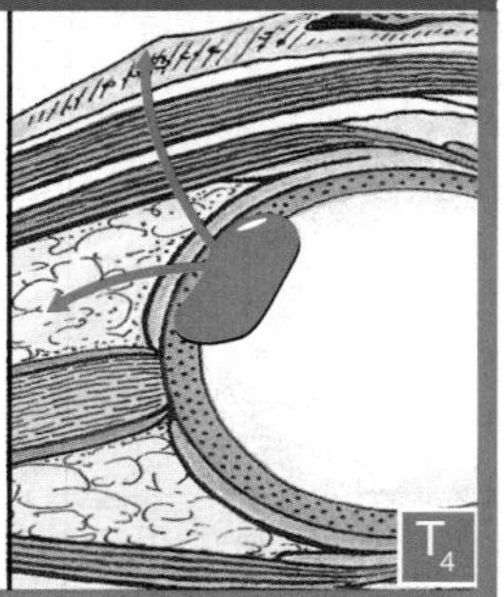

N1
Regional lymph node involvement (preauricular, submandibular, or cervical)

N2
Distant lymph node involvement

M1
Metastasis to central nervous system and/or bone, bone marrow, or other sites

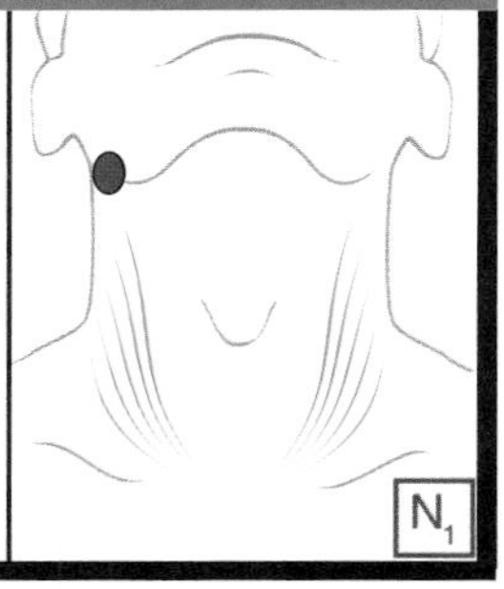

Figure 60.2 TNM staging criteria are color coded bars for T advancement: T0, yellow; T1, green; T2, blue; T3, purple; T4, red; and metastatic black.

TABLE 60.1	Histopathologic Types of Retinoblastomas
Retinoblastoma, NOS	
Retinoblastoma, differentiated	
Retinoblastoma, undifferentiated	
Retinoblastoma, diffuse	

NOS, not otherwise specified.
Used with permission from Greene FL, Page DL, Fleming ID, et al., eds. *AJCC Cancer Staging Manual*. 6th ed. New York: Springer; 2002:373.

Retinoblastoma conforms to the two-hit Knudson's hypothesis, in which two chromosomal mutational events are necessary to cause cancer. In the hereditary form, the mutational event affects a germ cell and thus all cells in the body, whereas in nongerminal cell cases, a single retinal cell is affected. The normal allele at the retinoblastoma locus is currently thought to act as a controller gene or suppressor of the malignant retinoblastoma growth. Thus, both alleles must be lost before malignant growth can ensue. In the hereditary cases, all cells have lost one normal allele, and the chance of several retinal cells losing the second allele is quite high, resulting in bilateral or multicentric tumor growth at an earlier age (median, 14 months). In the nonhereditary or somatic form, one retinal cell has lost one allele and must lose the second before a unicentric, unilateral tumor arises, usually at a later age (median, 23 months). Thus, in nongerminal cases, the chance of bilateral mutations (two hits) on two separate retinal cells is low, and the chance that a bilateral tumor would be nongerminal or somatic is equally low. Because 50% of the offspring of germinal retinoblastoma patients are affected, prenatal or presymptomatic diagnosis is crucial. A few laboratories have developed diagnostic tests to identify the retinoblastoma gene in this group of patients. Detection of the gene in the 15% of patients with unilateral disease that have the germinal mutation is also important because they carry a lifelong risk of secondary malignancies. Healthy parents who have a single affected child can expect an attack rate of 6% among their other offspring. An unaffected sibling of a child with sporadic retinoblastoma, like one of his parents, may be a carrier; however, the risk is extremely low (<1%). If retinoblastoma occurs more than once in a given pedigree, there is a 40% to 48% chance that the affected members of this pedigree will have offspring with retinoblastoma. The unaffected members have a chance of only 5% to 20%.

Retinoblastoma usually arises from the posterior portion of the retina and consists of small, closely packed, round or polygonal cells with dark staining nucleus and scanty cytoplasm (Table 60.1). In many cases, the tumor cells are arranged in rosettes, but their absence does not necessarily exclude this diagnosis. Histopathologic classification of retinoblastoma permits a certain amount of separation between more and less differentiated tumor varieties. The more differentiated tumors show small rosettes that are thought to represent differentiated spongioblasts (neuroepitheliomas). The tumor often outgrows its blood supply. Areas of necrosis are common and are responsible for the formation of calcium deposits. Rarely, the tumor may become so necrotic as to destroy itself entirely, giving rise to the rare instance of spontaenous regression. The necrotizing tendency of the tumor is one of the factors responsible for the occasional intense ocular inflammation that may be highly misleading clinically.

TNM Staging Criteria

The tumor spreads readily within the eye (Fig. 60.1). Trilateral retinoblastoma occurs when both eyes are involved and pineoblastoma occurs in the pineal gland. This rare but interesting combination illustrates that the pineal or third eye shares the same developmental anlage as the retina. This diagnosis must be considered in a patient with bilateral retinoblastoma who subsequently develops headache or lethargy.

There have been numerous changes to the subgrouping under each stage (Fig. 60.2). T1 is localized to retina, vitreous or subretinal space (contained in retinal layer); T2 is minimal invasion of optic duct/nerve/coats, whereas T3 indicates significant invasion of optic duct/nerve/coats. T4 is massive extraocular extension into orbit, subarachnoid space, brain, and optic chiasm. There are numerous attempts to stage retinoblastoma; the most frequently utilized is the Reese-Ellsworth system (Table 60.2).

Summary of Changes

T1, T2, T3, have redefined with division into subcategories a, b, c, M1a and M1b.

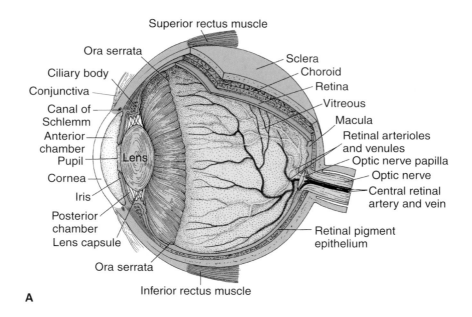

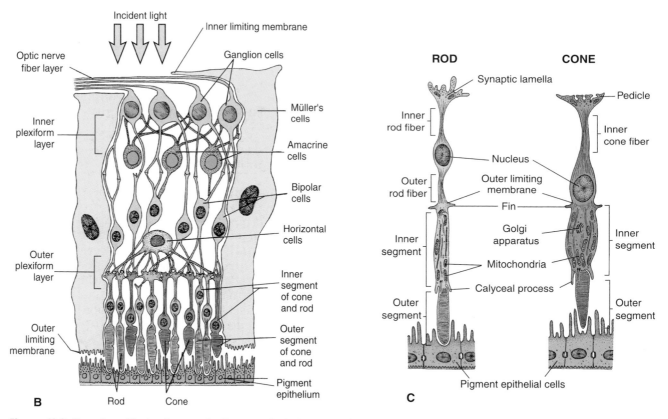

Figure 60.3 **Overview: Photomicrograph diagram. A.** Retina: Inner layer. Schematic diagram illustrating the internal structures of the human eye. The retina consists of photosensitive and nonphotosensitive regions that differ in their function. Note that the photosensitive region of the retina occupies the posterior part of the eye and terminates anteriorly along the ora serrata. The nonphotosensitive region of the retina is located anterior to the ora serrata and lines the inner aspect of the ciliary body and the posterior surface of the iris. The other layers of the eyeball as well as the attachment of two of the extraocular muscles to the sclera are also shown. **B.** Ultrastructure of retina. Schematic drawing of the layers of the retina. The interrelationship of the neurons is indicated. Light enters the retina and passes through the inner layers of the retina before reaching the photoreceptors of the rods and cones that are closely associated with the pigment epithelium. **C.** Ultrastructure of rod and cones. Schematic diagram of the ultrastructure of rod and cone cells. The outer segments of the rods and cones are closely associated with the adjacent pigment epithelium.

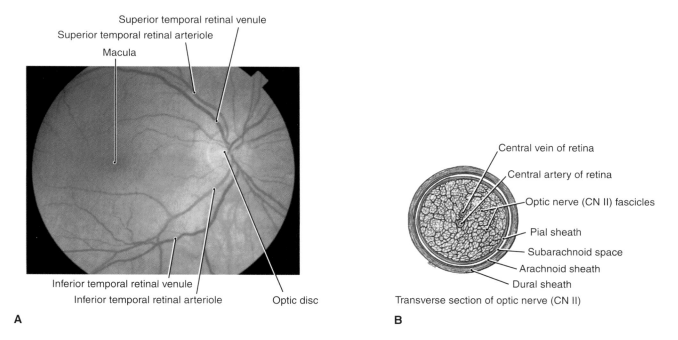

Superior temporal retinal venule
Superior temporal retinal arteriole
Macula

Inferior temporal retinal venule
Inferior temporal retinal arteriole
Optic disc

A

Central vein of retina
Central artery of retina
Optic nerve (CN II) fascicles
Pial sheath
Subarachnoid space
Arachnoid sheath
Dural sheath

Transverse section of optic nerve (CN II)

B

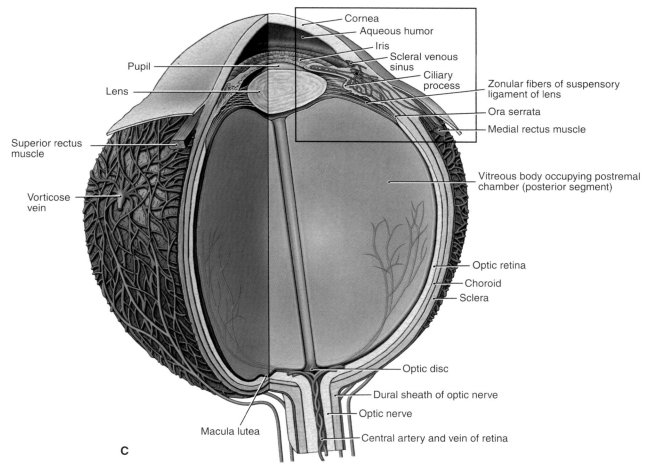

Cornea
Aqueous humor
Iris
Scleral venous sinus
Ciliary process
Zonular fibers of suspensory ligament of lens
Ora serrata
Medial rectus muscle

Pupil
Lens
Superior rectus muscle
Vorticose vein

Vitreous body occupying postremal chamber (posterior segment)

Optic retina
Choroid
Sclera

Optic disc
Dural sheath of optic nerve
Optic nerve
Central artery and vein of retina

Macula lutea

C

Figure 60.4 **Three-planar T-oncoanatomy. A.** Right ocular fundus, ophthalmoscopic view. Retinal venules (wider) and retinal arterioles (narrower) radiate from the center of the oval optic disc, formed in relation to the entry of the optic nerve into the eyeball. The *round, dark area* lateral to the disc is the macula; branches of vessels extend to this area, but do not reach its center, the fovea centralis, a depressed spot that is the area of most acute vision. It is avascular but, like the rest of the outermost (cones and rods) layer of the retina, is nourished by the adjacent choriocapillaris. **B.** Transverse section of optic nerve. Note the subarachnoid space that surrounds the optic nerve and lies between the pial and arachnoid sheath, both of which are surrounded by the dura. **C.** Sagittal and transverse cross-section of eyeball. The aqueous humor is produced by the ciliary processes and provides nutrients for the avascular cornea and lens; the aqueous humor drains into the scleral venous sinus (also called the *sinus venosus sclerae* or *canal of Schlemm*). If drainage of the aqueous humor is reduced significantly, pressure builds up in the chambers of the eye (glaucoma).

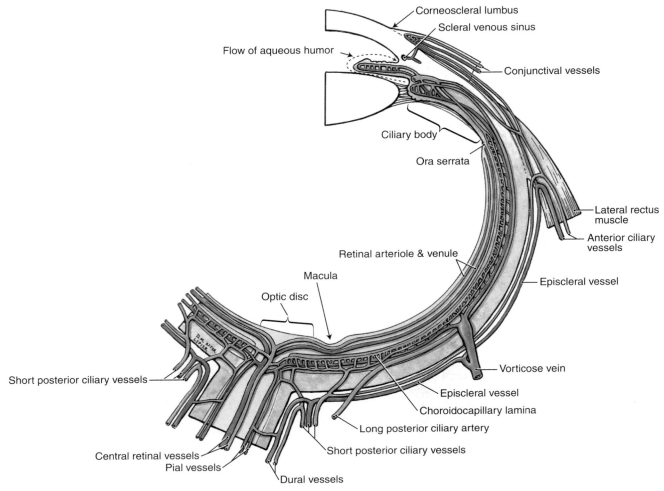

Figure 60.5 M-oncoanatomy of the eye. The choroid is drained by posterior ciliary veins, and four to five vorticose veins drain into the ophthalmic veins.

TABLE 60.2	The Reese-Ellsworth System of Classifying Retinoblastoma

Group I: Very favorable
A. Solitary tumor, <4DD* in diameter, at or behind the equator
B. Multiple tumors, none >4DD in diameter, all at or behind the equator

Group II: Favorable
A. Solitary tumor, 4–10 DD in diameter, at or behind the equator
B. Multiple tumors, 4–10 DD in diameter, all at or behind the equator

Group III: Doubtful
A. Any lesion anterior to the equator
B. Solitary tumors >10 DD in diameter, behind the equator

Group IV: Unfavorable
A. Multiple tumors, some >10 DD in diameter
B. Any lesion extending anterior to the ora serrata

Group V: Very unfavorable
A. Massive tumors involving more than half of the retina
B. Vitreous seeding

*The optic nerve's exit (the optic nerve head or disc) is approximately 1.5 mm in diameter. The disc diameter (DD) often is used as a measure of tumor dimensions.
Used with permission from Halperin EC, Constine LS, Tarbell, NJ, et al. *Pediatric Radiation Oncology*. 4th ed. Philadelphia: Lippincott Williams & Wilkins; 2005:144.

TABLE 60.3	Imaging Modalities Eye and Orbit	
Method	Diagnosis and Staging Capability	Recommended for Use
CT	Provides excellent anatomic detail of globe, orbital content and bony orbit; can distinguish smooth, round cysts from infiltrative tumors versus pseudotumors and detect bone destruction and sinus invasion	Yes
Primary tumor ultrasonography and fine-needle aspiration biopsy	A and B scans can be used to screen intraocular and orbital tumors and cysts, especially melanomas	No
MRI	Provides excellent 3D view, orbital fat hyperintense and vitreous hypointense in tumor (T1) and reverse in T2; can detect tumors versus pseudotumors and cysts; may be superior for diagnosis of vascular lesions, demyelinating disease	Yes
Endoscopy	Orbital endoscopy with fiber optic lights is used in conjunction with CT and/or MRI for obtaining core biopsy	Yes, when indicated
Standard orbital view	Useful for assessing optic nerve foramen and supraorbital fissure, but supplanted by CT; can detect intraocular calcification	No
Orbital phlebography	Venography particularly useful for detecting orbital varices, but is less efficient and more invasive than CT	No
Carotid angiography	Useful in diagnosis of vascularized tumors and aneurysms, but replaced by CT/MRI	No
Fluorescein angiography	Sometimes used in diagnosis of ocular melanoma	No
Biopsy	Usually an incisional or excisional biopsy is indicated to confirm malignant versus pseudotumors; directed stereotactically by CT/MRI; contraindicated for melanomas owing to high risk of seeding	Yes, if indicated

CT, computed tomography; 3D, three-dimensional; MRI, magnetic resonance imaging.
Used with permission from Rubin P. *Clinical Oncology.* 7th ed. Philadelphia: WB Saunders; 1993:300.

Overview

Layers of the retina includes the interrelationships of the neurons and the supporting cells are variously defined as many different types of neurons and multiple synapses but are classified in three categories: (i) Photoreceptors—retinal rods and cones, (ii) conducting neurons—bipolar and ganglion cells, and (iii) association with other neurons—horizontal, centrifugal amacrine supporting cells. The ultrastructure of the rod and cone is an (i) inner fiber, (ii) inner segment, and, (iii) outer segment (Fig. 60.3).

T-oncoanatomy

The retina is the innermost layer of the eye and its posterior (75%) portion is photosensitive and is stimulated by light. Anteriorly, it ends at the ora serrata. The photo receptor cells are rods (color) and cones (black and white). Leaving the retina are nerve fibers that form the optic disc and nerve and pass signals to the brain. There are sight strata of cells; in addition to the optic disc, there is the macula and an array of retinal arterioles and venules that characterize the eye grounds (Fig. 60.4).

Author	Year	No. of Eyes Irradiated	Groups I–V		Groups I–III	
			RT (%)	RT and Salvage (%)	RT (%)	RT and Salvage (%)
Cassady	1969	223	49	69	—	73
Egbert	1978	38	—	58	—	80
Schipper	1985	54	41	81	54	94
Foote	1989	25	29	79	40	80
Fontanesi	1995, 1996	7*	71	71	67	67
		13†	67	76	60	100
Toma	1995	67	72	93	69	92
Blach	1996	67‡	38	71	37	81
Scott	1999	113§	65	78	84	94

TABLE 60.4   Reported Eye Preservation Rates After Lens-Sparing External Beam Radiation Therapy

* >1 year old.
† <1 year old.
‡Anterior lens-sparing technique or modified lateral beam technique.
§ Modified lateral beam technique.
Used with permission from Halperin EC, Constine LS, Tarbell, NJ, et al. *Pediatric Radiation Oncology.* 4th ed. Philadelphia: Lippincott Williams & Wilkins; 2005:152.

N-oncoanatomy

The eye globe is immunologically privileged and has no lymphatics or regional lymph nodes.

M-oncoanatomy

It can seed itself throughout the interior of the eye and include the iris and anterior chamber (Fig. 60.5). Distant spread of retinoblastoma commonly occurs along the optic nerve. Here the tumor can spread readily along the meningeal spaces of the optic sheath and soon reach the subarachnoid space and seed out the cerebrospinal fluid. Distant spread can also occur though the bloodstream, most commonly to bone, lungs, and liver. The causes of death in this tumor are interesting. More than 90% of the patients have intracranial involvement; in almost 50% of all deaths, disease is confined to the cranial cavity and spinal cord; the remaining half have distant metastases. Distant metastasis occurs with equal incidence ($\approx$50%) of spread to lymph nodes, skull bones, distant bones, and viscera.

Rules for Classification and Staging

Clinical Staging and Imaging

Examination under anesthesia is most desirable and if simple orbital radiographs show calcification in the child's globe, it is pathognomonic for retinoblastoma (Table 60.3). Enhanced computed tomography is the preferred cross-sectional imaging, although magnetic resonance imaging is complimentary for extraocular soft tissue extension and especially to assess for optic nerve invasion. With multiple lesions, ultrasound identification of their location with detailed retinal drawings. In bilateral cases, each eye should be staged separately. Distance of tumor from disc, fovea, and ora serrata should noted in millimeters or estimated in terms of size of optic nerve disc (e.g., 1.5 × 1 or 2, etc.).

Pathologic Staging

If eye is sacrificed and enucleated, tumor size, invasion of optic nerve, and margins, if there is extraocular spread, need notation.

Cancer Statistics and Survival

The eye and orbit only account for 2,090 new diagnoses excluding carcinomas of the eyelids. Deaths attributed to ocular malignancy are <10% of the entire group (<200 patients/year). Some of the most elegant proton and three-dimensional conformal radiation stereotactic techniques allow for cure of choroidal melanomas and retinoblastoma with preservation of vision, the majority with eye preservation (Table 60.4). Survival remains impressive; 90% reach long-term survival.

- Retinoblastomas are highly curable; with radiation, >90% local tumor control is achieved with vision conservation. Those that relapse can still be cured by enucleation.
- In Africa and Asia, retinoblastoma is the most common primary intraocular malignancy.

61

Lacrimal Gland and Orbit

The lacrimal apparatus consists of 3 parts: Lacrimal gland, canaliculi and naso-lacrimal duct.

Perspective and Patterns of Spread

Lacrimal gland tumefactions tend to be associated with salivary gland infiltrations in Mikulicz disease and in lymphomas, referred to as Mikulicz syndrome. The lacrimal gland is one of the least common sites for adenocarcinomas. Curiously, investigations at the AFIP provided a histopathologic classification, which is similar to salivary gland neoplasms.

There are two entirely different groups of malignancy, one in the pediatric age group, mainly embryonal rhabdomyosarcomas (ERMS); in adults, there is the very uncommon adenocarcinoma of the lacrimal gland (Tables 61.1 and 61.2). Although ERMS can occur in multiple sites, the occurrence in orbits is not a common site (9%), but is often dramatic in presentation with sudden swelling, proptosis, discoloration, and dystopia owing to limited extraocular motion. The histopathology is characteristic with blastin cells that tend to differentiate into striated muscle with a tendency to cross-striations in 30% of patients. Most often cells are fusiform or stellate, but when undifferentiated they can be diffuse in pattern akin to primitive noncommitted mesenchymal cell. There can be other associated pediatric abnormalities and genetic defects.

TNM Staging Criteria

Lacrimal gland cancer remain confined to gland: T1, <2.5 cm; T2, <5 cm, but with extraglandular invasion; T3, in periosteum; and T4, into orbital soft tissues, optic nerve, globe and brain.

The embryonal RMS can invade the orbit and progresses to involve the globe, optic nerve, and even bone (Fig. 61.1). However, size is the dominant criteria in the staging system: Early with T1, <15 mm; T2, >15 mm; T3, limited invasion of orbital tissue and bone wall; and T4, extensive invasion into the globe and periorbital tissues, central nervous system, and brain (Fig. 61.2).

Overview

Lacrimal apparatus consists of three parts, as do the tears: (i) The lacrimal gland secretions are watery, the glands of the tarsal plate provide a waxy sebaceous secretion (Merbomian) and an oily film (Zeis and Moll), which is collected by (ii) canaliculi, the inner canthus into a lacrimal sac, and (iii) a lacrimal canal that vertically descends into the inferior nasal meatus below the inferior concha (Fig. 61.3).

T-oncoanatomy

The isocenter of the boney wall of the orbit, the eye socket, is through the optic nerve exiting at the optic foramen in its posterior wall. The orbital content anteriorly is the location of the lacrimal gland on its superior lateral wall (Fig. 61.4).

- *Coronal*: The true content is posterior to the globe where the extraocular muscles and their innervation by cranial nerves III, IV, and VI, which enter through the medially placed optic nerve as well as cranial nerve VI and the nasociliary nerve.
- *Sagittal*: The extraocular muscles and fat are appreciated in relation to the boney eye socket.
- *Axial*: Provides the medial entry of cranial nerves particularly the optic nerve offer access to the subarachnoid space and accounts of blurring of optic disc when intracranial metastatic disease occurs. Note the lateral superior location of the lacrimal gland.

N-oncoanatomy

The eyelids and conjunctiva drain predominantly into the preauricular nodes except for its medial margin, which follow medial lymphatics into the submandibular nodes (Fig. 61.5).

M-oncoanatomy

The pterygoid plexus of veins drain the fine veins of the eyelids into the internal jugular vein (Fig. 61.6).

Rules for Classification and Staging

Clinical Staging and Imaging

Careful examination is undertaken, preferably under anesthesia if deep in orbit. Imaging essential to

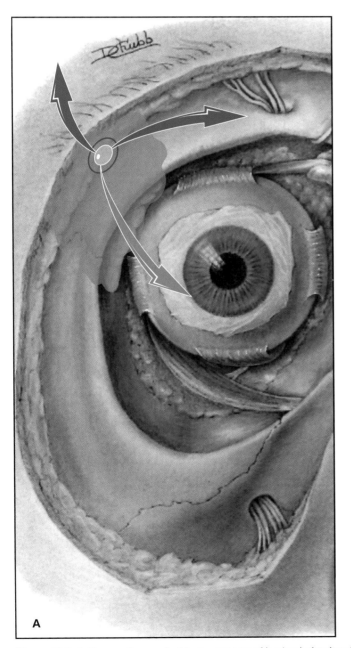

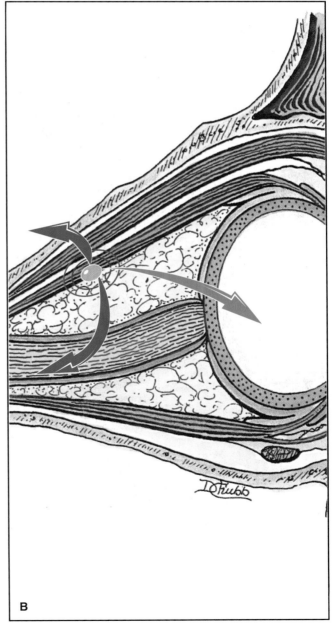

Figure 61.1 **Patterns of spread.** Primary cancers of lacrimal gland and orbit are color coded for progression: T0, yellow; T1, green; T2, blue; T3, purple; T4, red. **A.** Lacrimal gland. **B.** Orbit.

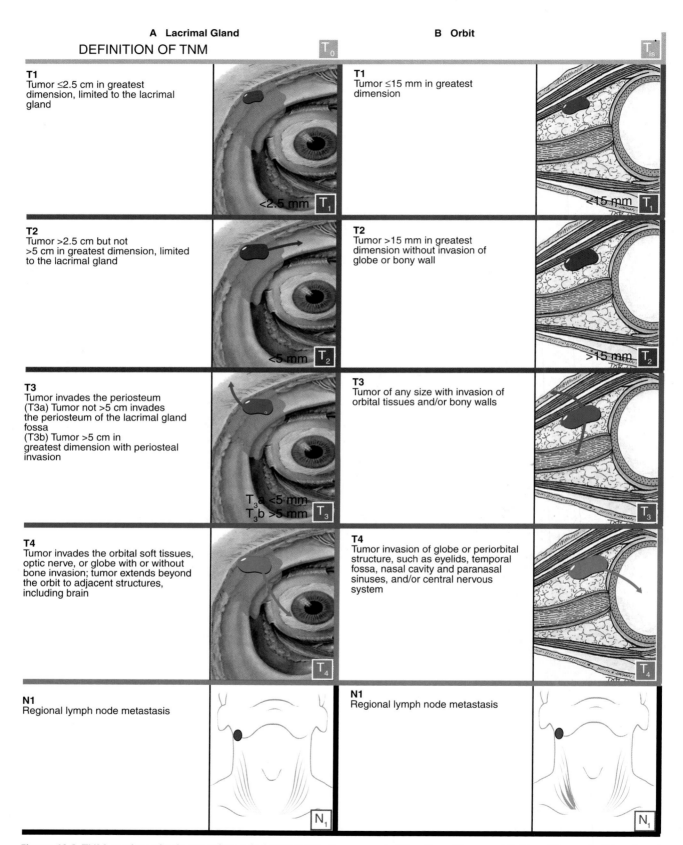

Figure 61.2 **TNM staging criteria are color coded bars for T advancement:** T0, yellow; T1, green; T2, blue; T3, purple; T4, red; and metastatic, black. **A.** Lacrimal gland. **B.** Orbit.

TABLE 61.1	Histopathologic Types of Sarcomas of the Orbit
Malignancies of the orbit primarily include a broad spectrum of malignant soft tissue tumors	

Used with permission from Greene FL, Page DL, Fleming ID, et al., eds. *AJCC Cancer Staging Manual.* 6th ed. New York: Springer; 2002:382.

determine if orbital mass is primary or metastatic. Cross-sectional imaging as enhanced computed tomography and magnetic resonance imaging are worthwhile. Ultrasound-guided biopsy deserves consideration (Table 61.3).

Pathologic Staging

For lacrimal gland cancer resections, complete specimen should be studied for margins. Perineural and sentinel preauricular/parotid node evaluation need to be recorded if positive.

Cancer Statistics and Survival

The eye and orbit only account for 2,090 new diagnoses excluding carcinomas of the eyelids. Deaths attributed to ocular malignancy are <10% of the entire group (<200 patients/year). Some of the most elegant proton and three-dimensional conformational radiation stereotactic techniques allow for cure of choroidal melanomas and retinoblastoma with preservation of vision (Fig. 61.7). Survival remains impressive; 90% reach long-term survival.

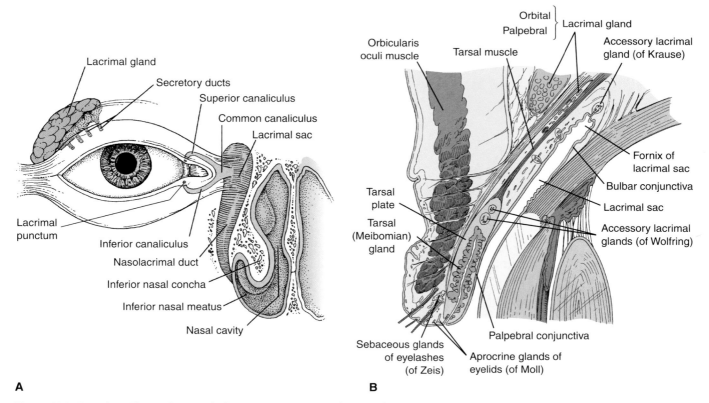

A   **B**

Figure 61.3 **Overview: Photomicrograph diagram.** **A.** Anterior. Schematic diagram of the eye and lacrimal apparatus. This drawing shows the location of the lacrimal gland and components of the lacrimal apparatus, which drains the lacrimal fluid into the nasal cavity. **B.** Lateral. Structure of the eyelid. This schematic drawing of the eyelid shows the skin, associated skin appendages, muscles, tendons, connective tissue, and conjunctiva. Note the distribution of multiple small glands associated with the eyelid and observe the reflection of the palpebral conjunctiva in the fornix of the lacrimal sac to become the bulbar conjunctiva.

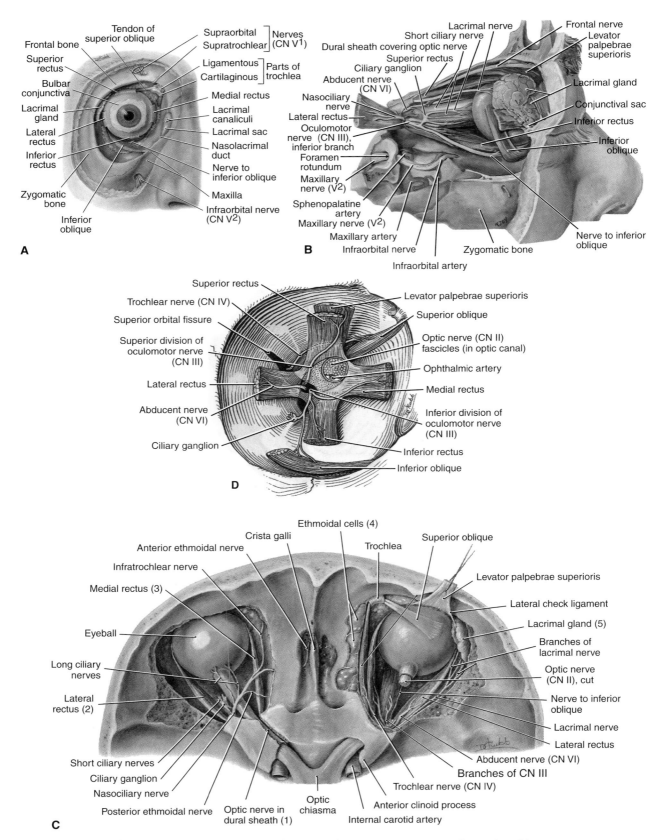

Figure 61.4 **Three-planar T-oncoanatomy. A.** Coronal. **B.** Sagittal. **C.** Transverse. **D.** Inset of posterior orbit.

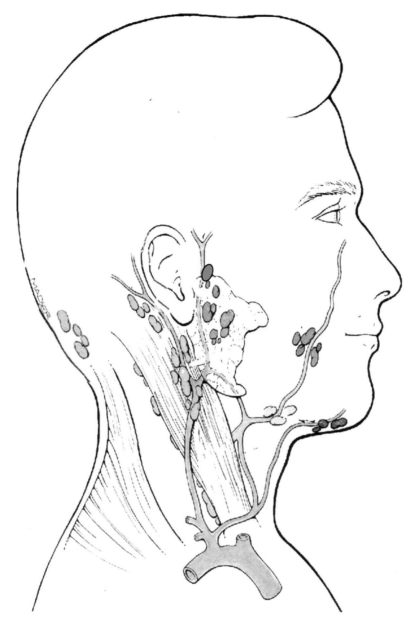

Figure 61.5 **N-oncoanatomy.** The sentinel node is the preauricular node.

TABLE 61.2	Histopathologic Types of Carcinoma of the Lacrimal Gland

Malignant mixed tumor (carcinoma arising in pleomorphic adenoma), which includes adenocarcinoma and adenoid cystic carcinoma arising in a pleomorphic adenoma (benign mixed tumor).

    Adenoid cystic carcinoma, arising de novo
    Adenocarcinoma, arising de novo
    Mucoepidermoid carcinoma
    Squamous cell carcinoma

Used with permission from Greene FL, Page DL, Fleming ID, et al., eds. *AJCC Cancer Staging Manual.* 6th ed. New York: Springer; 2002:378.

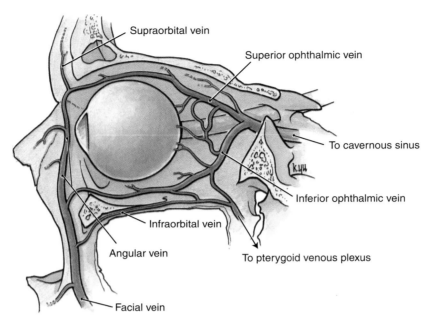

Figure 61.6 **M-oncoanatomy of eye.** Retinal arteries and veins.

TABLE 61.3	**Imaging Modalities: Eye and Orbit**	
Method	**Diagnosis and Staging Capability**	**Recommended for Use**
CT	Provides excellent anatomic detail of globe, orbital content and bony orbit; can distinguish smooth, round cysts from infiltrative tumors versus pseudotumors and detect bone destruction and sinus invasion	Yes
Primary tumor ultrasonography and fine-needle aspiration biopsy	A and B scans can be used to screen intraocular and orbital tumors and cysts, especially melanomas	No
MRI	Provides excellent 3D view, orbital fat hyperintense and vitreous hypointense in tumor (T1) and reverse in T2; can detect tumors versus pseudotumors and cysts; may be superior for diagnosis of vascular lesions, demyelinating disease	Yes
Endoscopy	Orbital endoscopy with fiber optic lights is used in conjunction with CT and/or MRI for obtaining core biopsy	Yes, when indicated
Standard orbital view	Useful for assessing optic nerve foramen and supraorbital fissure, but supplanted by CT; can detect intraocular calcification	No
Orbital phlebography	Venography particularly useful for detecting orbital varices, but is less efficient and more invasive than CT	No
Carotid angiography	Useful in diagnosis of vascularized tumors and aneurysms, but replaced by CT/MRI	No
Fluorescein angiography	Sometimes used in diagnosis of ocular melanoma	No
Biopsy	Usually an incisional or excisional biopsy is indicated to confirm malignant versus pseudotumors; directed stereotactically by CT/MRI; contraindicated for melanomas owing to high risk of seeding	Yes, if indicated

CT, computed tomography; 3D, three-dimensional; MRI, magnetic resonance imaging.
Used with permission from Rubin P. *Clinical Oncology*. 7th ed. Philadelphia: WB Saunders; 1993:300.

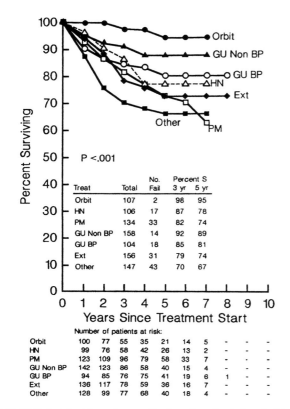

Treat	Total	No. Fail	Percent S	
			3 yr	5 yr
Orbit	107	2	98	95
HN	106	17	87	78
PM	134	33	82	74
GU Non BP	158	14	92	89
GU BP	104	18	85	81
Ext	156	31	79	74
Other	147	43	70	67

Number of patients at risk:

Orbit	100	77	55	35	21	14	5	-	-	-
HN	99	76	58	42	26	13	2	-	-	-
PM	123	109	96	79	58	33	7	-	.	-
GU Non BP	142	123	86	58	40	15	4	-	-	-
GU BP	94	85	76	75	41	19	6	1	-	-
Ext	136	117	78	59	36	16	7	-	.	-
Other	128	99	77	68	40	18	4	-	-	-

Figure 61.7 Survival by primary site for all patients treated in IRS III. Orbital rhabdosarcomas are the most curable rhabdosarcomas. Ext, extremities; GU BP, genitourinary tract (bladder or prostate); GU Non BP, genitourinary tract (nonbladder, nonprostate); HN, head and neck; nonparameningeal; PM, parameningeal sites.

- Optic nerve gliomas are extremely curable by stereo-tactic radiation therapy. The University of Pittsburgh group reports 96%, 90%, and 90% survivals at 5, 10, and 15 years, respectively; 86% retain vision.
- Orbital lymphomas and orbital rhabdomyosarcomas are 100% locally controlled with chemoradiation.
- Curiously, lymph node metastases were noted at >12 different sites with the sole exception of the orbit in IRS I and IRS II, which totaled 592 cases. The range of nodal metastases was 3% to 26%, averaging 14%. The most recent IRS (IV) has achieved a 100% successful outcome compared with 83% in IRS III.

Appendix A: Recommended Reading and References

The gains in survival and excellence in outcomes are due not only to improvements in each treatment modality, but to the multidisciplinary approach that has been adopted. Goals include eradication of the cancer and conservation of normal tissues, cosmesis with maintenance of physiologic function, and the need to achieve a socially acceptable result. Reference to multi-authored, multidisciplinary oncology textbooks presents the progress detailed in cooperative group clinical trials and the gains in practice due to evidence-based medicine over the past five decades. There are an equal number of single- or dual-authored monographs on upper aerorespiratory and digestive tract cancers.

Perspective and Patterns of Spread

American Cancer Society. *Cancer Facts & Figures*. Atlanta: Author; 2004.

Fearon ER, Vogelstein B: A genetic model for colorectal tumor genesis. *Cell* 1990;61:759.

Hedinger C. Histological typing of thyroid tumours. In: *International Histological Classification of Tumors*. 2nd ed. New York: Springer; 1988.

Maruyama M, Hamada T: *Diagnosis of gastric cancer in Japan*. In Feeney PC, Stevenson GW [eds]: *Alimentary Tract Radiology*, 5th ed. St. Louis, Mosby-Year Book, 1994, pp 349–428.

McDivitt RW, Stewart FW. *Tumors of the Breast*. Washington, DC: Armed Forces Institute of Pathology; 1968.

Nakanishi K. Alveolar epithelial hyperplasia and adenocarcinoma of the lung. *Arch Pathol Lab Med* 1990;114:363.

Ries LAG, Eisner MP, Kosary CL, et al, eds. *SEER Cancer Statistics Review, 1975–2001*. Bethesda, MD: National Cancer Institute. Available: http://seer.cancer.gov/csr/1975_2001/2004.

TNM Staging Criteria

American Joint Committee on Cancer (AJCC). *AJCC Cancer Staging Manual*. 6th ed. New York: Springer; 2002.

International Union against Cancer (UICC). *TNM Classification of Malignant Tumours*. 6th ed. New York: Wiley-Liss; 2002.

Martini N, Melamed MR. Multiple primary lung cancers. *J Thorac Cardiovasc Surg* 2002.

Sobotta. *Atlas of Human Anatomy, Head, Neck, and Upper Limb*. Vol. 1. 13th ed. Philadelphia: Lippincott Williams & Wilkins; 2000.

Tobias MJ. *Anatomy of the Human Lymphatic System: A Compendium Translated From the Original "Anatomie des Lymphatiques de l'Homme" by H. Rouviere Rearranged for the Use of Students and Practitioners*. Ann Arbor: Edward Bros; 1938.

Rules for Classification and Staging (Imaging)

American Joint Committee on Cancer (AJCC). *AJCC Cancer Staging Manual*. 6th ed. New York: Springer; 2002.

Bragg DG, Rubin P, Hricak H. *Oncologic Imaging*. 2nd ed. Philadelphia: WB Saunders; 2002.

Husband JES, Reznek RH. *Imaging in Oncology*. Oxford: Isis Medical Media; 1998.

International Union against Cancer (UICC). *TNM Classification of Malignant Tumours*. 6th ed. New York: Wiley-Liss; 2002.

Patz EF Jr, Rush VW, Heelan R. The proposed new international TNM staging system for malignant pleural mesothelioma: application to imaging. *Am J Roentgenol* 1996;166:323–327.

Rush VW. The international Mesothelioma Interest Group: a proposed new international TNM staging system for malignant pleural mesothelioma. *Chest* 1995;108:1122–1128.

Schwartz SI, Shires GT, Spencer FC. *Principles of Surgery*. New York: McGraw-Hill; 1989.

Cancer Statistics and Survival

Aisner J, Arrigada R, Green MR, eds. *Comprehensive Textbook of Thoracic Oncology*. Baltimore: Williams and Wilkins; 1996.

Al-Sarraf M, Martz K, Herskovic A, et al. Progress report of combined chemoradiotherapy vesus radiotherapy alone in patients with esophageal cancer: an intergroup study. *J Clin Oncol* 1997; 15:277.

American Cancer Society (ACS). *Cancer Facts & Figures*. Atlanta: Author; 2004.

Ang KK, Garden AS. *Radiotherapy for Head and Neck Cancers*. 2nd ed. Philadelphia: Lippincott Williams & Wilkins; 2002.

Bartlett D, Ramanathan R, Deutsch M, *Cancer of the Biliary Tree*. In DeVita V, Hellman S, Rosenberg SE [eds]: *Cancer Principles and*

Practice of Oncology. 7th ed. Philadelphia: Lippincott Williams & Wilkins; 2004, p 1031.

DeVita V, Hellman S, Rosenberg SE. *Cancer Principles and Practice of Oncology.* 6th ed. Philadelphia: Lippincott Williams and Wilkins; 2001.

DeVita V, Hellman S, Rosenberg SE. *Cancer Principles and Practice of Oncology.* 7th ed. Philadelphia: Lippincott Williams & Wilkins; 2004.

Gunderson LL, Martenson JA, Smalley SR, et al. Upper gastrointestinal cancers: rationale, results, and techniques of treatment. *Front Radiat Ther Oncol* 1994;28:121–139.

Gunderson LL, Martenson JA, Smalley SR, et al. Lower gastrointestinal cancers: rationale, results, and techniques of treatment. *Front Radiat Ther Oncol* 1994;28:140–154.

Haegensen DC. *Diseases of the Breast.* 3rd ed. Philadelphia: W.B. Saunders; 1986.

Harris JR, Lippman ME, Morrow M, et al. *Diseases of the Breast.* 3rd ed. Philadelphia: Lippincott Williams & Wilkins; 2005.

Herskovic A, Martz K, Al-Sarraf M, et al. Combined chemotherapy and radiotherapy compared with radiotherapy alone in patients with cancer of the esophagus. *N Engl J Med* 1992;326:1593.

HHS/HRSA/OSP/DOT and UNOS. 2000 Annual Report of the U.S. Scientific Registry Transplant Recipients and the Organ Procurement and Transplantation Network: Transplant Data: 1989–1998. 2004. Rockville, MD and Richmond, VA, 2-16-2001.

Johnson DH, ed. Lung cancer. *Semin Oncol* 1997;24:387–499.

Libutti S, Saltz L, Rustgi A, Tepper J. *Cancer of the Colon.* In DeVita V, Hellman S, Rosenberg SE [eds]: *Cancer Principles and Practice of Oncology.* 7th ed. Philadelphia: Lippincott Williams & Wilkins; 2004, p 1087.

Libutti S, Tepper J, Saltz L, Rustgi A. *Cancer of the Rectum.* In DeVita V, Hellman S, Rosenberg SE [eds]: *Cancer Principles and Practice of Oncology.* 7th ed. Philadelphia: Lippincott Williams & Wilkins; 2004, p 1117.

MacDonald JS, Smalley S, Bendetti J, et al. Chemoradiotherapy after surgery compared with surgery alone for adenocarcinoma of the stomach or gastroesophageal junction. *N Engl J Med* 2001;345:725.

Martenson JA, Gunderson LL. External radiation therapy without chemotherapy in the management of anal cancer. *Cancer* 1993;71:1736.

Mountain CE. A new international staging system for lung cancer. *Chest* 1986;89(suppl):225.

Nouguchi M, Morikawa A, Kawasaki M, et al. Small adenocarcinoma of the lung. Histologic characteristic and prognosis. *Cancer* 1995;75:2844.

Pass HI, Carbone DP, Johnson DH, et al. *Lung Cancer: Principles and Practice.* 3rd ed. Philadelphia: Lippincott-Raven; 2005.

Paulson DH. The "superior sulcus" lesion. In: Delarue NC, Eschapasse H, eds. *International Trends in General Thoracic Surgery. Vol. 1: Lung Cancer.* Philadelphia: WB Saunders; 1985:185–121.

Paulson DL. Technical considerations in stage III disease: the "superior sulcus" lesion. In Delarue NC, Eschapasse H, eds. *International Trends in General Surgery.* Philadelphia: WB Saunders, 1985:121–131.

Perez CA, Brady LW, Halperin EC, et al. *Radiation Oncology.* 4th ed. Philadelphia: Lippincott Williams & Wilkins; 2003.

Posner M, Forastiere A, Minsky B, ch. 29.1 Pg. 887.

Roth JA, Ruckdeschel JC, Weisenburger TH. *Thoracic Oncology.* Philadelphia: WB Saunders; 1995.

Rubin P. *Clinical Oncology.* 8th ed. New York: Elsevier; 2001.

Sohn TA, Yeo CJ, Cameron JL, et al. Resected adenocarcinoma of the pancreas-616 patients: results, outcomes, and prognostic indicators. *J Gastrointest Surg* 2000;4:567.

Wang CC. *Radiation Therapy for Head and Neck Neoplasms.* 3rd ed. New York: John Wiley; 1996.

Appendix B: Figure and Table Credits

Section 1 (Chapters 1–12)

Modified from Agur A, Dalley A, eds. *Grant's Atlas of Anatomy*. 11th ed. Philadelphia: Lippincott Williams & Wilkins; 2005. Figures 1.1, 1.2, 1.4C–E, 1.5, 1.6, 2.1–2.6, 3.1–3.5, 4.1–4.5, 5.1–5.5, 6.1–6.5, 7.1–7.5, 8.1–8.5, 9.1–9.5, 10.1–10.5, 11.1–11.5, 12.1–12.5.

Used with permission from Bragg DG, Rubin P, Hricak H, eds. *Oncologic Imaging* 2nd ed. Philadelphia: Elsevier; 2002:465. Table 1.5.

Modified from Eroschenko VP, ed. *di Fiore's Atlas of Histology with Functional Correlations*. 10th ed. Philadelphia: Lippincott Williams & Wilkins; 2005. Figure 1.3.

Used with permission from Reis LAG, Eisner MP, Kosary CL, et al., eds. *SEER Cancer Statistics Review, 1975–2001*. Bethesda, MD: National Cancer Institute. Available at http://seer.cancer.gov/csr/1975_2001/,2004. Tables XII-4, XIX-4, 1.6, 1.7, 9.2 and 12.2.

Used with permission from Rubin P, Williams J, eds. *Clinical Oncology: A Multidisciplinary Approach for Physicians and Students*. 8th ed. Philadelphia: Elsevier; 2001:408. Tables 2.1, 3.1, 5.1, 7.1, 8.1, 9.1, 10.1, and 11.1.

Used with permission of the American Joint Committee on Cancer (AJCC), Chicago, Illinois. The original source for this material is the *AJCC Cancer Staging Manual*. 6th ed. New York: Springer-Verlag; 2002. Tables 4.1, 6.1, and 12.1.

Section 2 (Chapters 13–22)

Used with permission from Movsas B, Langer CJ, Goldberg M, eds. *Controversies in Lung Cancer. A Multidisciplinary Approach*. New York: Marcel Dekker, Inc., 2001: p 244. Figure 14.7.

Modified from Agur A, Dalley A, eds. *Grant's Atlas of Anatomy*. 11th ed. Philadelphia: Lippincott Williams & Wilkins, 2005. Figures 13.1, 13.2, 13.3A–C, 13.5A, 13.6, 14.1–14.6, 15.1–15.4, 16.1–16.4, 17.1–17.4, 17.6, 18.1–18.4, 19.1–19.4, 20.1–20.4, 21.1–21.6, 22.3, and 22.4.

Modified from Eroschenko VP, ed. *di Fiore's Atlas of Histology with Functional Correlations*. 10th ed. Philadelphia: Lippincott Williams & Wilkins; 2005. Figure 13.3G.

Modified from Mountain, CF: Revisions in the international system for staging lung cancer. *Chest* 1997;111: 1710–1717. Table 15.3.

Used with permission of the Mayo Foundation for Medical Education and Research. Lymph node classification adapted from Mountain CF, Dresler CM. Regional lymph node classification for lung cancer staging. *Chest* 1977;111:1718–1723. Figure 13.5B. Table 14.2.

Used with permission from Constine LS, Rubin P, Qazi R. Malignant lymphomas. In Rubin P, ed. *Clinical Oncology*. 7th ed. Philadelphia: WB Saunders; 1993:217–250. Figure 13.5C.

Used with permission of the American Joint Committee on Cancer (AJCC), Chicago, Illinois. The original source for this material is the *AJCC Cancer Staging Manual*. 6th ed. New York: Springer-Verlag; 2002. Figure 13.5D. Tables 20.1, 21.1, and 22.1.

With kind permission of Springer Science and Business Media from Bates M, ed. *Bronchial Carcinoma. An Integrated Approach to Diagnosis and Management*. Berlin: Springer-Verlag; 1984. Figure 13.7.

Used with permission from Line DH, Deeley TJ. The necropsy findings in carcinoma of the bronchus. *Br J Dis Chest* 1971;62:238–242. Table 13.5.

Used with permission from Mountain CF. A new international staging system for lung cancer. *Chest* 1986;89(suppl):225. Tables 13.8, 13.9.

Used with permission from Ross MH, Kaye GI, Pawlina W, eds. *Histology: A Text and Atlas.* 5th ed. Philadelphia: Lippincott Williams & Wilkins; 2006. Figures 13.3 D–F.

Used with permission from Rubin P, Williams J, eds. *Clinical Oncology: A Multidisciplinary Approach for Physicians and Students.* 8th ed. Philadelphia: Elsevier; 2001. Figure 21.7.

Used with permission from Travis WD, Travis LB, DeVessa SS. Lung cancer. *Cancer* 1995;75(1 suppl): 191–198. Table 15.4.

Modified from Akiyama H, Tsurumaru M, Kawamura T. Principles of surgical treatment of carcinoma of the esophagus: Analysis of lymph node involvement. *Ann Surg* 1981;194(4):438–446. Figure 22.5.

Used with permission from Bragg DG, Rubin P, Youker JE, eds. Breast cancer. In: *Oncologic Imaging.* Elmsford, New York: Pergamon Press; 1985:271. Table 21.3.

Section 3 (Chapters 23–34)

Data from ACS and Cancer Facts and Figures 2005. Table 24.4.

From Sindelar WF: Cancer of the small intestine. In: DeVita VT Jr, Hellman S, Rosenberg SA (eds) *Cancer, Principles and Practice of Oncology,* 3rd ed, Philadelphia: JB Lippincott Co; 1989: 875–894. Table 32.1.

Reprinted with permission from Kadish SL, Kochman ML. *Oncology* 1995;9(10):967–983. Figure 23.7.

Used with permission of the American Joint Committee on Cancer (AJCC), Chicago, Illinois. The original source for this material is the *AJCC Cancer Staging Manual.* 6th ed. New York: Springer-Verlag; 2002. Tables 23.1, 24.1, 31.1, 33.1, and 34.1.

Used with permission from Robinson P. Liver. In Husband JSS, Reenek, eds. *Imaging in Oncology.* Oxford: ISI Medical Media; 1998:787. Table 23.5.

Used with permission from Rubin P, Williams J, eds. *Clinical Oncology: A Multidisciplinary Approach for Physicians and Students.* 8th ed. Philadelphia: Elsevier; 2001. Table 26.1.

Used with permission from Carriaga MT, Henson DE. Liver, gallbladder, extrahepatic bile ducts, and pancreas. *Cancer* 1995;75(1 suppl):171. Table 27.1.

Section 4 (Chapters 35–42)

Data from ACS and Cancer Facts and Figures 2005. Table 35.5.

Modified from Agur A, Dalley A, eds. *Grant's Atlas of Anatomy.* 11th ed. Philadelphia: Lippincott Williams & Wilkins; 2005. Figures 35.1, 35.3(A), 35.6, 36.1, 36.2, 36.4–36.6, 37.1, 37.2, 37.4–37.5, 38.1, 38.2, 38.4–38.6, 39.1, 39.2, 39.4–39.6, 40.1, 40.2, 40.4–40.5, 41.1, 41.2, 41.4, 41.5, 42.1, 42.2, and 42.4.

Used with permission from Bragg DG, Rubin P, Hricak H, eds. *Oncologic Imaging.* 2nd ed. Philadelphia: Elsevier; 2002. Tables 35.4, 39.3, and 41.3.

Used with permission of the American Cancer Society. *Cancer Facts and Figures 2005.* Atlanta: American Cancer Society; 2005. Tables 35.5, 36.4, and 43.5.

Used with permission from Reis LAG, Eisner MP, Kosary CL, et al., eds. *SEER Cancer Statistics Review, 1975–2001.* Bethesda, MD: National Cancer Institute. Available at http://seer.cancer.gov/csr/1975_2001/,2004. Tables XI, XXIII, XXV, XXVII, 35.6, and 36.4.

Used with permission from Rubin P, Williams J, eds. *Clinical Oncology: A Multidisciplinary Approach for Physicians and Students.* 8th ed. Philadelphia: Elsevier; 2001. Table 36.1.

Used with permission of the American Joint Committee on Cancer (AJCC), Chicago, Illinois. The original source for this material is the *AJCC Cancer Staging Manual.* 6th ed. New York: Springer-Verlag; 2002. Tables 37.1, 38.1, 39.1, 40.1, 41.1, and 42.1.

Used with permission from Ross MH, Kaye GI, Pawlina W, eds. *Histology: A Text and Atlas.* 5th ed. Philadelphia: Lippincott Williams & Wilkins; 2006: Figures 35.3B–F.

Section 5 (Chapters 43–50)

Data from ACS and Cancer Facts and Figures 2005. Table 43.5.

Used with permission of the American Cancer Society. *Cancer Facts and Figures 2005.* Atlanta: American Cancer Society; 2005:4. Table 43.5.

Used with permission from Reis LAG, Eisner MP, Kosary CL, et al., eds. *SEER Cancer Statistics Review, 1975–2001.* Bethesda, MD: National Cancer Institute. Available at http://seer.cancer.gov/csr/1975_2001/,2004, Tables V, XII, XXI, and 43.6.

Used with permission of the American Joint Committee on Cancer (AJCC), Chicago, Illinois. The original source for this material is the *AJCC Cancer Staging Manual*. 6th ed. New York: Springer-Verlag; 2002. Tables 44.1, 45.1, 47.1, 47.2, 49.1, and 50.1.

Used with permission from Rubin P, Williams J, eds. *Clinical Oncology: A Multidisciplinary Approach for Physicians and Students*. 8th ed. Philadelphia: Elsevier; 2001. Table 46.1.

Used with permission from Bragg DG, Rubin P, Hricak H, eds. *Oncologic Imaging*. 2nd ed. Philadelphia: Elsevier; 2002:465. Table 48.1.

Used with permission from Ross MH, Kaye GI, Pawlina W, eds. Histology: *A Text and Atlas*. 5th ed. Philadelphia: Lippincott Williams & Wilkins; 2006. Figures 43B–G.

Section 6 (Chapters 51–56)

Modified from Eroschenko VP, ed. *di Fiore's Atlas of Histology with Functional Correlations*. 10th ed. Philadelphia: Lippincott Williams & Wilkins; 2005. Figures 51.1–51.7, 52.3, 53.3B, 54.3, and 56.5.

Used with permission from Rubin P, Williams J, eds. *Clinical Oncology: A Multidisciplinary Approach for Physicians and Students*. 8th ed. Philadelphia: Elsevier; 2001. Figures 51.8.

Modified from Agur A, Dalley A, eds. *Grant's Atlas of Anatomy*. 11th ed. Philadelphia: Lippincott Williams & Wilkins; 2005. Figures 54.4–54.6, 55.1, and 55.2.

Modified from Ross MH, Kaye GI, Pawlina W, eds. *Histology: A Text and Atlas*. 5th ed. Philadelphia: Lippincott Williams & Wilkins; 2006. Figures 52.3B, 52.3D, 52.4, 53.3A, 53.4, and 55.7.

Used with permission from Ross MH, Kaye GI, Pawlina W, eds. *Histology: A Text and Atlas*. 4th ed. Philadelphia: Lippincott Williams & Wilkins; 2003. Figure 52.3C.

Used with permission of the American Joint Committee on Cancer (AJCC), Chicago, Illinois. The original source for this material is the *AJCC Cancer Staging Manual*. 6th ed. New York: Springer-Verlag; 2002. Figure 56.8. Tables 53.1, 53.2, 55.1, 56.1–56.3, and 56.5.

Used with permission from Rubin P. *Dynamic Classification of Bone Dysplasia*. Chicago: Yearbook Medical Pub.; 1964. Figures 55.3–55.6.

Used with permission from Kaplan HS. *Hodgkin's Disease*.

2nd ed. Cambridge: Harvard University Press; 1980. Figures 56.1, 56.2, and 56.4.

Used with permission from Bragg DG, Rubin P, Hricak H, eds. *Oncologic Imaging*. 2nd ed. Philadelphia: Elsevier, 2002. Figure 56.6.

Section 7 (Chapters 57–61)

Modified from Ross MH, Kaye GI, Pawlina W, eds. *Histology: A Text and Atlas*. 5th ed. Philadelphia: Lippincott Williams & Wilkins; 2006. Figures 57.1, 57.2B, 57.2 D–H, 57.3A–D, 57.5B, 58.3A, 59.3A and B, 60.3 A–C, and 61.3A and B.

Modified from Eroschenko VP, ed. *di Fiore's Atlas of Histology with Functional Correlations*. 10th ed. Philadelphia: Lippincott Williams & Wilkins; 2005. Figures 57.2C and 58.3B.

Modified from Agur A, Dalley A, eds. *Grant's Atlas of Anatomy*. 11th ed. Philadelphia: Lippincott Williams & Wilkins, 2005. Figures 57.2A, 57.3E, 57.4, 57.5A, 58.1A and B, 58.2A, 58.4–58.6, 59.1A and B, 59.2A, 59.4, 59.5, 60.1, 60.2, 60.4, 60.5, 61.1A and B, 61.2A and B, and 61.4–61.6. Table 58.1.

Used with permission from Rubin P, Williams J, eds. *Clinical Oncology: A Multidisciplinary Approach for Physicians and Students*. 8th ed. Philadelphia: Elsevier; 2001. Figure 59.6. Tables 57.2, 57.5, 58.2, 59.2, and 61.3.

Used with permission from Rubin P. *Clinical Oncology*. 7th ed. Philadelphia: W.B. Saunders, 1993:300. Table 60.3.

Reprinted with permission from the American Society of Clinical Oncology from Crist W, Gehan EA, Ragab AH, et al. The Third Intergroup Rhabdomyosarcoma Study. *J Clin Oncol* 1995;13:610–630. Figure 61.7.

Used with permission from Halperin EC, Constine LS, Tarbell NJ, et al. *Pediatric Radiation Oncology*. 4th ed. Philadelphia: Lippincott Williams & Wilkins; 2005:144. Table 60.2.

Used with permission from Halperin EC, Constine LS, Tarbell NJ, et al. *Pediatric Radiation Oncology*. 4th ed. Philadelphia: Lippincott Williams & Wilkins; 2005:152 Table 60.4.

Used with permission of the American Joint Committee on Cancer (AJCC), Chicago, Illinois. The original source for this material is the *AJCC Cancer Staging Manual*. 6th ed. New York: Springer-Verlag; 2002. Tables 59.1, 60.1, 61.1, and 61.2.

Index

Note: Page numbers followed by *f* indicate figures; page numbers followed by *t* indicate tables.